CHIROPRACTIC TECHNIQUE
Principles and Procedures

CHIROPRACTIC TECHNIQUE
Principles and Procedures

Thomas F. Bergmann, D.C.
Clinic Faculty
Center for Clinical Studies
Northwestern College of Chiropractic
Bloomington, Minnesota
Editor-in-chief
Journal of Chiropractic Technique
Mendota Heights, Minnesota

David H. Peterson, D.C.
Associate Professor
Division of Chiropractic Science
Department of Chiropractic
Western States Chiropractic College
Portland, Oregon

Dana J. Lawrence, D.C., F.I.C.C.
Professor
Department of Chiropractic Practice
Director
Department of Editorial Review and Publication
National College of Chiropractic
Editor
Journal of Manipulative and Physiological Therapeutics
Lombard, Illinois

With illustrations by Nicholas Lang, M.A.M.S.

 CHURCHILL LIVINGSTONE
New York, Edinburgh, London, Madrid, Milan, Melbourne, Tokyo

Library of Congress Cataloging-in-Publication Data

Bergmann, Thomas F.
    Chiropractic technique : principles and procedures / Thomas F.
Bergmann, David H. Peterson, Dana J. Lawrence ; with illustrations
by Nicholas Lang.
        p.   cm.
    Includes bibliographical references and index.
    ISBN 0-443-08752-0
    1. Chiropractic. 2. Manipulation (Therapeutics)   I. Peterson,
David H., date.   II. Lawrence, Dana J.   III. Title.
    [DNLM: 1. Chiropractic—methods.   WB 905 B499c]
    RZ255.B47 1993
    615.5'34—dc20
    DNLM/DLC
    for Library of Congress   92-48893
                                                                      CIP

Distributed in the United Kingdom by Churchill Livingstone, Robert Stevenson
House, 1–3 Baxter's Place, Leith Walk, Edinburgh EH1 3AF, and by associated companies, branches, and representatives throughout the world.

The Publishers have made every effort to trace the copyright holders for borrowed
material. If they have inadvertently overlooked any, they will be pleased to make the
necessary arrangements at the first opportunity.

Acquisitions Editor: *Leslie Burgess*
Copy Editor: *Elizabeth Bowman-Schulman*
Production Designer: *Jody L. Ouellette*
Production Supervisor: *Jeanine Furino*
Cover Design: *Paul Moran*

Printed in the United States of America

First published in 1993   7 6 5 4 3 2

With love to our families
for their support, patience, and sacrifice
during the long hours of work
that were necessary to produce this text.

Foreword

The opportunity to write a foreword for a new textbook defining the art and science of chiropractic adjustive procedures presents itself rarely. I am grateful indeed to the authors for this privilege.

Chiropractic Technique: Principles and Procedures is probably the first work to define rationally those clinically successful chiropractic adjustive techniques that originated largely from anecdotal evidence, since the 1947 James, Houser, and Wells classic *Chiropractic Principles and Technic.* It presents a thoroughly researched literature base of joint anatomy, joint biomechanics, principles of joint assessment, and adjustive technique as these apply to the spine and peripheral articulations. This literature support is relatively current, impressive, and encouraging because it agrees with scientific knowledge or incorporation by a consensus of experts. If for no other reason than the authors' dedication to scientific principles to understand and support their premises, this work is an important landmark for chiropractic education and clinical practice.

The adjustment — of the spine, pelvis, and extremities — is the primary therapeutic procedure used by chiropractic physicians. When combined with a broad range of diagnostic skills, it is effective for a wide range of clinical conditions.

I am particularly proud to have known Dr. Peterson when he was a student and to recognize some of the traditional concepts I have fostered for longer than I can remember in his in-depth contributions to this remarkable textbook. As for Drs. Bergmann and Lawrence, I have been a witness to their scholarship for many years. I am convinced that as long as scientific aptitude such as all three possess continues, then chiropractic clinical care will continue to demonstrate its efficacy.

I would be remiss not to comment on the final chapter, which deals with research and validation. Having presented a scholarly scientific approach to spinal adjustive procedures, the authors do not want to leave their readers with any misconceptions about the "status quo" for those procedures.

Rather, they want their audience not to subscribe to the "status quo" and accompanying anecdotal evidence and suggest three research directions; no doubt there are more, but those recommended will challenge the profession's resources for some time. The challenge can and will be met.

A fourth century quote from the Babylonian Talmud says, "I have learned much from my teachers, and from my colleagues more than from my teachers, and from my students more than from all." And without this hierarchy, all scholarship would come to an end.

Herbert J. Vear, D.C., F.C.C.S., L.L.D.
President Emeritus
Western States Chiropractic College
Portland, Oregon
Dean Emeritus
Canadian Memorial Chiropractic College
Toronto, Ontario, Canada

Preface

Chiropractic Technique: Principles and Procedures describes procedures fundamental to the application of chiropractic adjustive technique and provides a rationale for their selection and use. It was written to fill a void in the literature relating to the use of manipulative therapy, particularly the chiropractic adjustment. It is designed to be a practical guide for the evaluation and use of manual treatment of joint dysfunction/subluxation.

A wide variety of adjustive methods exist, many with significantly different attributes and applications. The goal of this text is to review the basic principles (anatomic, biomechanical, and pathophysiologic) necessary to evaluate, select, and apply specific adjustive procedures. Fundamental to the effective application of adjustive techniques is an understanding of joint and body mechanics coupled with knowledge of and skills in the use of joint evaluative tests and procedures. With this goal in mind, we have covered the major adjustive methods but have not attempted to be exhaustive.

The book is organized so that each chapter can stand on its own; it is not essential to have read the information in one chapter to understand the material in another. As a result, some information may be repeated from chapter to chapter, as well as from section to section within chapters. We hope that this design will eliminate the need to frequently refer to other parts of this book to identify information or concepts fundamental to a given section.

The book is divided into seven chapters. The first briefly outlines the past, present, and future developments in manipulative therapy generally, and chiropractic specifically. The second establishes a foundation, with information about the anatomy and biomechanics of the numerous joint systems composing the human upright locomotor complex. Chapter 3 explores and describes the specific evaluative procedures used to identify characteristics of the manipulable lesion (subluxation/joint dysfunction). Chapter 4 develops the mechanical principles necessary for understanding the differences between, and the application of, adjustive procedures. The next two chapters discuss specific adjustments for spinal and extremity joint dysfunction, including regional anatomy, joint assessment procedures, indications, position of doctor and patient, contact points, and vectors of force. The final chapter, attempting to provide a rationale for the use of manipulative therapy in health and disease, discusses research studies and methods for validating manipulative therapy.

Although this book was written with the student in mind it should also be useful to practicing clinicians of chiropractic, osteopathy, and physical therapy. Mastery of chiropractic technique requires diligent practice and learning by example. However, we hope we have provided a clear textual exposition that will help all students and practitioners evaluate their practice of those techniques.

Thomas F. Bergmann, D.C.
David H. Peterson, D.C.
Dana J. Lawrence, D.C., F.I.C.C.

Acknowledgments

The authors wish to acknowledge the role of many individuals in the production of this book: Glenn Gumaer for his photographic talent and Nick Lang for the artwork; Dr. Janice Justice, Dr. Fred Rhead, Dr. Janet Preckel, Dr. Lolin Fletcher, and Dr. Andrew Baca for serving as models; the Lloyd Table Company (Lisbon, IA) for contributing photographs of a variety of adjusting tables.

Appreciation and gratitude is expressed to the following faculty members at Western States Chiropractic College for their willing editorial evaluation and comments. Dr. Ed Rothman, Dr. Dave Panzer, Dr. Dick Stonebrink, Dr. Fred Colley, Mark Kaminski, Dr. Joanne Nyiendo, and Rich Gillette.

Special recognition goes to Dr. Mitch Haas for the discussion on joint fixation, Rich Gillette for his contributions to the discussion of the neurobiologic effects of spinal adjusting, and Dr. Ed Rothman for submitting the section on surface electromyography.

Contents

1
General Overview of the Chiropractic Profession

Dana J. Lawrence

The chiropractic profession is only a century old, but manipulation has been used to treat human ailments since antiquity. Though no single origin is noted, manual procedures are evident in Thai artwork dating back 4,000 years. Ancient Egyptian, Chinese, Japanese, and Tibetan records describe the use of manual procedures to treat disease. Manipulation was also a part of the North and South American Indian cultures. Certainly, Hippocrates was known to use manual medical procedures in treating spinal deformity, and the noted physicians Galen, Celsies, and Orbasius alluded to manipulation in their writings. The nineteenth century witnessed a rise in popularity of American and English "bonesetters," the most well known being Mr. Hutton, who influenced the thoughts and writing of Sir James Paget and Wharton Hood.

It was not until the days of D.D. Palmer and Andrew Taylor Still, the founders of chiropractic and osteopathy, that these procedures were codified into a system. The early days of chiropractic and osteopathy represented major attempts to place manual procedures on firmer ground, and while the major developments in manual manipulative procedures in the late nineteenth century were largely American, developments were also occurring in other locations around the globe. At the same time, bonesetters were working in the United States and England and continued to do so into the early parts of the twentieth century. While chiropractic was developing under the leadership of the Palmers, medical manipulators were also making significant advances, as were early osteopathic researchers. The works of Mennell, Cyriax, Paget, and others are important in this regard.

Both chiropractic and osteopathy chose to focus on the musculoskeletal system, although in philosophically divergent ways. Andrew Still placed great emphasis on the somatic component of disease, largely involving the musculoskeletal system, and on the relationship of structure to function. Palmer postulated that subluxation, or improper juxtapostition of a vertebra, could interfere with the workings of the human nervous system and with innate intelligence, that power within the body to heal itself. Both emphasized the role the musculoskeletal system played in health and disease.

THE PAST

Daniel David Palmer (1845 to 1913) came to the United States from Port Perry, Ontario, Canada, in 1865. He spent the next 20 years in such various occupations as farming, beekeeping, and store sales. In 1885, he opened a practice as a magnetic healer in the city of Davenport, Iowa, though he had no formal training in any healing art. His formulation of chiropractic practice and theory purportedly developed from his application of a manual thrust, which he called *an adjustment,* to Harvey Lillard in September 1895 (coincidentally and significantly, the same year that Roentgen discovered the x-ray). This event has moved beyond that of a simple tale to an apocrypha. As the story goes, this manual adjustment was directed to the fourth thoracic vertebrae and resulted in the restoration of Mr. Lillard's lost hearing. From the reasoning used to devise this treatment, Palmer then applied similar lines of thought to other individuals with a variety of problems, each time using the spinous process of a vertebra as a lever to produce the adjustment. Palmer was the first to claim use of the spinous and transverse processes of the vertebrae as levers for manual adjustment of the spine, in effect, short lever contacts. This constituted the initiation of chiropractic as an art, a science, and a profession.

From this nearly chance opportunity came the outlines of the profession. Palmer developed the concept of a "subluxation" as a causal factor in disease through the pressure such "displacements" would cause to nerve roots. Within 2 years of the initial discovery, Palmer had started the Chiropractic School and Cure and soon had his first student enrolled. By the year 1902, Palmer's son, Bartlett Joshua (usually referred to as B.J.), had enrolled in his father's school and 2 years later had gained operational control of the institution, becoming president in 1907. He maintained this post until his death in 1961.

Animosity between the father and the son developed, and the elder Palmer left the school of his name and traveled around the country, forming at least four other chiropractic colleges (in California, Oregon, and Oklahoma). He was also placed in jail for a short time, for the crime of practicing medicine without a license, through the action of the Board of Medical Examiners. Although he might have been able to avoid jail by paying a small fine, he felt he had a more important principle to uphold. Palmer was not the last to be jailed for this "crime."

D.D. Palmer died in 1913 after enjoying only a short reconciliation with his son. B.J. had by that time led the original Palmer College for nearly 7 years. In 1906, D.D. Palmer had already forsaken education at the original Palmer College. That year was also significant because it marked the first philosophical differences within the fledgling chiropractic profession. John Howard, one of the first graduates of the Palmer School, was unable to accept many of the philosophical beliefs, relative to health care, that B.J. Palmer was now openly espousing. B.J. had by then begun to preach that subluxation was the cause of all disease, in opposition to his father's initial beliefs. Howard, therefore, left the Palmer School and founded the National School of Chiropractic not far from Palmer's school in Davenport.

As Beideman had noted,[1] Howard wanted to teach chiropractic "as it should be taught" and, therefore, moved the school to Chicago, feeling that chiropractic education required course work in the basic and clinical sciences, including access to laboratory, dissection, clinics, etc., to develop proper chiropractic care. These two schools (now colleges) still exist today.

By this time, other chiropractic colleges were being founded all over the country, and there was more and more internecine warfare among practitioners. B.J. Palmer had set himself up as the protector of a fundamental form of chiropractic (today referred to as "straight" chiropractic). During the years 1910 to 1926, Palmer lost many important administrators, most of whom went to form their own colleges. Furthermore, from 1924 to his death in 1961, he was a titular leader only, keeping the flame for a fundamentalist minority and battling with most of the profession, which he saw as inevitably following the osteopathic moth into the seductive medical flame.[2] Regardless of the philosophical issues debated then, and that still divide the profession today, it is possible that without B.J. Palmer's missionary zeal and entrepreneurial brilliance, the chiropractic profession would not exist as it is today. B.J.'s role as the "developer" of chiropractic was honestly earned.

THE PRESENT

Today, chiropractic is approved under federal law in all 50 states of the nation and is licensed as well in an increasing number of foreign countries. Chiropractic is included under Medicare and Medicaid laws, as well as insurance equity laws. The doctor of chiropractic (DC) degree is an approved degree through the U.S. Department of Education, and chiropractic colleges are accredited through professional accrediting bodies, as well as regional bodies through the Council on Postsecondary Education. Most chiropractors practice in private practices.

The chiropractic model of health care is one of holism, viewing health as a complex process integrating all parts and systems of the body in the dynamic procedure of change and adaptation resulting from the influences of the internal and external environments. The human body is viewed as being imbued at birth with the innate ability (innate intelligence) to respond to the environment, which was seen by earlier health-care pioneers as proof of the healing power of nature, *vis medicatrix naturae*. This concept emphasized the inherent recuperative powers of the body in the restoration and maintenance of health. It must be relegated, however, to a belief system, because there is no appropriate method of testing its existence.

D.D. Palmer and his early followers emphasized health and the absence of disease over the management of disease once it was present. Therefore, evaluation and treatment of neuromusculoskeletal disorders relating structure to function in the body became the focus. Moreover, patients were required to become active in their health care. Although many of the early forebears in chiropractic postulated a "one cause, one cure" approach to health, the monocausal theory of disease has now been rejected. Today, chiropractic has many theories for the role of manipulation in human ailments, and through its science, chiropractic is attempting to examine further the role it should play in national health care.

Clinically, the musculoskeletal system remains a neglected component of the body, although musculoskeletal disorders are common and account for significant amounts of lost time at work and recreation. The musculoskeletal system therefore deserves full consideration and evaluation whenever patients are seen, regardless of the complaint causing them to seek care. The musculoskeletal system should be viewed as part of the whole body and therefore subject to the same intensive diagnostic evaluation as any other system in the body. The musculoskeletal system is involved in so many alterations of function that it demands such attention and should not be "removed" from consideration in diagnosis, even when the initial problem appears removed from the musculoskeletal system. Moreover, the human musculoskeletal system, while accounting for more than half of its mass, is also the body's greatest energy user. The musculoskeletal systems require large amounts of energy, which must be supplied through the other systems in the body. If the musculoskeletal system increases its activity, an increased demand is placed on all the other body systems to meet the new, higher energy demands. Chiropractic notes that the presence of joint subluxation and dysfunction may interfere with the ability of the musculoskeletal system to act efficiently, which in turn requires greater work from the other systems within the body.

A preeminent principle of chiropractic is that the nervous system is highly developed in the human being, influences all other systems in the body, and therefore plays a role in health and disease. Though the exact nature of the relationship between dysfunction of the musculoskeletal system and changes in neurologic input to other body systems is not known, an enduring basic principle of chiropractic is that some aberration in structure (musculoskeletal) affects function (neurologic) and hence the body's sense of well-being. This is demonstrated by the nervous system's effects on the body's ability to fight disease through the immune response.[3]

The nervous system also interplays with the endocrine system to maintain a state of homeostasis defined simply as physiologic stability. This tendency of the body to maintain a steady state or to seek equilibrium despite external changes, referred to as *ponos* by Hippocrates, is the underlying theme in Palmer's concept of innate intelligence influencing health. Manual procedures and, specifically, the adjustment are thought to improve the body's ability to self-regulate through affecting the nervous system and hence all other systems, thereby allowing the body to seek homeostasis. In Haldeman's outline of this process, manipulative therapy can cause a change in the musculoskeletal system, which then causes a change in the nervous system, which in turn affects an organ dysfunction, tissue pathology, or symptom complex.[4] Reflex mechanisms that support these ideas have indeed been documented, though the effects of manipulation on these reflexes have yet to be adequately assessed.[5–8]

Palmer developed his model of the effects on the nervous system through the belief that subluxation affects the tone of the body. By *tone*, he referred to the efficiency of the nervous system and to the ability of the body to self-regulate its processes properly. This view was in opposition to the medical thought of the day, which focused on the germ theory and its relationship to disease.

Although chiropractors today certainly accept the existence and reality of germs, they reconceptualize the role of germs in creating disease.[9] Both the chiropractic and medical paradigms mandate that a susceptible host must be present along with a germ. Furthermore, the host's susceptibility depends on a multitude of factors. The chiropractic model, however, states that one such factor may be the presence of subluxation. A subluxation can serve as a noxious irritant to the body and its removal, therefore, becomes necessary for optimal health.

Although organized medicine rejected chiropractic from its outset, occurrences within medicine had a major impact on the development of the chiropractic profession. The Flexner Report, released in 1910, had a profound effect on chiropractic education.[10] This report was highly critical of the status of medical education in the United States. It recommended that medical colleges affiliate with universities to gain educational support. As Beideman has noted, it took the chiropractic profession nearly 15 years from the time of that report to begin the same types of changes that medicine underwent to improve its education.[11]

The changes were not long in coming, however, once their need was recognized. These improvements ultimately led to the creation of the Council on Chiropractic Education (CCE), which later was recognized by the U.S. Department of Education (then, the Department of Health, Education and Welfare) as the accrediting agency for the chiropractic profession.

John Nugent was largely responsible for ensuring that educational improvements would occur within the chiropractic profession. In 1935, Nugent was made the first Director of Education for the National Chiropractic Association (NCA). Nugent reported to the NCA that there were 37 active chiropractic colleges, all of which were proprietary and apparently followed different educational standards. It took Nugent the better part of the next two decades to begin to standardize the chiropractic educational process. Part of this standardization process included the initiation in 1947 of the CCE. In 1963, the NCA reformed itself as the American Chiropractic Association (ACA). By the late 1960s, the CCE had required its accredited colleges to use a 2-year preprofessional educational experience as a requirement for matriculation. In 1968, the DC degree became a recognized first professional degree, and in 1971, the CCE became an autonomous body.

This educational process allowed the chiropractic colleges to upgrade their professional standards to an unprecedented degree. The requirements of the CCE govern the entire educational spectrum of chiropractic education, mandating that certain information must be imparted to the student body, and providing a way to monitor compliance and to provide guidance to an individual college. The effect has been salubrious. Today, all CCE-accredited colleges teach a comprehensive program, incorporating elements of basic science (e.g., physiology, anatomy, and biochemistry); clinical science (e.g., laboratory diagnosis, radiographic diagnosis, orthopedics, nutrition, etc.); and clinical experience (providing experience in patient management involving therapeutic intervention).

What is interesting in this approach is that although the curriculum is standardized, assuring the public that most graduates of CCE colleges have been provided competent educations, each college does not necessarily teach its students the same chiropractic manipulative techniques. That is, each college must teach its students to adjust, but the procedures taught at one college may differ from those taught at other colleges. Although all these forms of chiropractic adjustive techniques have many elements in common, their approaches may differ substantially. A graduate of one college may find it difficult to share information with the graduate of a different college that teaches some alternate form of an adjustive procedure. Furthermore, a plethora of techniques are available in the form of postgraduate seminars, many of which are not governed by a regulatory body or accrediting procedure that would ensure an adequate scholastic level.

The majority of chiropractic technique systems were started by interested and probing doctors who noticed a regularity in their results and began to ask why those results occurred. This was largely a bootstrapping effort; the impetus to gain new knowledge and then disseminate it was largely self-driven. These approaches typically developed into systems of diagnosis and treatment ("system techniques"). The limitation of many of these system approaches is that the evaluative procedure linked to the manipulative procedure is often singular and simplistic. The human body, however, is a very complex and integrated organism, and to rely on a single evaluative tool for the sole application of a therapeutic intervention is not considered sound clinical practice. Some forms of chiropractic technique systems are summarized in Appendix 1, and a list of most of the named chiropractic techniques is provided in Appendix 2.

THE FUTURE

The chiropractic profession has labored long and hard to get to where it is. What does the future portend for the chiropractic profession? There are both the chance for opportunity and advancement and the chance to lose many hard-gained privileges. Recent occurrences will have a large impact on our future.

The outcome of the Wilk Trial on February 7, 1990, in the Seventh Circuit U.S. Court of Appeals found the American Medical Association (AMA) guilty of an illegal conspiracy to destroy the competitive profession of chiropractic. This decision arose from a suit brought by five chiropractors alleging that the AMA, along with several other organizations involved in health care, conspired to restrain the practice of chiropractic through a sustained and unlawful boycott of the chiropractic profession. This was despite the fact that chiropractic care had been found to be, in many cases, more effective in treating certain kinds of health problems.

The boycott severely limited the potential effectiveness of chiropractic in offering itself as a viable alternative to allopathic medical care. The trial took over 12 years to complete and was recently upheld by the U.S. Supreme Court in their refusal to hear arguments in the case, thus upholding the decision of Judge Susan Getzendanner in the Seventh Circuit Court.

This decision opens many avenues of health care long thought closed to chiropractors. Although inroads had already been made in gaining hospital privileges for individual chiropractors, the decision makes it easier for this to occur. However, although the Joint Commissions on the Accreditation of Hospitals was named in the original suit, it was soon separated from the suit. Thus, it is entirely possible that pressure could still be brought to bear on any hospital that accepts a chiropractor on staff. Indeed, it seems likely that this will occur, at least during the short term.

The effects of medical propaganda on chiropractors will take many years to overcome; that it will be overcome, we have no doubt. Suits are still being brought by chiropractors against medical practitioners who refuse to have anything to do with the chiropractic profession. In one notable case, the use of RICO laws has been proposed to punish several medical doctors who successfully caused the removal of a neurosurgeon from a hospital because of his association with a local chiropractor. The burden, however, rests mainly with the chiropractic profession, and over the long term, more and more chiropractors likely will gain hospital privileges.

This must come, in part, by our successfully defending our techniques and by our testing and refining them. This is a process in its infancy. The profession is now involved in developing standards of care; these standards have a mechanism for testing chiropractic methods and then classifying them as experimental, mainstream, etc. In early 1990, the profession held its first Consensus Conference on the Validation of Chiropractic Methods.[12] The conference brought together researchers, academicians, technique developers, politicians, and others from all walks of chiropractic life to develop systems to test the validity of chiropractic procedures. The process is a continuous process. In this program, the first day was given over to invited speakers talking on a variety of topics relating to technique, while the second day had several roundtable and panel discussions relating to the way such validation might occur. It is exciting to see how many technique developers were involved. The history of chiropractic technique is largely one of individual drive rather than hard scientific research before the release of information.

At a second Consensus Conference, held in 1991, techniques used within the profession were discussed using generic terms based on the contacts taken and characteristics of the thrust procedure.[13] This was done with the broad intention of developing a means to classify different technique systems in a generic format for research and validation procedures. For instance, the category of short-lever, specific contact using a high-velocity low-amplitude thrust would include many of the techniques in the Diversified and Gonstead Techniques, whereas the category of mechanically assisted, short-lever, specific contact with a high-velocity and low-amplitude thrust would include Thompson and Pierce-Stillwagon Techniques. This conference set the scene for the need to validate individual technique procedures and to develop comparison studies as to the effectiveness of one technique procedure over another.

The science of chiropractic is now beginning to investigate the art of chiropractic. The profession will then be better able to define itself for the coming debate regarding national health insurance. Without doubt, the potential to lose all that was won in the Wilk case exists with the emerging national health debate. The nation has become increasingly cost conscious, and many decisions regarding health care no longer rest with those involved in delivering that care. Instead, these decisions rest with insurance company executives, politicians, and governmental agencies. These groups are not likely to support inclusion of health-care methods that lack scientific credibility in a national health insurance plan. The need to continue scientific research is paramount to maintaining chiropractic practice rights. The process initiated by the Consensus Conference must be ongoing.

If national health insurance becomes a reality, we must ensure that chiropractic procedures are covered by the plan. A book such as this is only one method to ensure that they are.

The chiropractic profession is rapidly gaining acceptance. It now has a body of credible research to document much of what it claims, it supports several fine scientific journals (at least one of which is indexed worldwide), it has an increasing number of high-quality textbooks, it has developing teaching techniques in its educational curriculum (many of which are moving toward problem-based learning), and it has increasing legislative clout.

A challenge for the future is to classify and place all chiropractic technique into a framework that allows us to determine which ones have a basis in fact. The profession can then begin to weed out unacceptable procedures that are promoted largely on the strength of the cult of personality that arises around the founder of the system. We can all appreciate the effort and drive that led so many chiropractic pioneers to devise their system, but to allow those systems to flourish solely because of those efforts is to do a grave disservice to those who follow. Serious investigation into many of these systems is underway.

The techniques in this book are not those of any particular system but represent a collection of procedures from many different systems, thus providing information about adjusting a wide range of areas in the body. Taken as a whole, they are a fair cross-representation of what the chiropractic profession has to offer.

REFERENCES

1. Beideman RP: Seeking the rational alternative: The National College of Chiropractic from 1906 to 1982. Chiro History 3:17, 1983

2. Gibbons RW: The evolution of chiropractic: medical and social protest in America. p. 3. In Haldeman S (ed): Modern Developments in the Principles and Practice of Chiropractic. Appleton Century Crofts, East Norwalk, CT, 1980

3. Brooks WH, Cross RJ, Roszman TL, Markesbery WR: Neuroimmunomodulation: neural anatomical basis for impairment and facilitation. Ann Neurol 12:56, 1982

4. Haldeman S: The clinical basis for discussion of mechanisms of manipulative therapy. p. 4. In Korr IM (ed): The Neurobiologic Mechanisms of Manipulative Therapy. Plenum, New York, 1978

5. Sato A: Physiological studies of the somatoautonomic reflexes. p. 93. In

Haldeman S (ed): Modern Developments in the Principles and Practice of Chiropractic. Appleton Century Crofts, East Norwalk, CT, 1980

6. Coote JH: Central organization of the somatosympathetic reflexes. In Haldeman S (ed): Modern Developments in the Principles and Practice of Chiropractic. Appleton Century Crofts, East Norwalk, CT, 1980

7. Beal MC: Viscerosomatic reflexes: a review. JAOA 85:786, 1985.

8. Proceedings: The Central Connection: Somatovisceral/Viscerosomatic Interaction, 1989. International Symposium, Cincinnati, 1989

9. Caplan R: Chiropractic. In Salmon J (ed): Alternative Medicines. Tavistock Publications, New York, 1984

10. Flexner A: Medical education in the United States and Canada. Carnegie Foundation Advancement Teaching Bull No. 4, 1910.

11. Beideman RP: A short history of the chiropractic profession. In Lawrence DJ (ed): Fundamentals of Chiropractic Diagnosis and Management. Williams & Wilkins, Baltimore, 1947.

12. Proceedings, 1990 Consensus Conference on Validation of Chiropractic Technique, Seattle. J Chiro Tech 2(3):71, 1990

13. Proceedings, 1991 Consensus Conference on Validation of Chiropractic Technique, Monterey. J Chiro Tech 4(1):1, 1991

14. Janse J, Hauser RH, Wells BF: Chiropractic Principles and Technique. National College of Chiropractic, Chicago, 1947

15. Kirk CR, Lawrence DJ, Valvo NL (eds): The States Manual of Spinal, Pelvic and Extravertebral Technique. National College of Chiropractic, Lombard, IL, 1985

16. Garrow JS: Kinesiology and food allergy. Br Med J 296:1573, 1988

17. Rybeck CH, Swenson RS: The effect of oral administration of refined sugar on muscle strength. J Manipulative Physiol Ther 3:155, 1980

18. Triano JJ: Muscle strength testing as a diagnostic screen for supplemental nutrition testing: a blind study. J Manipulative Physiol Ther 5:179, 1982

19. Van Rumpt R: Directional non-force technique. In Kfoury PW (ed): Catalogue of Chiropractic Techniques. Publisher unknown

20. Fuhr A, Smith DB: Accuracy of piezoelectric accelerometers measuring displacement of a spinal adjusting instrument. J Manipulative Physiol Ther 9:15, 1986

2

Joint Anatomy and Basic Biomechanics

Dana J. Lawrence
Thomas F. Bergmann

FUNDAMENTAL CONCEPTS, PRINCIPLES, AND TERMS

This chapter provides an academic picture of the applied anatomy and biomechanics of the musculoskeletal system. The human body may be viewed as a machine formed of many different parts that allow motion. These motions occur at the many joints formed by the specific parts composing the body's musculoskeletal system. Although there is some controversy and speculation among those who study these complex activities, the information presented here is considered to be essential for understanding clinical correlations and applications. Biomechanical discussions require specific nomenclature, which enables people working in a wide variety of disciplines to communicate (see Appendix 3).

Mechanics is the study of forces and their effects. *Biomechanics* is the application of mechanical laws to living structures, specifically to the locomotor system of the human body. *Kinematics* is a branch of mechanics that deals with the geometry of the motion of objects including displacement, velocity, and acceleration, without taking into account the forces that produce the motion. *Kinetics*, however, is the study of the relations between the force system acting on a body and the changes it produces in body motion. Forces have vector characteristics whereby a specific direction is delineated at the point of application. Moreover, forces can vary in magnitude, which will affect the acceleration of the object to which the force is applied. Knowledge of joint mechanics and structure as well as the effects that forces will exert on the body has important implications for the use of manipulative procedures and, specifically, chiropractic adjustments. Therefore, biomechanics concerns the interrelations of the skeleton, muscles, and joints. The bones form the levers, the ligaments surrounding the joint form a hinge, and the muscles provide the forces for moving the levers about the joints.

The *lever* is a rigid bar revolving about a fixed point called the *axis* or

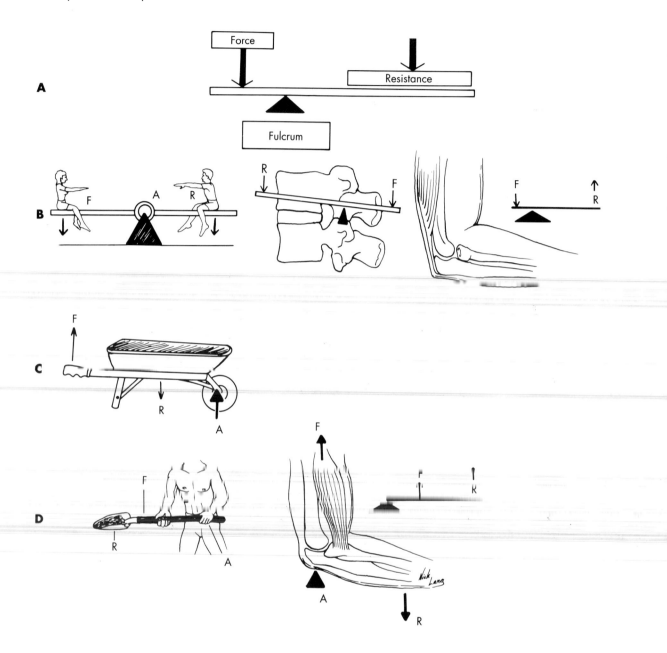

Figure 2.1 (**A**) Lever system. (**B**) First-class lever system. (**C**) Second-class lever system. (**D**) Third-class lever system. A, axis (fulcrum); F, force; R, resistance.

fulcrum. Force is applied from muscles at some point along the lever so as to move the body part; this is called *resistance.* The lever is one of the simplest of all mechanical devices that can be called a machine. The relationship of fulcrum to force to resistance distinguishes the different classes of levers.

In a first-class lever, the axis (fulcrum) is located between the force and resistance; in a second-class lever, the resistance is between the axis and the force; and in a third-class lever, the force is between the axis and the resistance (Fig. 2.1). Every bone in the body acts alone or in combination, forcing a network of lever systems characteristic of the first- and third-

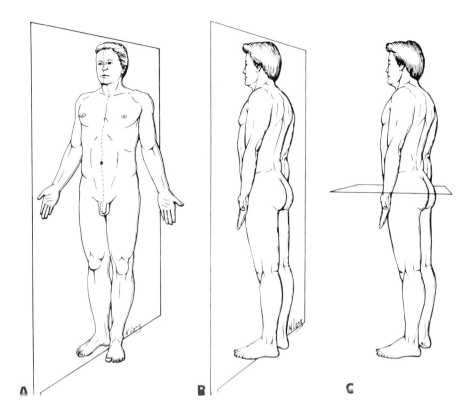

Figure 2.2 **(A)** Midsagittal plane. A "sagittal axis" lies in the sagittal plane and extends horizontally from front to back. The movements of abduction and adduction take place about this axis in a coronal plane. **(B)** Coronal plane. A "coronal axis" lies in the coronal plane and extends horizontally from side to side. The movements of flexion and extension take place about this axis in a sagittal plane. **(C)** Transverse plane. A "longitudinal axis" is vertical, extending in a cranial-caudal direction, and permits medial and lateral rotation movements.

class levers. There are virtually no second-class levers in the body, though opening the mouth against resistance is an example.

With a first class lever, the longer the lever arm, the less force required to overcome the resistance. The force arm may be longer, shorter, or equal to the resistance arm, but the axis will always be between these two points. An example of a first-class lever in the human body is the forearm moving at the elbow through contraction of the triceps muscle.

Third-class levers are the most common type in the body because they allow the muscle to be inserted near the joint and can thereby produce increased speed of movement, although at a sacrifice of force. The force must be smaller than the resistance arm, and the applied force lies closer to the axis than the resistance force. An example of a third-class lever is the forearm moving at the elbow through contraction of the biceps muscle.

It is also necessary to delineate the specific body planes of reference as they will be used to describe structural position and directions of functional movement. The standard position of reference or anatomic position has the body facing forward, the hands at the sides of the body, with the palms facing forward, and the feet pointing straight ahead. The body planes are derived from dimensions in space and are oriented at right angles to one another. The sagittal plane is vertical and extends from front to back, or from anterior to posterior. Its name is derived from the direction of the human sagittal suture in the cranium. The median sagittal plane, also called

Table 2.1 Body Planes of Movement

Plane of Movement	Axis	Joint Movement
Sagittal	Coronal	Flexion and extension
Coronal	Sagittal (anteroposterior)	Abduction and adduction
Transverse	Longitudinal (Vertical)	Medial and lateral rotation

the *midsagittal plane*, divides the body into right and left halves (Fig. 2.2A) (Table 2.1).

The coronal plane is vertical and extends from side to side. Its name is derived from the orientation of the human coronal suture of the cranium. It may also be referred to as the *frontal plane,* and it divides the body into anterior and posterior components (Fig. 2.2B).

The transverse plane is a horizontal plane and divides a structure into upper and lower components (Figure 2.2C).

An axis is a line around which motion occurs. Axes are related to planes of reference and the *cardinal axes* are oriented at right angles to one another. This is expressed as a three-dimensional coordinate system with "x, y, and z" used to mark the axes (Fig. 2.3). The significance of this coordinate system is in defining or locating the extent of the types of movement possible at each joint—rotation, translation, and curvilinear. All movements that occur about an axis are considered *rotational,* whereas linear movements along an axis and through a plane are called *translational.* Curvilinear motion occurs when rotational movements are accompanied by a translational movement.

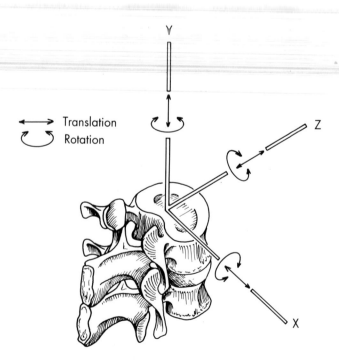

Figure 2.3 The three-dimensional coordinate system.

Joint Motion

Motion can be defined as a continuous change in position of an object. *Specific motions* or *resultant positions* are defined by the axis around which movement takes place and the plane through which movement occurs. The coronal axis (x-axis) lies in the coronal plane and extends from one side of the body to the other. The motions of flexion and extension occur about this axis and through the sagittal plane. Flexion is motion in the anterior direction for joints of the head, neck, trunk, upper extremity, and hip. Flexion of the knee, ankle, foot, and toes refers to movement in the posterior direction. Extension is motion in the direct opposite manner from flexion (Fig. 2.4A).

The sagittal axis (z-axis) lies in the sagittal plane and extends horizontally from anterior to posterior. Movements of abduction and adduction as well as lateral flexion of the spine occur around this axis and through the coronal plane. Lateral flexion is then a rotational movement and is used to denote lateral movements of head, neck, and trunk in the coronal plane (Fig. 2.4B). In the human, lateral flexion is usually combined with some element of rotation. Abduction and adduction are also motions in a coronal plane. Abduction is movement away from the body, and adduction is movement toward the body; the reference here is to the midsagittal plane of the body. This would be true for all parts of the extremities excluding the thumb, fingers, and toes. For these structures, reference points are to be found within that particular extremity.

The longitudinal axis (y-axis) is vertical, extending in a head to toe direction. Movements of medial and lateral rotation as well as axial rotation in the spine occur around it and through the transverse plane. Axial rotation is used to describe this type of movement for all areas of the body except the scapula and clavicle. Rotation occurs about an anatomic axis except in the case of the femur, which rotates around a mechanical axis.[1] In the human extremity, the anterior surface of the extremity is used as a reference area. Rotation of the anterior surface toward the midsagittal plane of the body is medial (internal) rotation, and rotation away from the midsagittal plane is lateral (external) rotation (Fig. 2.4C).

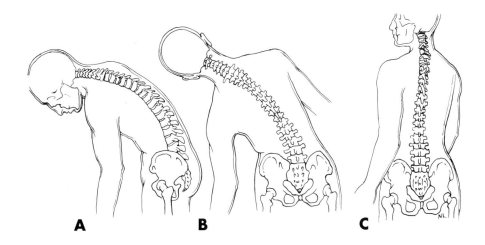

Figure 2.4 (**A**) Sagittal plane movement of flexion. (**B**) Coronal plane movement of lateral flexion. (**C**) Transverse plane movement of axial rotation.

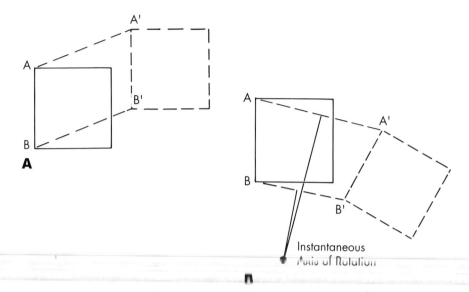

Figure 2.5 **(A)** Translational movement. **(B)** Curvilinear movement, a combination of translation and rotation movements.

Because the head, neck, thorax, and pelvis rotate about longitudinal axes in the midsagittal area, rotation cannot be named in reference to the midsagittal plane. Rotation of the head, spine, and pelvis is described as rotation of the anterior surface toward the right or left. *Rotation of the scapula* refers to movements about a sagittal axis, rather than about a longitudinal axis. The terms *clockwise* or *counterclockwise* are used (Table 2.1).

Translational movements are linear movements, or simply, movement in a straight line. Gliding movements of the joint are translational in character. The arthrokinematic term *slide* has also been used in referring to translational movements between joint surfaces. Anterior to posterior and posterior to anterior glide (anterolisthesis and retrolisthesis) are translational movements through the sagittal plane. Lateral to medial and medial to lateral glide (laterolisthesis) translate through the coronal plane. Distraction and compression (altered interosseous spacing) translate through the transverse plane along the vertical axis (y-axis). Curvilinear motion combines both rotational and translational movements and is the most common motion produced by the joints of the body (Fig. 2.5).

Moreover, the potential exists for each joint to exhibit three translational movements and three rotational movements constituting 6 degrees of freedom. The extent of each movement is based more or less on the joint anatomy and specifically the plane of the joint surface. This is especially important in the spinal joints. Each articulation in the body should then exhibit, to some degree, flexion, extension, right and left lateral flexion, right and left axial rotation, anterior to posterior glide, posterior to anterior glide, lateral to medial glide, medial to lateral glide, compression, and distraction.

Joints are classified first by their functional capabilities and then are subdivided by their structural characteristics. Synarthroses allow very little,

Table 2.2 Joint Classification

Functional Type	Structural Type	Example
Synarthroses	Fibrous	
	Suture—nearly no movement	Cranial sutures
	Syndesmosis—some movement	Distal tibular–fibular
	Cartilaginous	
	Synchondrosis—temporary	Epiphyseal plates
	Symphysis—fibrocartilage	Pubes, intervertebral discs
Diarthroses	Uniaxial	
	Ginglimus (hinge)	Elbow
	Trochoid (pivot)	Atlantoaxial
	Condylar	Metacarpophalangeal
	Biaxial	
	Ellipsoid	Radiocarpal
	Sellar (saddle)	Carpometacarpal of the thumb
	Multiaxial	
	Triaxial	Shoulder
	Spheroid (ball and socket)	Hip
	Plane (nonaxial)	Intercarpals, posterior facet joints in spine

if any, movement; diarthroses, or true synovial joints, allow significant amounts of movement. The structural characteristics of these joints are detailed in Table 2.2.

Synovial Joints

Synovial joints are the most common joint of the human appendicular skeleton, representing highly evolved movable joints. Though these joints are considered freely movable, the degree of possible motion will vary according to the individual structural design, facet planes, and primary function (motion vs. stability). The components of a typical synovial joint include the bony elements, subchondral bones, articular cartilage, synovial membrane, and fibroligamentous joint capsule. An understanding of the basic anatomy of a synovial joint forms the foundation for developing an appreciation of clinically significant changes in the joint that lead to joint dysfunction.

The bony elements provide the supporting structure that gives the joint its capabilities and individual characteristics by forming lever arms to which intrinsic and extrinsic forces are applied. Bone is actually a form of connective tissue that has an inorganic constituent (lime salts). A hard, outer shell of cortical bone provides structural support and surrounds the cancellous bone, which contains marrow and blood vessels that provide nutrition. Trabecular patterns develop in the cancellous bone corresponding to mechanical stress applied to and required by the bone (Fig. 2.6). Bone also has the important role of hemopoiesis (formation of blood cells). Furthermore, bone stores calcium and phosphorous, which it exchanges with blood and

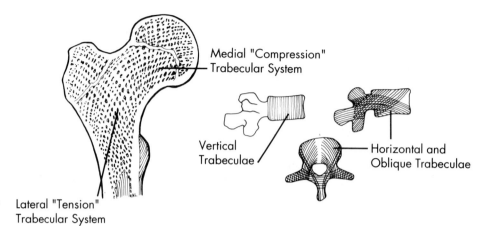

Figure 2.6 Trabecular patterns corresponding to mechanical stresses in the hip joint and vertebra. (Modified from Hertling and Kessler,[5] with permission.)

Medial "Compression" Trabecular System

Vertical Trabeculae

Horizontal and Oblique Trabeculae

Lateral "Tension" Trabecular System

tissue fluids. Finally, bone has the unique characteristic of repairing itself with its own tissue as opposed to fibrous scar tissue, which all other body tissues use.

Articular cartilage covers the articulating bones in synovial joints and helps to transmit loads and reduce friction. It is bonded tightly to the subchondral bone through the zone of calcification, which is the end of bone visible on x-ray. The joint space visualized on x-ray is composed of the synovial cavity and noncalcified articular cartilage. In its normal composition, articular cartilage has four histologic areas or zones (Fig. 2.7). These zones have been further studied and refined so that a wealth of newer information regarding cartilage has developed.

The outermost layer of cartilage is known as the gliding zone, which itself contains a superficial layer (outer) and a tangential layer (inner). The outer segment is made up solely of collagen randomly oriented into flat bundles. The tangential layer consists of densely packed layers of collagen, which are oriented parallel to the surface of the joint.[2] This orientation is along the lines of the joint motion, which implies that the outer layers of collagen are stronger when forces are applied parallel to the joint motion rather than perpendicular to it.[3] This particular orientation of fibers provides a great deal of strength to the joint in normal motion. The gliding zone also has a role in protecting the deeper elastic cartilage.

The transitional zone lies beneath the gliding zone. It represents an area where the orientation of the fibers begins to change from the parallel orientation of the gliding zone to the more perpendicular orientation of the radial zone; thus, fiber orientation is more or less oblique and, in varying angles, formed from glucuronic acid and N-acetyl-galactosamine with a sulfate on either the fourth or sixth position. The keratin compound is formed with galactose and N-acetyl-galactosamine. All of this occurs in linked, repeating units (Fig. 2.8).

Articular cartilage is considered to be mostly avascular. Therefore, it must rely on other sources for nutrition. One role of the highly vascularized

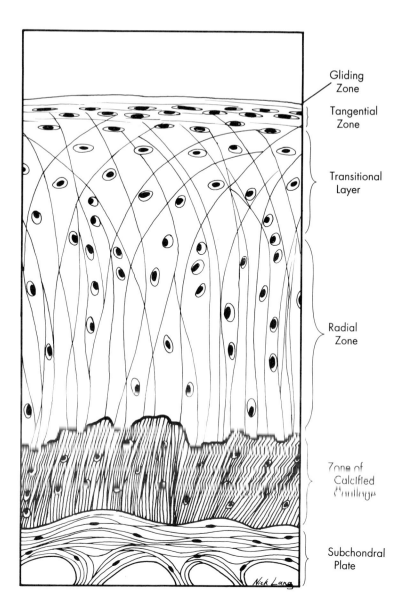

Gliding
Zone

Tangential
Zone

Transitional
Layer

Radial
Zone

Zone of
Calcified
Cartilage

Subchondral
Plate

Figure 2.7 Microscopic anatomy of articular cartilage. (Modified from Albright and Brand,[33] with permission.)

synovium is believed to be a supply of nutrition for the articular cartilage it covers. Direct contact is made with the articular cartilage superficially, with diffusion and imbibition serving as mechanisms for the deeper layers. Therefore, intermittent compression and distraction (loading and unloading) is necessary for adequate exchange of nutrients and waste products. Although the exact role of synovial fluid is still unknown, it is thought to serve as a joint lubricant or at least to interact with the articular cartilage to decrease friction between joint surfaces. This is of clinical relevance, because immobilized joints have been shown to undergo degeneration of the articu-

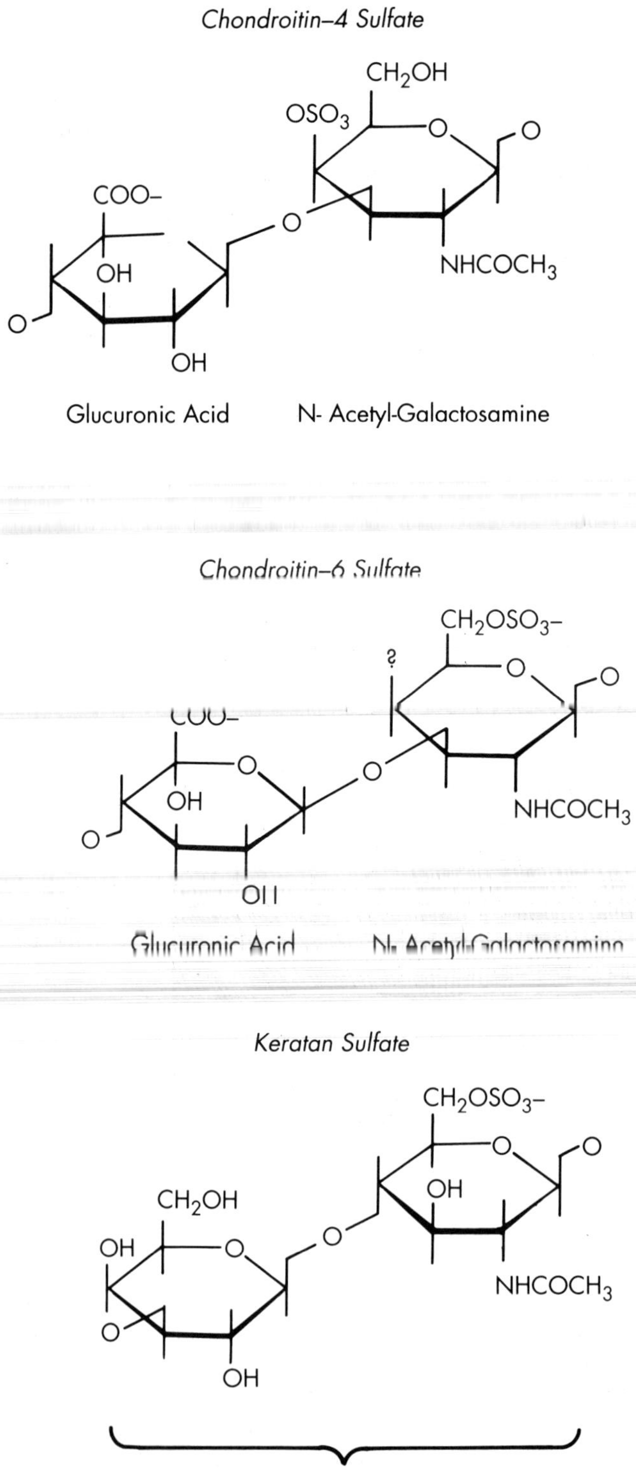

Figure 2.8 Structure of chondroitan and keratin compounds.

lar cartilage.[4] Synovial fluid is similar in composition to plasma with the addition of mucin (hyaluronic acid), which gives it a high molecular weight and its characteristic viscosity. Three models of joint lubrication exist. The controversy lies in the realization that no one model of joint lubrication applies to all joints under all circumstances.

According to the hydrodynamic model, synovial fluid fills in spaces left by the incongruent joint surfaces. With joint movement, synovial fluid is attracted to the area of contact between the joint surfaces, resulting in the maintenance of a fluid film between moving surfaces. This model was the first to be described and works well with quick movement but would not provide adequate lubrication for slow movements and movement under increased loads.

The elastohydrodynamic model is a modification that considers the viscoelastic properties of articular cartilage whereby deformation of joint surfaces occurs with loading, creating increased contact between surfaces. This would effectively reduce the compression stress to the lubrication fluid. Although this model allows for loading forces, it does not explain lubrication at the initiation of movement or the period of relative zero velocity during reciprocating movements.[5]

In the boundary lubrication model, the lubricant is adsorbed in the joint surface, which would reduce the roughness of the surface by filling the irregularities and effectively coating the joint surface. This model can allow for initial movement and zero velocity movements. Moreover, boundary lubrication combined with the elastohydrodynamic model, creating a mixed model, meets the demands of the human synovial joint (Fig. 2.9).

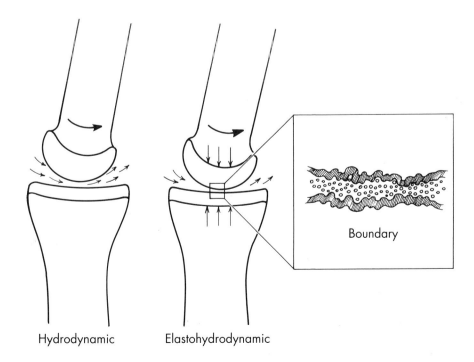

Hydrodynamic   Elastohydrodynamic

Boundary

Figure 2.9 Lubrication models for synovial joints. (Modified from Hertling and Kessler,[5] with permission.)

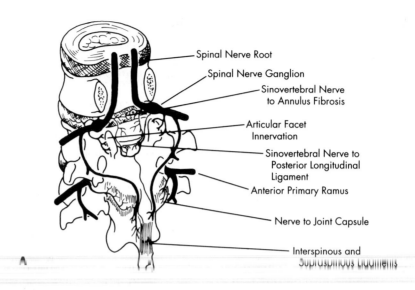

Spinal Nerve Root

Spinal Nerve Ganglion

Sinovertebral Nerve
to Annulus Fibrosis

Articular Facet
Innervation

Sinovertebral Nerve to
Posterior Longitudinal
Ligament

Anterior Primary Ramus

Nerve to Joint Capsule

Interspinous and
Supraspinous Ligaments

A

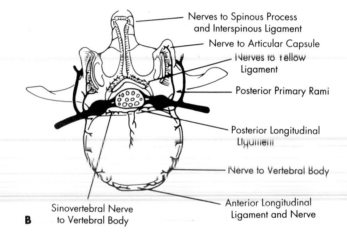

Nerves to Spinous Process
and Interspinous Ligament

Nerve to Articular Capsule

Nerves to Yellow
Ligament

Posterior Primary Rami

Posterior Longitudinal
Ligament

Nerve to Vertebral Body

Anterior Longitudinal
Ligament and Nerve

Sinovertebral Nerve
to Vertebral Body

B

Figure 2.10 Innervation of the outer fibers of the disc and facet joint capsule by the sinuvertebral nerve. (A) Side view. (B) Top view. (Modified from White and Panjabi,[12] with permission.)

Articular neurology gives invaluable information on the nature of joint pain, the relation of joint pain to joint dysfunction, and the role of manipulative procedures in affecting pain from a joint. Synovial joints are innervated by three or four varieties of neuroreceptors with a wide variety to their parent neurons. The parent neurons differ in diameter and conduction velocity, representing a continuum from the largest heavily myelinated A α-fibers to the smallest unmyelinated C fibers. All are derived from the dorsal and ventral rami, as well as the recurrent meningeal nerve of each segmental spinal nerve (Fig. 2.10). Information from these receptors spread among many segmental levels because of multilevel ascending and descending primary afferents. The receptors are divided into the four groups according to their neurohistologic properties, which includes three corpuscular mechanoreceptors and one nociceptor.[6]

Type I receptors are confined to the outer layers of the joint capsule and are stimulated by active or passive joint motions. Their firing rate is inhibited with joint end approximation, and they have a low threshold, making them very sensitive to movement. Some are considered static receptors in that they will fire continually even with no joint movement. Because they are slow adapting, the effects of movement are long lasting. Stimulation of type I receptors is involved with the following:

1. Reflex modulation of posture, as well as with movement (kinesthetic sensations), through constant monitoring of outer joint tension
2. Perception of posture and movement
3. Inhibition of centripetal flow from pain receptors via an enkephalin synaptic interneuron transmitter
4. Tonic effects on lower motor neuron pools involved in the neck, limbs, jaw, and eye muscles

Type II mechanoreceptors are found within the deeper layers of the joint capsule. They are also low threshold and again are stimulated with even minor changes in tension within the inner joint. Unlike type I receptors, however, type II receptors are very rapidly adapting and quickly cease firing when the joint stops moving. Type II receptors are completely inactive in immobilized joints. Functions of the type II receptors are likely to include the following:

1. Movement monitoring for reflex actions and perhaps perceptual sensations
2. Inhibition of centripetal flow from pain receptors via an enkephalin synaptic interneuron neutral transmitter
3. Phasic effects on lower motor neuron pools involved in the neck, limbs, jaw, and eye muscles

The type III mechanoreceptors are absent from all of the synovial spinal joints (some have been identified in cervical discs) but are found in the intrinsic and extrinsic ligaments of the peripheral joints. These receptors are very slow adaptors with a very high threshold because they are innervated by large myelinated fibers. They seem to be the joint version of the Golgi tendon organ in that they impose an inhibitory effect on motoneurons. Although the functions of type III receptors are not completely understood, it is likely that they achieve the following:

1. Monitor direction of movement
2. Create a reflex effect on segmental muscle tone, providing a "braking mechanism" against movement that overdisplaces the joint
3. Recognize potentially harmful movements

Type IV receptors are composed of a network of free nerve endings as well as unmyelinated fibers. They are associated with pain perception and include many different varieties with large ranges of sensations, including itch and tickle. They possess an intimate physical relationship to the mechanoreceptors and are present throughout the fibrous portions of the joint capsule and ligaments. They are absent from articular cartilage and synovial linings, though they have been found in synovial folds.[7,8] They are very high-threshold receptors and are completely inactive in the physiologic joint. Joint capsule pressure, narrowing of the intervertebral disc, fracture of a vertebral body, dislocation of the zygapophyseal joints, chemical irritation, and interstitial edema associated with acute and/or chronic inflammation may all activate the nociceptive system. The basic functions of the nociceptors include the following:

1. Evoke pain
2. Tonic effects on neck, limb, jaw, and eye muscles
3. Central reflex connections for pain inhibition
4. Central reflex connections for a myriad of autonomic affects

A relationship exists between mechanoreceptors and nociceptors such that when the mechanoreceptors can function correctly, an inhibition of nociceptor activity occurs. The converse also holds true; when the mechanoreceptors fail to function correctly, inhibition of nociceptors will occur less and pain will be perceived.

Discharges from the articular mechanoreceptors are polysynaptic and produce coordinated facilitory and inhibitory reflex changes in the spinal musculature. This provides a significant contribution to the reflex control of these muscles.[6] Gillette suggests that a chiropractic adjustment produces sufficient force to coactivate a wide variety of mechanically sensitive receptor types in the paraspinal tissues.[7] The A-δ-mechanoreceptors and C-polymodal nociceptors, which can generate impulses during and after stimulation, may well be the most physiologically interesting component of the afferent bombardment initiated by high-velocity, low-amplitude manipulations. For normal function of the joint structures, an integration of proprioception, kinesthetic perception, and reflex regulation is absolutely essential.

Pain-sensitive fibers also exist within the annulus fibrosis of the disc. Malinsky demonstrated a variety of free and complex endings in the outer one-third of the annulus.[8] Posteriorly, the disc is innervated by the recurrent meningeal nerve (sinuvertebral nerve) and laterally by branches of the grey rami communicantes. During evaluation of disc material surgically removed before spinal fusion, Bogduk found abundant nerve endings with various morphologies. The varieties of nerve endings included free terminals, complex sprays, and convoluted tangles.[9] Furthermore, many of these endings contain substance P, a putative transmitter substance involved in nociception.

Shinohara reported the presence of such nerve fibers accompanying granulation tissue as deep as the nucleus in degenerated discs.[10] The postulated function of encapsulated disc receptors is proprioception, though this remains to be proven. Abundant evidence, however, shows that the disc can be painful, supporting the ascribed nociceptive function of the free nerve endings.[10a-f]

Because structure and function are interdependent, the study of joint characteristics should not isolate structure from function. The structural attributes of a joint are defined as the anatomic joint, consisting of the articular surfaces with the surrounding joint capsule and ligaments as well as any intra-articular structures. The functional attributes are defined by the physiologic joint, consisting of the anatomic joint plus the surrounding soft tissues including the muscles, connective tissue, nerves, and blood vessels (Fig. 2.11).

To describe the relationship of structure to function, the term *arthrokinematics* is used to examine what happens between joint surfaces when a joint undergoes movement. Consideration of the motion between bones alone or osteokinematic movement is insufficient, because no concern is given to what occurs at the joint and because movement commonly involves coupling of motion around different axes. It is, therefore, important to relate osetokinematic movement to arthrokinematic movement when evaluating joint motion (Fig. 2.12). This involves determining the movement of the mechanical axis of the moving bone relative to the stationary joint surface. The mechanical axis of a joint is defined as a line that passes through the moving bone to which it is perpendicular while contacting the center of the stationary joint surface (Fig. 2.13). MacConnail and Basmajian[11] use the term *spin* to describe rotational movement around the mechanical axis, which is possible as a pure movement only in the hip, shoulder, and proximal radius. Any

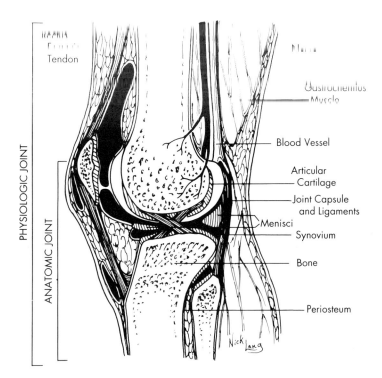

Figure 2.11 Structures that make up the anatomic joint and the physiologic joint.

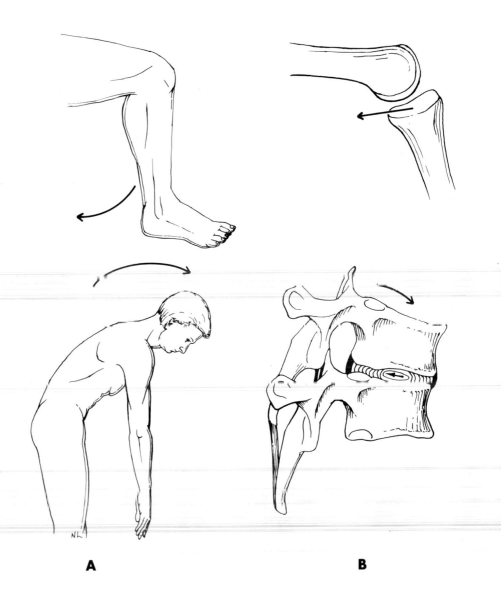

Figure 2.12 (A) The osteokinematic movement of knee and trunk flexion. (B) The arthrokinematic movements of tibiofemoral and T6–T7 joint flexion.

A

B

movement of a joint that is not pure spin is called *swing,* which can occur alone or in combination with spin.

When one joint surface moves relative to the other, roll, or slide, or both occur. Roll occurs when points on the surface of one bone contact points at the same interval of the other bone. Slide occurs when only one point on the moving joint surface contacts various points on the opposing joint surface (Fig. 2.14). In most joints of the human body, these two motions occur simultaneously. The concave–convex rule relates to this expected coupling of rotational (roll) and translational (slide) movements. When a concave surface moves on a convex surface, roll and slide movements should

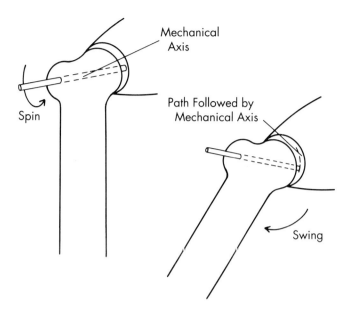

Mechanical
Axis

Spin

Path Followed by
Mechanical Axis

Swing

Figure 2.13 The mechanical axis of a joint and MacConnail and Basmajian's[11] concept of spin and swing. (Modified from Hertling and Kessler,[5] with permission.)

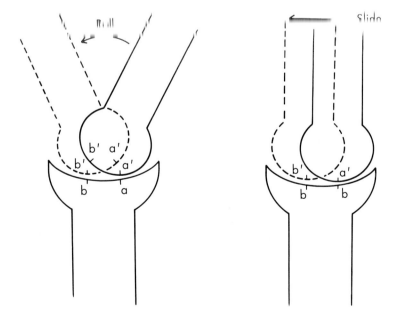

Roll

Slide

b' a'

b'   a'

b   a

b'   a'

b   'b

Figure 2.14   The arthrokinematic movements of roll and slide. (Modified from Hertling and Kessler,[5] with permission.)

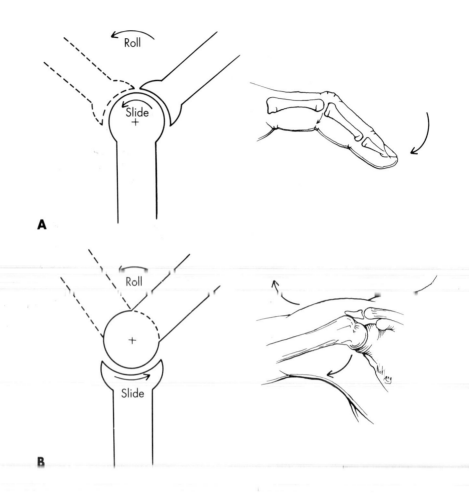

Figure 2.15 The concave–convex rule. (A) Movement of concave surface on a convex surface. (B) Movement of a convex surface on a concave surface.

occur in the same direction. When a convex surface moves on a concave surface, however, roll and slide should occur in opposite directions (Fig. 2.15). Pure roll movement tends to result in joint dislocation, whereas pure slide movement causes joint surface impingement. Moreover, coupling of roll and slide is important anatomically because less articular cartilage is necessary in a joint to allow for movement and may also decrease wear on the joint (Fig. 2.16). These concepts are instrumental in clinical decision making regarding the restoration of restricted joint motion.

Additionally, when an object moves, the axis around which the movement occurs can vary in placement from one instant to another. The term *instantaneous axis of rotation (IAR)* is used to denote this location point. Asymmetric forces applied to the joint can cause a shift in the IAR. Furthermore, vertebral movement is more easily analyzed as the IAR becomes more completely understood (Fig. 2.17). White and Panjabi point out that the beauty of this concept is that any kind of plane motion can be described relative to the IAR. Complex motions are simply regarded as many very

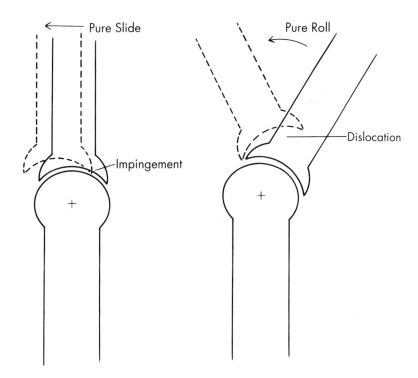

Figure 2.16 The consequences of pure roll or pure slide movements. (Modified from Hertling and Kessler,[5] with permission.)

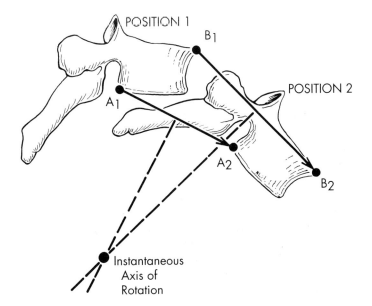

Figure 2.17 The instantaneous axis of rotation. (Modified from White and Panjabi,[12] with permission.)

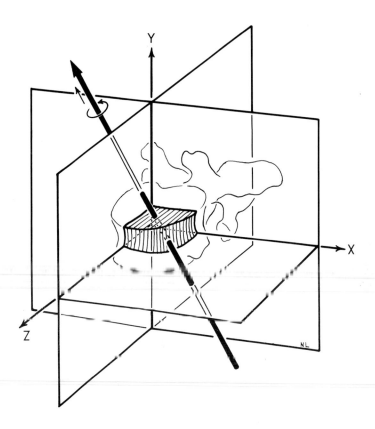

Figure 2.18 Helical axis of motion. (Modified from White and Panjabi,[12] with permission.)

small movements with many changing instantaneous axes of rotation.[12] This concept is designed to describe plane movement, or movement in two dimensions. When three-dimensional motion occurs between objects, a unique axis in space is defined called the *helical axis of motion* (HAM), or *screw axis of motion* (Fig. 2.18). HAM is the most precise way to describe motion occurring between irregularly shaped objects, such as anatomic structures, because it is difficult to consistently and accurately identify reference points for such objects.

Clearly, most movements occur around and through several axes simultaneously, so pure movements in the human frame rarely occur. The nature and extent of individual joint motion is determined by the joint structure and, specifically, by the shape and direction of the joint surfaces. No two opposing joint surfaces are perfectly matched, nor are they perfectly geometric. All joint surfaces have some degree of curvature, which is not constant but changing from point to point. Because of the incongruence between joint surfaces, some joint space and "play" must be present to allow free movement. This "joint play" is an accessory movement of the joint that is essential for normal functioning of the joint.

The resting position of a joint, or its "neutral" position, occurs when the joint capsule is most relaxed and the greatest amount of play is possible. When injured, a joint often seeks this maximum loose-packed position to allow for swelling. The close-packed position occurs when the joint capsule and ligaments are maximally tightened. Moreover, there is maximal contact between the articular surfaces, making the joint very stable and difficult to move or separate.

Joint surfaces will approximate or separate as the joint goes through a range of motion. This is the motion of compression and distraction. A joint moving toward its close-packed position is undergoing compression while movement toward the open-packed position undergoes distraction. All joint motion involves movement toward and away from the close-packed position[11] (see Table 2.3).

Each joint can undergo, more or less, five types of movement. From the neutral close-packed position, joint play should be present. This is followed by a range of active movement that is under the control of the musculature. The passive range of motion is produced by the examiner and includes the active range plus a small degree of movement into the elastic range. The elastic barrier of resistance is then encountered, which exhibits the characteristic movement of end feel. Movement of the joint beyond the paraphysiologic barrier of end feel takes the joint beyond its limit of anatomic integrity and into a pathologic zone of movement. Should a joint enter the pathologic zone, there will be damage to the joint structures including the osseous and soft tissue components (Fig. 3.16).

Table 2.3 Close-Packed Positions for Each Joint

Region	Specific Joint	Close-Packed Position
Fingers	Distal interphalangeal joints	Maximal extension
	Proximal interphalangeal joints	Maximal extension
	Metacarpophalangeal joints	Maximal flexion
Hand	Intermetacarpal joints	Maximal opposition
Wrist	Intercarpal joints	Maximal dorsiflexion
Forearm	Radioulnar joints	5 degrees supination
Elbow	Ulnohumeral joint	Extension in supination
	Radiohumeral joint	Flexion in supination
Shoulder	Glenohumeral joint	Abduction and external rotation
	Acromioclavicular joint	90 degrees of abduction
	Sternoclavicular joint	Maximal elevation
Toes	Distal interphalangeal joints	Maximal extension
	Proximal interphalangeal joints	Maximal extension
	Metatarsophalangeal joints	Maximal extension
Foot	Intermetatarsal joints	Maximal opposition
Ankle	Tarsometatarsal joints	Maximal inversion
	Tibiotalar joint	Maximal dorsiflexion
Knee	Tibiofemoral joint	Maximal extension and external rotation
Hip	Coxofemoral joint	Maximal extension, internal rotation, and abduction
Spine	Three-joint complex	Maximal extension

Both joint play and end-feel movements are thought to be necessary for the normal functioning of the joint. A loss of either movement can result in a restriction of motion, pain, and most likely, both. Active movements can be influenced by exercise; passive movements, by traction and some mobilization; but end-feel movements are affected when the joint is taken quickly to the elastic barrier, creating a sudden yielding of the joint and a characteristic cracking noise. This action can be accomplished with a high-velocity, low-amplitude manipulative thrust.

MECHANICAL PROPERTIES OF SYNOVIAL JOINT COMPONENTS

Whereas an understanding of structure is needed to form a foundation, understanding the dynamics of the components of the joint will aid in the explanation of joint injury and repair. Functionally, the most important properties of bone are its strength and stiffness, which become significant qualities when loads are applied (Fig. 2.19). Living bone will be subjected to many different combinations of loading force throughout the requirements of daily living. Though each type of loading force is described individually, most activities produce varying amounts and combinations of all of them.

Tensile loading is a "stretching action" that creates equal and opposite loads outward from the surface and tensile stress and strain inward. These forces can pull apart the cement from the osteons resulting in fractures (the most common of which is at the base of the fifth metatarsal from the pull of the peroneus brevis). Calcaneal fractures from the pull of the Achilles tendon also occur through this mechanism.

Compression loading on bone creates equal and opposite loads toward the surface and compressive stress and strain inward, causing the structure to become shorter and wider. Compression fractures of the vertebral bodies are examples of failure to withstand compressive forces.

Shear loading causes the structure to deform internally in an angular manner owing to loads applied parallel to the surface of the structure. Cancellous bone is most prone to fracture from shear loading, with the femoral condyles and tibial plateaus often falling victim.

Bending loads are a combination of tensile and compressive loads. The magnitude depends on the distance of the forces from the neutral axis. Fractures to long bones frequently occur through this mechanism.

Torsional loads are produced through a twisting force applied about the bone's axis, creating torque within the structure. Spiral fractures are examples of the results from torsional loads.

The response of connective tissue to various stress loads contributes significantly to the soft tissue component of joint dysfunction. Within the past several decades, a great deal of scientific investigation has been directed to defining the physical properties of connective tissue.

Connective tissue is made up of various densities and spacial arrangements of collagen fibers embedded in a matrix of protein-polysaccharide, which is commonly called *ground substance*. Collagen is a fibrous protein that has a very high tensile strength. Collagenous tissue is organized into many

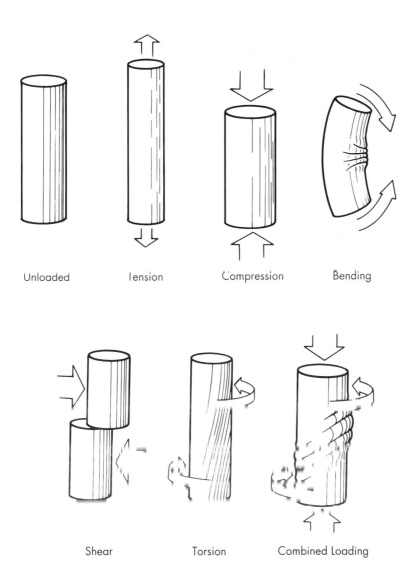

Unloaded   Tension   Compression   Bending

Shear   Torsion   Combined Loading

Figure 2.19 Loads that bone may be subject to.

different higher order structures, including tendons, ligaments, joint capsules, aponeuroses, and fascial sheaths. The principle sources of passive
resistance at the normal extremes of joint motion include ligaments, tendons, and muscles. Thus, under normal and pathologic conditions, the
range of motion in most body joints is predominately limited by one or more
connective tissue structures. The relative contribution of each to the total
resistance varies with the various body joints. Following trauma or surgery,
the connective tissue involved in the body's reparative process frequently
impedes function, because it may abnormally limit the joint range of motion.
Scar tissue, adhesions, and fibrotic contractures are common types of pathologic connective tissue that must be dealt with during chiropractic manipulative procedures.

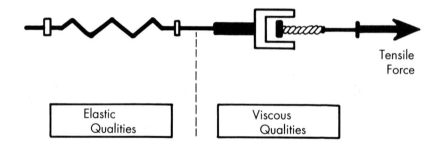

Tensile
Force

Elastic
Qualities

Viscous
Qualities

Figure 2.20 Model of connective tissue properties.

All connective tissue has a combination of two qualities, elastic stretch and plastic (viscous) stretch (Fig. 2.20). The term *stretch* refers to elongation of a linear deformation that increases in length. Stretching, then, is the process of elongation. Elastic stretch represents spring-like behavior with the elongation produced by tensile loading being recovered after the load is removed. It is, therefore, also described as *temporary, or recoverable, elongation*. Plastic (viscous) stretch refers to putty-like behavior; the linear deformation produced by tensile stress remains even after the stress is removed. This is described as *nonrecoverable, or permanent, elongation*.

The term *viscoelastic* is used to describe tissue that represents both viscous and elastic properties. The viscous properties permit time-dependent plastic or permanent deformation. Elastic properties, on the other hand, result in elastic or recoverable deformation. This allows it to rebound to the previous size, shape, and length.

Different factors influence whether the plastic or elastic component of connective tissue is predominantly affected. These include the amount of applied force and the duration of the applied force. Therefore, the major factors affecting connective tissue deformation are force and time. Given equal amounts of force great enough to overcome joint resistance, applied over a short period of time elastic deformation occurs and applied over a long time plastic deformation occurs.

When connective tissue is stretched, the relative proportion of elastic and plastic deformation can vary widely, depending on how and under what conditions the stretching is performed. When tensile forces are continuously applied to connective tissue, the time required to stretch the tissue a specific amount varies inversely with the force used. Therefore, a low-force stretching method requires more time to produce the same amount of elongation as a higher force method. However, the proportion of tissue lengthening that remains after the tensile stress is removed is greater for the low-force, long-duration method. Of course, high force and long duration will also cause stretch and possibly rupture of the connective tissue.

When connective tissue structures are permanently elongated, some degree of mechanical weakening occurs even though outright rupture has not occurred. The amount of weakening depends on the way the tissue is stretched as well as how much it is stretched. For the same amount of tissue elongation, however, a high-force stretching method produces more structural weakening than a slower, lower force method.

Because plastic deformation involves permanent changes in connective tissue, it is important to know when plastic deformity is most likely to occur. The greatest impact will occur when positions of stress are maintained for long periods. Awkward sleep postures and standing stationary for extended periods can create plastic changes that have the potential for skeletal misalignment, joint dysfunction, and instability.

Acute trauma is generally considered to be a result of a high force of short duration, influencing primarily the elastic deformation of the connective tissue. If the force is beyond the elastic range of the connective tissue, it enters the plastic range. If the force is beyond the plastic range, tissue rupture occurs. More commonly encountered by the chiropractor is the microtrauma seen in postural distortions, repetitive minor trauma occurring in occupational and daily living activities, and joint dysfunction as a result of low gravitational forces occurring over a long period, thus creating plastic deformation.

The role of muscles is to move bone and allow the human body to perform work. In the normal man, muscle accounts for about 40 to 50 percent of body weight. For the woman, this falls to approximately 30 percent of total body weight. Three types of muscle are in the body: striated skeletal muscle,

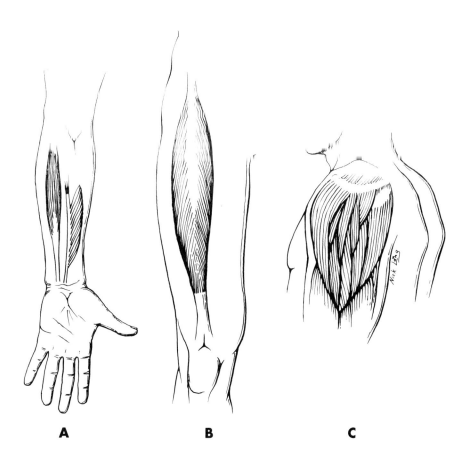

Figure 2.21 **(A)** Unipennate, **(B)** bipennate, and **(C)** multi-pennate muscles.

A   **B**   **C**

nonstriated smooth involuntary muscle, and cardiac muscle. Only the skeletal muscle is under voluntary control.

There are three gross morphologic muscle types (Fig. 2.21). Parallel muscles have fibers that run parallel throughout the length of the muscle and end in a tendon. This type of muscle is essentially designed to rapidly contract, though it typically cannot generate a great deal of power. Pennate muscles are those in which the fibers converge onto a central tendon. A muscle of this type is unipennate if the fibers attach to only one side of a central tendon, and it is bipennate if the muscle attaches to both sides of a central tendon. Finally, there is a multipennate muscle, in which the muscle fibers insert on the tendon from a variety of differing directions. This form of muscle can generate large amounts of power, though it will perform work slower than a parallel muscle.

Muscle comprises three layers (Fig. 2.22). An epimysium formed of connective tissue surrounds the muscle; a perimysium separates the muscle cells into various bundles, and an endomysium surrounds the individual muscle cells. The muscle wall also has three layers. The outermost layer is formed of collagen fibers. A basement membrane layer comprises polysaccharides and protein and is approximately 500 Å thick. The innermost layer, the sarcolemma, forms the excitable membrane of a muscle. Muscle fibers contain columns of filaments of contractile proteins. In striated muscle, these molecules are interrelated layers of actin and myosin molecules. An extensive system of sacs and tubules is arranged in the sarcoplasm. A sarcoplasmic reticulum functions in calcium ion equilibrium. A transverse tubular system transmits membrane depolarization from the muscle cell to the protein.

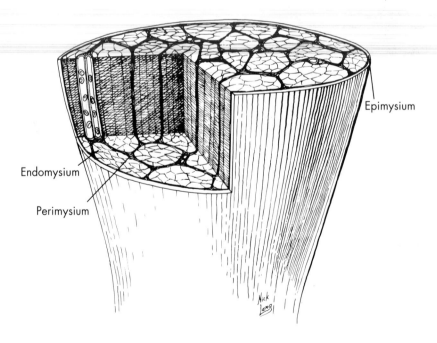

Figure 2.22 Composition of a muscle.

Also, located within the sarcoplasm, is the protein myoglobin that is necessary for oxygen binding and oxygen transfer.

Skeletal muscle occurs in two forms, originally known as *white* and *red muscle*. The white muscle is a fast-twitch, or phasic, muscle. It has a rapid contraction time and contains a large amount of glycolytic enzyme. Essentially, this muscle allows for rapid function in short periods of time. Red muscle is slow-twitch, or tonic, muscle. It contracts much slower than does white muscle and contains a great deal more myoglobin and oxidative enzymes. Red muscle is more important in static activities that require sustained effort over longer periods of time. Standing is a good example. In the human body, each individual muscle is composed of a mix of both types of muscle.

When a stimulus is delivered to a muscle from a motor nerve, all fibers in the muscle will contract at once.[13] Two types of muscle contractions have been defined. During an isotonic contraction, a muscle shortens its fibers under a constant load. This allows work to occur. During an isometric contraction, the length of the muscle does not change. This produces tension, but no work. No muscle can perform a purely isotonic contraction, because each isotonic contraction must be initiated by an isometric contraction.

Muscles can perform various functions because of their ability to contract and relax. One property is that of shock absorption, another is acceleration, and a third is deceleration. Each is very important to the overall understanding of the biomechanics of the body and will be discussed separately.

The predominant responsibility for the dissipation of axial compression shocks rests with the muscular–tendon system. As a result, shock causes many musculoskeletal complaints. Shin splints, plantar fasciitis, achilles tendinitis, lateral epicondylitis, as well as some forms of back pain can result from the body's inability to absorb and dissipate shock adequately.

Muscle contraction refers to the development of tension within the muscle, not necessarily creating a shortening of the muscle. When a muscle develops enough tension to overcome a resistance so that the muscle visibly shortens, moving the body part, concentric contraction is said to occur. *Acceleration* is thus the ability of a muscle to exert a force (concentric contraction) on the bony lever to produce movement around the fulcrum to the extent intended.

When a given resistance overcomes the muscle tension so that the muscle actually lengthens, the movement is termed an *eccentric contraction*. Deceleration is the property of a muscle being able to relax (eccentric contraction) at a controlled rate. There are numerous clinical applications of the eccentric contraction of muscles, particularly in posture.

Though the muscular system is the primary stabilizer of the joint, if the muscle breaks down, the ligaments take up the stress. This is often seen in an ankle sprain, when the muscles cannot respond quickly enough to protect the joint, and the ligaments become sprained or torn. If the ligaments are stretched but not torn completely through, this can lead to a chronic instability of the joint, especially if the surrounding musculature is not adequately rehabilitated. When the muscles fail and the ligaments do not maintain adequate joint stability, the stress cannot be fully absorbed by those tissues, and the stress is taken up by the bone and its architecture. Wolf's law indicates that the bones model according to imposed demands; that is, they will conform with changes in their external contour and internal architecture owing to the mechanical stresses to which they are habitually subjected.

Forces applied to joints in any position may cause damage to the bony structure, ligaments, and muscles. Because the closed packed position has the joint surfaces approximated and capsular structures tight, an inappropriate force may cause fracture of the bone, dislocation of the joint, or tearing of the ligaments. Kaltenborn states that it is important to know the closed packed position for each joint because testing of joint movements and manipulative procedures cannot be done to the joint in its closed packed position[14] (Table 2.3). When an inappropriate force is applied in the open packed position, the joint laxity and loss of stability may allow damage to the ligaments and supporting musculature.

Facet Joints

The one common factor in all of the spinal segments from the atlanto occipital joint to the sacroiliac joint is the fact that each has two posterior spinal articulations. These paired components have been referred to as *the zygapophyseal (meaning an "oval offshoot") joints* and are enveloped in a somewhat baggy capsule, which has some degree of elasticity. Each of the facet facings is lined with articular cartilage, as is the case with all contact-bearing joint surfaces, with the exception of the temporomandibular joint and the sternoclavicular joint. These joints have intracapsular fibrocartilaginous discs that separate the joint surfaces.

When compared to what has been studied with respect to the intervertebral disc, the facet joints have been the focus of very little biomechanical research. Yet these structures must control patterns of motion, protect the disc from shear forces, and provide support of the spinal column.

Because these joints are true diarthrodial (synovial) articulations, they have a synovial membrane that supplies the joint surfaces with synovial fluid. The exact role of synovial fluid is still unknown, though it is thought to serve as a joint lubricant or, at least, to interact with the articular cartilage to decrease friction between joint surfaces. Additionally, the synovium may be a source of nutrition for the avascular articular cartilage. Intermittent compression and distraction of the joint surfaces must occur for an adequate exchange of nutrients and waste products to occur.[15] Furthermore, as mentioned, immobilized joints have been shown to undergo degeneration of the articular cartilage.[16] Certainly, the nature of synovial joint function and lubrication are of interest because there is evidence that the facet joints sustain considerable stress and undergo degenerative changes.

Although the posterior joints were not designed to bear much weight, they can share up to about one-third of this function with the intervertebral disc. Moreover, as a part of the three joint complex, if the disc undergoes degeneration and loses height, more weight-bearing function will fall on the facets. During long periods of axial loading, the disc loses height through fluid loss, thereby, creating more weight bearing on the facets on a daily basis.

The posterior joints also have been found to contain fibroadipose meniscoids, whose clinical significance remains controversial. Bogduk and Engel

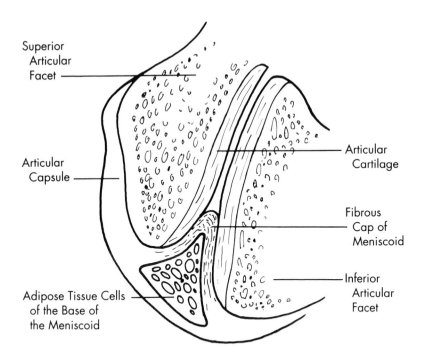

Figure 2.23 Fibroadipose meniscoid in a lumbar facet joint. (Modified from Bogduk and Engel,[17] with permission.)

provide an excellent review of the menisci of the lumbar zygapophyseal joints.[17] Although the genesis of their article was as a literature review to support the contention that the menisci could be the cause of an acute locking of the low back as a result of entrapment, the article also provided a comprehensive review of the anatomic considerations of lumbar menisci. The menisci appear to be synovial folds continuous with the periarticular tissues and with both intracapsular and extracapsular components. Microscopically, the tissue consisted of loose connective and adipose tissue, mixed with many blood vessels (Fig. 2.23). The menisci could present in various shapes including annular menisci found in the thoracic region, with linguiform menisci and filiform menisci commonly found in the lumbar region.[18]

These meniscal structures can project into the joint space when the joint surfaces of articular cartilage are not in contact. Bogduk and Engel noted two groups of menisci: one located along the dorsal and ventral margins of the joint and one located at the poles of the joint. In their view, only the ones located along the dorsal and ventral borders of the joint represented a true meniscus. Functionally, Bogduk and Engel feel these structures may help to provide greater stability to a lumbar zygapophyseal joint by helping to distribute the load over a wider area. In their words, the meniscus plays a space-filling role.[17]

Clinically and theoretically, these menisci may become entrapped.[19] Entrapment of the meniscus itself is not believed to be painful, though pain can be created by traction on the joint capsule through the base of the meniscus. This could, through a cascade of events, lead to more pain and reflex muscle spasm, known as *acute locked low back,* which is amenable to manipulative therapy.

Giles and Taylor examined the innervation of synovial folds in the lumbar zygapophyseal joints, using both light microscopy and transmission electron microscopy.[20,21] The authors removed part of the posteromedial joint capsule along with adjacent ligamentum flavum and synovial folds following a laminectomy, fixed these specimens in various solutions, and prepared them for microscopy. They demonstrated the neurologic structures located in the areas studied. Nerves seen in the synovial fold were 0.6 to 12 μm in diameter. These neurologic structures may give rise to pain.

Adams and Hutton examined the mechanical function of the lumbar apophyseal joints on spines taken from cadavers.[22] The authors wanted to examine various loading regimens on the function of these joints. They found that the lumbar zygapophyseal joints can resist most of the intervertebral shear force only when the spine is in a lordotic posture. These joints also can aid in resisting the intervertebral compressive force and can prevent excessive movement from damaging the intervertebral discs. The facet surfaces protect the posterior annulus, whereas the capsular ligament helps to resist the motion of flexion. The authors noted that in full flexion the capsular ligaments provide nearly 40 percent of the joint's resistance. They conclude, "the function of the lumbar apophyseal joints is to allow limited movement between vertebrae and to protect the discs from shear forces, excessive flexion and axial rotation.[22]

Taylor and Twomey studied how age affected the structure and function of the zygapophyseal joints.[23] They took transverse sections of the lumbar spine from cadavers ranging in age from fetus to 84 years and prepared them in staining media. They noted that fetal and infant lumbar zygapophyseal joints are coronally oriented, which only later (in early childhood) change to become curved or biplanar joints. In the adult, the joint has a coronal component in the anterior medial third of the joint and a sagittal component in the posterior two-thirds of the joint. The joint is generally hemicylindrical.

The structures located in the anterior third of the joint, primarily articular cartilage and subchondral bone, tend to show changes that are related to loading the joint in flexion. The posterior part of the joint shows a variety of different changes related to age. There may be changes from shearing forces. The subchondral bone will thicken as it ages and is wedge shaped. These changes occur as a result of loading stresses from flexion.[23]

Taylor and Twomey are careful to note they could make no clinical correlations with their findings, which is one of the problems with cadaveric studies of this sort. They believe that this work has biomechanical implications; they feel that the lumbar zygapophyseal joints limit the forward translational component of flexion. Indeed, they feel this fact may be the most important component limiting forward flexion.

Intervertebral Discs

The intervertebral discs are fibrocartilaginous mucopolysaccharide structures that lie between adjoining vertebral bodies. In the adult, there are 23 discs, each given a numeric name based on the segment above. Thus, the L5 disc lies between the fifth lumbar segment and the sacrum, and the L4 disc lies between the fourth and fifth lumbar segments. In the early years of life, the discs between the sacral segments are replaced with osseous tissue but remain as rudimentary structures, generally regarded as having no clinical significance.

The unique and resilient structure of the disc allows for its function in weight bearing and motion. The anterior junction of two vertebra is an amphiarthrodial, symphysis articulation formed by the two vertebral end plates and the intervertebral disc. The discs are responsible for approximately one-fourth of the entire height of the vertebral column. A disc has three distinct components: the annulus fibrosis, the nucleus pulposis, and the cartilaginous end plates.

The cartilaginous end plates are composed of hyaline cartilage that separate but also help attach the disc to the vertebral bodies. There is no closure of cortical bone between the hyaline cartilage and the vascular cancellous bone of the vertebral body. The functions of the end plates are to anchor the disc, to form a growth zone for the immature vertebral body, and to provide a permeable barrier between the disc and body. This role allows the avascular disc material to receive nutrients and repair products.

The annulus fibrosis is a fibrocartilage ring that serves to enclose and retain the nucleus pulposis, though the transition is gradual with no clear distinction between the innermost layers of the annulus and outer aspect of the nucleus. The fibrous tissue of the annulus is arranged in concentric, laminated bands, which appear to cross one another obliquely, each forming an angle of about 30 degrees to the vertebral body (Fig. 2.24). The annular

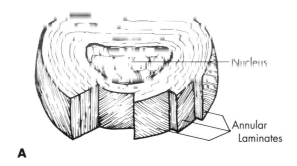

A

Nucleus

Annular Laminates

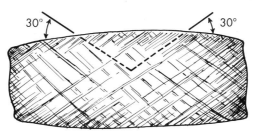

30°   30°

B

Figure 2.24 Intervertebral disc. **(A)** nucleus pulposus and annulus fibrosis. **(B)** Orientation of annular fibers. (Modified from White and Panjabi,[12] with permission.)

fibers of the inner layers are attached to the cartilaginous end plates, while the outer layers attach directly into the osseous tissue of the vertebral body by means of Sharpey's fibers.[24] Superficially, the fibers are reinforced by the anterior longitudinal ligament and the posterior longitudinal ligament (PLL). The PLL is significant clinically in that as it courses caudally, its width narrows until covering only about 50 percent of the central portion of the lower lumbar discs. The weakest area of the annulus and, hence, the most likely area for injury, is the posterolateral aspect. This is the most likely spot for a disc herniation in the lumbar spine.[25]

The annulus fibrosis contains little elastic tissue, and the amount of stretch is limited to only 1.04 times its original length, with further stretch resulting in a tearing of fibers. The functions of the annulus fibrosis includes enclosing and retaining the nucleus pulposis, absorbing compressive shocks, forming a structural unit between vertebral bodies, and allowing as well as restricting motion.

The nucleus pulposis is the central portion of the disc and is the embryologic derivative of the notochord. It accounts for about 40 percent of the disc and is a semifluid gel that will deform easily but is considered incompressible. The nucleus is composed of a loose network of fine fibrous strands that lie in a mucoprotein matrix containing mucopolysaccharides, chondroitin sulphate, hyaluronic acid, and keratin sulphate. These large molecules are strongly hydrophilic, capable of binding nearly nine times their volume of water and are, therefore, responsible for the high water content of the disc. In young adults, the water content approaches 90 percent and maintains an internal pressure of about 30 pounds per square inch.[12] The water content, however, steadily decreases with age. The composition of the nucleus produces a resilient spacer, which allows motion between segments, and although it does not truly function as a shock absorber, it does serve as a means to distribute compressive forces.

The intervertebral disc is a vital component for the optimum, efficient functioning of the spinal column. In conjunction with the vertebral bodies, the discs form the anterior portion of the functional unit responsible for bearing weight and dissipating shock. In so doing, it distributes loads, acts as a flexible buffer between the rigid vertebrae, and permits adequate motion at low loads while providing stability at higher loads.

The simple compression test of the disc has been one of the most popular experiments owing to the importance of the disc as a major load-carrying element of the spine. Axial compression forces continually affect the disc during upright posture. The nucleus bears 75 percent of this force initially but redistributes some to the annulus.

Furthermore, the ability of the disc to imbibe water causes it to "swell" within its inextensible casing. Thus, the pressure in the center or the nucleus is never zero in a healthy disc. This is termed a *preloaded state*. The preloaded state gives the disc a greater resistance to forces of compression.

With age and exposure to biomechanical stresses, the chemical nature of the disc changes and becomes more fibrous. This reduces the imbibition effect and, in turn, the preloaded state. As a result, flexibility is lost, and more pressure will be exerted on the annulus and peripheral areas of the

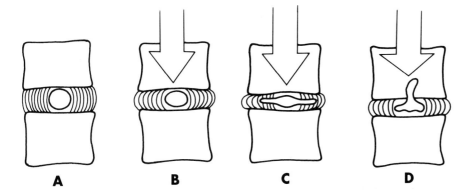

Figure 2.25 **(A)** Normal disc height. **(B)** Normal disc under load, showing slight approximation of bodies. **(C)** Diseased disc under load, showing significant loss of disc height. **(D)** End-plate fracture from axial load causing a Schmorl's node.

end plate. A disc that has been injured will deform more than a healthy one.

The preloaded state also explains the elastic properties of the disc. When the disc is subjected to a force, the disc exhibits dampened oscillations over time. If the force is too great, however, the intensity of the oscillations can destroy the annulus, thus accounting for the deterioration of intervertebral discs that have been exposed to repeated stresses.

Compressive forces are transmitted from end plate to end plate by both the annulus and the nucleus. When compressed, the disc bulges in the horizontal plane. A diseased disc will compress more and, as this occurs, stress is distributed differently to other parts of the functional unit, notably the apophyseal articulations. Because the disc is prepared for axial compressions, it should be noted that the vertebral body will collapse or the end plate will fracture under large loads (Schmorl's node) (Fig. 2.25).

Axial tensile stresses are also produced in the annulus during the movements of flexion, extension, and lateral flexion. This produces axial compression stresses ipsilaterally and tensile stresses contralaterally. This causes a bulging (buckling) on the concave side and a contraction on the convex side (Fig. 2.26). Axial rotation of the spine also produces tensile stresses in the disc. Studies have shown that the greatest tensile capabilities of the disc are in the anterior and posterior regions, with the center portion being the weakest. When the disc is subjected to torsion, shear stresses are produced in the horizontal as well as the axial plane. Shear stresses act in the horizontal plane, perpendicular to the long axis of the spine. It has been found that torsional and, hence, shear forces are the major injury causing load factors.

All viscoelastic structures, which includes the disc, exhibit a phenomenon called *hysteresis*. It represents the loss of energy when the disc or other viscoelastic structures are subjected to repetitive loads. For example, when a person jumps up and down, the shock energy is absorbed on the way from the feet to the head. The larger the load, the larger the hysteresis, but when the load is applied for a second time, the hysteresis decreases. This implies that the discs are less protected against repetitive loads.

Cadaveric studies allowed Twomey and Taylor to study creep and hysteresis in the lumbar spine.[26] *Creep* is the progresive deformation of a structure

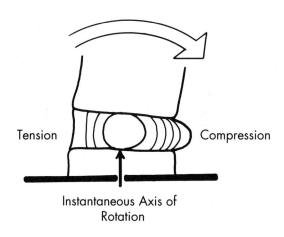

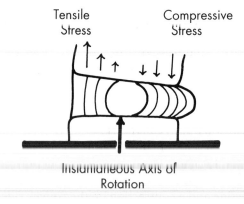

Figure 2.26 Disc stresses with bending movements of flexion, extension, and lateral flexion. Tension is produced on the convex side, whereas compression and buckling occur on the concave side.

under constant load, while *hysteresis* is the absorbtion or dissipation of energy by a distorted structure. As might be expected, the creep and hysteresis created in differing types of load forces (e.g., flexion loading vs. extension loading) may differ, but this has not been quantified for the lumbar spine.

Because the disc is under the influence of the preloaded state of the nucleus, movements will have specific effects on the behavior of the nucleus and annular fibers. When a distraction force is applied, the tension on the annular fibers increases and the internal pressure of the nucleus decreases. When an axial compression force is applied symmetrically, the internal pressure of the nucleus increases and transmits this force to the annular fibers. The vertical force is transformed into a lateral force, applying pressure outward. During the asymmetric movements of flexion, extension, and lateral flexion, a compressive force is applied to the side of movement and a tensile force occurs on the opposite side. The tension transmitted from the nucleus to the annular fibers helps to restore the functional unit to its original position. During axial rotation, some layers of the annulus are stretched while others are compressed (slackened). Tension forces reach a maximum within the internal layers of the annulus. This has a strong compressive force on the nucleus and causes an increased internal pressure proportional to the degree of rotation. Various maneuvers will increase the pressure within the disc. Standing in the upright posture is used as the standard for comparison.

Kurowski and Kubo investigated how degeneration of the intervertebral disc influenced the loading conditions on the lumbar spine.[27] Because disc degeneration is common, almost inevitably, it will contribute to low back dysfunction in many different ways. One way is by influencing motion and load bearing at each individual level. But what effect does degeneration have? Kurowski and Kubo examined load transmission through the lumbar spine with differing amounts of disc degeneration and used fine element analysis to study stress transmission. In healthy discs, they found the highest effective stresses in the center of the end plate of the vertebra, but in an unhealthy and degenerated disc, they found these stresses in the lateral aspects of the end plates as well as in the cortical wall and vertebral body rims.

MODELS OF SPINE FUNCTION

Understanding the overall function of the human spine has proved to be difficult and frustrating. It is important to view the spine as an integrated unit capable of functioning as a unit. It must be remembered, however, that the spine is also a part of the locomotor system. If consideration is not given to this, whole being the potential for clinical failures results.

Many models of spine function have been developed, each attempting to define spine function according to new and different parameters. Gracovetsky proposed a model of the spine based on the concept that spinal joints contain stress sensors that drive a feedback mechanism.[28] He believes that this mechanism creates an arrangement that can react to loads by modifying muscular action to decrease or minimize stress at those joints and cut the risk of injury. This model depicts the spine in terms of stresses, forces, and moments acting at the intervertebral joints.

As Gracovetsky notes, mathematical models of erector spinae muscles demonstrate that these muscles cannot support more than 50 kg of weight, so other or additional mechanisms must explain human ability to carry loads greater than that.[28] To explain this feature of the human spine, Gracovetsky theorizes that the interaction between the erector spinae group and the abdominal mucles is of "fundamental importance" in understanding spinal function. He later uses this theory to show how posture and behavior may produce spinal injury.

One of the major problems with this model is that no such monitoring system of stress sensors has been delineated by neurophysiologic research. Gracovetsky shows how the system would have to work if such sensors did exist, and thus, this model of the spine is based on the demarcation of stress, loads, and moments.[28] With such a mathematical model in place, it is possible to determine automatic diagnosis of spinal disability.

Aspden[29] notes that many theories of the spine tend to fall into two broad categories: those that treat the spine as a cantilever and those that perform an elastic analysis of the system. When treating the spine as a cantilever system, which is connected to a series of free bodies, forward-bending moments are balanced by the movement created by the spinal mucles acting about the sacrum. However, in using such a model to make mathematical calculations, the forces generated are extremely high and may be dangerous. Furthermore, they probably do not exist, indicating that the cantilever model is incomplete.

Aspden's model to explain the static behavior of the human spine looks at the spine as an arch rather than as the more accepted cantilever system. According to Aspden, if the spine is considered an arch, one can describe its mechanical stability and can calculate the forces developed along the spinal axis for any given posture or load.

Aspden notes that the human spine shares many characteristics with a masonry arch and that a masonry arch can be analyzed using plasticity theory. The plasticity theory describes the behavior of a structure once it has been loaded beyond its limits, and it describes how these materials flow in response to stress. To reduce stress, the structure deforms. Also, the theory helps provide the limits to elastic behavior. In normal erect posture, the lumbar lordosis forms an arch, which is convex anteriorly, and this brings the vertebral bodies almost directly into the center of the body. When we flex our spine, this arch will flatten and even reverse, so it is concave anteriorly, and a single arch is formed with the thoracic and lower cervical vertebrae. Body weight is transmitted along the spinal axis. The forces generated can then be calculated. Muscle forces can be overlaid on this, and then forces can be recalculated. Aspden shows how this can be calculated for a spine placed in certain configurations. Having this information, it is then possible to predict failure when these criteria are violated. Using these procedures, Aspden demonstrates that compressive forces developed in the spine may not be as high as was previously believed. He also demonstrated that normal spinal curvatures are necessary for proper load-bearing function. The presence of the normal lumbar lordosis, coupled with intra-abdominal pressure, helps to provide the spine with strength and to protect the spine from injury during heavy-load lifting.

The human spine, with its musculature removed, cannot carry normal physiologic loads. This fact led Panjabi and co-workers to devise a model of spinal stability and intersegmental muscle force.[30] Those authors note that muscles are necessary to stabilize the spine and to allow the spine to carry out its other physiologic functions. This stabilization feature is in addition to the obvious need for a muscle to move body parts. Their experiment simulated intersegmental muscle forces on spinal instability subjecting cadaveric lumbar functional spinal units (FSUs) to biomechanical tests of increasing muscle forces. Compressive preload and six physiologic movements were applied to a series of FSU to determine three-dimensional motion of the spine. The FSUs were also then given a series of injuries and incremental intersegmental muscle forces were applied to the upper vertebra of the FSUs. The same tests were then repeated on the injured segments. The injuries included (1) division of the supraspinous and interspinous ligaments, (2) left medial facetectomy, and (3) bilateral medial facetectomy. Some biomechanical parameters were then calculated including range of motion and neutral zone.

When the muscle forces were applied, range of motion increased, and neutral zone increased in flexion loading, while both decreased in extension loading.[30] With lateral bending, neither of these parameters was affected by applying the muscle forces. With rotation, the range of motion was significantly decreased, while the neutral zone was essentially unaffected. Panjabi and associates concluded that the action of the intersegmental muscle forces is to maintain or decrease intervertebral motions after injury, with the exception of flexion range of motion, which increased with the application of the muscle force. The neutral zone may be a better indicator of spinal instability than range of motion.

Louis examined spinal stability from an entirely different perspective, that of the three-column spine.[31] He notes there exists an axial and a transverse stability in the spine. The axial stability is maintained along a vertical column system consisting of two columns at the C1–C2 level and three columns from C2 to the sacrum (Fig. 2.27). These three columns consist of one anterior column (formed by the vertebral bodies and the disc) and two posterior columns (formed by the posterior joints). The transverse stability present is due to coupling of bony buttresses and ligamentous brakes.

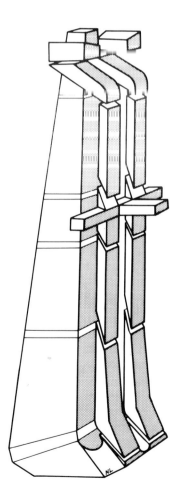

Figure 2.27 The three-column spine model, representing vertebral bodies and articular pillars. (Modified from Louis,[31] with permission.)

Louis sees the C1 vertebra as two lateral masses jointed by two arches. He sees the C2 vertebra as three pillars: "a vertical conical pillar lying medially and anteriorly (dens and body) and two lateral oblique pillars."[31] These three pillars are fused above in the body of C2 and then diverge below that area. The three resultant pillars run down to the sacrum, where three points of contact support the pillars at the sacral base and at the two sacral faces. Of these three pillars, the anterior one (as compared to the two posterior ones) is by far the larger. It takes on the characteristics of a quadrangular pyramid that is formed by alternating vertebral bodies and intervertebral discs down on the sacral base. In this model, the spinous processes and transverse processes do not contribute to spinal stability. Louis believes this three-column model of the spine provides the simplest and most efficient system of stability.[31]

Gracovetsky and Farfan use system theory to describe a model of the human spine.[32] After a great deal of discussion of the evolutionary considerations of the human spine, they make the point that intervertebral joints are essential for our survival as a species. They describe the mechanical behavior of the intervertebral joint and then use that information to calculate spinal motion and muscular action. This allows the authors to ultimately devise a new theory of human locomotion, which also allows for the calculation of safe loads for the spine. This article provides one of the most detailed and important papers concerning mathematical modeling of the human spine.

By incorporating the types of research noted here, a more complete picture of spinal biomechanics is developed, one in which pathologic changes may ultimately be better studied, as well.

REFERENCES

1. Kendall HO, Kendall FP, Wadsworth GE: Muscles Testing and Function. 2nd Ed. Williams & Wilkins, Baltimore, 1971

2. Weiss C, Rosenberg L, Helfet AJ: An ultrastructural study of normal young adult human articular cartilage. J Bone Joint Surg [Am] 50:663, 1968

3. Woo SLY, Adeson WH, Jemmott GF: Measurements of nonhomogeneous directional mechanical properties of articular cartilage in tension. J Biomech 9:785, 1976

4. Akeson WH, Amiel D, LaViolette D: The connective tissue response to immobility. Clin Orthop 51:183, 1967

5. Hertling D, Kessler RM: Management of Common Musculoskeletal Disorders, Physical Therapy Principles and Methods. 2nd Ed. JB Lippincott, Philadelphia, 1990

6. Wyke BD: Articular neurology and manipulative therapy. In Glasgow EF, Twomey LT, Scull ER, Kleynhans AM, Idczak RM (eds): Aspects of Manipulative Therapy. Churchill Livingstone, Edinburgh, 1985

7. Gillette RG: A speculative argument for the coactivation of diverse somatic receptor populations by forceful chiropractic adjustments. Manual Med 3:1, 1987

8. Malinsky J: The ontogenetic development of nerve terminations in the intervertebral discs of man. Acta Anat (Basel) 38:96, 1959

9. Bogduk N: The innervation of the lumbar intervertebral discs. p. 146. In Grieve G (ed): Modern Manual Therapy of the Vertebral Column. Churchill Livingstone, Edinburgh, 1986

10. Shinohara H: A study on lumbar disc lesions. J Jap Orthop Assoc 44:553, 1970

10a. Rabischong P, Louis R, Vignaud J, Massare C: The intervertebral disc. Anat Clin 1:55, 1978

10b. Roofe PG: Innervation of the annulus fibrosis and posterior longitudinal ligament. Arch Neurol Psychiatry 44:100, 1940

10c. Bogduk N, Tynan W, Wilson AS: The nerve supply to the human lumbar intervertebral discs. J Anat 132:39, 1981

10d. Hirsch C, Ingelmark BE, Miller M: The anatomical basis for low back pain. Acta Orthop Scand 33:1, 1963

10e. Jackson HC, Winkelmann RK, Bickel WH: Nerve endings in the human lumbar spinal column and related structures. J Bone Joint Surg 48A:1272, 1966

10f. Malinsky J: The ontogenetic development of nerve terminations in the intervertebral discs of man. Acta Anat 38:96, 1959

11. MacConnail MA, Basmajian JV: Muscles and Movements: A Basis for Human Kinesiology. Williams & Wilkins, Baltimore, 1969

12. White AA, Panjabi MM: Clinical Biomechanics of the Spine. JB Lippincott, Philadelphia, 1978

13. Astand O, Rodahl K: Textbook of Work Physiology. McGraw-Hill, New York, 1970

14. Kaltenborn FM: Mobilization of the Extremity Joints—Examination and Basic Treatment Principles. 3rd Ed. Olaf-Norlis-Bokhandel, Oslo, 1980

15. Nordin M, Frankel VH: Basic Biomechanics of the Musculoskeletal System. 2nd Ed. Lea & Febiger, Philadelphia, 1989

16. Akeson WH, Amiel D, LaViolette D: The connective tissue response to immobility. Clin Orthop 51:183, 1967

17. Bogduk N, Engel R: The menisci of the lumbar zygapophyseal joints: a review of their anatomy and clinical significance. Spine 9:454, 1984

18. Zaccheo D, Reale E: Contributo alla conoscenza delle articolazioni tra i processi articolari delle vertebre dell'uomo. Arch Anatomica 61:1, 1956

19. Kos J, Wolf J: Les menisques intervertebraux et leur role possible dans les blocages vertebraux. Ann Med Phys 15:2, 1972

20. Giles LGF, Taylor JR: Human zygapophyseal joint capsule and synovial fold innervation. Br J Rheumatol 26:93, 1987

21. Giles LGF, Taylor JR: Innervation of lumbar zygapophyseal joint synovial folds. Acta Orthop Scand 58:43, 1987

22. Adams MA, Hutton WC: The mechanical function of the lumbar apophyseal joints. Spine 8:327, 1983

23. Taylor JR, Twomey LT: Age changes in the lumbar zygapophyseal joints: observations on structure and function. Spine 11:739, 1986

24. Danbury R: Functional anatomy of the intervertebral disc. Man Med 6:128, 1971

25. Farfan HF: Mechanical Disorders of the Lumbar Spine. Lea & Febiger, Philadelphia, 1973

26. Twomey L, Taylor J: Flexion creep deformation and hysteresis in the lumbar vertebral column. Spine 7:116, 1982

27. Kurowski P, Kubo A: The relationship of degeneration of the intervertebral disc to mechanical loading conditions on lumbar vertebrae. Spine 11:726, 1986

28. Gracovetsky S: Function of the spine. J Biomed Eng 8:217, 1986

29. Aspden RM: The spine as an arch: a new mathematical model. Spine 14:266, 1989

30. Panjabi M, Abumi K, Duranceau J, Oxland T: Spinal stability and intersegmental muscle forces: a biomechanical model. Spine 14:194, 1989

31. Louis R: Spinal stability as defined by the three-column spine concept. Anat Clin 7:33, 1985

32. Gracovetsky S, Farfan H: The optimum spine. Spine 11:543, 1986

33. Albright JA, Brand RA: The Scientific Basis of Orthopaedics. Appleton-Century-Crofts, East Norwalk, CT, 1979

34. Soderberg GL: Kinesiology: Application to Pathological Motion. Williams & Wilkins, Baltimore, 1986

3
Joint Assessment Principles and Procedures

David H. Peterson
Thomas F. Bergmann

The doctor of chiropractic views the human being as a dynamic, integrated, and complex creature having an innate capacity for self-healing.[1-6] Chiropractic health care focuses on the evaluation and treatment of neuromusculoskeletal-based disorders but does not disregard the multiple potential causes of ill health and the complex nature of health maintenance.[7,8]

In keeping with this philosophy and the responsibility as "port-of-entry" health-care providers, doctors of chiropractic must maintain broad and thorough diagnostic skills. The chiropractic physician who chooses to limit therapeutic alternatives must still possess the skills necessary to determine if patients have a health-care problem amenable to the specific treatment offered.[9]

This chapter focuses on the knowledge, principles, and evaluation procedures central to the process of assessing joint function. Although joint assessment is a critical prerequisite to the application of manual or adjustive therapy, it is only one aspect of the diagnostic skills chiropractors must employ to maintain primary contact privileges.

THE MANIPULABLE LESION

Before employing therapy, the physician must first ascertain if there is a clinical basis for treatment. The chiropractic physician considering manual or adjustive therapy must establish if conditions exist which support this treatment.

Manual therapy has been proposed as an effective treatment for a wide variety of conditions, but it is most commonly associated with disorders that have their origins in pathomechanical or pathophysiologic alterations of the locomotor system and its synovial joints. As a result, manual therapy is based on assessment procedures that take into consideration both functional and structural alteration of the neuromusculoskeletal (NMS) system. Haldeman[10] has referred to this process as *the identification of a manipulable lesion*.

The identification of the common functional and structural components of the manipulable lesion is critical to the management of these conditions, but it has also contributed to the misconception that all manipulative disorders have the same pathologic basis. The overwhelming percentage of disorders effectively treated with chiropractic adjustments do display joint and somatic functional alterations, but many pathologic processes can induce joint dysfunction.

A diagnosis of joint dysfunction identifies local altered mechanics, but it does not identify the underlying nature of the dysfunction. Although joint derangements may present as independent clinical syndromes, they are more commonly associated with other identifiable disorders and injuries of the NMS system.[11–15] If doctors of chiropractic limit their examination to the identification of structural or functional signs of joint derangement, they may minimize the extent of the disorder and the effectiveness of their treatment. For example, both the patient with acute disc herniation and the patient with acute facet syndrome present with clinical signs of joint dysfunction. An evaluation confined to the detection of joint dysfunction might not uncover the underlying pathomechanical and pathophysiologic differences between these two conditions and the distinctions in therapy that might be necessary. Furthermore, spinal malpositions or fixations may be induced by other disease states or traumatic events that would contraindicate adjustive therapy.

A singular diagnosis of joint dysfunction should be reserved for when it is determined to be the sole identifiable lesion; the term should not be used as a category for all conditions treated with adjustive therapy. Moreover, the potential relationship of joint dysfunction to other identifiable disorders of the NMS system should be determined and so stated. When joint dysfunction is perceived as the sole cause of the disorder being considered for treatment, adjustive therapy may stand alone. However, when dysfunction is secondary to other disorders, then therapy directed to treat the source of the problem should be provided or made available to the patient. Determination of the appropriateness of adjustive therapy should not be based on the presence of a fixation, malposition, or spinal listing alone. The cause of the altered mechanics indicates whether adjustive therapy or some other form of therapy is in order.[15]

SUBLUXATION

Within the chiropractic profession, the manipulable lesion has been equated primarily with the term *joint subluxation*. Historically, joint subluxation was defined predominantly in structural terms.[1,2,15–20] The founder of chiropractic, D.D. Palmer, defined subluxation as a "partial or incomplete separation: one in which the articulating surfaces remain in partial contact."[21] Central to Palmer's original subluxation hypothesis was the concept that vertebral subluxations could impinge on the spinal nerve roots as they exit through the intervertebral foramina. This was postulated to obstruct the flow of vital nerve impulses from the central nervous system to the periphery and to induce lowered tissue resistance and potential disease in the segmentally innervated tissues.[1,2,8,19,21–25] Palmer went as far as to suggest that the primary cause of all disease could be related to subluxations and interruption of normal "tone—nerves too tense or to slack."[8,26] The most impassioned supporter of this concept was D.D. Palmer's son B.J. Palmer. Throughout his career, B.J. Palmer ardently promoted a monocausal concept of disease,[8,17,18,27,28] specifically stating that chiropractic is "A *science* with provable knowledge of *one cause of one* disease being an *internal* interference of the *internal* flow of abstract mental impulses or nerve force flow supply, from *above down, inside out*."[27]

Although the profession today emphasizes the important relationship between health and the structure and function of the neuromusculoskeletal system,[4–7,22–25,29,30] it does not promote a monocausal concept of subluxation-induced disease.[7–9,28–31] The monocausal concept runs contrary to the profession's recent literature[24,25,28–30] and to the view held by the overwhelming majority of practicing chiropractors.[8] It is not taught at any of the Council on Chiropractic (CCE) accredited chiropractic colleges, and it is disavowed by the profession's national associations.[9,31]

Beginning with the published work of Gillet,[32–37] Illi,[38] and Mennell,[39,40] and later through the writings of Sandoz[15,20,41,42] and Faye,[43,44] the importance of the dynamic characteristics of joint subluxation moved to the forefront. As a result, joint integrity was defined not only in structural terms but also in functional terms.[15,20,24,25,32–47] Within this context, joint subluxation took on a broader definition, and joint malposition became a possible sign of disturbed joint function, not absolute confirmation.

This view provided a more dynamic perspective and suggests that minor joint misalignment does not necessarily predict the presence or absence of joint dysfunction, or the direction of possible restricted movement.[15,20,41–45] Joints can be fixed in a neutral position or can have multiple planes of joint restriction.[15,20,41,48,49] As a consequence, treatment decisions concerning adjustive therapy and adjustive vectors, once based predominately on the direction of malposition, would now require an assessment of joint mobility and the directions of possible joint fixation.[32–46] Today, consideration is given to both the static and functional components of spinal subluxations.[15,22,24,45]

Other health-care providers within the field of manual medicine also struggle with multiple definitions and explanations for manipulable lesions. Table 3.1 contains a list of terms and definitions commonly used to describe functional or structural disorders of the synovial joints.

VERTEBRAL SUBLUXATION COMPLEX

As a consequence of continued professional debate and increasing scientific inquiry, a trend toward defining subluxations as complex clinical phenomenon has unfolded.[15,16,20,23–25,30,46,47] Although the profession has yet to reach a formal consensus on a clinical description of joint subluxations, it is moving toward a broader perspective. Rather than a condition definable by one or two characteristics, subluxation is emerging as a clinical syndrome identified

Table 3.1   Definitions of Terms Describing Functional or Structural Disorders of the Synovial Joints

---

Orthopedic Subluxation
A partial or incomplete dislocation (Taber's Cyclopedia Medical Dictionary. 15th Ed., 1985)

Subluxation
(Chiropractic definition)
  A. The alteration of the normal dynamic, anatomic, or physiologic relationships of contiguous articular structures
  B. An aberrant relationship between two adjacent articular structures that may have functional or pathologic sequelae, causing an alteration in the biomechanical and/or neurophysiologic reflections of these articular structures, and/or body systems that may be directly or indirectly affected by them (Index Synopsis of ACA Policies on Public Health and Related Matters. 1987)

Joint Dysfunction
Joint mechanics showing area disturbances of function without structural change—subtle joint dysfunctions affecting quality and range of joint motion. Definition embodies disturbances in function that can be represented by decreased motion, increased motion or aberrant motion[253]
  A. Joint hypomobility: decreased angular or linear joint movement
  B. Joint hypermobility: Increased angular or linear joint movement; aberrant joint movements are typically not present
  C. Clinical joint instability: Increased linear and aberrant joint movement; the instantaneous axis's of rotation (centroids) and patterns of movement are disturbed

Somatic Dysfunction
Impaired or altered function of related components of the somatic (body framework) system; skeletal, arthrodial, and myofascial structures; and related vascular, lymphatic, and neural elements. (Hospital Adaption of the International Classification of Disease. 2nd Ed. 1973)

Osteopathic Lesion
A disturbance in musculoskeletal structure and/or function as well as accompanying disturbances of other biologic mechanisms. A term used to describe local stress or trauma and subsequent effects on other biologic systems (e.g., effects mediated through reflex nerve pathways including autonomic supply of segmentally related organs). (Ward M: Glossary of Osteopathic Terminology. AOA 1981)

Joint Fixation
The state whereby an articulation has become temporarily immobilized in a position that it may normally occupy during any phase of physiologic movement. The immobilization of an articulation in a position of movement when the joint is at rest, or in a position of rest when the joint is in movement.[20]

---

by its presenting symptoms and physical signs.[15,16,24,25,30,41–47] Gitelman, and later Faye, were the first to promote this broader model and its theoretical components.[44,47,50,51] Although this model and its components have a pathomechanical and pathophysiologic basis, many aspects have yet to be experimentally verified.[24,25,30]

The potential pathologic effects of the vertebral subluxation complex (or syndrome) (VSC) may be broadly divided into mechanical, inflammatory–vascular, and neurobiologic categories. Although the divisions are modeled after those proposed by previous authors, they are not identical categories, and they do not represent an established professional convention. The following categories and topics represent an overview of the effects of the VSC and are not intended to be an inclusive or exhaustive treatise on the subject.

Mechanical Components

The mechanical category of the VSC includes derangements or disorders of the somatic structures of the body that lead to altered joint structure and function. Derangement of the articular soft tissues and mechanical joint dysfunction may result from acute injury, repetitive use injury, faulty posture or coordination, aging, immobilization, static overstress, congenital or developmental defects, or other primary disease states.[11–16,20,24,41–45,47,52–71]

Joint Fixation

A commonly proposed source of joint fixation (hypomobility) and dysfunction is articular soft tissue injury with its resultant fibrosis and loss of elasticity and strength.[11–14,45,47,52–54] Soft tissue injury and fibrosis may result from acute or repetitive trauma to muscular, tendinous, myofascial, or ligamentous tissue.[11–13,45,47,52–54,58] Regardless of the mechanism of injury, an ensuing inflammatory response is triggered.[48] This process is considered to be nonspecific and often excessive in the case of traumatic NMS injuries.[11,56] As a consequence, early conservative management is often directed at limiting the extent of the inflammatory response. By limiting the degree of inflammatory exudates, decreasing pain and muscle spasm, and promoting pain-free mobility, it may be possible to encourage flexible repair and speed the recovery process.[56,60–62,71–85]

The exudates that form as a byproduct of injury and inflammation set the stage for the next step in the process of connective tissue repair. They provide the matrix for the development of granulation tissue and scar formation. The formation of granulation tissue is predominately carried out by the proliferation of fibroblasts and the synthesis and deposition of collagen tissue. The collagen is initially very poorly organized and must add additional collagen cross-linkages and reorganize along planes of stress to improve the tensile strength of the injured area. This process of repair and remodeling may take months and may result in less than optimum restoration and extensibility of the involved tissue, especially in the presence of progressive immobilization.[52,53,60–71]

If the repair process leads to decreased flexibility in the periarticular soft tissues, then therapies such as articular adjustments should be directed toward the restoration of joint motion.[11,56,59,74]

Degenerative change within osseous articular structures (osteoarthrosis) may also induce altered joint mechanics characterized by decreased, increased, or aberrant joint motion.[42] These may develop as a product of the effects of altered joint mechanics, developmental or congenital defect, immobility, joint instability, inflammatory or metabolic joint disease, excessive loading, acute trauma or repetitive motion injury.[11–13,16,42,45,47,65,69,71,82–94] Adjustive and manual therapy directed in these circumstances is unlikely to reverse marked bony structural derangement; rather, it is directed at decreasing symptoms and maximizing function within the patients structural limitations.

Painful conditions capable of triggering persistent muscle spasm are additional sources of restricted joint motion (Fig. 3.1). Muscle contraction, once initiated, may become a self-perpetuating source of pain and muscle spasm.[24,42,45,47,53,95–99] Reactive splinting in the joint's intrinsic muscles may further accentuate this process by blocking passive joint movement and the pain-inhibiting qualities of joint mechanoreceptor stimulation.[100] Maladies capable of producing acute muscle contraction are wide ranging; they include trauma, structural inadequacies, visceral disease, emotional distress, and exposure to cold.[101,102]

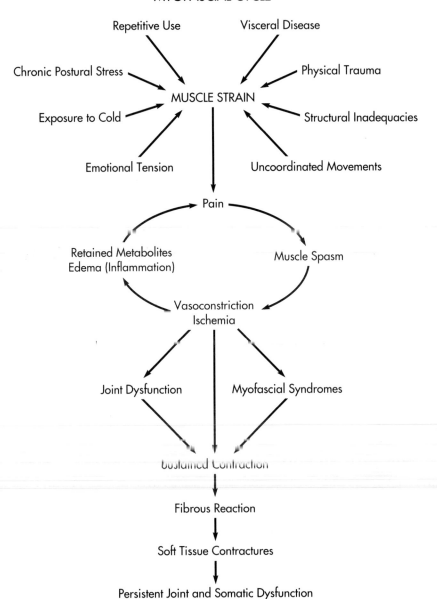

MYOFASCIAL CYCLE

Figure 3.1 Myofascial conditions are triggered by many causes and can become a self-perpetuating source of pain, muscle spasm, and joint dysfunction.

Many internal joint derangements have also been submitted as probable causes of joint locking and back pain. They include internal derangements of the intervertebral disc (interdiscal block)[41,42,53,58,103–110] and interarticular entrapment of joint meniscoids and synovial folds (intermeniscoid block).[41,42,111–129] They are hypothesized to induce mechanical blockage to movement and unleveling of the motion segment with resultant tension on the joint capsule, annulus, or both (Fig. 3.2). The joint capsule and posterior

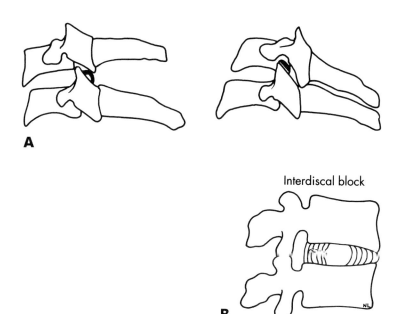

Interdiscal block

Figure 3.2 **(A)** Meniscoid entrapment and **(B)** interdiscal block are probable causes of joint locking and joint pain.

annulus are pain-sensitive structures, and tension on these elements may induce additional painful muscle splinting, further accentuating the mechanical blockage and joint restriction.

Clinical Joint Instability and Hypermobility

Joint dysfunction resulting from soft tissue injury or degeneration does not necessarily result in joint hypomobility. Disturbances of function of the vertebral column also include joint hypermobility and instability. The distinction between clinical joint instability and segmental hypermobility is controversial. The two are most typically distinguished by the degree of pathologic change in the joints' stabilizing structures. Hypermobile joints demonstrate increased segmental mobility, but the pattern of movement may be normal. The hypermobility may be only in one plane and not associated with any abnormal translational movements. The functional changes are considered to be potentially reversible in hypermobile joints, and they typically maintain their stability and function normally under physiologic loads.[130]

In contrast, clinically unstable joints have more advanced and purportedly nonreversible changes in the joints' stabilizing structures. Damage to these structures leads to abnormal patterns of coupled and translational movements and multiple planes of aberrant joint movement. Clinical joint instability should not be equated with gross orthopedic instability resulting from fracture or fracture dislocation.

Models of Spinal Dysfunction and Degeneration

The profession places significant emphasis on the mechanical components of joint dysfunction and subluxation. Mechanical joint dysfunction is considered to be a significant and frequent cause of spinal pain and a potential source of spinal degeneration.[11,16,23–25,30,36,41–45,52,53] The spine is viewed as an interdependent organ system inextricably connected with the rest of the locomotor system. Altered mechanics in one component of the motion segment are perceived to have unavoidable mechanical effects on other functional elements of the motion segment and spine.[16,24,36,41–45,48,52]

Gillet's model

Gillet[32–36,44] considers the process of mechanical joint dysfunction to develop through three different phases of joint fixation: muscular, ligamentous, and articular. The muscular fixation was considered to be a product of segmental muscle hypertonicity and contraction; ligamentous fixations, the product of contracture and shortening in the joint capsule and its periarticular ligaments; and articular fixations, the product of fibrous interarticular adhesions between articular surfaces. The end stage of articular adhesions is the potential progression to full bony ankylosis and irreversible fixation.

Muscular fixations are identified by the palpation of taut and tender muscle fibers and restricted joint mobility. The end feel is restricted but has a rubbery and giving quality. Ligamentous fixations demonstrate restricted joint movement and a hard abrupt leathery end feel. Articular fixations demonstrate the same quality of restriction but in all planes of motion.

Gillet maintains that ligamentous or articular fixations are the most significant. He considered muscular fixations as secondary compensations to marked fixations at other levels. As a result, he presented an approach that stressed the identification and treatment of the patient's *major* fixations.

Gillet classified major fixations as those demonstrating the most dramatic blockages to movement. He contended that the major fixations were frequently not the most symptomatic sites but were the key to inhibiting pain-free spinal function. Although his ideas are intriguing and have had a profound effect on the profession, they have yet to be experimentally confirmed.

Kirkaldy-Willis' model

Kirkaldy-Willis[131,132] presents a pattern of spinal degeneration founded on the principle that spinal degeneration often begins with local mechanical derangement in the absence of structural alteration. He postulates that the process is often initiated with the development of individual motion segment dysfunction secondary to alteration in segmental mucle tone and function. Although the disorders that are postulated to initiate dysfunction are extensive, most share as a consequence the potential to develop joint hypomobility.[16]

Joint hypomobility is speculated to initiate the degenerative cycle through the development of altered segmental biomechanics.[16,24,30,41–45,47,52,130] If mechanical derangement persists, repetitive abnormal loading eventually leads to fatigue and attenuation of the articular soft tissues. Local joint

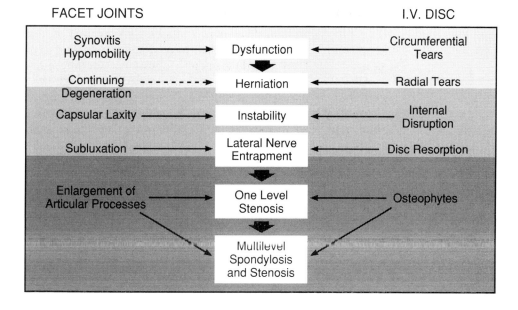

FACET JOINTS   I.V. DISC

Figure 3.3 The proposed sequence of pathologic changes in the facet joints and disc as a consequence of the degenerative process. (From Kirkaldy-Willis,[131] with permission.)

instability develops as a result of capsular laxity and internal disruption of the intervertebral disc.[16,131,132] Consequently, if the derangement is of sufficient magnitude, osseous structural alteration will result and degenerative joint disease becomes radiographically visible (Fig. 3.3).[131]

The final effect of this degenerative cycle is the restabilization of the joint through soft tissue fibrosis and bony exostosis.[131,132] As a consequence, the incidence of spinal pain may decrease during the later stages of stabilization. However, bony entrapment of the nerve roots and/or stenosis of the spinal canal are of increasing frequency, and this may lead to an increased frequency of leg pain and neurologic deficits.[131,132]

The presented models of motion-segment degeneration and the compensational adaptations initiated are not necessarily limited to the involved joint. Not only is it possible for joint hypomobility, instability, and degenerative joint disease all to occur at the same motion segment, it is also possible for compensatory dysfunction and degenerative changes to develop at other spinal levels or other joints within the locomotor system.[16,24,37,42–44,52]

Certainly, not all joint dysfunction fits this pattern of progression. A large percentage of dysfunction is self-limiting or so minor that the individual adapts and compensates to the change with limited structural or functional alteration. If dysfunction persists, however, the processes of local and distant joint degeneration may ensue. A point of emphasis and concern for the chiropractic profession is, therefore, to detect persistent mechanical dysfunction at an early stage of alteration and strive to eliminate it before it develops into irreversible or permanent disorders.

Inflammatory and Vascular Components

The inflammatory and vascular components of the VSC may be initiated by joint injury, chronic mechanical joint derangement, or joint immobilization.[24,45,47,52] They include vascular congestion, ischemia, and inflammation.

All inflammatory reactions are accompanied by cellular and humoral components that act as an intrinsic source of pain and vasodilation.[133] The accompanying pain may initiate local reflex mucle contraction, which over time, may lead to local ischemia and potentially more pain and muscle splinting. The end result, as described previously, is a self-perpetuating cycle of pain and continued muscle spasm.[24,42,45,47,53,95-99]

The inflammatory reaction as described is identical to that initiated by a foreign object or infection. Although it is a normal protective response, it may accentuate the pain response, slow the recovery time, and perpetuate joint dysfunction. If the muscle contraction persists, it may eventually develop into a muscle contracture as the myofascial structures become shortened and infiltrated with fibrotic tissue.[191-194] The resulting soft tissue derangements and contractions that develop must be dealt with therapeutically or they will serve as a source of continued pain and reoccurring joint subluxation–dysfunction.

Additionally, chronic joint inflammation may lead to synovial tissue hyperplasia and thickening as a result of persistent irritation and secretion of synovial fluid.[90,135] Synovial tags may develop as a hyperplastic reaction to chronic inflammation, and they in turn may become further impediments to joint movement.[134,136] Eventually, fibrous invasion of the synovial connective tissue layer may induce an attendant loss of vascularity and subsequent loss of synovial fluid secretion.[91]

Some degree of joint or soft tissue inflammation should be suspected when the patient's pain is constant. Clinical signs include muscle splinting, soft tissue swelling, and temperature alteration. Inflammation associated with spinal joint injuries or dysfunction is unlikely to produce palpable swelling at the surface. Some have suggested, however, that joint dysfunction may be associated with a local sympathetic reflex alteration capable of inducing a slight boggy feeling in overlying segmental tissues.

Neurobiologic Components

Historically, the profession has emphasized spinal nerve root compression as the significant neurologic disorder accompanying vertebral subluxations.[1-3,17-29] Spinal subluxations were hypothesized to induce nerve root compression as a result of either direct anatomic compression of neural elements or indirectly through disruption of neural blood supply (non-impulsed based model). The resulting nerve root compression was subsequently hypothesized to induce dysfunction of the somatic or visceral tissues they supplied.[2,3,17-25,27-29]

This model has induced considerable skepticism outside the profession and less than universal endorsement within the profession.[25,29,137] In the absence of degenerative joint or disc disease, it seems unlikely that joint subluxation could produce enough distortion to produce direct anatomic compression of spinal nerve roots. The spinal nerve roots, however, do lack the epineural covering of peripheral nerves and are more susceptible to pressure, inflammation, and ischemia.[138,139] They receive a significant portion of their nutrition through the cerebrospinal fluid, and local inflammatory reactions may be sufficient to obliterate their source of nutrition.[140] Therefore, some have speculated that subluxations may induce alterations in the vascular dynamics of the intervertebral foramen (IVF) sufficient to alter nerve root function.[25,141]

This hypothesis remains largely untested. Although the nerve roots may be susceptible to vascular ischemia, they actually gain a dural covering at their point of entry to the IVF and therefore become more resistant to direct compression.[139,142] Furthermore, lumbar and cervical derangements are commonly associated with paresthesia and radicular pain syndromes. These findings run contrary to the model of marked nerve root compression and are more indicative of nerve root inflammation and ischemia secondary to traction, irritation, or compression.[25]

In the absence of evidence to confirm the nerve compression hypothesis and as a result of growing skepticism about this paradigm, the profession has assembled a potentially more plausible model of subluxation-induced neurologic alterations (impulsed based model).[22–25,28–30] This hypothesis envisions vertebral joint dysfunctions—and their associated mechanical alterations, pain, and potential local inflammation—as lesions capable of inducing chronically altered nociceptive and proprioceptive input. The persistent altered afferent input is then theorized to produce sensitization of local spinal neuron pools and the establishment of abnormal somato-somato or somatovisceral reflexes. The reflexes, once established, become the potential driving source of altered somatic or visceral function.[22–25,28–30,143–144] Thus, joint subluxation/dysfunction may result as a product of disease or dysfunction in other somatic or visceral structures or initiate secondary dysfunction in tissues with shared segmental innervation.

The segmental muscle spasm that is associated with joint dysfunction is characteristic of a somato-somatic reflex. It may accentuate local joint locking or trigger compensatory dysfunction at adjacent sites. Additionally, midthoracic joint dysfunction associated with dyspepsia is an effective example of a somatovisceral disorder. In this example, joint dysfunction is theorized to induce somatovisceral reflexes, which initiate functional alterations in gastric equilibrium and induce symptoms of dyspepsia.

The proposed joint subluxation/dysfunction-induced neurologic phenomena may be clinically manifested by the presence of pain, altered temperature regulation, hyperesthesia, or altered somatic and/or visceral function.

SPINAL LISTINGS

As the chiropractic profession has evolved, it has developed various abbreviated descriptions for designating abnormal joint position or movement. The result is a profession laden with redundant nomenclatures describing spinal subluxations and fixations. As new descriptive terms are introduced, old ones are not replaced. It is not uncommon for each technique approach to have its own unique listing system.

As part of the process to include chiropractic in Medicare, there was an attempt to standardize listing systems at the 1977 American Chiropractic Assocation (ACA) conference in Houston. Although the parties did succeed in developing a common nomenclature for Medicare claims, it unfortunately did not form a basis for larger professional consensus. There is still significant variation between chiropractors and state board examinations as to preferred listing systems.

To the student's continual frustration, the colleges are left in a position of teaching repetitive and often contradictory methods of describing joint malpositions and fixations. Presently, the common systems used to describe abnormal position are Medicare, Palmar-Gonstead, and National. In an attempt to reduce the confusion and redundancy, this book emphasizes standard kinesiologic terms and the Medicare listing system. When deviations in position are described, the term *malposition* is applied, and when limitations to movement are described, the term *restriction* is employed (Fig. 3-4).

All motion segment malpositions are described with the position of the upper vertebra compared to the lower vertebrae. For example, a *flexion malposition* describes a vertebrae that has deviated into a position of flexion relative the vertebrae below, and a *flexion restriction* describes a limitation or loss of joint flexion.

Trunk and neck movements are described in kinesiologic terms. They are based on vertebral body movement, not spinous process movement. *Left rotation of the trunk* is defined by left posterior vertebral body rotation not by right rotation of the spinous process.

CLINICAL EVALUATION OF SUBLUXATION/DYSFUNCTION

Therapeutic decisions on where, when, and how to apply adjustive therapy are typically based on the evaluation of the integrity of the NMS and on the presence or absence of associated joint subluxation/dysfunction. As mentioned previously, the presence or absence of subluxation or dysfunction alone does not determine the need for adjustive therapy. The nature of the dysfunction must be evaluated before therapy is administered. This necessitates an evaluation directed toward determining the cause and the pathomechanical and pathophysiologic components of the suspected problem.

The diagnosis of joint dysfunction alone may identify a painful clinical syndrome that may respond to manual therapy, but its likely cause and mechanical components must be determined before adjustive treatment is delivered. The chiropractor must determine if the dysfunction is a product of joint hypermobility or hypomobility. The site, side, and directions of immobility, aberrant movement, or hypermobility must also be determined. Therefore, before instituting treatment, the doctor must elicit a case history, perform a physical examination, and complete any other appropriate imaging or laboratory procedures.

The diagnosis of subluxation/dysfunction is primarily a clinical diagnosis based on the patient's presentation and on physical findings. Often, it is suspected after other conditions with a similar presentation have been excluded. With the exception of radiographic evaluation, the majority of the commonly applied examination procedures devoted to assessing joint structural and functional integrity are physical examination procedures. The profession uses both standard and unique physical diagnostic methods of observation, palpation, percussion, and auscultation. Of these, observation and palpation are the most commonly applied. They include postural and gait evaluation, soft tissue and bony palpation, global range of motion, and segmental range of motion assessment.[46,149–152]

Diagnostic Criteria

Modifying the acronym PARTS from Bourdillon and Day,[153] Bergmann identifies the five diagnostic criteria for the identification of joint dysfunction.[154] The physical signs indicative of joint subluxation/dysfunction are pain, abnormalities in alignment, joint mobility, and tissue texture:

Pain and Tenderness

The perception of pain and tenderness is evaluated in terms of location, quality, and intensity. Most primary musculoskeletal disorders manifest by a painful response. The patient's description of the pain and its location is obtained. Furthermore, the location and intensity of tenderness produced by palpation of osseous and soft tissue are noted. Pain and tenderness findings are identified through observation, percussion, and palpation.

Asymmetry

Asymmetric qualities are noted on a sectional or segmental level. This includes observation of posture and gait, as well as palpation for misalignment of vertebral segments and extremity joint structures. Asymmetry is identified through observation (posture and gait analysis), static palpation, and static radiography.

Range of Motion Abnormality

Changes in active, passive, and accessory joint motions are noted. These changes may be reflected by increased, decreased, or aberrant motion. It is thought that a decrease in motion is a common component of joint dysfunction. Range of motion abnormalities are identified through motion palpation and stress radiography.

Tone, Texture, and Temperature Abnormality

Changes in the characteristics of contiguous and associated soft tissues, including skin, fascia, muscle, and ligaments, are noted. Tissue tone, texture, and/or temperature changes are identified through observation, palpation, instrumentation, and tests for length and strength.

Special Tests

Finally, diagnosis may require testing procedures that are specific to a technique system.

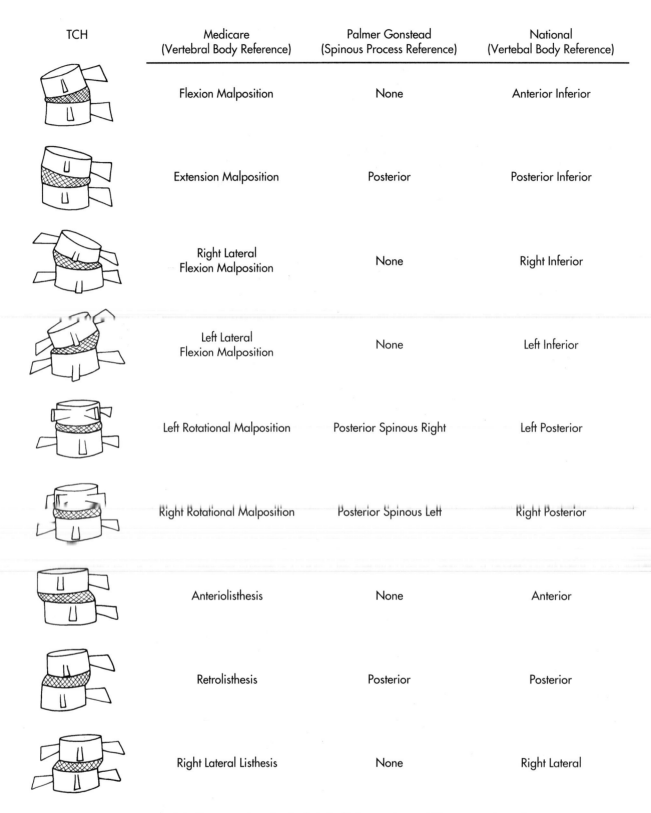

TCH	Medicare (Vertebral Body Reference)	Palmer Gonstead (Spinous Process Reference)	National (Vertebal Body Reference)
	Flexion Malposition	None	Anterior Inferior
	Extension Malposition	Posterior	Posterior Inferior
	Right Lateral Flexion Malposition	None	Right Inferior
	Left Lateral Flexion Malposition	None	Left Inferior
	Left Rotational Malposition	Posterior Spinous Right	Left Posterior
	Right Rotational Malposition	Posterior Spinous Left	Right Posterior
	Anteriolisthesis	None	Anterior
	Retrolisthesis	Posterior	Posterior
	Right Lateral Listhesis	None	Right Lateral

Figure 3.4 Comparative chart of static listing systems. (*Figure continues.*)

TCH	Medicare (Vertebral Body Reference)	Palmer Gonstead (Spinous Process Reference)	National (Vertebal Body Reference)
	Left Rotational Malposition Left Lateral Flexion Malposition	Posterior Right Superior Spinous	Left Posterior Inferior
	Left Rotational Malposition Right Lateral Flexion Malposition	Posterior Right Inferior Spinous	Left Posterior Superior
	Right Rotational Malposition Right Lateral Flexion Malposition	Posterior Left Superior Spinous	Right Posterior Inferior
	Right Rotational Malposition Left Lateral Flexion Malposition	Posterior Left Inferior Spinous	Right Posterior Superior

Restriction — limitation to movement. Describes the direction of limited movement in subluxated and/or dysfunctional joints.

Listing (dynamic) — designation of the abnormal movement of one of the vertebra in relation to subadjacent segments, e.g.:

Dynamic Listing Nomenclature

1. Flexion restriction
2. Extension restriction
3. Lateral flexion restriction (right or left)
4. Rotational restriction (right or left)

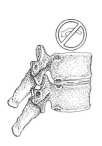 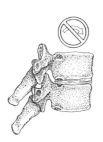 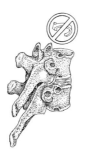 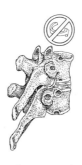 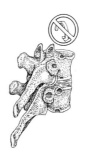 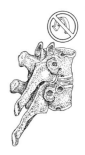

| Extension restriction | Flexion restriction | Right rotational restriction | Left rotational restriction | Right lateral flexion restriction | Left lateral flexion restriction |

Fig. 3.4 (*Continued*). (Modified from the ACA Council on Technic,[253] with permission.)

Reliability of Joint Assessment Procedures

The detection of dysfunction is not an exact science, and any of the examination procedures used to detect subluxation/dysfunction may produce false-positive, false-negative, and equivocal results. Although the effectiveness of chiropractic adjustive therapy for treating back pain has been demonstrated[155-161] and patient satisfaction has been well established,[162-164] the reliability and validity of many of the procedures used to detect joint subluxation/dysfunction have not been confirmed.[149,165-170]

Palpation for bony and soft tissue tenderness,[165,168,169,171,172] global range of motion assessment,[173-181] and postural assessment[182-184,185] have demonstrated satisfactory reliability. Palpation for spinal motion segment mobility[165,168-170,172,186-196] and leg length assessment[165,197-201] have demonstrated poor to satisfactory reliability.

Haas[165] reviewed the literature on the reliability of chiropractic joint assessment procedures and concluded that many of the studies had questionable design and statistical analyses. Additionally, nearly all the studies tested the reliability of only one procedure at a time. This leaves the question of combined reliability unanswered; the procedures may very well demonstrate higher reliability when used in conjunction with each other.[168,202]

Based on the present data, it seems prudent to refrain from drawing any firm conclusion on the independent reliability of many of the procedures commonly applied in the assessment of joint dysfunction. Definitive statements await further professional investigation.

Validity of Joint Assessment Procedures

Assessment of the validity of physical examination procedures for the detection of segmental joint subluxation/dysfunction is quite limited. One of the first investigations in this area was performed by Brunarski.[203] This study evaluated the validity of selected physical examination procedures in the identification of myofascial low back pain. Postural assessment and global range of motion assessment were identified as valid screening procedures for distinguishing myofascial low back pain subjects from a control group of normal subjects. However, this study did not address the value of these procedures in determining a level of joint dysfunction.

Falltrick and Pierson[204] tested the ability of leg length evaluation coupled with cervical rotation to see if this procedure could distinguish individuals with cervical dysfunction. The authors divided the subjects into two groups, depending on the presence or absence of cervical lesions. They then placed the patients in the prone position and instructed them to rotate their heads in one direction, then the other as their leg length was monitored for any change. The assumption was that those with cervical lesions would show changes in leg length that would set them apart from the lesioned group. The outcome did not confirm this hypothesis. The authors found no difference between groups and concluded that this procedure was not valid for identifying cervical lesions. Their results must be seriously questioned, however, because of experimental design flaws: there were no criteria for defining what constituted cervical lesions, and the testing procedures did not represent established standards for determining cervical dysfunction.

Perhaps the most noteworthy study on spinal joint assessment by physical examination was conducted by Jull et al.[205] They investigated the accuracy of manual examination procedures to locate painful cervical joints that had been confirmed by diagnostic nerve blocks. Using a combination of accessory and physiologic joint movements, a group of therapists identified the appropriate individuals and levels of abnormal painful cervical joints with 100% sensitivity and specificity. These results are quite dramatic and should stimulate further investigation.

The chiropractic profession is not the only health-care profession lagging in reliability and validity assessment.[170,206–209] Other health disciplines also suffer from significant variations in the application of diagnostic tests, and many lack experimental evaluation and conformation.[210–213]

There is no doubt that further investigation will lead to technologic advances and refinement of those procedures used to evaluate spinal and extremity joint function. It is likely, however that examination procedures dependent on human evaluation will always carry some error. The chiropractic physician must be aware of these limits yet constructively use the physical evaluation to help gain the patient's confidence and compliance. Physical examination procedures placed within proper clinical perspective still provide a significant cost-effective contribution to the formation of a clinical impression. Within this context, it is important not to rely excessively on any one procedure but rather to use a combination of diagnostic procedures and allow the weight of evidence to build a clinical impression of the patient's problem.

Symptoms of Joint Subluxation/ Dysfunction

Pain is an important sign of joint subluxation/dysfunction, but joint dysfunction cannot be excluded or confirmed by the presence or absence of pain. Joint dysfunction is not necessarily symptomatic, and the nature and cause of joint pain and dysfunction cannot be determined from the pain pattern alone. Joint pain will not discriminate between joint hypomobility, hypermobility, and clinical instability. Furthermore, all structures of the synovial joint are not pain sensitive. Some are very poorly innervated, and some are not innervated at all. The articular cartilage, nucleus pulposus, and cartilaginous end plates are devoid of nociceptive innervation.[214] Thus, pathologic change within certain articular structures may be insidious and well advanced before it becomes symptomatic.

Spinal or extremity joint pain is often poorly localized, and sites of pain and pathology may not necessarily correspond. Disorders of the musculoskeletal system are often associated with areas of referred pain and hypalgesia.[215,216] The referred pain is sclerogenic, ill-defined, deep, and achey. It is referred from the deep somatic tissues of the involved joint to the corresponding sclerotome. The anatomic sites of referred pain correspond to tissues that share the same segmental innervation (Fig. 3.5).

Sites of referred pain may be more painful to palpation and of greater intensity than the site of injury. The common phenomena of interscapular pain with cervical joint derangement or disc herniation illustrates this point.

The body is also more adept at discriminating sensations on the surface than pain originating in deep somatic structures and joints.[215,216] Ordinarily, the closer the effected tissue is to surface of the body, the better the pain

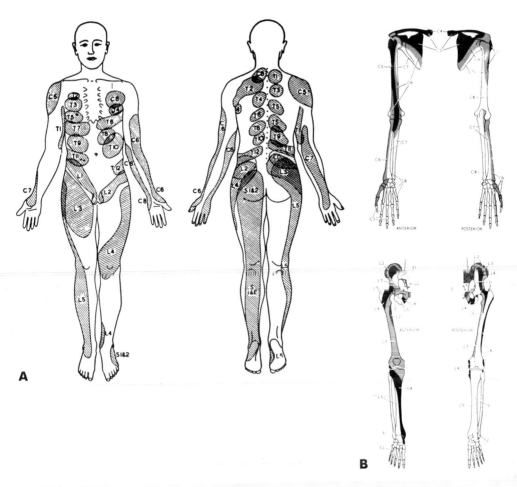

Figure 3.5 Segmental areas of pain of deep somatic origin: **(A)** interspinous ligament injection—Kellgren. (From Lewis,[15] with permission.) **(B)** Sclerotome pain patterns. (From Grieve,[306] with permission.)

coincides to the site of injury. It is therefore essential to subject all painful joint disorders to physical examination, and to rule out contraindications, before considering adjustive therapy.

Joint pain of mechanical origin characteristically has pain-free intervals, whereas joint pain associated with inflammation is more constant. Mechanical joint pain is often aggravated by joint movement and the activities of daily living. Although it is often alleviated by deceased activity, total immobilization may accentuate the pain response. Pain questionnaires and diagrams, algometers, visual analog scales, and functional capacity questionnaires are very helpful measures in the examination and quantification of painful complaints[217–223] (Fig. 3.6).

Patient Observation

The examination of any regional complaint begins with superficial observation and an investigation for any signs of trauma or inflammation. These signs include abrasions, lacerations, scars, discoloration, bruises, erythema,

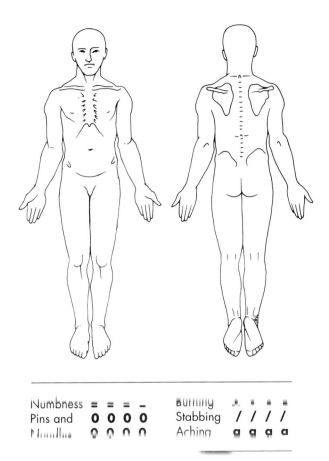

Numbness = = = –   Burning   ⋅ ⋅ ⋅ ⋅
Pins and   O O O O   Stabbing / / / /
Needles   O O O O   Aching   a a a a

Scoring Sheet for Pain Drawing

Writing anywhere	1
Unphysiologic pain pattern	1
Unphysiologic sensory change	1
More than one type of pain	1
Both upper and lower areas of the body involved	1
Markings outside the body	1
Unspecified symbols	1

A   Score: 1 = Normal. 5 or more = Very bad.

Figure 3.6 Tools to objectify pain: **(A)** pain diagram. (Adapted from Mooney and Robertson,[309] with permission.) (*Figure continues.*)

VISUAL ANALOG PAIN SEVERITY SCALE

INSTRUCTIONS: Please make a mark on the line provided below that corresponds to how you presently feel.

B NO PAIN ━━━━━━━━━━━━━━━━━━━━━━ WORST PAIN EVER

Fig. 3.6 (*Continued*). **(B)** Visual analog scale. (*Figure continues.*)

The Robert Jones and Agnes Hunt Orthopaedic Hospital, Oswestry, Shropshire
Department for Spinal Disorders

Name _____   Address _____   Date _____

Date of birth _____ Age _____   _____

Occupation _____   _____ Hospital No _____

How long have you had back pain? _____ Years _____ Months _____ Weeks

How long have you had leg pain? _____ Years _____ Months _____ Weeks

Please read:
This questionnaire has been designed to give the doctor information as to how your pain has affected your ability to manage in everyday life. Please answer every section, and mark in each section only the *one box* which applies to you. We realise you may consider that two of the statements in any one section relate to you, but please just *mark the box which most closely describes your problem.*

Section 1 — Pain Intensity
❏ I can tolerate the pain I have without having to use pain killers.
❏ The pain is bad but I manage without taking pain killers.
❏ Pain killers give complete relief from pain.
❏ Pain killers give moderate relief from pain.
❏ Pain killers give very little relief from pain.
❏ Pain killers have no effect on the pain and I do not use them.

Section 2 — Personal Care (Washing, Dressing, etc)
❏ I can look after myself normally without causing extra pain.
❏ I can look after myself normally but it causes extra pain.
❏ It is painful to look after myself and I am slow and careful.
❏ I need some help but manage most of my personal care.
❏ I need help every day in most aspects of self care.
❏ I do not get dressed, wash with difficulty and stay in bed.

Section 3 — Lifting
❏ I can lift heavy weights without extra pain.
❏ I can lift heavy weights but it gives extra pain.
❏ Pain prevents me from lifting heavy weights off the floor, but I can manage if they are conveniently positioned, eg on a table.
❏ Pain prevents me from lifting heavy weights but I can manage light to medium weights if they are conveniently positioned.
❏ I can lift only very light weights.
❏ I cannot lift or carry anything at all.

Section 4 — Walking
❏ Pain does not prevent me walking any distance.
❏ Pain prevents me walking more than 1 mile.
❏ Pain prevents me walking more than ½ mile.
❏ Pain prevents me walking more than ¼ mile.
❏ I can only walk using a stick or crutches.
❏ I am in bed most of the time and have to crawl to the toilet.

Section 5 — Sitting
❏ I can sit in any chair as long as I like.
❏ I can only sit in my favourite chair as long as I like.
❏ Pain prevents me sitting more than 1 hour.
❏ Pain prevents me from sitting more than ½ hour.
❏ Pain prevents me from sitting more than 10 mins.
❏ Pain prevents me from sitting at all.

Section 6 — Standing
❏ I can stand as long as I want without extra pain.
❏ I can stand as long as I want but it gives me extra pain.
❏ Pain prevents me from standing for more than 1 hour.
❏ Pain prevents me from standing for more than 30 mins.
❏ Pain prevents me from standing for more than 10 mins.
❏ Pain prevents me from standing at all.

Section 7 — Sleeping
❏ Pain does not prevent me from sleeping well.
❏ I can sleep well only by using tablets.
❏ Even when I take tablets I have less than six hours sleep.
❏ Even when I take tablets I have less than four hours sleep.
❏ Even when I take tablets I have less than two hours sleep.
❏ Pain prevents me from sleeping at all.

Section 8 — Sex Life
❏ My sex life is normal and causes no extra pain.
❏ My sex life is normal but causes some extra pain.
❏ My sex life is nearly normal but is very painful.
❏ My sex life is severely restricted by pain.
❏ My sex life is nearly absent because of pain.
❏ Pain prevents any sex life at all.

Section 9 — Social Life
❏ My social life is normal and gives me no extra pain.
❏ My social life is normal but increases the degree of pain.
❏ Pain has no significant effect on my social life apart from limiting my more energetic interests, eg dancing, etc.
❏ Pain has restricted my social life and I do not go out as often.
❏ Pain has restricted my social life to my home.
❏ I have no social life because of pain.

Section 10 — Travelling
❏ I can travel anywhere without extra pain.
❏ I can travel anywhere but it gives me extra pain.
❏ Pain is bad but I manage journeys over two hours.
❏ Pain restricts me to journeys of less than one hour.
❏ Pain restricts me to short necessary journeys under 30 minutes.
❏ Pain prevents me from travelling except to the doctor or hospital.

Comments _____

_____

C

Fig. 3.6 (*Continued*). (**C**) Functional capacities questionnaires. (Adapted from Fairbank et al.,[310] with permission.) (*Figure continues.*)

NECK DISABILITY INDEX

This questionnaire has been designed to give the doctor information as to how your neck pain has affected your ability to manage everyday life. Please answer every section and mark in each section only the ONE box that applies to you. We realize you may consider that two of the statements in any one section relate to you, but please just mark the box that most closely describes your problem.

Section 1— Pain Intensity
- ☐ I have no pain at the moment.
- ☐ The pain is very mild at the moment.
- ☐ The pain is moderate at the moment.
- ☐ The pain is fairly severe at the moment.
- ☐ The pain is very severe at the moment.
- ☐ The pain is the worst imaginable at the moment.

Section 2 — Personal Care (Washing, Dressing, ect.)
- ☐ I can look after myself normally without causing extra pain.
- ☐ I can look after myself normally but it causes extra pain.
- ☐ It is painful to look after myself and I am slow and careful.
- ☐ I need some help but manage most of my personal care.
- ☐ I need help every day in most aspects of self care.
- ☐ I do not get dressed, wash with difficulty, and stay in bed.

Section 3 — Lifting
- ☐ I can lift heavy weights without extra pain.
- ☐ I can lift heavy weights but it causes extra pain.
- ☐ Pain prevents me from lifting heavy weights off the floor, but I can manage if they are conveniently positioned, for example on the table.
- ☐ Pain prevents me from lifting heavy weights, but I can manage light to medium weights if they are conveniently positioned.
- ☐ I can lift only very light weights.
- ☐ I cannot lift or carry anything at all.

Section 4 — Reading
- ☐ I can read as much as I want with no pain in my neck.
- ☐ I can read as much as I want with slight pain in my neck.
- ☐ I can read as much as I want with moderate pain in my neck.
- ☐ I can't read as much as I want because of moderate pain in my neck.
- ☐ I can hardly read at all because of severe pain in my neck.
- ☐ I cannot read at all.

Section 5 — Headaches
- ☐ I have no headaches at all.
- ☐ I have slight headaches, which come infrequently.
- ☐ I have moderate headaches, which come infrequently.
- ☐ I have moderate headaches, which come frequently.
- ☐ I have severe headaches, which come frequently.
- ☐ I have headaches almost all the time.

Section 6 — Concentration
- ☐ I can concentrate fully when I want with no difficulty.
- ☐ I can concentrate fully when I want with slight difficulty.
- ☐ I have a fair degree of difficulty in concentrating when I want.
- ☐ I have a lot of difficulty in concentrating when I want.
- ☐ I have a great deal of difficulty in concentrating when I want.
- ☐ I cannot concentrate at all.

Section 7 — Work
- ☐ I can do as much work as I want.
- ☐ I can only do my usual work, but no more.
- ☐ I can do most of my usual work, but no more.
- ☐ I cannot do my usual work.
- ☐ I can hardly do any work at all.
- ☐ I can't do any work at all.

Section 8 — Driving
- ☐ I can drive my car without any neck pain.
- ☐ I can drive my car as long as I want with slight pain in my neck.
- ☐ I can drive my car as long as I want with moderate pain in my neck.
- ☐ I can't drive my car as much as I want because of moderate pain in my neck.
- ☐ I can hardly drive at all because of severe pain in my neck.
- ☐ I can't drive my car at all.

Section 9 — Sleeping
- ☐ I have no trouble sleeping.
- ☐ My sleep is slightly disturbed (less than 1 hr. sleepless)
- ☐ My sleep is mildly disturbed (1–2 hrs. sleepless)
- ☐ My sleep is moderately disturbed (2–3 hrs. sleepless)
- ☐ My sleep is greatly disturbed (3–5 hrs. sleepless).
- ☐ My sleep is completely disturbed (5–7 hrs. sleepless).

Section 10 — Recreation
- ☐ I am able to engage in all my recreation activities with no neck pain at all.
- ☐ I am able to engage in all my recreation activities with some pain in my neck.
- ☐ I am able to engage in most, but not all of my usual recreation activities because of pain in my neck.
- ☐ I am able to engage in only a few of my usual recreation activities because of pain in my neck.
- ☐ I can hardly do any recreation activities because of pain in my neck.
- ☐ I can't do any recreation activities at all.

C

Fig. 3.6 (**C**) (*Continued*).

For each section, scores fall on a zero (0) to five (5) scale, with the higher values representing greater disability. The sum of the 10 scores is expressed as a percentage of the maximum score. If a patient fails to complete a section, the percentage is adjusted accordingly.

For each section, the possible score is 5; if the first statement is marked the section score = 0; if the last statement is marked the section score = 5. The sections are then totaled, divided by the possible score, and multiplied by 100 to obtain a percentage.

OSWESTRY LOW BACK PAIN DISABILITY QUESTIONNAIRE
SCORING

0 to 5%	= no disability
6 to 20 %	= minimal (mild) disability
21 to 40%	= moderate disability
41 to 60%	= severe disability
over 60%	= the patient is severely disabled by pain in several areas of life

NECK DISABILITY INDEX
SCORING

0 to 10%	= no disability
11 to 30 %	= minimal (mild) disability
31 to 50%	= moderate disability
51 to 70%	= severe disability
over 70%	= completely disabled by pain in several areas of life

Fig. 3.6 (**C**) (*Continued*).   **C**

pallor, swelling, or misalignment. Acute injury, congenital or developmental defects, and many systemic diseases of the NMS are often represented by abnormalities observed in posture or gait.

The observational evaluation of NMS function routinely incorporates a detailed assessment of patient symmetry, posture, and locomotion. The examination is based on the premise that there is a postural ideal that can be used as a comparative standard, and that deviations in posture, gait, or movement may identify or predispose an individual to neuromusculoskeletal disease or dysfunction.

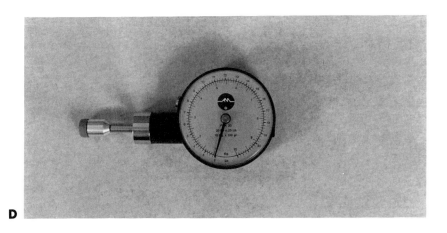

Fig. 3.6 (*Continued*). (**D**) Algometer.

Ample evidence supports the association of painful disorders of the NMS with restrictions to joint motion and abnormalities in posture.[181,185,203,224–234] Evidence also suggests that deviations from "ideal posture" may predilect an individual to neuromusculoskeletal dysfunction and possible joint degeneration.[235–240] However, the degree of deviation necessary to impact a patient's health has not been established. Individual biologic variation and adaptability certainly play a role in limiting the development and morbidity of joint dysfunction and degenerative joint disease. Those that would set a narrow standard for posture and range of motion ignore the mounting evidence that suggests a range of normal individual variation.[15,229,237,241–249] This does not discount the value of postural and movement evaluation in the assessment of spinal dysfunction but reinforces the need to balance the assessment with the patient's symptoms and function.

Gait Evaluation

Gait evaluation is conducted formally during the physical examination but begins as the patient walks to the examination room. Locomotion involves integrated activity of numerous components of the motor system and therefore becomes an efficient method for screening neuromusculoskeletal function.

The objectives of gait analysis are to identify deviations and to obtain information that may assist in determining the cause of the deviations and provide a basis for the use of therapeutic procedures or supportive devices to improve the walking pattern.[250] There are two basic phases of the normal pattern of gait, one involving a weight-bearing period (stance phase), the other a non-weight-bearing period (swing period) (Fig. 3.7). Disease or dysfunction may effect one phase and not the other, necessitating careful evaluation of both components.

Evaluation begins with a general impression of locomotion: is it guarded, or painful? Is the patient protective of any part and/or unwilling to put equal weight on each leg?

The movements of the upper and lower extremity are noted. Length of stride, degree of pronation or supination, tilt of pelvis, adaptational movements of the shoulder girdle, and pendulousness of the arms are

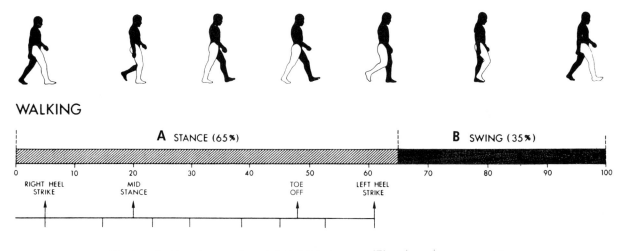

WALKING

Figure 3.7 The phases of gait: (A) stance phase, (B) swing phase. (Modified from Adelaar,[308] with permission.)

assessed. Specific components of gait evaluation are listed in Table 3.2, and disorders that may alter gait are listed in Table 3.3

Apparent abnormal findings or deviations from the expected pattern identified with gait analysis must be supported or validated by other test procedures including muscle tests for strength, length, tone and texture, as well as tests for joint function.

Postural Evaluation

Like all physical examination skills, postural evaluation must be learned and practiced. Reliable and accurate assessment is founded on attention to proper technique. The room must be appropriately lit to clearly illuminate the parts being examined and to prevent shadows from projecting false contours. The doctor must be oriented to the patient so that the dominant

---

Table 3.2 Components of Gait Evaluation

Alignment and symmetry of the head, shoulders, and trunk

Gross movements of the arms and legs, looking for reciprocal and equal amplitude of movement

Symmetry of stride from side to side for length, timing, and synchronization

Assessment of body vertical oscillations at an even tempo

Assessment of pelvic transverse rotation, anterior to posterior rotation, lateral tilt, and lateral displacement through the phases of gait

Assessment to determine if the lower extremities medially rotate then laterally rotate going from swing to stance

Assessment to determine if the knees have two alterations of extension and flexion during a single-gait cycle

Assessment to determine if the ankles go from maximum dorsiflexion to maximum plantar-flexion when going from the stance phase to the swing phase

Table 3.3 Disorders That May Induce Altered Gait

Pain or discomfort during the weight-bearing phase

Muscle weakness and imbalance

Limitation of joint motion—active, passive, and/or accessory

Incoordination of movement due to neurologic condition (e.g., cerebral vascular accident, Parkinson's syndrome, etc.)

Changes and deformities in bone or soft tissues

eye is located in the midline between the landmarks being compared.[251] If observing the patient while he or she is supine or prone, the doctor stands on the side of eye dominance. Table 3.4 outlines the procedures for determining one's dominant eye.

When combining observation and palpation of asymmetry, it is important that the doctor's hands and eyes are on the same reference plane. For example, when evaluating the relative heights of the iliac crests, the doctor places hands on each crest, and positions the dominant eye in the midline on the same plane as the doctor's hands.

The assessment of symmetry, locomotion, and posture are critical in the evaluation of NMS dysfunction. They are objective signs supportive of NMS disease or injury,[203] but they are not specific tests for the determination of articular dysfunction/subluxation. Regional asymmetry should trigger further evaluation of that area, but asymmetry alone does not confirm or rule out the presence of segmental subluxations or dysfunction.

Postural asymmetry is a challenge to homeostatic regulation and may indicate potential areas of imbalance including bony asymmetry and mechanical stress. Its relationship to initiating, predisposing, or perpetuating segmental dysfunction should not be overlooked. In our rush to find the specific level of spinal subluxation, we often overlook significant postural decompensations that may be predisposing the patient to pain and dysfunction. The patient with extremity or spinal complaints may not respond to local therapy until gait and postural stresses are removed.

Spinal postural evaluation

During standing postural assessment, the patient is instructed to assume a relaxed stance, looking straight ahead with feet approximately 4 to 6 inches apart. The patient should be in a gown or undergarments and should not

Table 3.4 Determination of Dominant Eye

1. Bring both hands together to form a small circle with the thumbs and index fingers.
2. Straighten both arms out and with both eyes open, sight through the small circle an object at the other end of the room
3. Close one eye. If the object is still seen, the open eye is dominant. For example, if the right eye is closed and the object is still seen, the left eye is dominant. If the right eye is closed and the object is no longer seen, the right eye is dominant.

be wearing shoes. If the patient has orthotics or corrective footwear, posture is assessed with the patient's shoes both off and on. The evaluation is conducted from the posterior and anterior to determine distribution of weight and symmetry of landmarks in the coronal plane, and from the side to evaluate posture and landmarks relative to the center of gravity line. In addition, the upper and lower extremities are surveyed for deformity, pronation or supination, and internal or external rotation.

The examination should include a determination of the carriage of the center of gravity and symmetry of key bony and soft tissue landmarks. The flexibility (Adams sign) of the curve is determined, and any associated rib humps are noted. The evaluation of spinal posture may be aided by the use of a plumb line (Fig. 3.8) and devices such as the posturometer, scoliometer (Fig. 3.9), and bilateral weight scales.

In a patient with suspected scoliosis, an assessment for potential leg length inequality and a screen for anatomic or functional leg length discrepancy should be included. Suspected anatomic discrepancy should be measured and radiographically confirmed if clinically significant.

Range of Motion Assessment

Both active and passive joint range of motion are assessed. During active range of motion assessment, the patient performs the movement, and during passive motion assessment the examiner produces the movement. When acute joint pain and muscle splinting are involved, the patient may be unable to relax sufficiently to allow for true passive assessment.

During both active and passive motion assessment, the physician is evaluating the total range of movement, symmetry of movement, pattern of movement, and muscle tone. Any painful limitations, abnormal movements, or painful arcs should be recorded. Unless contraindicated by joint injury or disease, additional "overpressure" should be applied at the end of passive movement to assess for pain and end feel.

Significant limitation and asymmetry of movement is considered to be evidence of neuromusculoskeletal impairment.[252] Noted reductions in joint movement, however, must be placed within the context of the normal variations that exist between sexes and age groups. This increases the importance of making a bilateral comparison of joint and spinal mobility.

Many different methods of measurement are employed in the evaluation of joint and spinal range of motion. They range from visual estimates, goniometric and inclinometric measurements, to the more technical approaches of computerized digitation.[177,181] The use of inclinometers for spinal range of motion and inclinometers or goniometers for extremity range of motion is becoming a minimal standard.[252] For the spine, the two-inclinometer method as described by Mayer et al.[181] is a reliable, inexpensive, and efficient technique. It can be applied in the measurement of all spinal movements except trunk rotation (Figs. 3.10 and 3.11).

Spinal and extremity joint motion are measured in degrees relative to the zero or starting position. In a patient demonstrating 50 degrees of cervical extension and 55 degrees of cervical flexion, the motion would be recorded as EXT/FL 50–0–55. All physiologic movements, on both sides of the zero position (0 degrees), should be measured and recorded. Table

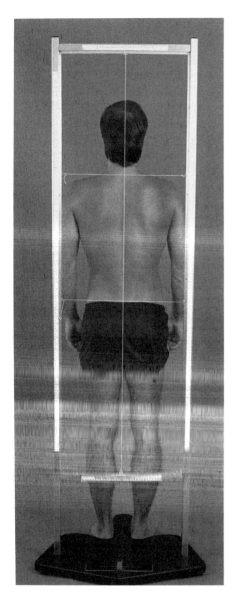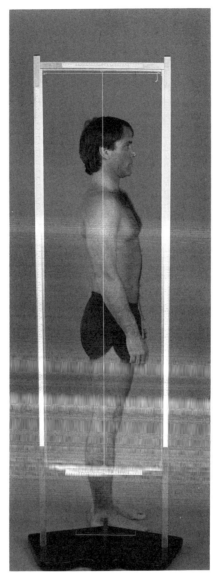

Figure 3.8 Plumb-line evaluation of spinal posture.

3.5 outlines the common format for recording spinal and extremity range of motion.

In joints with quite limited range of motion, actual quantitative measurement may be unfeasible (e.g., spinal joints). In such circumstances, motion is estimated by manual palpation procedures; the motion of one spinal joint is compared to motion at the contralateral and adjacent joints. Methods for estimating the quality and quantity of individual spinal and extremity joint motion are covered regionally in Chapters 5 and 6, respectively.

Range of motion abnormalities are potential signs of dysfunction in both the extremity and spinal joints, but regional restrictions to spinal movement do not confirm the presence or absence of segmental spinal joint dysfunction. Spinal injuries or disease may affect the nonsegmental somatic tissues

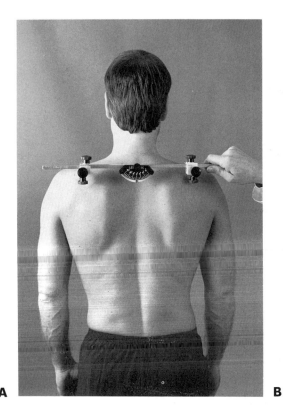 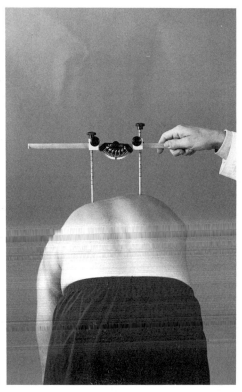

Figure 3.9 Scoliometer used for measuring **(A)** shoulder heights and **(B)** rib deformity seen with scoliosis in the Adams position.

Table 3.5 Assessment of Spinal and
Extremity Motion

Spinal Motion
Extension-0-flexion
Right lateral bending-0-left lateral bending
Right·rotation-0-left rotation
Extremity Motion
Extension-0-flexion
Abduction-0-adduction
External rotation-0-internal rotation
Supination-0-pronation
Radial deviation-0-ulnar deviation
Inversion-0-eversion
Valgus-0-varus

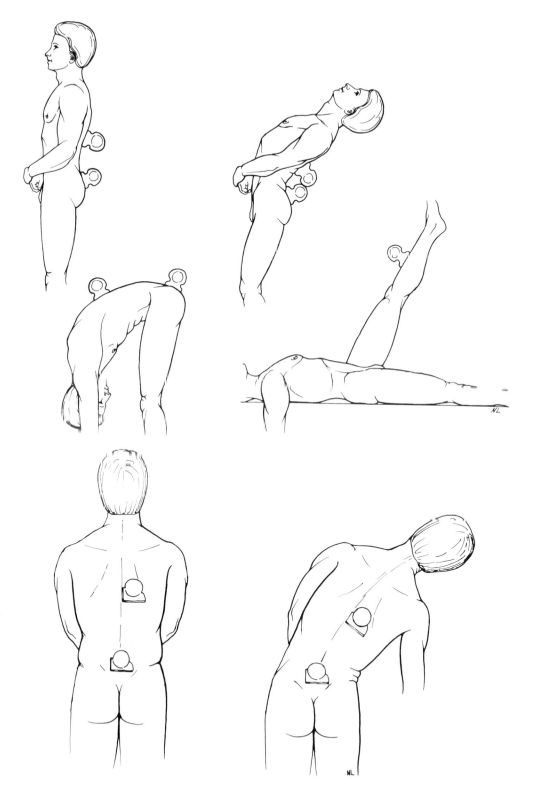

Figure 3.10 Measurement of lumbar ranges of motion using dual inclinometers. (Modified from American Medical Association,[252] with permission.)

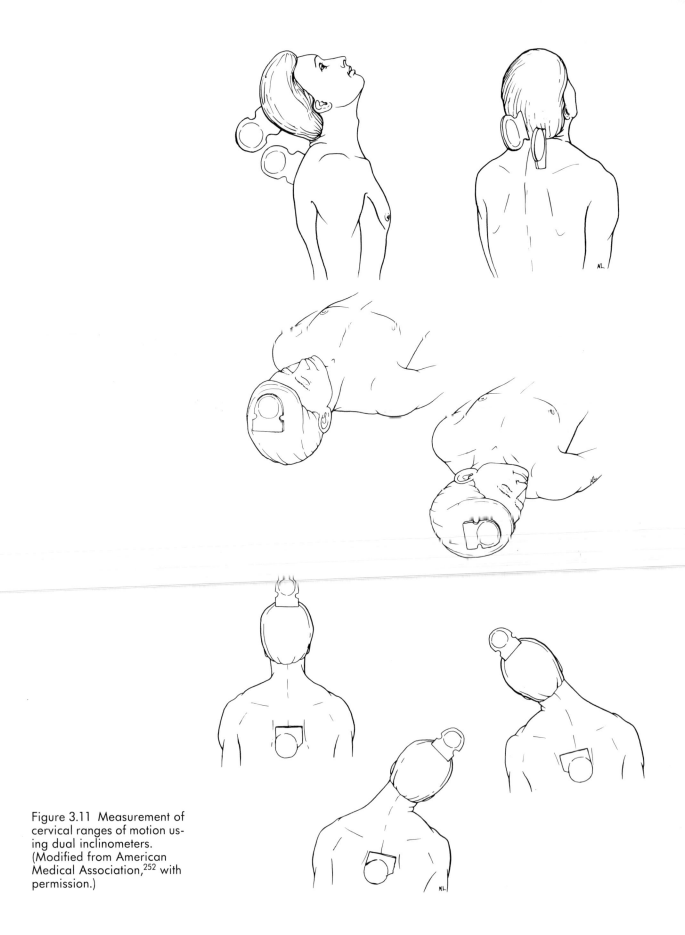

Figure 3.11 Measurement of cervical ranges of motion using dual inclinometers. (Modified from American Medical Association,[252] with permission.)

and spare the vertebral joints. In these circumstances, altered regional movements are present, and individual segmental range of joint movement may be limited. However, the loss of mobility is uniform, and the individual spinal motion segments demonstrate normal joint play and end feel.

Conversely, disorders that produce individual spinal joint restrictions may still demonstrate normal regional movements, as individual joint restriction is concealed by compensatory hypermobility at adjacent joints. Spinal abnormalities in global range of motion therefore are more valuable in identifying general NMS dysfunction and the possibility of segmental dysfunction than they are in confirming a specific level of dysfunction.

Disorders capable of altering individual joint and regional spinal movements are extensive. They include joint subluxation, dislocation, effusion, joint mice, myofibrosis, periarticular fibrosis, muscle hypertrophy, degenerative joint disease, muscle guarding, and fracture. Other nontraumatic disease states with pathologic effects on somatic structures or the nervous system also produce abnormalities in movement.

Palpation

Palpation is the application of variable manual pressures, through the surface of the body, to determine the shape, size, consistency, position, and inherent motility of the tissues beneath.[253] Palpation is the oldest examination technique employed by chiropractors to detect subluxation/dysfunction and is still the most emphasized clinical finding supportive of subluxation/dysfunction.[149-152]

Like observational skills, palpation skills are learned tasks that take hours of devotion and practice. Good palpation skills are the result of both physical abilities and mental concentration. The skilled palpator is one who has developed an improved ability to tactually discriminate and mentally focus.

Palpatory procedures are commonly divided into static and motion components. Static palpation is performed with the patient in a stationary position, and is often further subdivided into bony and soft tissue palpation. Motion palpation is performed during active or passive joint movement and also involves the evaluation of accessory joint movements. Motion palpation procedures have been an integral part of chiropractic since its inception; but only through the cultivation of Gillet,[32-36] Faye,[43] and Schafer and Faye[44] have formalized techniques been widely disseminated.

Bony Palpation

The major goal of bony palpation is to locate bony landmarks and assess bony contour for any joint malpositions, anomalies, or tenderness. Typically, the palmer surfaces of the fingers or thumbs are used because they are richly endowed with sensory receptors. Light pressure is used for superficial structures, gently increasing pressure for deeper landmarks.

During spinal palpation, the pelvis, lumbar, and thoracic regions are customarily evaluated with the patient in the prone position and the patient's cervical spine in the sitting or supine position. The spinous processes, transverse processes in the thoracic spine, articular pillars in the cervical spine, and mammillary processes in the lumbar spine are palpated for tenderness and compared for contour and alignment (Fig. 3.12). Individual motion

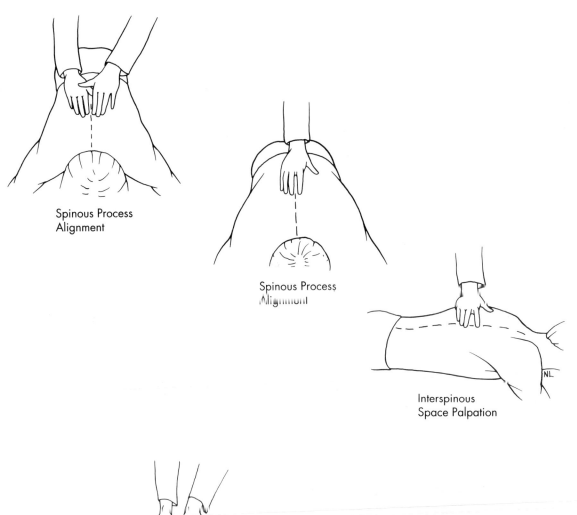

Spinous Process
Alignment

Spinous Process
Alignment

Interspinous
Space Palpation

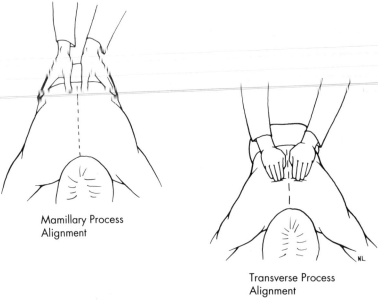

Mamillary Process
Alignment

Transverse Process
Alignment

Figure 3.12 Bony palpation of segmental spinal landmarks.

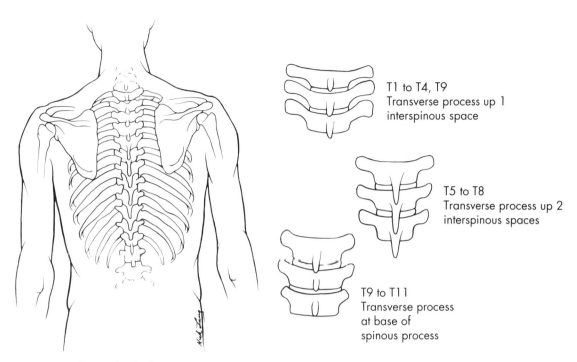

T1 to T4, T9
Transverse process up 1
interspinous space

T5 to T8
Transverse process up 2
interspinous spaces

T9 to T11
Transverse process
at base of
spinous process

Figure 3.13 The structural relationship between thoracic spinous processes and
transverse processes.

segments are often located relative to these bony landmarks, and it is important to appreciate the anatomic relationship of the transverse process to the corresponding spinous processes (Fig. 3.13).

Tenderness and misalignment of articular landmarks are important potential signs of joint subluxation. Misaligned articular structures do suggest joint subluxation/dysfunction, but apparent joint malpositions may result from anomaly or compensation without dysfunction. Spinal landmarks, especially the spinous process, are prone to congenital or developmental malformation. Disrelationship between adjacent spinous process can be falsely positive and cannot be relied on to represent true misalignment. Furthermore, the spine functions as a kinetic chain, and disease or dysfunction at one level may force adaptational alterations in neutral alignment at adjacent levels. These sites of compensational change may palpate as being malpositioned (out of ideal neutral alignment) yet have normal pain-free function. Static bony palpation does not ascertain joint mobility or the full extensibility of the articular soft tissues and cannot distinguish normal compensation from joint subluxation/dysfunction.

Tenderness to pressure at bony landmarks that are close to articulations is another proposed empirical sign of joint dysfunction. In the spine, the spinous process and interspinal spaces are commonly palpated for tenderness to screen for a possible level of segmental pathology or dysfunction. The relationship between spinous and interspinous tenderness and dysfunction is speculated to result from reflex sensitivity in tissues with shared segmental innervation, or as a result of mechanical deformation in structures attaching at these bony sites.

Remember that bony tenderness may result from many different pathologic processes such as bone infection, neoplasia, osteoporosis, and fractures. Additionally, the spinous process may be tender whether the joint is hypomobile, hypermobile, or unstable. For the previously outlined reasons, suspected malpositions and/or bony tenderness must be associated with other clinical signs before an impression of joint subluxation or dysfunction is formed.

Soft Tissue Palpation

The major function of soft tissue palpation is to determine the contour, consistency, quality, and the presence or absence of pain in the dermal, subdermal, and deeper "functional" tissue layers. The dermal layer incorporates the skin, subdermal layer, subcutaneous adipose, fasciae, nerves, and vessels. The functional layer consists of the muscles, tendons, tendon sheaths, bursae, ligaments, fasciae, vessels, and nerves

Palpation of the dermal layer is directed toward the assessment of temperature, moisture, motility, consistency, and tissue sensitivity (e.g., hyperesthesia, tenderness, etc.). Palpation techniques involve light, gentle exploration of the skin with the palmar surfaces of the fingers or thumbs. When manually assessing temperature of superficial tissues, the dorsum of the hands are typically used (Fig. 3.14). Motility and sensitivity of the dermal layer may also be assessed by the technique of skin rolling (Fig. 3.14).

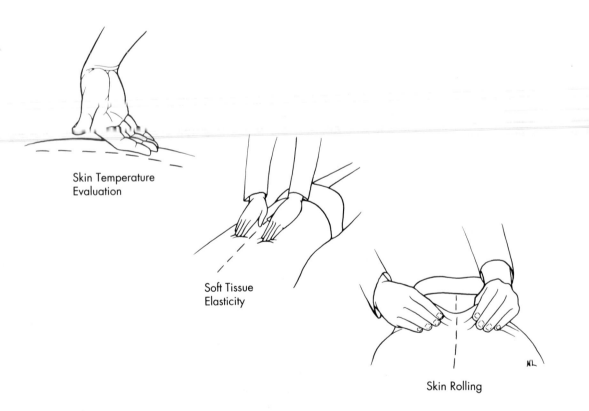

Skin Temperature Evaluation

Soft Tissue Elasticity

Skin Rolling

Figure 3.14 Assessment techniques for the superficial layer of the soft tissues.

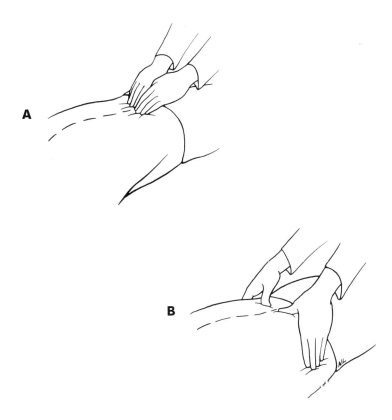

Figure 3.15 Assessment techniques for the deep functional layer of the soft tissues using (**A**) fingertips or (**B**) thumbs.

The subcutaneous and deeper functional layers are explored for internal arrangement, contour, consistency, flexibility, and response to pressure. The deeper soft tissues are usually investigated with the fingertips or thumbs (Fig. 3.15). Palpation of paraspinal soft tissues is customarily performed immediately following bony palpation. The cervical spine is customarily examined with the patient in the supine or sitting position and the lumbopelvic and thoracic regions in the prone position.

The palpatory investigation of the functional layer is decisive in the soft tissue investigation for signs of joint dysfunction. The presence of soft tissue pain, asymmetric tone, and/or consistency are regarded as important indicators of joint dysfunction. Grieve[254] suggests it may be the objective findings of muscle abnormality (palpable nodules, bands, stringiness) and the presence of muscle tenderness that represent external evidence of changes in peripheral tissues related to joint problems. Furthermore, muscle pain is sometimes acute and surprisingly quite unknown to the asymptomatic patient until made manifest by careful localized palpation.

In health, normal neuromuscular coordination is accepted as unremarkable; only in dysfunction does the underlying complexity of movement become apparent, and the disturbance of reciprocal muscle action become manifest.[254] Moreover, abnormal soft tissues patterns and presentations may persist after joint function has been restored. Although chronic muscle imbalance has a role in initiating and perpetuating joint problems and

Table 3.6 How to Use Your Palpation Tools

Use the least pressure possible. Your touch receptors are designed to respond only when not pressed on too firmly; experiment with decreasing pressure instead of increasing pressure, and your tactile perception may improve.

Try not to cause pain if possible. Pain may induce protective muscle splinting and make palpation more difficult.

Try not to lose skin contact before you are done with the palpation of the area.

Use broad contacts whenever possible. For deep palpation, use broad contacts to reach the desired tissue, then palpate with your palpation finger, keeping the overlying tissue from expanding with the other fingers of your palpation hand.

Close your eyes to increase your palpatory perception.

somatic pain, it may be secondary to stresses imposed by ligamentous failure, denervation, or reflex inhibition from pain. Adjustment of the joint without attention to the supporting and controlling effects of the soft tissues will likely result in recurrence of joint dysfunction.

Suppleness and flexibility of muscle and connective tissues are important and necessary for proper functioning of the joint systems of the body. With trauma and longstanding occupational or postural stress, the imposed asymmetry to the soft tissues results in increased fibroblastic activity and the production of more collagen. The connective tissue elements will occupy more space and possibly encroach on the space occupied by nerves and blood vessels. Furthermore, the affected tissues will lose elasticity, which restricts movement as well as create pain when activity is required. Janda,[255] Gatterman,[98] and Travell[256] have written and described much concerning the muscular and myofascial factors in the pathogenesis of somatic and joint pain syndromes.

Soft tissue asymmetries may also result from congenital or developmental variations or be the product of nonmanipulative disorders. Accordingly, any noted soft tissue abnormalities must be assessed within the context of a broader examination to be clinically significant. Instructions and tips on the application of static bony and soft tissue palpation are included in Tables 3.6 and 3.7.

Table 3.7 Palpation Hints and Comments

Concentrate on the area and/or structure you want to palpate; do not palpate casually.

Do not let your attention be carried away by unrelated sensations.

Concentrate on your fingers; do not feel what you see or expect to feel.

Keep an open mind and do not deceive yourself; never let your mind "out palpate" your fingers.

Establish a palpation routine and stay with it.

Take every opportunity to add to your tactile "vocabulary" through comparative experiences.

Motion Palpation

Adjustive therapy is often directed at restoring pain-free joint movement. The effective practitioner must be able to identify alterations in range and quality of joint movement. Motion palpation is a skill that depends not only on psychomotor training but also on an understanding of the local functional anatomy, biomechanics, and pathomechanics. Each individual extremity joint and spinal region has its unique patterns and ranges of motion that must be learned if the student is to master the art of motion palpation.

Motion palpation covers a collection of manual examination procedures that are customarily divided into techniques designed to assess active, passive, and accessory joint movements. Active movements are internally driven and are the result of voluntary muscle contraction. During active movement assessment, the doctor may help guide the patient through a given motion, but the patient provides the muscular effort necessary to induce joint movement. The range of active joint movement is determined by its articular design and the inherent tension and resilience in its associated muscular, myofascial, and ligamentous structures. The end point of active joint movement has been labeled by Greenman as *the physiologic barrier*[251] (Fig. 3.16).

In contrast, passive joint movements are involuntary movements. With the patient in a relaxed position, the examiner carries the joint through its

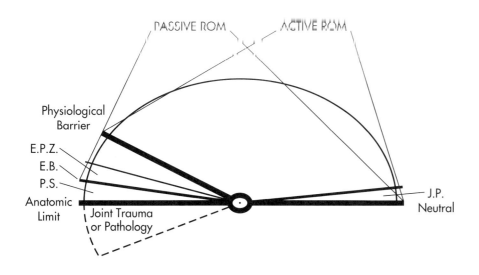

E.P.Z. = End Play Zone
E.B. = Elastic Barrier
J.P. = Joint Play
P.S. = Paraphysiological Space

Figure 3.16 Joint motions: The diagram represents joint motion in one plane starting from a neutral position. Joint play occurs in the neutral position, followed by the active and passive ranges of motion. The passive range of motion goes beyond the active range of motion entering the joint's elastic limit and encountering the elastic barrier. Following cavitation, the paraphysiologic space extends the passive range of motion. If the joint is carried beyond its anatomic limit, trauma results.

arc of available motion. The range for passive joint movement is somewhat greater than the range for active joint movement because of decreased muscle tension (Fig. 3.16). The range of passive joint movement also depends on articular design and flexibility of related articular soft tissues.

As the limits of passive joint movement are approached, additional resistance is encountered as the joints elastic limits are challenged. Movement into this space (end play zone) (Fig. 3.16) may be induced by forced muscular effort by the patient, or by additional overpressure (end play) applied by the examiner. If the forces applied at this point are removed, the joint springs back from its elastic limits. Movements into this region are valuable in assessing the elastic properties of the joint capsule and its periarticular soft tissues.

Movement beyond the end play zone is possible, but only after the fluid tension between synovial surfaces has been overcome. This process is typically associated with an articular crack (cavitation). Sandoz[11] has labeled this as the zone of paraphysiologic movement and identified its boundaries as the elastic and anatomic barriers (Fig. 3.16). Although the paraphysiologic space aptly identifies an area of increased movement available after cavitation, it is still within the joint's elastic range. One must guard against the misleading assumption that movement beyond the elastic barrier is movement beyond the joint's elastic limits.

Movement into this space does not induce joint injury. Adjustive therapy is typically directed at inducing this movement by producing joint cavitation.[41] However, if the outer boundaries (anatomic limits) of the paraphysiologic space are breached, then plastic deformation and joint injury will occur (Fig. 3.17).

Restrictions to joint motion may occur at any point within the joint's range of motion. They may be minor or major in nature and encountered within the joint's active or passive range. Restrictive barriers encountered within the joint's active range of motion are due primarily to myofascial shortening.[251] This may be a product of muscle splinting, hypertrophy, aging, or contracture. Restrictive barriers to movement at the end range of passive movement are more indicative of shortening in the joint capsule and periarticular soft tissues.

During the performance of motion palpation, the examiner characteristically uses one hand to palpate joint movement (palpation hand) while the other hand (indifferent hand) produces or guides movement. The palpation hand establishes bony or soft tissue contacts over the joint as attention is directed to the assessment of joint range, pattern, and quality of movement (Fig. 3.18). When assessing joint motion, the palpator is evaluating the quality and quantity of movement from the starting or zero point to the end range of passive movement.

In spinal evaluation, the landmarks commonly used in spinal evaluation are the spinous processes, articular pillars, transverse process, and mamillary processes.

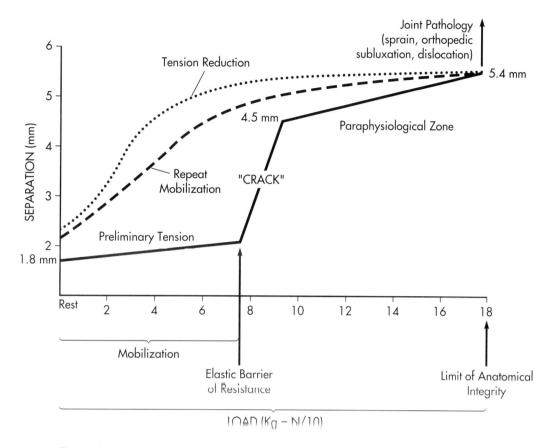

Figure 3.17 Graph representing the effects of joint separation and cavitation. If the anatomic limits are breached, plastic deformation of soft tissues and joint injury will occur.

Accessory Joint Motion

Accessory joint movements are also involuntary movements and represent the small give or play within a joint that is necessary for normal function. Joint surfaces do not form true geometric shapes with matching articular surfaces. As a result, movement occurs around a shifting axis, and the joint capsule must allow sufficient play and separation between articular surfaces to avoid abnormal joint friction.

Accessory joint movements are evaluated by the procedures of joint play and end play (feel).[39,44] End-play evaluation is the qualitative assessment of resistance at the end point of passive joint movement, and joint play is the assessment of resistance from a neutral and/or loose-packed joint position.[253] Both motions depend on the flexibility (play) of the articular soft tissue and are therefore not distinguished by some authors.[39,44] Rather, end play is considered to be joint play delivered at the end range of joint motion.

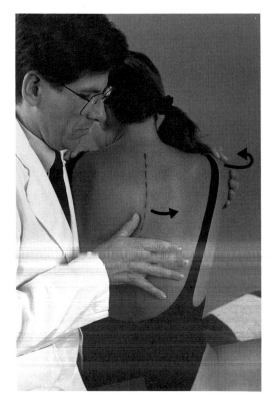

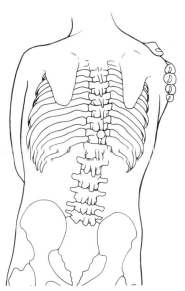

Figure 3.18 Assessment of segmental range of motion, e.g., midthoracic left axial rotation. The circle represents the location of the thumb contact traversing the spinous processes.

End play

During end-play assessment, the physician is concerned with the qualitative assessment of motion through the end play zone (Fig. 3.16). The end play zone is characterized by a sense of increasing resistance as it is approached (first stop) and a second firmer resistance (second stop) as its limits are approached (Fig. 3.19).

End-play is assessed by applying additional overpressure to the specified joint at the end range of passive movement. A gentle springing force is induced through the palpation and indifferent hand contacts (Fig. 3.19). To execute end feel, evaluate the point at which resistance is encountered, the quality of that resistance, and whether there is any associated tenderness. End-play evaluation is critical to the assessment of joint function. In spinal joints where individual joint movement is limited, qualitative end-play assessment may be more informative than procedures designed to assess the full range of passive joint motion.[257]

Each spinal region or extremity joint has characteristic end-play qualities that are determined by the local bony and soft tissue anatomy (physiologic end feel). For example, elbow extension has a hard bony end feel produced by the bony impact of the olecranon on the humerus, while elbow flexion has a soft springy end feel produced by the impact of soft tissues of the arm

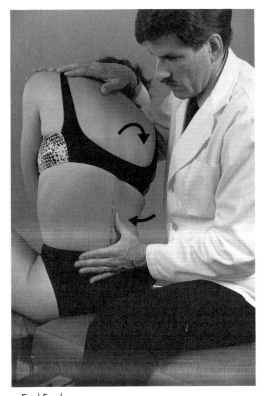

End-Feel

Zone

ꭥꭥꭥꭥꭥꭥ a

Final   First
Stop   Stop

Start

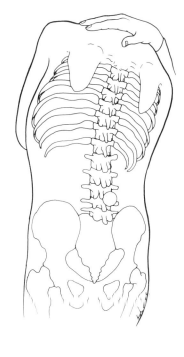

Figure 3.19 Assessment of lateral flexion end feel motion. Circle represents the location of the thumb contact against the lateral surface of the spinous process.

and forearm. What may be a normal end play at one joint may be a pathologic end play at another. A hard bony end play to elbow flexion might indicate a fracture or an intra-articular blockage, and a soft springing end play to elbow extension might indicate joint effusion. Physiologic and pathologic end plays have been tabulated for the spine and extremity joints and are outlined in Table 3.8.

Loss of anticipated end-play elasticity is thought to be indicative of disorders within the joint, its capsule, or periarticular soft tissue. Encountered end-play resistance is a significant finding in the determination of joint dysfunction and adjustive vector orientation. Adjustive therapy is commonly applied along planes of encountered resistance in an attempt to restore normal mobility.

Cyriax[14] has suggested that end-play assessment is particularly valuable in isolating the integrity of the joint capsule. He has proposed that injuries or disorders that lead to contractures of the joint capsule will lead to predictable patterns of end-play restrictions in multiple ranges. Each joint purportedly has its own characteristic capsular pattern of restricted movement that indi-

Table 3.8 Normal and Abnormal End Feels

Capsular
Firm but giving; resistance builds with lengthening, like stretching a piece of leather
    Example: close-packed position of the joint; external rotation of shoulder
    Abnormal example: capsular fibrosis and/or adhesions leading to a capsular pattern of abnormal end feels

Ligamentous
Like capsular but may have a slightly firmer quality
    Example: knee extension
    Abnormal example: noncapsular pattern of abnormal resistance due to ligamentous shortening

Soft Tissue Approximation
Giving, squeezing quality; results from the approximation of soft tissues; typically painless
    Example: elbow flexion
    Abnormal example: muscle hypertrophy, soft tissue swelling

Bony
Hard, nongiving abrupt stop
    Example: elbow extension
    Abnormal example: bony exostosis, articular hypertrophic changes

Muscular
Firm but giving, builds with elongation; not as stiff as capsular or ligamentous
    Normal example: hip flexion

Muscle Spasm
Guarded, resisted by muscle contraction; should feel muscle reaction. The end feel cannot be assessed because of pain and/or guarding
    Abnormal example: protective muscle splinting that is due to joint or soft tissue disease or injury

Interarticular
Bouncy springy quality
    Abnormal example: meniscal tear, joint mice

Empty
Normal end feel resistance is missing; end feel is not encountered at normal point, and/or the joint demonstrates unusual give and deformation
    Abnormal example: joint injury or disease leading to hypermobility or instability

cates capsular involvement (Table 3.9). Injuries or contractures in only one aspect of the capsule do not necessarily follow this typical pattern and may effect movement in only one direction.

Loss of normal end-play resistance (empty end feel) is also clinically significant, because it is a potential manifestation of joint hypermobility or instability. Injuries or disorders that lead to elongation of the joint's stabilizing structures may lead to a loss of normal end-range resistance. Although an empty end feel is indicative of possible clinical joint instability, its presence may be masked by segmental muscle splinting, especially in the symptomatic patient.

Table 3.9 Capsular Patterns

Joint	Pattern
Spine	Ipsilateral rotation and contralateral lateral flexion
Hip	Internal rotation–abduction–Flexion–Extension–Adduction–External Rotation
Knee	Flexion (great)–extension (slight)
Ankle	Dorsiflxion–plantar flexion
Metatarsophalangeal	Flexion–extension
Interphalangeal	Flexion–extension
Shoulder	External rotation–abduction–internal rotation–flexion
Elbow	Flexion–Extension (pronation and supination–full range)
Distal radioulnar	Pronation–supination
Radioulnacarpal	Flexion–extension
Midcarpal	Extension–flexion
Thumb carpometacarpal	Abduction–extension
Metacarpophalangeal	Flexion–extension
Interphalangeal	Flexion–extension

Patterns are in order of decreasing stiffness (exception, the spine, where either is possible).

Joint play

Joint play assessment is the qualitative evaluation of the joint's resistance to movement when it is in its neutral or loose-packed position. The loose-packed position allows for the greatest possible play between the joint surfaces and the best opportunity to isolate the joint capsule from the periarticular muscles (see Fig. 3.16). Joint play assessment therefore is helpful in the isolation and differentiation of articular-based pain and dysfunction from nonarticular soft tissue disorders. It has also been proposed as an evaluative procedure for the clinical assessment of joint instability; it is purportedly valuable in detecting excessive translational movements that result from derangement of the joint's stabilizing structures.[130]

Joint play is assessed by placing the tested joint in its loose-packed position, establishing palpating contacts over the joint, and inducing gentle shallow springing movements (Fig. 3.20). The true loose-packed position may not always be achievable in the acutely injured or pathologic joint, and attempts to force a loose-packed position should be avoided. In such circumstances, attempt to find the loosest possible position. Joint play movements are small in magnitude and vary by spinal region or extremity joint. It is therefore essential that the examiner, through practice, develop an appreciation for the regional and specific qualitative differences.

Joint play procedures include methods where the palpatory contacts are established on one side, both sides, or across the tested joint. Methods that involve contacts on both sides of the joint typically involve the generation of opposing counterstabilizing or springing movements in attempts to specifically isolate a particular plane of increased or restricted glide (Fig. 3.21).

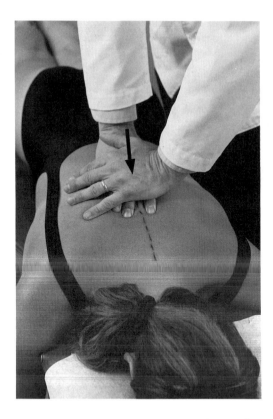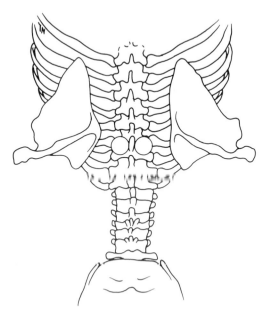

Figure 3.20 Assessment of joint play movement: posterior to anterior glide, midthoracic segment. Circles indicate location of fingers over joints to be assessed.

During the performance of joint play, check for the presence or absence of pain, the quality of movement, and the degree of encountered resistance. Joint play should not induce pain; some resistance to movement should be encountered, but the joint should yield to pressure, producing short-range gliding and distracting movements. Increased resistance to joint play movements suggests articular soft tissue contractures.

The assessment of pain during the application of joint play is often referred to as *joint challenging*. It is commonly applied to isolate joint pain and pathology and determine which segmental tissues placed under tension may be sensitive to mechanical deformation. It often involves methods that attempt to isolate a given joint by applying counterpressures across the joint.

In the spine the counteropposing pressures are commonly applied against the spinous processes. During this procedure, the joint is stressed in different directions from its neutral position and directions of increased pain and decreased pain are noted. Pain during movement is theorized to result from increased tension on injured or inflamed articular tissue. The absence of pain during movement indicates that tissues tractioned (challenged) in the direction of movement are not injured.

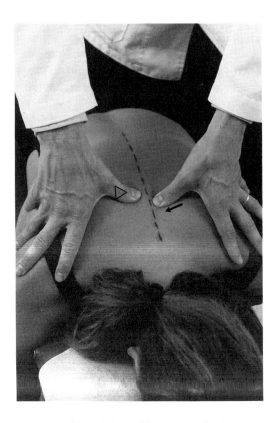
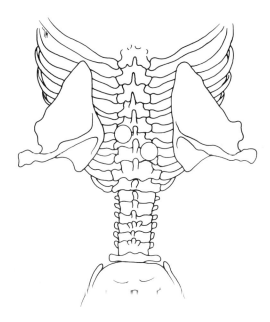

Figure 3.21   Assessment of joint play movement in motion between T4 and T5. Circles indicate placement of thumb contacts on adjacent spinous processes.

Additionally, this procedure has been proposed as a method for determining the alignment of joint subluxations and direction of appropriate adjustment. The assumption is that pain is increased when subluxated vertebrae are pushed in directions that increase the misalignment (into lesion) and that pain is decreased in the direction that reduces the misalignment (out of lesion). For example, pressure exerted against the left side of a right-rotated T4 spinous (body posterior on left) purportedly would increase the misalignment and induce pain (Fig. 3.21). Pressure exerted against the right side of the T4 spinous would decrease the misalignment and not elicit discomfort. This approach has value in the evaluation and treatment of the acutely injured patient when the physician is trying to determine how to induce joint distraction or reduce a traumatic subluxation without causing more tissue damage.

Whether this principle applies equally in all cases of joint subluxation/ dysfunction is questionable. If the rule of pain-free manipulation were applied in the case of post-traumatic joint dysfunction resulting from periarticular soft tissue contractures, would it accurately determine the appropriate direction on adjustment? Manual therapy applied in this scenario would logically be directed to stretch the shortened and contracted tissue.

However, tensile stretch applied to contracted and inelastic tissue commonly induces some discomfort. Applying the rule of pain-free manipulation in this scenario would lead to the application of an adjustment in the direction opposite the restriction. In this circumstance, the adjustment should be applied in the direction of encountered joint restrictions even if it is associated with some tenderness. Without attention to patient history and directions of encountered abnormal resistance, proper adjustive care may be missed.

From this discussion, the following generalizations about adjustive treatment for established joint dysfunction can be made:

Adjustments should never be made in directions of marked pain and splinting.

Adjustments may be delivered in directions of increased tenderness if associated with abnormal increased resistance.

Adjustments may be delivered in the nonpainful direction if directed to reduce joint subluxation or induce cavitation and pain relief.

The procedures of segmental motion palpation have focused on the detection of joint pain and mobility, and although restricted joint and accessory joint motion may be indicative of joint dysfunction and sufficient evidence for joint manipulation, one must guard against perceiving it as a diagnostic panacea. Isolation of a painful joint does not determine the cause of the pain or possible disease. Motion palpation cannot be applied in all clinical situations (i.e., acute joint pain or injury), and certain disease states capable of producing joint restrictions may produce pathophysiologic change that contraindicate adjustive therapy. As mentioned previously, segmental motion palpation is also subject to error and therefore should not be applied in isolation. The determination of dysfunction must be made in conjunction with other clinical findings. No one evaluative tool should be the sole source for therapeutic decisions.

Goals, principles, and tips for conduction of motion palpation are outlined in Tables 3.10 to 3.12.

Table 3.10 Goals of Motion Palpation

To assess the following:

Quantity: How much does the joint move?

Quality: How does the joint move through its range of motion?

End feel: At what point is end feel encountered, what is the quality of resistance, and at what point does the motion stop?

Joint play: What is the quality of resistance? Is there too much or too little?

Symptoms: Are there changes in the amount or the location during assessment and motion?

Table 3.11 Principles of Motion Palpation

Joint movement is tested by assessing how two bony joint partners and their soft tissues move in relation to each other.

When evaluating segmental movement test *one* movement, at *one* joint, around *one* axis, in *one* plane, on *one* side of neutral whenever possible.

Develop a pattern, and test each motion segment being evaluated in sequence.

Move through the entire available range of motion; start and end at neutral. The singular assessment of end feel is an exception to this principle.

Motion must be performed slowly and smoothly with the minimal force necessary.

Compare mobility to the contralateral side and adjacent segments.

Radiographic Analysis

Radiographic assessment and determination of joint subluxation has been an integral part of chiropractic evaluation since the early 1900s.[249,258,259] Relative to the assessment of biomechanical relationships, the primary focus has been on the measurement and description (listing) of spinal joint malpositions. To that end, the profession and many of its individual technique innovators have developed specific radiographic measurement techniques (spinography) designed to quantify and classify spinal malpositions and subluxations[22,109,259–264] (Fig. 3.22).

Spinal X-Rays

Proponents of radiographic evaluation for the detection of spinal subluxations, claim that x-rays are the best method for accurately determining the level and direction of vertebral malposition.[258] They contend that chiropractors who do not use radiography to evaluate spinal subluxations are at a disadvantage in determining and delivering the appropriate adjustment

---

Table 3.12 Motion Palpation Tips

Do not let soft tissue movement and tension changes fool you. They are important indicators of the amount of underlying joint movement, but it takes experience to evaluate them.

Concentrate and be alert from the beginning; valuable information is often gained early in the range of motion.

Where possible, contacting both joint partners of the joint being evaluated is an advantage. This can be done by using two fingers of the same hand, one finger of each hand, or one finger palpating both joint partners simultaneously, thereby crossing the joint space.

Your patient has to feel comfortable, relaxed, and safe.

Do not produce too much movement with your palpation hand. It helps focus your palpation forces, but it must also be free to palpate.

Your palpating finger applies minimal pressure; applies enough pressure so as not to lose firm contact with the bony prominence on the moving joint partner; and is an impartial observer.

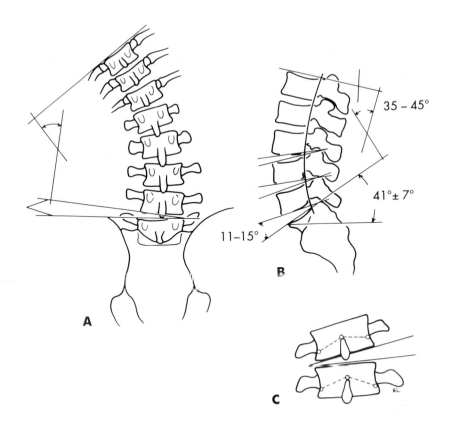

Figure 3.22 Examples of radiographic marking methods for spinal misalignment. (A) lateral curve evaluation, (B) anterior to posterior curve evaluation and measurement of lumbosacral and sacral base angles, and (C) segmental rotation and lateral flexion measurements.

This view has produced a policy requiring chiropractors to demonstrate radiographically the presence of spinal subluxations to receive direct reimbursement for Medicare patients.

Spinal x-rays are routinely taken with the patient in upright weight-bearing positions and may include the selection of full-spine anterior to posterior views.[22,109,258] Full-spine radiographs are used primarily for biomechanical evaluation including the assessment of individual motion segment alignment. Traditionally, the alignment of the upper vertebrae is compared relative to the lower vertebrae, and any malpositions are recorded accordingly. Full-spine evaluations do provide an integrated view of spinal biomechanics and are the method of choice in the evaluation of spinal scoliosis. Full-spine radiographs, however, compromise bony detail and should not be used as a routine procedure for the assessment of suspected local pathology.[265–267] "The clinical justification for the full-spine radiograph must insure that the benefit to the patient is greater than the radiation hazard. The film must be of such quality the presence or absence of pathology can be determined."[266] Furthermore, when indicated, full-spine films should be taken with a posterior to anterior projection to improve visualization of the lumbar intervertebral disc spaces and to minimize exposure to the ovaries and breasts.[259,268]

Though some form of radiographic measurement and assessment of spinal subluxation is used by the majority of the profession, there is considerable controversy as to whether radiographic evaluation should play a significant role in the diagnosis of spinal subluxations.[249,259,260,266,269] Claims of accuracy in detecting minor joint malpositions may not be supportable against the technical limitations of radiography.[249,259,260,266,270–272] Inherent radiographic magnification and distortion, patient positional errors, and the exactness of the marking procedures are common concerns.

Interrater and intrarater reliability have been investigated on only a few of the profession's unique spinographic procedures, and the results are mixed.[165,249,261,270,273–280] Although recent attempts have been made to address issues of spinographic reliability, very little has been done to investigate the validity of radiographic measurement in diagnosing and treating spinal dysfunction.[249,274,275,280] This process is complicated by the lack of a consensus on the definition, pathophysiology, and pathomechanics of spinal subluxations.

Functional X-Rays

The potential limitations of static radiographs in determining joint dysfunction has lead to increased use of functional x-ray studies.[42,281–284] The principle attraction of function x-rays is the ability to assess joint mobility and identify disturbances in function that might not be represented by static films. Functional x-ray studies involve the evaluation of regional and segmental spinal movements by comparing range and pattern of movement at each segmental level. A series of three views are typically taken for each plane of movement evaluated: a neutral view and end range view in each direction. These views are then used to measure and evaluate restricted or aberrant segmental movements. Methods for measuring and classifying segmental motion abnormalities in the lumbar spine, and for measuring and templating cervical flexion and extension, are in common use.[12,281–283,285–289] (Figs. 4-24 and 4-25)

Though the use of dynamic x-rays overcome some concerns about the inability to functionally assess the spine with static x-rays, there remains considerable controversy as to their contribution in predicting back pain or differentiating those individuals with or without back pain.[244,246,247,283,284] Early investigation into the value of functional radiography did identify its merit in the diagnosis of sciatica,[290] although abnormal lumbar motion was also noted in asymptomatic patients. Vernon[284] concluded that there was a higher prevalence of abnormal lateral bending patterns in symptomatic subjects, but Phillips et al. failed to demonstrate a relationship between abnormal spinal motion and patients suffering from low back pain.[243]

Those investigating the relationship between spinal pathology and segmental movement have demonstrated supportive evidence for the application of flexion–extension studies in the detection of spinal instability.[281,285] Additionally, lateral bending radiography has been helpful in identifying the level of disc involvement in those patients with suspected herniation.[224] However, the relationship between motion alterations and the subsequent development of pathology needs to be further investigated before the value of stress x-rays is clearly established.

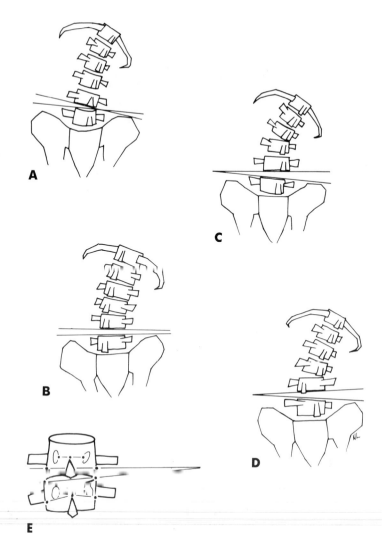

Figure 3.23 Evaluation of functional lateral bending radiographs in the lumbar spine demonstrating movement patterns. **(A)** Type I, lateral bending with contralateral rotation. **(B)** Type II, lateral bending with ipsilateral rotation. **(C)** Type III, contralateral bending with contralateral rotation. **(D)** Type IV, contralateral bending with ipsilateral rotation. **(E)** Segmental measurements for rotation in millimeters and lateral flexion in degrees. (Figs. A–D from Journal of Manipulative and Physiological Therapeutics[307]; Fig. E from Haas et al.,[305] with permission.)

Videofluoroscopy

Videofluoroscopy of the spine is another radiographic procedure that has been proposed as a potential tool for the assessment of segmental spinal motion. It has the capabilities to measure the full arch of motion and therefore provides information on the quality of motion in addition to the range of motion. This technology has made significant advances, and the new techniques of digital videofluoroscopy (DVF) have dropped the exposure rates considerably below those of the conventional x-ray.[291,292] Furthermore, when appropriate equipment and calibration are used, the procedure has demonstrated promising inter- and intraobserver reliability, with measurement accuracy between 1 and 2 degrees.[291–293] Although DVF holds significant promise in the assessment of spinal mechanics, it is presently in the investigational stage, without established clinical protocols for use.

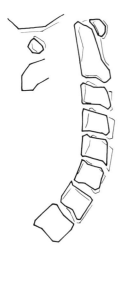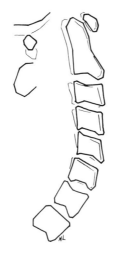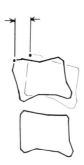

Figure 3.24 Evaluation of flexion and extension radiographs in the cervical spine.

Clinical Utility of X-Ray

The clinical utility of static and functional radiographs might be improved if these procedures were placed in proper clinical perspective and considered to be a component of evaluation and not a pathognomonic indicator of joint dysfunction/subluxation. With further refinement, they may eventually parallel a role provided by specialized imaging techniques in the structural detection of intervertebral disc (IVD) derangement.

For example, the presence of IVD derangement on computed tomography (CT) or magnetic resonance imaging (MRI) indicates the presence of anatomic derangement of the IVD, but it does not confirm that the disc derangement is of clinical significance. The degree that IVD derangement can be present and not be associated with symptoms is unknown. The incidence of radiographically detected disc derangement in asymptomatic patients is significant (24 to 37 percent), suggesting that there is a poor correlation between mechanical disc derangement and morbidity.[294] Within this context, it becomes apparent that the imaging findings must be matched to the clinical presentation and physical findings before a final impression is established.

The role of x-ray, in the evaluation of spinal subluxations, should play a similar role. Radiographic findings alone cannot identify whether a given malposition or joint dysfunction is clinically relevant and worthy of treatment. They must be placed within the context of the physical exam and patient complaints.

The discussion on the use and application of radiography has been directed toward its relationship to the detection of spinal subluxations and joint dysfunction. This is not meant to imply that chiropractors only take x-rays to detect subluxations. They are commonly taken to investigate for fracture, pathology, and biomechanical integrity. A rational for use of plain film imaging in the chiropractic office is, first, to rule out the presence of pathology that contraindicates manipulative therapy; second, to identify any anomalies or structural changes that may influence how an adjustment will be applied; and last, to obtain static and functional biomechanical relationships that may have clinical relevance to the patient's symptoms or health.

Percussion

Percussion plays a secondary role in the assessment of joint dysfunction. The area of greatest application in this regard is probably the spine, where a positive response may help localize a painful motion segment. Spinal percussion may be applied by the pisiform of the doctor's hand or with a reflex hammer (Fig. 3.25). In both circumstances, apply a gentle percussive force sequentially to the spinous processes. A marked or persistent painful response to percussion may indicate underlying fracture or nonmechanical pathology, whereas a mild pain response may indicate local irritation and dysfunction. When the response indicates a potentially serious disease, additional radiographic and/or laboratory procedures are necessary to differentiate a manipulative lesion from a nonmanipulative one.

Muscle Testing

Resisted muscle tests are performed to assess the strength and sensitivity of muscle and its tendinous attachments (Fig. 3.26). Pain with muscle testing may indicate either a muscle injury a joint injury or a combined muscle and joint injury. Pain, with isometric contraction, generally indicates that a muscle injury rather than a capsular injury has been sustained.[14]

Isometric muscle contraction, however, may still produce some degree of joint compression and capsular tension. Therefore, to differentiate a purely muscular injury from a capsular injury, passive joint movement and compression must be performed and compared to the response elicited during isometric muscle contraction.[11,14] A capsular injury will produce pain with passive and active movements as the capsule is elongated. A purely muscular injury produces pain with muscle contraction and muscle elongation, but passive shortening of myofascial tissue should not be painful.

Motor changes are characteristic of many neuromuscular conditions, making tests for muscle length and strength an integral part of the examination process. The testing of muscle structure and function requires a knowledge of joint motion, origin and insertion of muscles, agonistic and antagonistic actions, and the ability to palpate the muscle or its tendinous attachments for tone and texture changes. Muscle testing procedures have been described for isolating specific muscle function to determine length and strength.[295]

Muscle weakness results in a loss of movement, which is due to an inability of the muscle to contract sufficiently, determined through testing for strength and graded on a 5-point system where normal strength (can overcome or maintain position with examiner-applied resistance) is graded 5, and no palpable or perceivable muscle contraction is graded 0. Loss of movement may also be due to muscle shortening or contracture, which is identified through tests for muscle length. Regardless of whether changes

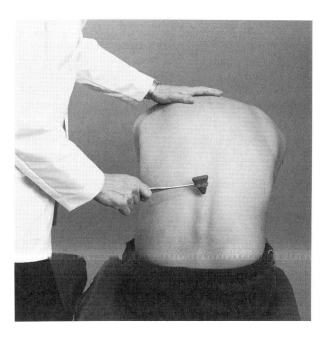

Figure 3.25 Percussion of the spinous processes with hammer.

occur in muscle strength or length, the result will be asymmetric tension across the joint, leading to faulty alignment and dysfunctional movement.

Instrumentation

With considerable same enthusiasm for the use of radiographic marking procedures the chiropractic profession has sought an instrument that would objectively measure and quantify the presence of subluxation dysfunction

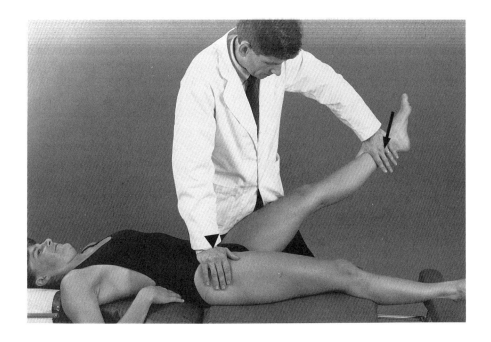

Figure 3.26 Resisted muscle tests evaluate strength as well as sensitivity at the tendinous attachments, e.g., left psoas muscle test.

Of these, surface temperature-detecting instruments are the most commonly used.

Thermography

Local temperature regulation comes from the interaction of the multilevel spinal reflexes with the central autonomic control mechanism. Control of the thermal regulatory system is under the influence of the sympathetic nervous system via vasomotor reflex mechanisms.[296] In a healthy individual, paraspinal temperature radiation is regionally symmetric to within 0.5 to 1 degree centigrade.[297,298] Additionally, the human body is segmented, tracing back to embryologic derivatives. This somatic segmentation is extrapolated from the distribution of the segmented nerves from the spinal cord. It is postulated that spinal subluxation and dysfunction may produce a local inflammatory reaction or reflex alteration in sympathetic tone, which in turn alters this segmental symmetry.

In an attempt to measure temperature asymmetries, numerous devices have been developed using infrared, contact thermistors or thermocouples as a means to determine paraspinal temperature variations. With thermocouples, the temperature differential is usually displayed on a calibrated galvanometer or plotted on a strip graph. Deflection of the needle or the graph will be to the relatively warmer side. Segmental dysfunction, however, may cause a sympathetic vasoconstriction leading to a cooling of the skin in the neurologically related area. Moreover, the sympathetics have suprasegmental and infrasegmental connections and influence so that a temperature change at one level may be due to irritation at another location.[299] Some have suggested that heat-detecting instruments be used to monitor effects of manual treatment rather than as a conclusive method of localizing the area of dysfunction.[300]

Liquid crystal and electronic thermography have been recently developed and introduced as means to identify aberrations in the body wall. Thermography is described as imaging physiologic changes resulting from pathophysiologic stimuli to the sensory or sympathetic nerves, providing complementary information to most other diagnostic tests.[296] Meeker and Gahlinger,[301] in a comprehensive review of the literature, found thermography to be highly sensitive, with high negative predictive value, but less specific and with a lower positive predictive value. Furthermore, it compared favorably to other diagnostic tests (myelography, electromyography, and CT) for accuracy and sensitivity in determining the level of radiculopathy while demonstrating high correlation with these tests, which are more invasive. Thermography gives a picture that depicts physiologic changes, and it has been postulated that abnormalities may provide objective evidence to support painful complaints. However, further research is needed to confirm or refute the theories, indications, and limitations of this unique diagnostic tool.

Galvanic Skin Response

Galvanic skin response (GSR) measures the cutaneous conduction or resistance that fluctuates with the level of perspiration. Sweat gland function is under the influence of cholinergic postganglionic sympathetic fibers, but both central and spinal mechanisms are responsible for control of perspiration. Therefore, neurologic malfunction may result in a change in GSR. An irritative lesion that increases peripheral autonomic activity results in increased skin conductance. The converse also holds that a condition inhibitory to autonomic activity will result in a decrease in skin conductance.[302]

Surface Electromyography

A recent method to assess spinal dysfunction is *paraspinal electromyography scanning*. It has garnered enthusiasm in the profession; however, the use of surface paraspinal electromyography must be questioned. The profession, in attempting to document intersegmental dysfunction, has jumped too quickly onto an unproven technology.[303]

Surface-scanning paraspinal electromyography gives a rough estimation of transient muscle activity. It cannot give information about specific muscles, because the recording electrodes are placed over the skin and not into a muscle. The muscle activity that is recorded by the various paraspinal scanning machines are relative values relating to resting and contractile muscles states. Muscle unit action potentials are amplified by the electromyographic machine. The responses are filtered and rectified by the instrument. These rectified responses are bidirectional waves of depolarization and repolarization along cell membranes. They are integrated over time, and analog signals are converted to digital signals.

The signal recorded by the apparatus is a transient signal. The interpretation of these signals by associated computer software programs is questionable. There are a number of technical problems, including low signal/noise ratios, movement signal artifacts introduced into surface electrodes are not fixed to the skin, and other sources of signal artifacts such as cardiac.

Aside from these hardware problems, we must question the need for an examination that tells the doctor there is some local muscle spasm. Chiropractic doctors have sufficient training and palpation skills to assess contracted muscles, and the cost generated by this technology may not be warranted.

CLINICAL DOCUMENTATION

Practice efficiency is enhanced when manual examination findings are recorded with symbols or on charts. One of the less rewarding aspects of practice is the time spent writing reports. Accurate and legible chart notes make that process more efficient and less painful. A method that is quick and accurate can take the drudgery out of note taking and free the doctor to concentrate on patient care. Figure 3.27 outlines a set of symbols used to record the location of pain and other bony and soft tissue abnormalities. Figure 3.28 contains examples of methods that can be used to record abnormalities in range of motion and joint play and end play. There are many different methods, and each doctor usually makes modifications to fit his or her style. We hope that these examples will be of value in the search and development of a method of charting.

The total management of the patient includes clinical assessment, application of necessary treatment, and patient education. Clinical assessment pro-

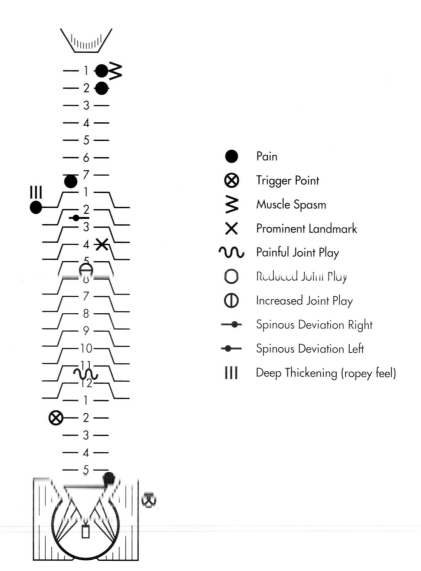

●	Pain
⊗	Trigger Point
≷	Muscle Spasm
✕	Prominent Landmark
∿	Painful Joint Play
O	Reduced Joint Play
◐	Increased Joint Play
—●	Spinous Deviation Right
●—	Spinous Deviation Left
‖‖	Deep Thickening (ropey feel)

Figure 3-22 Examples of symbols and recording method for charting and tracking joint assessment findings.

cedures are performed to identify appropriate case management; that is, frank acceptance and sole responsibility for care; acceptance with consultation from other health care professionals; and frank referral transferring responsibility for immediate care to another health-care professional. Assessment procedures are necessary to identify the nature, extent, and location of the problem as well as to determine the course of action in treatment. Lastly, these same procedures must be used to monitor the effects of care. It is an important process to record adequately the various aspects of this ordeal.

Errors in recording that have been identified include failure to record findings all together, illegible handwriting, obscure abbreviations, improper terminology, and bad grammar. It is imperative that though the clinical

Diagram for Segmental Motion Palpation Findings

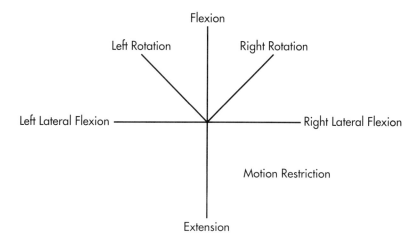

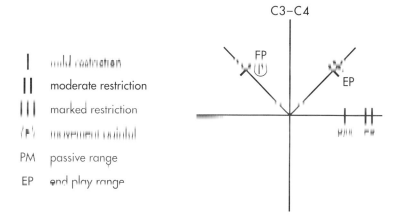

	mild restriction
I	mild restriction
II	moderate restriction
III	marked restriction
(P)	movement painful
PM	passive range
EP	end play range

Figure 3.28 Diagram for recording segmental motion palpation findings.

record comprises the physician's personal notations, it must be complete and translatable. If it is not written down, it was not done.

A systematic and accurate record of evaluation facilitates quick reference to salient findings during treatment. When findings either modify or contra-indicate some aspect of treatment, this should be noted in a conspicuous location on the patient's record so that it is readily seen before each visit.

It should be noted and emphasized that it is unacceptable to use and assign a diagnosis for convenience. Most clinical entities have specific and expected signs and symptoms. These findings need to be identified and recorded. Although it is nearly impossible to have complete certainty as to the nature and extent of the clinical problem, the compilation of clinical findings is necessary to influence the clinical judgment used in applying interventions in patient care. Furthermore, it must be clearly understood that third-party payers reimburse for problems (they provide "disease" insurance not "health" insurance). The reporting of problems to third-party payers must be substantiated in the clinical record.

In 1973, the New Zealand Commission on chiropractic reported:

> Chiropractors are the only health care practitioners who are necessarily equipped by their education to carry out spinal manual therapy.[304]

Chiropractors need to continue to develop skills and knowledge, both in the area of therapeutics and in recognition of patients at potential risk from manipulation. Furthermore, by recording clinical data in the form of history, examination findings, and treatment progress, information can be written for publication in journals available for intra- and interprofessional scrutiny.

REFERENCES

1. Palmer DD: Textbook of the Science, Art and Philosophy of Chiropractic. Portland Printing House, Portland, OR, 1910

2. Palmer DD, Palmer BJ: The Science of Chiropractic. Its Principles and Adjustments. The Palmer School of Chiropractic, Davenport, IA, 1906

3. Montgomery DP, Nelson JM: Evolution of chiropractic theories of practice and spinal adjustment, 1900–1950. Chiro Hist 5:71, 1985

4. Strasser A: The chiropractic model of health: a personal perspective. Dig Chiro Econ 31(2):12, 1988

5. Strasser A: The dynamics of human structure in the chiropractic model of health. Dig Chiro Econ 32(1):11 1990

6. Jamison JR. Chiropractic and medical models of health care—a contemporary perspective. J Manipulative Physiol Ther 8(1):17, 1985

7. Sandoz R: A perspective for the chiropractic profession. J Can Chiro Assoc 21(3):107, 1977

8. Quigley WH: Chiropractic's monocausal theory of disease. J Am Chiro Assoc 8(6):52, 1981

9. Indexed Synopsis of ACA Policies on Public Health and Related Matters 1989–1990. American Chiropractic Association, Des Moines, IA

10. Haldeman S: Spinal manipulative therapy. A status report. Clin Orthop 179:62, 1983

11. Stonebrink RD: Evaluation and Manipulative Management of Common Musculo-Skeletal Disorders. Western States Chiropractic College, Portland, OR, 1990

12. Grieve GP: Aetiology in general terms. p. 175. Pathological changes—general. p. 197. Manipulation in general terms. pp. 524–532. In: Common Vertebral Joint Problems. Churchill Livingstone, Edinburgh, 1988

13. Kirkaldy-Willis WH: Pathology and pathogenesis (Ch. 5); and The three phases of the spectrum of degenerative disease (Ch. 8). Cassidy JD, Kirkaldy-Willis WH: Manipulation (Ch. 16). In: Kirkaldy-Willis WH (ed): Managing Low Back Pain. 3rd Ed. Churchill Livingstone, New York, 1992

14. Cyriax J: Textbook of Orthopedic Medicine. Vol I. Diagnosis of Soft Tissue Lesions. 8th Ed. Bailliere Tindall, London, 1982

15. Sandoz R: Some critical reflections on subluxations and adjustments. Ann Swiss Chiro Assoc 9:7, 1989

16. Sandoz R: The natural history of a spinal degenerative lesion. Ann Swiss Chiro Assoc 9:149, 1989

17. Palmer BJ: Fight to climb. Palmer School of Chiropractic, Davenport, IA, 1950

18. Palmer BJ: The Subluxation Specific—The Adjustment Specific. An Exposition of the Cause of All Disease. Palmer School of Chiropractic, Davenport, IA, 1934

19. Stephenson RW: Chiropractic Textbook. Palmer School of Chiropractic, Davenport, IA, 1948

20. Sandoz R: Classification of luxations, subluxations and fixations of the cervical spine. Ann Swiss Chiro Assoc 6:219, 1976

21. Vear HJ: An Introduction to the Science of Chiropractic. Western States Chiropractic College, Portland, OR, 1981

22. Hildebrandt RW: The scope of chiropractic as a clinical science and art: an introductory review of concepts. J Manipulative Physiol Ther 1(1):7, 1978

23. Janse J: History of the development of chiropractic concepts; chiropractic terminology. p. 25. In: The Research Status of Spinal Manipulative Therapy. NINCDS monograph no. 15. DHEW publication no. 76-988. U.S. Government Printing Office, Washington, DC, 1975

24. Lantz CA: The vertebral subluxation complex. ICA Rev 45(5):37, 1989

25. Leach RA: The Chiropractic Theories. A Synopsis of Scientific Research. 2nd Ed. Williams & Wilkins, Baltimore, 1986

26. Palmer DD: Textbook of the Science, Art and Philosophy of Chiropractic. pp. 7, 39. Portland Printing House, Portland, OR, 1910

27. Palmer BJ: Our Masterpiece. Palmer College of Chiropractic, Davenport, IA, 1966

28. Haldeman S, Hammerich K: The evolution of neurology and the concept of chiropractic. J Am Chiro Assoc 7:57, 1973

29. Homewood AE: The Neurodynamics of the Vertebral Subluxation. Valkyrie Press, St. Petersburg, FL, 1979

30. Dishman R: Review of the literature supporting a scientific basis for chiropractic subluxation complex. J Manipulative Physiol Ther 8(3):163, 1985

31. ICA Policy Handbook and Code of Ethics. International Chiropractors Assoc, Arlington, VA, 1990.

32. Gillet H: Vertebral fixations, an introduction to movement palpation. Ann Swiss Chiro Assoc 1:30, 1960

33. Gillet H: The anatomy and physiology of spinal fixations. J Nat Chiro Assoc Dec:22, 1963

34. Gillet H, Liekens M: A further study of spinal fixations. Ann Swiss Chiro Assoc 4:41,1969

35. Gillet H: Spinal and related fixations. Dig Chiro Econ 14(3):22, 1973

36. Gillet H, Liekens M: Belgian Chiropractic Research Notes. Motion Palpation Institute, Huntington Beach, CA, 1984

37. Gillet H: The history of motion palpation. Eur J Chiro 31:196, 1983

38. Illi FH: The Vertebral Column, Life-Life of the Body. National College of Chiropractic, Chicago, 1951.

39. Mennell J McM: Back Pain Diagnosis and Treatment Using Manipulative Techniques. Little, Brown, Boston, 1960

40. Mennell J McM: Joint Pain Diagnosis and Treatment Using Manipulative Techniques. Little, Brown, Boston, 1964

41. Sandoz R: Some physical mechanisms and affects of spinal adjustments. Ann Swiss Chiro Assoc 6:91, 1976

42. Sandoz R: Newer trends in the pathogenesis of spinal disorders. Ann Swiss Chiro Assoc 5:93, 1971

43. Faye LJ: Motion Palpation of the Spine: From MPI Notes and Review of Literature. Motion Palpation Institute, Huntington Beach, CA, 1981

44. Schafer RC, Faye LJ: Motion Palpation and Chiropractic Technique: Principles of Dynamic Chiropractic. Motion Palpation Institute, Huntington Beach, CA, 1989

45. Dishman RW: Static and dynamic components of the chiropractic subluxation complex: a literature review. J Manipulative Physiol Ther 11(2):98, 1988

46. Triano JJ: The subluxation complex: outcome measure of chiropractic diagnosis and treatment. J Chiro Tech 2(3):114, 1990

47. Gitelman R: The treatment of pain by spinal manipulation. p. 277. In: The Research Status of Spinal Manipulative Therapy. NINCDS monograph no. 15. DHEW publication no. 76-988. U.S. Government Printing Office, Washington, DC, 1975

48. Howe JW: Preliminary observations from cineroentgenological studies of the spinal column. J Am Chiro Assoc 4;565, 1970

49. Brantingham JW: A survey of literature regarding the behavior, pathology, etiology, and nomenclature of the chiropractic lesion. J Am Chiro Assoc 19(8):65, 1985

50. Faye LJ: Most people who erect theories come to believe them themselves. Dynamic Chiro Oct:4, 1984

51. Hubka MJ: Another critical look at the subluxation hypothesis. J Chiro Tech 2(1):27, 1990

52. Lantz CA: Immobilization degeneration and the fixation hypothesis of chiropractic subluxation. Chiro Research J 1(1):21, 1988

53. Rahlmann JF: Mechanisms of intervertebral joint fixation: a literature review. J Manipulative Physiol Ther 10(4):177, 1987

54. Lewit K: Manipulative Therapy in Rehabilitation of the Locomotor System. Butterworths, Boston, 1985

55. Maigne R: Orthopedic Medicine, A New Approach to Vertebral Manipulations. Charles C. Thomas, Springfield, IL, 1972

56. Kellet J: Acute soft tissue injuries—a review of the literature. Med Sci Sports Exerc 18(5):489, 1986

57. Oakes BW: Acute soft tissue injuries: nature and management. Austr Family Physician, (suppl.) 10:3, 1982

58. Cyriax J: Treatment of pain by manipulation. p. 271. In: The Research Status of Spinal Manipulative Therapy. NINCDS monograph no. 15, DHEW publication no. 76-988. U.S. Government Printing Office, Washington, DC, 1975

59. Stonebrink RD: Physiotherapy Guidelines for the Chiropractic Profession. J Am Chiro Assoc 9:65, 1975

60. Akeson W, Amiel D, Woo S: Immobility effects on synovial joints. The pathomechanics of joint contracture. Biorheology 17:95, 1980

61. Akeson WH, Amiel D, Mechanic GL et al: Collagen crosslinking alterations in joint contractures: changes in reducible crosslinks in periarticular connective tissue collagen after nine weeks of immobilization. Connect Tissue Res 5:15, 1977

62. Woo S L-Y, Matthews JV, Akeson WH: Connective tissue response to immobility. Correlative study of biomechanical and biochemical measurements of normal and immobilized rabbit knees. Arthritis Rheum 18(3):257, 1975

63. Akeson WH: An experimental study of joint stiffness. J Bone Joint Surg [Am] 43(7):1022, 1961

64. Noyes FR, Torvik PJ, Hyde WB et al: Biomechanics of ligament failure. J Bone Joint Surg [Am] 56(7):1406, 1974

65. Enneking WF, Horowitz M: The intra-articular effects of immobilization of the human knee. J Bone Joint Surg [Am] 54(5):973, 1972

66. Binkley JM, Peat M: The effects of immobilization on the ultrastructure and mechanical properties of the medial collateral ligament of rats. Clin Orthop 203:301, 1986

67. Amiel D, Woo S L-Y, Harwood F: The effect of immobilization on collagen turnover in connective tissue: a biomechanical–biomechanical correlation. Acta Orthop Scand 53:325, 1982

68. Akeson WH, Amiel D, Mechanic GL et al: Collagen cross-linking alterations in joint contractures: changes in the reducible cross-links in periarticular connective tissue collagen after nine weeks of immobilization. Connect Tissue Res 5:15, 1977

69. Baker W De C: Changes in the cartilage of the posterior intervertebral joints after anterior fusion. J Bone Joint Surg [Br] 51(4):736, 1969

70. Donatelli R: Effects of immobilization on the extensibility of periarticular connective tissue. J Orthop Sports Phys Ther 3(2):67, 1981

71. Videman T: Experimental models of osteoarthritis: the role of immobilization. Clin Biomech 2:223, 1987

72. Mabit C, Bellaubre JM, Charissoux JI et al: Study of the experimental biomechanics of tendon repair with immediate active mobilization. Surg Radiol Anat 8(1):29, 1986

73. Cornwall MW, Leveau B: The effect of physical activity on ligamentous strength: an overview. J Orthop Sports Phys Ther 5(5):275, 1984

74. Fitz-Ritson D: Chiropractic Management and Rehabilitation of Cervical Trauma. J Manipulative Physiol Ther 13(1):17, 1990

75. Waddell G: A new clinical model for the treatment of low-back pain. Spine 12(7):632, 1987

76. Mealy K, Brennan H, Fenelon GC et al: Early mobilization of acute whiplash injuries. Br Med J 292:656, 1986

77. Deyo RA: How many days of bed rest for acute low back pain. N Engl J Med 315:1064, 1986

78. Triano JJ, Schultz A: Biomechanical Considerations for Spinal Disorders. The Source Medicine Approach. Lea & Febiger, Philadelphia, 1988

79. Salter RB: The biologic concept of continuous passive motion of synovial joints. The first 18 years of basic research and its clinical application. Clin Orthop 242:12, 1989

80. Salter RB: Motion vs. rest: Why immobilize joints? J Bone Joint Surg [Br] 64:251, 1982

81. Van Royen BJ, O'Driscoll SW, Wouter JAD: Comparison of the effects of immobilization and continuous passive motion on surgical wound healing in the rabbit. Plast Reconstr Surg 78:360, 1986

82. Evans E, Eggers GWN, Buttler JK et al: Experimental immobilization and remobilization of rat knee joints. J Bone Joint Surg [Am] 42(5):737, 1960

83. Allen ME: Arthritis and adaptive walking and running. Rheum Dis Clin North Am 16(4):887, 1990

84. Frank C, Akeson WH, Woo S L-Y et al: Physiology and therapeutic value of passive joint motion. Clin Orthop 185:113, 1984

85. Korcok M: Motion, not immobility, advocated for healing synovial joints. JAMA 246:2005, 1981

86. Palmoski M, Colyer R, Brandt K: Joint motion in the absence of normal loading does not maintain normal articular cartilage. Arthritis Rheum 23(3):325, 1980

87. Troyer H: The effect of short-term immobilization on the rabbit knee joint cartilage. Clin Orthop 249, 1975

88. McDonough AL: Effects of immobilization and exercise on articular cartilage—a review of literature. J Orthop Sports Phys Ther 3:2, 1981

89. Trias A: Effect of persistent pressure on the articular cartilage. J Bone Joint Surg [Br] 43(2):376, 1961

90. Salter R: Textbook of Disorders and Injuries of the Musculoskeletal System. 2nd Ed. William & Wilkins, Baltimore, MD, 1983

91. Tillmann K: Pathological aspects of osteoarthritis related to surgery. Inflammation, 8 suppl.: 557, 1984

92. Howell D: Pathogenesis of Osteoarthritis. Am J Med 80, suppl 4B:24, 1986

93. Hochberg MC: Osteoarthritis: pathophysiology, clinical features, management. Hosp Pract Dec:41, 1984

94. Murray RO, Duncan C: Athletic activity in adolescence as an etiological factor in degenerative hip disease. J Bone Joint Surg [Br] 53(3):407, 1971

95. Maigne R: Orthopedic Medicine. A New Approach to Vertebral Manipulations. Charles C. Thomas, Springfield, IL, 1972

96. Korr IM: Proprioceptors and somatic dysfunction. JAOA 74:638, 1975

97. Kirkaldy-Willis WH (ed): Managing Low Back Pain. 3rd Ed. Churchill Livingstone, New York, 1992

98. Gatterman MI: Chiropractic Management of Spine Related Disorders. Williams & Wilkins, Baltimore, MD, 1990

99. Good AB: Spinal joint blocking. J Manipulative Physiol Ther 8(1):1, 1985

100. Melzack R, Wall PD: Pain mechanisms: a new theory. Science 150:971, 1965

101. Simons D: Myofascial pain syndromes due to trigger points. I. Principles, diagnosis and perpetuating factors. Manipulative Med 1:67, 1985

102. Travell J, Simons D: Myofascial pain and dysfunction. The trigger point manual. Williams & Wilkins, Baltimore, MD, 1983

103. Maigne R: Orthopedic Medicine. Charles C. Thomas, Springfield, IL 1972

104. Cyriax J: Treatment of pain by manipulation. p. 271. In: The Research Status of Spinal Manipulative Therapy. NINCDS monograph no. 15 DHEW publication no. 76-988. U.S. Government Printing Office, Washington, DC, 1975

105. de Seze S: Les accidents de la deterioration structurale du disque. Semin Hop Paris 1:2267, 1955

106. de Seze S: Les attitudes antalgique dans la sciatique discoradiculaire commune. Semin Hop Paris 1:2291, 1955

107. Cyriax JH: Lumbago, mechanism of dural pain. Lancet 1:427, 1945

108. Cassidy JD, Kirkaldy-Willis WH: Manipulation (Ch. 16). In: Kirkaldy-Willis WH (ed): Managing Low Back Pain. 3rd Ed. Churchill Livingstone, New York, 1992

109. Herbst R: Gonstead Chiropractic Science and Art. The Chiropractic Methodology of Clarence S. Gonstead, D.C. SCI-CHI Publications, Mt. Horeb, WI, 1980

110. Barge FH: Torticollis. Bawden Bros., Davenport, IA, 1979

111. Schmorl G, Junghans H: The Human Spine in Health and Disease. 2nd Ed. Grune & Stratton, New York, 1971

112. Maigne R: Orthopedic Medicine. A New Approach to Vertebral Manipulations. Charles C Thomas, Springfield, IL, 1972

113. Giles LGF: Anatomical Basis of Low Back Pain. Williams & Wilkins, Baltimore, MD, 1989

114. Giles LGF, Taylor JR: Intra-articular synovial protrusions in the lower lumbar apophyseal joints. Bull Hosp Joint Dis Orthop Inst 42:248, 1982

115. Giles LGF, Taylor JR, Cockson A: Human zygapophyseal joint synovial folds. Acta Anat 126:110, 1986

116. Giles LGF, Taylor JR: Innervation of lumbar zygapophyseal joint synovial folds. Acta Orthop Scand 58:43, 1987

117. Giles LGF: Lumbar apophyseal joint arthrography. J Manipulative Physiol Ther 7(1):21, 1984

118. Giles LGF: Lumbo-sacral and cervical zygapophyseal joint inclusions. Manipulative Med 2:89, 1986

119. Kos J, Wolf J: Les menisques intervertebraux et leur role possible dans les blocages vertebraux. Ann Med Phys 15:203, 1972

120. Kos J, Wolf J: Translation of reference 119 into English. J Orthop Sports Phys Ther 1:8, 1972

121. Lewit K: Manipulative Therapy in Rehabilitation of the Locomotor System. Butterworths, Boston, 1985

122. Bogduk N, Engel R: The menisci of the lumbar zygapophyseal joints. A review of their anatomy and clinical significance. Spine 9(5):454, 1984

123. Bogduk N, Jull G: The theoretical pathology of acute locked back: a basis for manipulation. Manipulative Med 1:78, 1985

124. Engel RM, Bogduk N: The menisci of the lumbar zygapophyseal joints. J Anat 135:795, 1982

125. Badgley CE: The articular facets in relation to low back pain and sciatic radiation. J Bone Joint Surg 23:481, 1941

126. Hadley LA: Anatmico-Roentgenographic Studies of the Spine, 5th Ed. Charles C. Thomas, Springfield, IL, 1964

127. Kraft GL, Levinthal DH: Facet synovial impingement. Surg Gynecol Obstet 93:439, 1951

128. Saboe L: Possible clinical significance of intra-articular synovial protrusions: a review of the literature. Manipulative 3:148, 1988

129. Jones T, James JE, Adams JN et al: Lumbar zygapophyseal joint meniscoids: evidence of their role in chronic intersegmental hypomobility. J Manipulative Physiol Ther 12(5):374, 1989

130. Muhlemann D: Hypermobility as a common cause for chronic back pain. Ann Swiss Chiro Assoc (accepted)

131. Kirkaldy-Willis WH: Pathology and prognosis of low back pain (Ch 5), and The three phases of the spectrum of degenerative disease (Ch 8). In: Managing Low Back Pain. 3rd Ed. Churchill Livingstone, New York, 1992

132. Kirkaldy-Willis WH, Wedge III, Yong-Hing MD et al: Pathology and pathogenesis of lumbar spondylosis and stenosis. Spine 3(4):319, 1978

133. Fields HL: Pain. McGraw-Hill, San Francisco, 1987

134. Janda V: Muscles, central nervous motor regulation and back problems. In: Koor IM (ed): The Neurobiologic Mechanisms in Manipulative Therapy. Plenum Press, New York, 1978

135. Ritchie AC: Boyd's Textbook of Pathology. 9th Ed. Vol. 2. Lea & Febiger, Philadelphia, 1990

136. Kirkaldy-Willis WH: Pathology and pathogenesis of low back pain. pp. 55–60. In: Kirkaldy-Willis WH (ed): Managing low back pain. 2nd Ed. Churchill Livingstone, New York, 1988

137. Crelin ES: A scientific test of the chiropractic theory. Am Sci 61:574, 1973

138. Sharpless SK: Susceptibility of spinal roots to compression block. p. 155. In: The Research Status of Spinal Manipulative Therapy. NINCDS monograph no. 15. DHEW publication no. 76-988. U.S. Government Printing Office, Washington, DC, 1975

139. Rydevik B, Brown M, Lundborg G: Pathoanatomy and pathophysiology of nerve root compression. Spine 9(1):7, 1984

140. Mooney V: Where is the pain coming from? Spine 12(8):754, 1987

141. Drum DC: The vertebral motor unit and intervertebral foramen. p. 63. In: The Research Status of Spinal Manipulative Therapy. NINCDS monograph no. 15.

DHEW publication no. 76-988. U.S. Government Printing Office, Washington, DC, 1975

142. Young S, Sharpless SK: Mechanisms protecting nerve against compression block. In: Suh CH (ed): Proceedings of the 9th Annual Biomechanics Conference on the Spine, International Chiropractors Association. Boulder, CO, 1978

143. Gillette RG: A speculative argument for the coactivation of diverse somatic receptor populations by forceful chiropractic adjustments. Manipulative Med 3:1, 1987

144. Coote JH: Somatic sources of afferent input as factors in aberrant autonomic, sensory and motor function. p. 91. In: Korr IM (ed): The Neurobiologic Mechanisms in Manipulative Therapy. Plenum, New York, 1978

145. Kiyomi K: Autonomic system reactions caused by excitation of somatic afferents: study of cutaneo-intestinal reflex. p. 219. In: Korr IM: The Neurobiologic Mechanisms in Manipulative Therapy. Plenum, New York, 1978

146. Sato A: The somatosympathetic reflexes: their physiological and clinical significance. p. 163. In: The Research Status of Spinal Manipulative Therapy. NINCDS monograph no. 15., DHEW publication no. 76-988. U.S. Government Printing Office, Washington DC, 1975

147. Appenzeller O: Somatoautonomic reflexology—normal and abnormal. p. 179. In: Korr IM (ed): The Neurobiologic Mechanisms in Manipulative Therapy. Plenum, New York, 1978

148. Sato A, Swenson R: Sympathetic nervous system response to mechanical stress of the spinal column in rats. J Manipulative Physiol Ther 7(3):141, 1984

149. Russell R: Diagnostic palpation of the spine: a review of procedures and assessment of their reliability. J Manipulative Physiol Ther 6(4):181, 1983

150. Cassidy DJ, Potter GE: Motion examination of the lumbar spine. J Manipulative Physiol Ther 2:151, 1979

151. Faucret B, Mao W, Nakagoua T et al: Determination of body subluxations by clinical, neurological and chiropractic procedures. J Manipulative Physiol Ther 3:165, 1980

152. Sandoz R: The choice of appropriate clinical criteria for assessing the progress of a chiropractic case. Ann Swiss Chiro Assoc 8:53, 1985

153. Bourdillon JF, Day EA: Spinal Manipulation. 4th Ed. William Heinemann Medical Books, London, 1987

154. Bergmann TF: The chiropractic spinal examination. In: Ferezy JS (ed): The Chiropractic Neurological Examination. Aspen, Gaithersburg, MD, 1992

155. Shekelle PG, Adams AH: The Appropriateness of Spinal Manipulation for Low-Back Pain: Project Overview and Literature Review. Rand Corp, Santa Monica, CA, 1991

156. American Chiropractic Association: Comparison of Chiropractic and Medical Treatment of Nonoperative Back and Neck Injuries 1976–77. American Chiropractic Association, Des Moines, IA, 1978

157. Brunarski DJ: Clinical trials of spinal manipulation: a critical appraisal and review of the literature. J Manipulative Physiol Ther 7:243, 1984

158. Nyiendo J: Chiropractic effectiveness, series no. 1. Oregon Chiropractic Physicians Association Legislative Newsletter. April 1991

159. Anderson R, Meeker WC, Wirick BE et al: A meta-analysis of clinical trials of spinal manipulation. J Manipulative Physiol Ther 15(3):181, 1992

160. Waagen GN, Haldeman S, Cook G: Short term trial of chiropractic adjustments for the relief of chronic low back pain. Manipulative Med 2:63, 1986

161. Meade TW, Dyer SD, Brown W: Low back pain of mechanical origin: randomized comparison of chiropractic and hospital outpatient treatment. Br Med J 300:1431, 1990

162. Kane RL, Leymaster C, Olsen D et al: Manipulating the patient: a comparison of the effectiveness of physician and chiropractor care. Lancet 1:1333, 1974

163. Cherkin DC, MacCornack FA: Health care delivery. Patient evaluations of low back pain care from family physicians and chiropractors. West J Med 150(3):351, 1989

164. Cherkin DC, MacCornack FA, Berg AO: The management of low back pain—a comparison of the beliefs and behaviors of family physicians and chiropractors. West J Med 149:475, 1988

165. Haas M: The reliability of reliability. J Manipulative Physiol Ther 14(3):199, 1991

166. Keating J: Several strategies for evaluating the objectivity of measurements in clinical research and practice. J Can Chiro Assoc 32(3):133, 1988

167. Keating J: Inter-examiner reliability of motion palpation of the lumbar spine: a review of quantitative literature. Am J Chiro Med 2(3):107, 1989

168. Keating JC, Bergmann TF, Jacobs GE et al: Interexaminer reliability of eight evaluative dimensions of lumbar segmental abnormality. J Manipulative Physiol Ther 13(8):463, 1990

169. Boline P, Keating J, Brist J et al: Interexaminer reliability of palpatory evaluations of the lumbar spine. Am J Chiro Med 1(1):5, 1988

170. Panzer DM: Lumbar motion palpation: a literature review. p. 171. In: Proceedings of the Sixth Annual Conference on Research and Education. Monterey CA, 1991

171. Johnston W, Allan BR, Hondra JI et al: Interexaminer study of palpation in detecting location of spinal segmental dysfunction. JAOA 82(11):839, 1983

172. Deboer KF, Harmon R, Tuttle C et al: Reliability study of detection of somatic dysfunctions in the cervical spine. J Manipulative Physiol Ther 8(1):9, 1985

173. Zachman Z, Traina AD, Keating JC et al: Interexaminer reliability and concurrent validity of two instruments for the measurement of cervical ranges of motion. J Manipulative Physiol Ther 12(3):205, 1989

174. Keeley J et al: Quantification of lumbar function. Part 5. Reliability of range-of-motion measures in the sagittal plane and an in vivo torso rotation measurement technique. Spine 11(1):31, 1986

175. Comperatein R, Gardner R, Nansel D: Procedure noscibe concordance of two methods of motion palpation with goniometrically-assessed cervical lateral flexion asymmetry. p. 15. In: Proceedings of the 1991 World Chiropractic Congress. Toronto, 1991

176. Tucci S, Hicks J et al: Cervical motion assessment: a new, simple and accurate method. Arch Phys Med Rehabil 67:225, 1985

177. Liebenson C: The reliability of range of motion measurements for lumbar spine flexion: a review. J Chiro Tech 1(3):69, 1989

178. Johnston W, Elkiss ML et al: Passive gross motion testing: part II. A study of interexaminer agreement. JAOA 8(5):304, 1982

179. Fitzgerald GK, Wynveen K et al: Objective assessment with establishment of normal values for lumbar spinal range of motion. Phys Ther 63(11):1776, 1983

180. Boone D, Azen S: Reliability of goniometric measurements. Phys Ther 58(11):1355, 1978

181. Mayer TG, Tencer AF et al: Use of noninvasive techniques for quantification of spinal range-of-motion in normal subjects and chronic low-back dysfunction patients. Spine 9(6):588, 1984

182. Vernon H: An assessment of the intra- and inter-reliability of the posturometer. J Manipulative Physiol Ther 6(2):57, 1983

183. Adams AA: Intra- and inter-examiner reliability of plumb line posture analysis measurements using a three dimensional electrogoniometer. Research Forum 4(3):60, 1988

184. D'Angelo MD, Grieve DW: A description of normal relaxed standing postures. Clin Biomechanics 2:140, 1987

185. Klausen K: The shape of the spine in young males with and without back complaints. Clin Biomech 1:81, 1986

186. Nanzel DD, Peneff AL et al: Interexaminer concordance in detecting joint-play asymmetries in the cervical spines of otherwise asymptomatic subjects. J Manipulative Physiol Ther 12(6):428, 1989

187. Mootz RD, Keating JC, Kontz HP: Intra- and interexaminer reliability of passive motion palpation of the lumbar spine. J Manipulative Physiol Ther 12(6):440, 1989

188. Herzog W, Read LJ, Conway PJ et al: Reliability of motion palpation to detect sacroiliac joint fixations. J Manipulative Physiol Ther 12:86, 1989

189. Love RM, Brodeur RR: Inter- and intraexaminer reliability of motion palpation for the thoracolumbar spine. J Manipulative Physiol Ther 10:1, 1987

190. Carmichael JP: Inter- and intraexaminer reliability of palpation for sacroiliac joint dysfunction. J Manipulative Physiol Ther 10:164, 1987

191. Bergstrom E, Courtis G: An inter- and intra-examiner reliability study of motion palpation of the lumbar spine in lateral flexion in the seated position. Eur J Chiro 34:121, 1986

192. Mior SA, King RS, McGregor M et al: Intra- and interexaminer reliability of motion palpation in the cervical spine. J Can Chiro Assoc 29:195, 1985

193. Wiles MR: Reproducibility and interexaminer correlation of motion palpation findings of the sacroiliac joints. J Can Chiro Assoc 24:59, 1980

194. Leboeuf C, Gardner V, Carter AL et al: Chiropractic examination procedures: a reliability and consistency study. J Aust Chiro Assoc 19(3):101, 1989

195. Johnston W, Hill JL, Sealey JW et al: Palpatory findings in the cervicothoracic region: variations in normotensive and hypertensive subjects. A preliminary report. JAOA 79(5):300, 1980

196. Gonnella C, Paris SV, Kutner M: Reliability in evaluating passive intervertebral motion. Phys Ther 62(4):436, 1982

197. DeBoer KF, Harmon RO, Savoie S et al: Inter- and intra-examiner reliability of leg length differential measurement: a preliminary study. J Manipulative Physiol Ther 6(2):61, 1983

198. Fuhr AW, Osterbauer PJ: Interexaminer reliability of relative leg length evaluation in the prone, extended position. J Chiro Tech 1(1):13, 1989

199. Venn EK, Wakefield KA, Thompson PR: A comparative study of leg length checks. Eur J Chiro 31:68, 1983

200. Shambaugh MS, Sclafani L, Fanselow D: Reliability of the Derifield-Thomas test for leg length inequality, and use of the test to determine cervical adjusting efficacy. J Manipulative Physiol Ther 11(5):396, 1988

201. Rhudy TR, Burk JM: Inter-examiner reliability of functional leg-length assessment. Am J Chiro Med 3(2):63, 1990

202. Haas M: Interexaminer reliability for multiple diagnostic test regimens. J Manipulative Physiol Ther 14(2):95, 1991

203. Brunarski DJ: Chiropractic biomechanical evaluations: validity in myofascial low back pain. J Manipulative Physiol Ther 5(4):155, 1982

204. Falltrick D, Pierson SD: Precise measurement of functional leg length inequality and changes due to cervical spine rotation in pain-free students. J Manipulative Physiol Ther 12(5):364, 1989

205. Jull G, Bogduk N, Marsland A: The accuracy of manual diagnosis for cervical zygapophysial joint pain syndromes. Med J Aust 148:233, 1988

206. Koran LM: The Reliability of Clinical Methods, Data and Judgments. N Engl J Med 293:642, 1975

207. Nelson MA, Allen P, Clamp SE et al: Reliability and reproducibility of clinical findings in low back pain. Spine 4:97, 1979

208. Alley RJ: The clinical value of motion palpation as a diagnostic tool. J Can Chiro Assoc 27:91, 1983

209. Waddell G, Main CJ, Morris EW et al: Normality and reliability in the clinical assessment of backache. Br Med J 284:1519, 1982

210. Shekelle PG: Current status of standards of care. J Chiro Tech 2(3):86, 1990

211. Chassin MR, Kosecoff J, Park RE et al: Does inappropriate use explain geographic variations in the use of health services? A study of three procedures. JAMA 258:2533, 1987

212. Brook RH, Lohr K, Chassin M et al: Geographic variations in the use of services: do they have any clinical significance? Health Aff 3(2):63, 1984

213. Guyatt G, Drummond M, Feeny D: Guidelines for the clinical and economic evaluation of health care technologies. Soc Sci Med 22(4):393, 1986

214. Giles LGF: Anatomical Basis of Low Back Pain. Williams & Wilkins, Baltimore, 1989

215. Lewis T: Pain. McGraw-Hill, New York, 1987

216. Kellgren JH: The anatomical source of back pain. Rheumatol Rehabil 16(3):3, 1977

217. Deyo RA: Measuring the functional status of patients with low back pain. J Chiro Tech 2(3):127, 1990

218. Vernon H: The neck disability index: a study of reliability and validity. J Manipulative Physiol Ther 14(7):409, 1991

219. Love A, LeBoeuf C, Crisp T: Chiropractic chronic low back pain sufferers and self-report assessment methods. Part I. A reliability study of the visual analogue scale, the pain drawing and the McGill Pain Questionnaire. J Manipulative Physiol Ther 12(2):21, 1989

220. Price DD, McGrath P, Rafii A et al: The validation of visual analogue scales as ratio scale measures for chronic and experimental pain. Pain 17:45, 1983

221. Price DD, Harkins SW: The combined use of visual analogue scales and experimental pain in proving standardized assessment of clinical pain. Clin J Pain 1:1, 1987

222. Nyiendo J: A comparison of low back pain profiles of chiropractic teaching clinic patients with patients attending private clinicians. J Manipulative Physiol Ther 13(6):437, 1990

223. Finch L, Melzack R: Objective pain measurement: a case for increased clinical usage. Physiother Can 34(6):1, 1982

224. Wietz EM: The lateral bending sign. Spine 6(4):119, 1981

225. Peters RE: The facet syndrome. J Aust Chiro Assoc 13(3):15, 1983

226. Giles LGF, Taylor JR: Low-back pain associated with leg length inequality. Spine 6(5):510, 1981

227. Enwemeka CS, Bonet IM et al: Postural correction in persons with neck pain. I. A survey of neck positions recommended by physical therapists. JOSPT 8(5):235, 1986

228. Enwemeka CS, Bonet IM, Ingle JA et al: Postural correction in persons with neck pain. II. Integrated electromyography of the upper trapezius in three simulated neck positions. JOSPT 8(5):240, 1986

229. Pope MH, Bevins T, Wilder DG: The relationship between anthropometric, postural, muscular, and mobility characteristics of males ages 18–55. Spine 10(7):644, 1983

230. Burton AK: Variation in lumbar sagittal mobility with low-back trouble. Spine 14(6):584, 1989

231. Triano JJ, Schultz A: Correlation of objective measure of trunk motion and muscle function with low-back disability ratings. Spine 12(6):561, 1987

232. Pearcy M, Portek I, Shepard J: The effect of low-back pain on lumbar spinal movement measured by three-dimensional x-ray analysis. Spine 10(2):150, 1985

233. Fairbank J, Pynsent P, Van Pootvlief JA et al: Influence of anthropometric factors and joint laxity in the incidence of adolescent back pain. Spine 9(5):461, 1984

234. Mellin G: Correlations of spinal mobility with degree of chronic low back pain after correction for age and anthropometric factors. Spine 12(5):464, 1987

235. Giles LGF, Taylor JR: Lumbar spine structural changes associated with leg length inequality. Spine 7(2):159, 1982

236. Giles LGF: Lumbosacral facetal "joint angles" associated with leg length inequality. Rheumatol Rehabil 20(4):233, 1981

237. Sandoz R: Principles underlying the prescription of shoe lifts. Ann Swiss Chiro Assoc 9:49, 1989

238. Papaioannou T, Stokes I, Kenwright J: Scoliosis associated with limb-length inequality. J Bone Joint Surg [Am] 64:59, 1982

239. Illi C, Sandoz R: Spinal equilibrium. Further developments of the concepts of Fred Illi. Ann Swiss Chiro Assoc 8:81, 1985

240. Korr IM, Wright HM, Thomas PE: Effects of experimental myofascial insults on cutaneous patterns of sympathetic activity in man. J Neural Transm 23(22):330, 1962

241. Dieck G, Kelsey J et al: An epidemiologic study of the relationship between postural asymmetry in the teen years and subsequent back and neck pain. Spine 10(10):872, 1985

242. Hansson T, Bigos S, Beecher P et al: The lumbar lordosis in acute and chronic low-back pain. Spine 10(2):154, 1985

243. Phillips R, Howe J, Bustin G et al: Stress x-rays and the low back pain patient. J Manipulative Physiol Ther 13(3):127, 1990

244. Bigos SJ, Battie MC, Spengler DM et al: A prospective study of work perceptions and psychosocial factors affecting the report of back injury. Spine 16(1):1, 1991

245. Battie MC, Bigo SJ, Fischer CD et al: The role of spinal flexibility in back pain complaints within industry. A prospective study. Spine 15(8):768, 1990

246. Haas M, Nyiendo J, Peterson C et al: Lumbar motion trends and correlation with low back pain. Part I. A roentgenological evaluation of coupled lumbar motion in lateral bending. J Manipulative Physiol Ther 15(3):145, 1992

247. Haas M, Nyiendo J: Lumbar motion trends and correlation with low back pain. Part II. A roentgenological evaluation of quantitative segmental motion in lateral bending. J Manipulative Physiol Ther 15(4):224, 1992

248. Nansel D, Peneff A, Cremata E et al: Time course considerations for the effects of unilateral lower cervical adjustments with respect to the amelioration of cervical lateral-flexion passive end-range asymmetry. J Manipulative Physiol Ther 13(6):297, 1990

249. Phillips R, Frymoyer J, MacPherson B et al: Low back pain: a radiographic enigma. J Manipulative Physiol Ther 9(3):183, 1986

250. Daniels L, Worthingham C: Muscle testing techniques of manual examination. 3rd Ed. W.B. Saunders, Philadelphia, 1972

251. Greenman PE: Principles of Manual Medicine. Williams & Wilkins, Baltimore, 1989

252. Guides to the Evaluation of Permanent Impairment. 3rd Ed. American Medical Association, Chicago, 1990

253. ACA Council on Technic: Chiropractic terminology: a report. J Am Chiro Assoc 25(10):46, 1988

254. Grieve GP: Pathological changes—general. pp. 235, 243. In: Common Vertebral Joint Problems. 2nd Ed. Churchill Livingstone, Edinburgh, 1988

255. Janda V: Muscles, central nervous system motor regulation and back problems. In Korr I (ed): The neurobiologic mechanisms in manipulative therapy. London, Plenum, 1978

256. Travell J, Rinzler SH: The myofascial genesis of pain. Postgrad Med 11:425, 1952

257. Haas M, Peterson D: A roentgenological evaluation of the relationship between segmental motion and mal-alignment in lateral bending. J Manipulative Physiol Ther (in press)

258. Hildebrandt R: Chiropractic spinography and postural roentgenology. Part I. History of development. J Manipulative Physiol Ther 3(2):87, 1980

259. Howe J: Some considerations in spinal x-ray interpretations. J Clin Chiro Arch spring:75, 1971

260. Howe JW: Facts and fallacies, myths and misconceptions in spionography. J Clin Chiro Arch winter:34, 1972

261. Plaugher G, Hendricks A: The inter- and intraexaminer reliability of the Gonstead Pelvic Marking System. J Manipulative Physiol Ther 14(9):503, 1991

262. Logan HB: Textbook of Logan Basic Methods. Logan Chiropractic College, St Louis, 1950

263. Gregory RR: Manual for Upper Cervical X-ray Analysis. National Upper Cervical Chiropractic Association, Monroe, MI, 1971

264. Blair WG: Blair clinic of Lubbock, Texas. Dig Chiro Econ 14(1):10, 1971

265. Hildebrant RW: Full spine radiography—a matter of clinical justification. J Chiro 23(8):56, 1986

266. Peterson C, Gatterman MI, Wei T: Chiropractic Radiology. p. 90. In: Gatterman MI. Chiropractic Management Of Spine Related Disorders. Williams & Wilkins, Baltimore, 1990

267. Sellers T: Diagnostic or non-diagnostic. J Am Chiro Assoc 22(8):71, 1988

268. Peterson C: Standards for Diagnostic Imaging. p. 170. In: Vear HJ (ed): Chiropractic standards of practice and quality of care. Aspen, Gaithersburg, MD, 1992

269. Howe JW: The chiropractic concept of subluxation and its roentgenological manifestations. J Clin Chiro 1969 Fall(vii), 1973

270. Sigler DC, Howe JW. Inter- and intraexaminer reliability of the upper cervical x-ray marking system. J Manipulative Physiol Ther 8:75–80, 1985

271. Schram SB, Hosek R, Silverman HL: Spinographic positioning errors in Gonstead pelvic x-ray analysis. J Manipulative Physiol Ther 4(4):179, 1981

272. Schram SB, Hosek RS: Error limitations in x-ray kinematics of the spine. J Manipulative Physiol Ther 5(1):5, 1982

273. Phillips RB: An evaluation of the graphic analysis of the pelvis on the A-P full spine radiograph. J Am Chiro Assoc 9:S139, 1975

274. Grostic JD, DeBoer KF: Roentgenographic measurement of atlas laterality and rotation: a retrospective pre- and postmanipulation study. J Manipulative Physiol Ther 5:63, 1982

275. Anderson RT: A radiographic test of upper cervical chiropractic theory. J Manipulative Physiol Ther 4:129, 1981

276. Jackson BL, Barker W, Bentz J et al: Inter- and intraexaminer reliability of the upper cervical x-ray marking system: a second look. J Manipulative Physiol Ther 10:157, 1987

277. Jackson BL, Barker WF, Gamble AG: Reliability of the upper cervical x-ray marking system: a replication study. Chiropractic Research J 1(1):10, 1988

278. Reinert OC: An analytical survey of structural aberrations observed in static radiographic examinations among acute low back cases. J Manipulative Physiol Ther 11:24, 1988

279. Keating JC, Boline PD: The precision and reliability of an upper cervical marking system: lessons from the literature. Chiropractic 1:43, 1988

280. Plaugher G, Cremata E, Phillips RB: A retrospective consecutive case analysis of pretreatment and comparative static radiological parameters following chiropractic adjustments. J Manipulative Physiol Ther 13(9):498, 1990

281. Sandoz RW: Technique and interpretation of functional radiography of the lumbar spine. Ann Swiss Chiro Assoc 3:66, 1965

282. Cassidy JD: Roentgenological examination of the functional mechanics of the lumbar spine in lateral flexion. J Can Chiro Assoc 20(2):13, 1976

283. Grice A: Radiographic, biomechanical and clinical factors in lumbar lateral flexion. Part I. J Manipulative Physiol Ther 2(1):26, 1979

284. Vernon H: Static and dynamic roentgenography in the diagnosis of degenerative disc disease: a review and comparative assessment. J Manipulative Physiol Ther 5(4):163, 1982

285. Dupuis PR, Yong-Hing K, et al: Radiologic diagnosis of degenerative lumbar spinal instability. Spine 10(3):262, 1985

286. Hviid H: Functional radiography of the cervical spine. Ann Swiss Chiro Assoc 3:37, 1963

287. Prantl K: X-ray examination and functional analysis of the cervical spine. Manual Med 2:5, 1985

288. Penning L: Normal movements of the cervical spine. Am J Reontgenol 130:317, 1978

289. Pennal GF, Conn GS, McDonald G et al: Motion studies of the lumbar spine. J Bone Joint Surg [Br] 54(3):442, 1972

290. Hasner E, Schalimtzek M, Snorrason E: Roentgenological examination of the function of the lumbar spine. Acta Radiol 37:141, 1952

291. Breen A, Allen R, Morris A: An image processing method for spine kinematics—preliminary studies. Clin Biomech 3:5, 1988

292. Humphreys K, Breen A, Saxton D: Incremental lumbar spine motion in the coronal plane; an observer variation study using digital videofluoroscopy. Eur J Chiro 38:56, 1990

293. Antos JC, Robinson GK, Keating JC et al: Interrater reliability of fluoroscopic detection of fixation in the mid cervical spine. J Chiro Tech 2(2):53, 1990

294. Boden SD, Davis DO et al: Abnormal magnetic-resonance scans of the lumbar spine in asymptomatic subjects. J Bone Joint Surg [Am] 72(3):403, 1990

295. Kendall HO, Kendall FP, Wadsworth GE: Muscles Testing and Function. 2nd Ed. Williams & Wilkins, Baltimore, 1971

296. Christiansen J: Thermographic anatomy and physiology. In: Christiansen J, Gerow G (eds): Thermography. Williams & Wilkins, Baltimore, 1990

297. Uemtsu S: Symmetry of skin temperature comparing one side of the body to the other. Thermology 1:4, 1985

298. Silverstein EB, Bahr GJM, Katan B: Thermographically measured normal skin temperature asymmetry in the human male. Cancer 36:1506, 1975

299. Normell LA: Distribution of impaired cutaneous vasomotor and sudomotor function in paraplegic man. Scand J Clin Lab Invest Suppl 33; 138:25, 1974

300. Pierce WV: Results. Chirp, Dravosburg, PA, 1981

301. Meeker WC, Gahlinger PM: Neuromusculoskeletal thermography: a valuable diagnostic tool? J Manipulative Physiol Ther 9:257, 1986

302. Triano JJ: The use of instrumentation and laboratory procedures by the chiropractor. In: Haldeman S (ed): Modern Developments in the Principles and Practice of Chiropractic. Appleton-Century-Crofts, East Norwalk, CT, 1980

303. Meeker W, Matheson D, Wong A: Lack of evidence for a relationship between low back pain and asymmetrical muscle activity using scanning electromyography.

304. Inglis BD, Fraser B, Penfold BR: Chiropractic in New Zealand: report of the Commission of Inquiry. PD Hasselberg, Government Printer, Wellington, NZ, 1979

305. Haas M, Nyiendo J, Peterson C: Interrater reliability of roentgenological evaluation of the lumbar spine in lateral bending. J Manipulative Physiol Ther 13(4):179, 1990

306. Grieve GP: Patterns of somatic nerve root supply. p. 172. In: Common Vertebral Joint Problems. 2nd Ed. Churchill Livingstone, Edinburgh, 1988

307. Journal of Manipulative and Physiological Therapeutics 2:18, 1979

308. Adelaar RS: The practical biomechanics of running. Am J Sports Med 14:497, 1986

309. Mooney V, Robertson J: The facet syndrome. Clin Orthop 115:149, 1976

310. Fairbank JCT, Davies JB, Mbaot JC, Eisenstein S, O'Brien JP: The Oswestry low back pain disability questionnaire. Physiotherapy 66: 1980

4

Principles of Adjustive Technique

David H. Peterson

Chiropractors must maintain the necessary diagnostic skills to support their role as primary contact providers. There is, however, a wide range of choice in the chiropractic physician's scope of practice. Therapeutic alternatives range from manual therapy and spinal adjustments to physiologic therapeutics and exercise, nutritional, and dietary counseling. Additionally, the right to provide minor surgery and obstetric care exists in a few states.[1] Major surgery and the prescription of drugs are the only therapies not allowed in any state. Although there is wide variation in scope of practice from state to state, nearly all chiropractors use a variety of manual therapies with an emphasis on specific adjustive techniques.[1–7]

The preceding chapter discussed the examination procedures used to determine joint dysfunction; this chapter focuses on the knowledge, principles, and psychomotor skills necessary to perform adjustive therapy.

CLASSIFICATION OF MANUAL THERAPIES

Manual therapy includes all procedures during which the hands are used to mobilize, adjust, manipulate, create traction, or massage the somatic or visceral structures of the body.[8] They may be broadly classified into joint manipulative procedures and soft tissue manipulative procedures (Fig. 4.1).

Joint Manipulative Procedures

Joint manipulative procedures (Table 4.1) are physical maneuvers designed to induce joint motion through either nonthrust techniques (mobilization) or thrust techniques. They are intended to treat disorders of the neuromusculoskeletal (NMS) system by improving joint alignment, range of motion, and quality of movement.

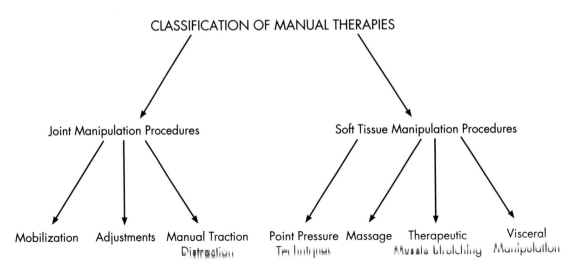

Figure 4.1 Classification of manipulative procedures. (This illustration is not intended to cover all possible manual therapies.)

Table 4.1 Joint Manipulative Procedures

Adjustment

The chiropractic adjustment is a specific form of articular manipulation using either long- or short-leverage techniques with specific contacts. It is characterized by a dynamic thrust of controlled velocity, amplitude, and direction.

1. Direct (short lever): Specific joint contact, high-velocity, low amplitude thrust
2. Semidirect: Combination of a specific joint contact with a long-lever contact; high-velocity low-amplitude thrust
3. Indirect (long lever): Nonspecific contact at points of leverage; high velocity, low-amplitude thrust
4. Characteristics of an adjustment
   a. Specific contact (exception, indirect method)
   b. Dynamic thrust of controlled depth and speed
   c. The thrust is delivered within the boundaries of the joint's anatomic integrity
   d. Usually associated with an audible articular click and subsequent improved joint mobility

Joint Mobilization

A form of manipulation applied within the physiologic range of joint motion and characterized by nonthrust passive joint manipulation.

1. Specific (segmental) mobilization: Manual procedure directed to maximize mobilization force to single joint
2. General (nonsegmental): Manual procedure directed to mobilize multiple spinal segments simultaneously

Manual Traction/Distraction

The manual production of a tractional or pulling force.

1. Cox technique (flexion distraction): Manual procedure designed to induce distraction of the lumbar spinal motion segments
2. McKenzie technique (extension distraction): Manual procedure designed to induce extension distraction of the lumbar spine
3. Leander technique: Manual procedure designed to induce distraction of the lumbar spine with the lordotic curve maintained and aided by motorized flexion and distraction

Muscle Energy (163)

Manual therapy procedure that involves the voluntary contraction of patient muscle in a precisely controlled direction, at varying levels of intensity, against a distinctly executed counterforce applied by the operator.

Joint manipulative procedures are delivered to induce joint movement. This leads to their common application in the treatment of suspected joint hypomobility (subluxation/dysfunction). When treating joint hypomobility, the adjustive thrust or mobilization is typically delivered in the direction of established joint restriction.

In some instances, however, the therapeutic force may be delivered in the relatively nonrestricted and pain-relieving direction. This is most common when acute joint pain and locking limit movement in one direction but still allow distraction of the joint capsule in another direction.[20–22] Under these circumstances, therapy is most commonly directed at inducing perpendicular separation of joint surfaces. The goal is to inhibit pain and muscle guarding and to promote flexible healing.

Adjustments

Adjustments are the most commonly applied chiropractic therapy.[2–4] They are perceived as the foundation of chiropractic practice and the most specialized and significant therapy employed by chiropractors.[2,3,9] Specific reference to adjustive therapy is incorporated in the majority of the state practice acts and is commonly cited as the key distinguishing feature of chiropractic practice.[10]

Unfortunately, the inextricable identification of adjustive therapy with chiropractic has not lead to a common professional definition and classification scheme.[10,11] At issue is whether the adjustment should be defined by therapeutic intention or defined and classified by physical characteristics.

Therapeutic intention

Historically, adjustive therapy has been distinguished on the basis of the doctor's therapeutic intentions and whether the therapy was directed toward reducing joint subluxation.[12,13] Based on this premise, any procedure directed to reduce joint subluxation and restore normal alignment is considered an adjustment. In other words, if you are a chiropractor attempting to adjust a patient, then you are performing an adjustment. Under these confusing circumstances, the goal defines the means, and the term *adjustment* is used interchangeably as a verb and a noun with very little basis for distinction.

The obvious problem with such an approach is the potential for a wide variety of significantly different physical procedures all to be classified as adjustments. The profession needs to objectively evaluate and compare the effectiveness of chiropractic therapeutic procedures. This cannot be accomplished without physical distinction and classification of these procedures. Furthermore, the identification and assessment of adjustive technique procedures would have to rely on an interview with the treating doctor to appraise his or her intentions and sincerity. Conceivably, this could result in a procedure that fits the physical characteristics of an adjustment but is determined not to be an adjustment because it was administered without the right intention.

We strongly feel that the profession must rectify this inconsistency and settle on a common definition that is distinct and void of dogma. Unless this issue is addressed, it will be very difficult for the profession to make further strides in the development of adjustive technique standards.

Adjustments delivered by the unskilled may be poor adjustments, dangerous, and delivered for the wrong reasons, but if they meet specified physical characteristics and are directed at inducing articular movement, they should still be considered adjustments. Separating the physical components of an adjustment from the rationale for its application does not diminish the profession. As stated by Levine,[14] "It is the reason why these techniques are applied and why they are applied in a certain manner, that distinguishes chiropractic from other healing disciplines, manipulative or not."

Chiropractic is a distinct profession not because it applies adjustive therapy but because it possesses unique health-care competencies and perspectives. The elements that make the profession distinct are the emphasis it places on the evaluation and treatment of disorders of the NMS system, the significance it places on the relationship between structure and function of the NMS system and overall health, and the characteristic rationale and skills it employs in the application of adjustive techniques.

Physical attributes

The basis for distinguishing and classifying adjustive procedures should incorporate its measurable characteristics and should not be based solely on therapeutic intention. The central physical feature distinguishing chiropractic adjustments from other manual procedures is the delivery of a precisely gauged *adjustive thrust* of controlled velocity, depth, and direction.[8,15] Although amplitude and velocity of the adjustive thrust may vary, it is a relatively high-velocity, low-amplitude force.

Adjustive contacts are usually established close to the joint being treated, and the thrust is delivered within the limits of anatomic joint integrity. Adjustive therapy is commonly associated with an audible articular "crack," but the presence or absence of joint cracking should not be the test for determining whether or not an adjustment has been performed.

Properly applied adjustments are usually painless though some minimal discomfort may be experienced by the patient who has long-standing dysfunction with some degree of periarticular soft tissue contracture. Adjustive procedures that induce increased pain should be considered only if they are directed at increasing joint mobility. Adjustments should not be forced when pain induces protective guarding and marked resistance.

Classification of adjustive procedures

Some attempt has been made to differentiate chiropractic adjustments by the degree of velocity or force delivered during their application. Unfortunately, the practice of differentiating adjustments as either high force or low force has developed individually, without any common underlying basis or protocol. Furthermore, this method does not confront the central issue of what constitutes an adjustment, nor does it address several other important qualities and potential distinguishing features such as patient positioning, contact points, or leverage.

In an attempt to be more precise in the distinction, classification, and validation of chiropractic procedures, Bartol and the Panel of Advisors to the American Chiropractic Association (ACA) Technic Council have proposed an algorithm for the categorization of chiropractic treatment procedures[11,16] (Appendix 4). Although these models were presented at the Sixth Annual Conference on Research and Education (CORE) and are laudable steps in the development of professional standards and consensus, they have yet to gain any official status or application.[17].

Recently, the application of mechanical devices designed to deliver a high-velocity short amplitude force also has increased. Where these devices fit in a classification scheme for adjustive therapy is unclear. The profession is working to establish criteria for defining and classifying adjustive procedures but has not yet ascertained whether mechanical "adjustments" produce physical forces and effects similar to manual adjustments. These devices are applied to both articular and nonarticular tissues, and their ability to cavitate synovial joints has not been investigated.[18] Until these issues are resolved, we suggest positioning these devices in a category labeled *mechanical thrust devices.*

Specific versus general adjustments

Specific adjustments involve procedures employed to focus the adjustive force as much as possible to one articulation or joint complex, whereas general adjustments are employed where a regional distraction of a group of articulations is desired. Additionally, specific adjustments involve the application of short-lever contacts, while general adjustments involve longer levers or multiple contacts.

The chiropractic profession has emphasized specific short-lever procedures, theorizing that these would be more precise in correcting local subluxation/dysfunction without inducing stress of possible injury to adjacent articulations. This may be especially pertinent in circumstances with adjacent joint instability. However, by applying principles of joint localization, long-lever procedures become more precise, and the assumption that short-lever adjustments are inherently more specific than long-lever adjustments may not always apply.

Chiropractic Technique

Technique refers to a method for accomplishing a desired aim. In chiropractic, the term is generally applied to manual therapeutic procedures directed at treating joint subluxation/dysfunction. Although it is most frequently applied to manual adjustive procedures, it is not unusual to see the term applied to other forms of chiropractic manual and nonmanual therapy.

Many chiropractic diagnostic and therapeutic procedures (techniques) have developed empirically in the profession by an individual or association of individuals. These techniques are commonly then assembled as a system incorporating theoretical models of dysfunction with procedures of assessment and treatment. Appendix 1 is an overview of selected system techniques.

Chiropractic *technique* should not be confused with chiropractic *therapy, or treatment,* which includes the application of all the primary and ancillary procedures appropriate in the management of a given health disorder. These are limited by individual state statutes but may include such procedures as joint mobilization, therapeutic muscle stretching, soft tissue manipulation, sustained and intermittent traction, meridian therapy, physical therapy modalities, application of heat or cold, dietary and nutritional counseling, therapeutic and rehabilitative exercises, and biofeedback and stress management.

Joint Mobilization

Joint mobilization in contrast to adjustive therapy does not employ a thrust component and is usually not associated with joint cavitation.[8,19] Joint mobilization is applied to induce movement through a series of graded movements of controlled depth and rate without a sudden increase in velocity. Furthermore, joint mobilization may involve active participation by the patient. The patient may assist the doctor by actively moving the involved joints during the mobilization procedure, whereas adjustive therapy always involves the application of the therapeutic force by the doctor. The patient, through muscular effort, may help position and prepare a joint for an adjustment, but the thrust itself is applied without patient assistance.

Manual Traction–Distraction

Manual traction–distraction is yet another form of manual therapy directed to mobilize articular tissues. The distinction between joint mobilization and manual traction–distraction is not clear, and the separation may be arbitrary. When the technique is applied to articular tissues, the goal is to develop sustained or intermittent separation of joint surfaces. In the field of manual therapy, traction–distraction is performed through contacts developed by the physician and is often aided by mechanized devices or tables.

Soft Tissue Manipulative Procedures

Soft tissue manipulative procedures (Table 4.2) are physical procedures using the application of force to improve health. This category includes techniques designed to manipulate, massage, or stimulate the soft tissues of the body.[8] "It usually involves lateral stretching, linear stretching, deep pressure, traction and/or separation" of connective tissue.[19] They may be applied to either articular or nonarticular soft tissues. Although joint movement may be produced or improved as a result of the application of soft tissue manipulative procedures, the induction of joint movement is not a necessary physical component of soft tissue procedures. The justification for a separate classification is to draw attention to their principal application in the treatment of soft tissue disorders. They are employed to alleviate pain; to reduce inflammation, congestion, and muscle spasm; and to improve circulation and soft tissue extensibility. In addition to their use as primary therapies, they are frequently used as preparatory procedures for chiropractic adjustments.

INDICATIONS FOR ADJUSTIVE THERAPY

The determination of a manipulative disorder depends largely on the doctor's physical examination skills and ability to diagnose conditions that have a noted positive response to adjustive therapy. The need for precision in evaluating disorders of the NMS system cannot be overstated. Differentiat-

Table 4.2 Soft Tissue Manipulative Procedures

Massage

The systematic therapeutic application of friction, stroking, percussion, and/or kneading to the body.

1. Effleurage
2. Petrissage
3. Friction
4. Pumping
5. Tapotement
6. Vibration

Therapeutic Muscle Stretching

A manual therapy procedure designed to stretch myofascial tissue, using the principles of postisometric muscular relaxation and reciprocal inhibition.

Point Pressure Techniques

Application of sustained or progressively stronger digital pressure. Involves stationary contacts or small vibratory or circulatory movements.

1. Nimmo (receptor tonus technique)
2. Accupressure
3. Shiatsu
4. Reflexology
5. Body wall reflex techniques (Chapman and Bennett)

Visceral Manipulation

Visceral manipulation is a manual method for restoring mobility (movement of the viscera in response to voluntary movement or to movement of the diaphragm in respiration) or motility (inherent motion of the viscera themselves) of an organ, using specific gentle forces.

(Adapted from Bergmann, Peterson, and Lawrence,[12] with permission.)

ing mechanical from nonmechanical conditions, determining the source of the presenting complaint, and understanding the pathomechanics and pathophysiology of the condition being considered for treatment are crucial to successful chiropractic care.

To determine if a given health complaint is manageable with chiropractic care, physicians must first form a clinical impression based on the patient's presentation, physical examination, and appropriate laboratory tests. Once an impression is formed, physicians must decide if their clinical experience and the current standard of care support chiropractic therapy for this condition.

Appropriate treatment decisions are founded on an understanding of the pathophysiology and natural history of the disorder considered for treatment and on an understanding of the physiologic effects of the considered therapy. If it is determined that the patient is suffering from a condition appropriately treated with chiropractic care, and other contraindications have been ruled out, then the presence of such conditions provide sufficient justification for a trial of adjustive therapy. If care is initiated, monitoring procedures must be maintained to assess whether the patient's condition is responding as expected or deteriorating. If treatment does not provide results within the expected period of time, it should be terminated and other avenues of therapy investigated.

Joint Subluxation/Dysfunction

Conditions inducing altered structure and/or function in the somatic structures of the body are the disorders most frequently associated with the application of manual and adjustive therapy. The component of these disorders that is conventionally associated with an indication for adjustive therapy is the identification of joint subluxation/dysfunction.

This is not to imply that chiropractors just treat joint subluxations or dysfunction. Joint dysfunction does not just happen; it results from alterations in function and structure of the NMS system. The causes and pathophysiologic changes that induce these alterations are varied, but those conditions successfully treated with adjustive therapy are assumed to incorporate joint subluxation/dysfunction as a central or complicating feature. If treatment reverses or ameliorates joint dysfunction, then one surmises that the care had a material effect on the underlying functional or structural pathophysiologic alterations.

Although the evaluation for joint subluxation/dysfunction is critical in determining whether to apply adjustive therapy, the identification of subluxation/dysfunction does not conclude the doctor's diagnostic responsibility. The physician must also determine if the dysfunction exists as an independent entity or as a product of other somatic or visceral disease. Joint subluxation/dysfunction may be the product of a given disorder rather than the cause, or it may exist as independent disorder, worthy of treatment, and still not be directly related to the patients chief complaint.

Before adjustive therapy is applied, the doctor must answer these questions and determine if the disorder and associated joint subluxation/dysfunction is negatively affecting the patient's health. If the answer is affirmative, and contraindications have been excluded, the doctor must decide whether adjustive therapy should be applied alone or in conjunction with other therapeutic procedures. If therapeutic procedures are indicated that are outside the doctor's scope of practice, then referral to another chiropractor or other health-care provider must be ensured.

Clinical Findings Supportive of Joint Subluxation/Dysfunction

The evaluation of primary joint subluxation/dysfunction is a formidable task complicated by the limited understanding of its pathomechanics and pathophysiology.[23] In the early stages of primary joint subluxation/dysfunction, functional change or minor structural alteration may be the only measurable events.[24] Evident structural alteration is often not present, or none is measurable with current technology, and a singular gold standard for detecting primary joint subluxation/dysfunction does not currently exist. Therefore, the diagnosis is based primarily on the presenting symptoms and physical findings without direct confirmation by laboratory procedures.[23] The physical findings conventionally associated with the detection of joint subluxation/dysfunction and the outcome measures for determining

Table 4.3 Clinical Features of Joint Dysfunction

1. Local pain: commonly changes with activity
2. Local tissue hypersensitivity
3. Altered alignment
4. Decreased, increased, or aberrant joint movement
5. Altered joint play
6. Altered end-feel resistance
7. Local palpatory muscle rigidity

successful treatment include pain, postural alterations, regional range of motion alterations, intersegmental motion abnormalities, tissue texture changes, muscle tone, hyperesthesia/hypesthesia, and functional capacity measures.[23] Although radiographic evaluation is commonly applied in the evaluation for joint subluxation, it must be incorporated with physical assessment procedures to determine the clinical significance of suspected joint subluxation/dysfunction.

At what point these specific physical measures are considered abnormal or indicative of joint dysfunction is controversial and a matter of ongoing investigation. The profession has speculated about the structural and functional characteristics of the optimum spine, but the degree of, or combination of, abnormal findings that are necessary to identify joint dysfunction has not been confirmed.[25–28] Professional consensus on the issue is further clouded by debates on how rigid a standard should be applied in the assessment of somatic and joint dysfunction and whether the standard should be set relative to optimum health or to the presence or absence of symptoms and disease.

Until a professional standard of care is established, each practitioner must use reasonable and conservative clinical judgment in the management of subluxation/dysfunction. The decision to treat must be weighed against the presence or absence of pain and the degree of noted structural or functional deviation. Minor structural or functional alteration in the absence of a painful presentation may not warrant adjustive therapy. The presentation, physical signs, and outcome measures used to detect and assess subluxation/dysfunction are presented in Tables 4.3 and 4.4.

The evaluation for the presence or absence of joint subluxation or dysfunction should not be the only means for determining the need for adjustive therapy. Patients presenting with acute spinal or extremity pain may be incapable of withstanding the physical examination procedures necessary to establish definitively the nature of the suspected dysfunction, yet they may be suffering from a disorder that would benefit from chiropractic care.

Table 4.4 Outcome Measures for Subluxation/Dysfunction

1. Regional mobility measures
2. Pain reporting instruments
3. Physical capacity questionnaires
4. Physical performance measures

(Modified from Triano,[23] with permission.)

A patient with an acute facet syndrome may present with just such a condition—a disorder that limits the doctor's ability to perform physical examination and joint assessment procedures yet potentially responds to adjustive therapy.[30]

The patient with acute facet syndrome typically presents with marked back pain and limited global movements. Radiographic evaluation is negative for disease and may or may not show segmental malalignment. The diagnostic impression is based on the patient's guarded posture, global movement restrictions, location and quality of palpatory pain, and elimination of other conditions that could account for a similar presentation.[30] The physical findings that often indicate the presence of local joint dysfunction (segmental motion palpation, end feel) are likely to be nonperformable because of pain and guarding.

The decision to implement treatment in such circumstances must then be based on a determination of whether this is a condition that may respond to adjustive therapy. If this is the case, as it may be in the patient with acute facet syndrome, then an evaluation to ensure that manipulation can be delivered without undue discomfort should be performed. This is accomplished by placing the patient in the position of anticipated adjustment and gently provoking the joint. If the patient is resistant or experiences undue discomfort during joint testing, consider other forms of manual or adjunctive care.

Once the patient has progressed to a point where full assessment is possible, a complete examination to determine the nature and extent of the disorder must be performed.

CONTRAINDICATIONS TO ADJUSTIVE THERAPY

As mentioned previously, the clinical corroboration of subluxation/dysfunction is not, in and of itself, an indication for adjustive therapy. Dysfunction may be associated with, or concomitant with, conditions that contraindicate forceful manipulation. Adjustive therapy is contraindicated when the therapy may produce an injury, worsen an associated disorder, or delay appropriate curative or life-saving treatment. Although certain conditions may contraindicate local adjustive therapy, they may not prohibit other forms of manual therapy or adjustments to other areas.[31,32] When manual therapy is not considered to be the sole method of care, it may still be appropriate and valuable in the patient's overall health management and quality of life. For example, although cancer patients are not primarily managed by manual therapy, they may still gain significant pain relief and an improved sense of well-being with appropriate chiropractic manual therapy. "Such palliative care should be rendered concomitantly and in consultation with the physician in charge of treating the malignancy."[31]

Serious injuries resulting from adjustive therapy are relatively uncommon.[33–37] Suitable adjustive therapy is less frequently associated with iatrogenic complications than many other health-care procedures. As a consequence, written consent is not required as a prerequisite to adjustive therapy.[38] The majority of spinal manipulative complications arise from misdiagnosis and improper technique, or are complications arising from cervical manipulation in the patient with vertebral artery insufficiency or in the lumbar spine as a complication of midline disc herniations.[34,35]

This does not release the doctor from the responsibility of informing the patient about the procedures to be performed and of any significant associated negative consequences.[38] The patient must understand the nature of the procedure and give verbal or implied consent before therapy is applied. Any unauthorized diagnostic evaluation or treatment is unacceptable and exposes the doctor to the potential charge of assault and battery.

Although the danger of injury from manipulation is low, it must be remembered that adjustments do carry some risk. In nearly all situations, injury can be avoided by sound diagnostic assessment and awareness of the complications and contraindications to manipulative therapy. Relative and absolute contraindications to adjustive therapy are listed in Table 4.5. A

Table 4.5 Relative and Absolute Contraindications to and Complications from Manipulative Therapy

Category	Condition		Complication
	Absolute Contraindications	Relative Contraindications	
Vascular	Vertebrobasilar insufficiency Aneurysm		Infarction in brain stem Hemorrhage
		Atherosclerosis	Thrombus formation, hemorrhage
		Anticoagulant therapy	Hemorrhage
Articular		Advanced osteoarthritis	Increased instability, neurologic compromise, increased pain
		Inflammatory arthritis (rheumatoid, psoriatic)	Transverse ligament rupture, increased inflammation
		Ankylosing spondylitis	Increased inflammation
		Joint instability, hypermobility	Increased instability, movement beyond physiologic limits
	Disc prolapse with neurologic deficit		Cauda equina syndrome, permanent neurologic loss
Trauma	Fracture		Delayed or improper healing, increased instability
	Dislocation		Increased instability, permanent soft tissue damage
		Severe sprains and strains	Increased instability, inflammation, and pain
Bone weakening disorders	Bone tumors		Pathologic fractures
	Bone infections (tuberculosis)	Osteomyelitis	Pathologic fracture
		Osteoporosis, osteomalacia	Pathologic fracture
Neurologic		Severe sacral nerve root compression	Cauda equina syndrome, permanent neurologic loss
		Vertigo	Stroke, paralysis
		Severe pain, patient intolerance	Unnecessary or increased pain
		Space-occupying lesion	Permanent neurologic loss
Psychological		Malingering	Secondary gain syndrome
		Hysteria	Prolonged treatment
		Hypochondriasis	Dependency on treatment

(Data from Kleynhans.[37])

relative contraindication is one for which caution should be used or technique modification should be made, because the potential for complication is higher. An absolute contraindication precludes manipulation therapy to the affected area.

Cervical Spine

Critics of manipulative therapy in general and chiropractic specifically emphasize the possibility of serious injury from cervical manipulation. It has required only the rare occurrence of manipulative related accidents to malign a therapeutic procedure that in experienced hands gives beneficial results with few side effects.[39]

Although it is difficult to unequivocally postulate a direct causal relationship between manipulative therapy and subsequent neural ischemia, the implication has become a reality. The vertebral arteries are inevitably linked with cervical spine syndromes because of their unusually tortuous course, close relationship to the cervical nerves and vertebrae, and their potential for causing bizarre and dramatic clinical manifestations.[40]

Hypotheses have been put forth to explain how vascular accidents may occur following manipulative procedures, though no procedure has been confirmed as the singular mechanism directly responsible. Brain stem ischemia is the described injury and is thought to occur from trauma to the arterial wall, producing either vasospasm, frank damage to the arterial wall, or both. Certainly, the anatomy of the cervical spine lends itself to developing a close relationship between the vertebral arteries and neighboring structures that have the potential for imparting mechanical compression and trauma.

When trauma occurs to the vertebral artery, the resultant damage or vasospasm produces a change in flow (hemodynamics) from either a decrease in volume or an increase in turbulence. The effects may be transient if the process is of short duration; however, an ischemic infarct may result if the damage is great or the duration long. With a decrease in flow or an increase in turbulence, a cascade mechanism is activated that results in fibrin deposition, leading to thrombus formation. The thrombus may then break away from the artery wall, becoming an embolism and eventually leading to infarct in the brain stem.

Head and neck movements have been associated with these vascular phenomena and therefore provide the link to cervical spine manipulative therapy. Studies on 20 cadavers showed that flow may be reduced more than 90 percent by movements of the head and neck well within the normal range of head motion.[41] The contralateral artery was compromised more often with rotation; however, when rotation was combined with extension, the ipsilateral artery was involved as frequently as the contralateral artery. Lateral flexion and extension movements individually were found to have little effect in altering flow. Rotation was the single most likely movement to cause occlusion. Other studies have corroborated these findings.[42,43]

Postulated sites and mechanisms for extraluminal vertebral artery obstruction associated with head movement include

1. Skeletal muscle and fascial bands at the junction of the first and second vertebral segments

2. Adjacent osteophyte, particularly at C4–5 and C5–6
3. Between the C1–2 transverse processes, where the relatively immobile vertebral arteries may be stretched with rotary movements
4. By the C3 superior articular facet on the ipsilateral side of head rotation

An evaluative procedure intended to identify patients at risk of vascular compromise has been developed and advocated.[44] Specific factors considered to be warning signs (Table 4.6) have also been identified, and their presence should suggest caution in the use of manipulative therapy to the cervical spine.[45] Unfortunately, any of these factors or tests, alone or in combination, do not specifically increase the chance of identifying the patient at risk. It would still be imprudent, however, to ignore significant factors that point to a possible predisposition to this injury.[46]

The intent of the screening procedure—which includes history, blood pressure, heart rate, auscultation, and provocational positional tests (Table 4.7)—is to identify people at risk and therefore decrease the likelihood of manipulative accidents. Despite these precautionary steps, a few people will no doubt still suffer from brain stem injury from iatrogenic stress forcefully applied to the head and neck.

Is it therefore absolutely imperative that the doctor be able to recognize when a vascular accident occurs and take the appropriate steps. Terrett believes that the signs and symptoms of a vertebrobasilar ischemia will usually occur after the first few cervical adjustments, although it is possible

Table 4.6 Warning Signs of Susceptibility to Vascular Insult[a]

Osseous Factors
    Cervical spine spondylosis
    Cervical spine osteophytes
    Abnormal bone structure

Injury
    Whiplash
    History of neck sprain

Vascular Factors
    History of positional vertigo
    Arteriosclerosis
    Transient ischemic attacks
    Hyper- or hypotension
    Cardiovascular disease
    Diabetes
    Medications (e.g., anticoagulants)

Neurologic Factors
    Headaches
    Visual disturbances
    Drop attacks
    Transient weakness in the legs
    Family history of stroke

Females Only
    Immediately postpartum
    Mid-30s, on the pill, especially if a smoker

Table 4.7 Screening Tests for Vertebrobasilar Ischemia

1. Blood pressure
2. Heart rate
3. Auscultation of the carotid arteries
4. At least one of the following provocational positional tests held for 10–40 sec, allowing the patient to express the associated clinical findings of vertigo, dizziness, nystagmus, nausea, vomiting, headaches, tinnitus, sensory disturbances, and/or fainting:
   A. **Maigne's test.** The patient is seated as the examiner brings the patient's head into extension and rotation. The patient's eyes are kept open and observed for the presence of nystagmus as well as the associated clinical findings.
   B. **Hautant's test.** The patient is seated with both arms stretched out forward and the hands supinated. The patient is then asked to close the eyes while the head is passively moved into extension and rotation. In addition to the associated clinical findings, the arms may drop into pronation.
   C. **DeKleyn's test.** The patient lies supine with the head over the end of the table in maximum cervical extension. The examiner holds the patient's head, turning the neck into rotation and observing the eyes for nystagmus or the presence of the associated clinical findings.
   D. **Underberger's test.** The patient stands, eyes closed and arms outstretched forward. The patient is then asked to march in place while bringing the head and neck into extension and rotation. A positive response is swaying or staggering so the examiner needs to stand close to the patient to assist in avoiding an impending fall.
5. The premanipulative position can be held for 5–10 sec on each visit, instructing the patient to express any problems before delivery of the adjustive thrust.

(Adapted from Terrett,[45] with permission.)

for symptoms to begin minutes to days later.[39] Significant signs and symptoms include nausea, vertigo, vomiting, difficulty walking, incoordination of the extremities, numbness, loss of consciousness, visual disturbances, tinnitus, and speech problems. These clinical findings are characteristic of an infarct in the dorsolateral area of the medulla oblongata, which is supplied by the posterior inferior cerebellar artery. The resultant clinical condition is called Wallenburg's syndrome. Most vertebral artery injuries result in complete recovery, or at least, in minimal residual neurologic deficit.

If a patient reports adverse effects following a cervical adjustment, it is important that specific steps be followed. The most important step is *do not administer another cervical adjustment.*[46] The remaining steps are listed in Table 4.8.

Other possible complications from cervical spine manipulation include dislocation of atlas on axis that is due to agenesis of the transverse ligament (common in Down syndrome); rupture of the transverse ligament (common in the inflammatory arthropathies); and agenesis of the odontoid process. These conditions can be identified with lateral cervical stress radiographs.

Thoracic Spine

The main complication from manipulative therapy in the thoracic spine is rib fracture. Sprain to the costovertebral and costotransverse articulations with concomitant strain to the intercostal muscles may also occur.[37] Additionally, transverse process fracture and hematomyelia have been identified in rare instances.[47] These problems are usually due to excessive force in

Table 4.8 Steps Following a Possible Vascular Injury[46]

1. **Do not** administer another cervical adjustment.
2. Do not allow patients to ambulate, keep them comfortable.
3. Note all physical and vital signs (pallor, sweating, vomiting, heart and respiratory rate, blood pressure, body temperature).
4. Check the pupils for size, shape, and equality.
5. Check eye light and accommodation reflexes.
6. Test the lower cranial nerves (facial numbness or paresis, swallowing, gag reflex, slurred speech, palatal elevation).
7. Test cerebellar function (dysmetria of extremities, nystagmus, tremor).
8. Test the strength and tone of the somatic musculature.
9. Test for somatic sensation to pinprick.
10. Test for muscle stretch and pathologic reflexes.

relation to the patient's size and physical condition. They can be avoided by appropriate technique selection and application as well as an adequate evaluation.

Lumbar Spine

The most frequently described complication from spinal manipulative therapy in the lumbar spine is compression of the cauda equina by a midline disc herniation at the level of the third, fourth, or fifth intervertebral disc.[47] The resultant cauda equina syndrome is characterized by paralysis, weakness, pain, reflex change, and bowel and bladder disturbances. Though there is a risk of precipitating a cauda equina compression syndrome through manipulative therapy, the general consensus is that an uncomplicated lumbar disc lesion can be effectively treated conservatively with manipulative therapy.[18] However, bilateral radiculopathies with distal paralysis of the lower limbs, sensory loss in the sacral distribution, and sphincter paralysis should be considered a surgical emergency.[49]

EFFECTS OF ADJUSTIVE THERAPY

Treatment of NMS dysfunction and disease has historically been the major category for which chiropractors are consulted[2,3,5-7] and NMS disorders are those most commonly recognized by insurance companies and government health-care programs as covered conditions.[2,7]

Chiropractic patients have repeatedly expressed satisfaction with the quality and effectiveness of chiropractic care. In comparative studies for the treatment of back pain, patients consistently rate chiropractic care as superior to medical care.[50-52] Furthermore, authors who have reviewed the literature on spinal manipulative therapy have concluded that sufficient evidence exists to support the use of spinal manipulation in the treatment of specific painful NMS conditions.[53-56] This is most notable in the case of low back pain; over 30 controlled clincial trials have consistently shown "spinal manipulation to be as effective or more effective than an array of other comparison treatments."[55] Although the number of low back pain trials is exhaustive, consensus on the issue of the appropriateness of spinal manipulation has been impeded by the criticism that a significant proportion of the research is flawed by methodologic design deficiencies, systematic bias, or statistical unsophistication.[34,54–56]

A recent review of the literature conducted by the RAND Corporation[34] concluded that the majority of the studies on spinal manipulation support manipulative treatment of patients with acute and subacute low back pain with or without minor neurologic findings; with the greatest benefit demonstrated in the early stages of care. The case for the manipulative treatment of chronic low back pain patients was less conclusive (Appendix 4-2). However, two randomized, controlled trials—one by Waagen and co-workers[57] and one by Meade and associates,[48]—specifically evaluated chiropractic manipulation and demonstrated significant benefit for chronic pain patients receiving chiropractic manipulative therapy. Waagen's study compared the effectiveness of chiropractic manipulation to that of a sham manipulation in patients with subacute or chronic low back pain. The group receiving manipulation demonstrated significant improvements in mobility and pain relief compared to those receiving the sham manipulation. Meade's study compared the effects of chiropractic treatment to hospital outpatient treatment on a large population of patients suffering from back pain of any duration. Patient's receiving chiropractic care demonstrated significant improvements relative to the medical care group. Not only was the care more effective initially, but it was also more effective in the long term, especially for patients with chronic or severe low back pain.

Furthermore, the chiropractic profession has demonstrated itself to be more cost-effective in the treatment of back pain. Since 1980, five out of seven studies conducted on workers compensation claimants have demonstrated lower compensation costs, and six out of seven have demonstrated fewer time loss days with chiropractic care than medical care.[55] In those states reporting higher treatment costs, it is suggested that a greater level of complicated or chronic cases exists in the chiropractic population.[55] Nyiendo[59] found a dramatic reduction in time loss for chronic back patients receiving chiropractic treatment rather than medical treatment, and both Meade and co-workers[58] and Greenwood[60] found that a higher proportion of patients initially attending the chiropractor's had chronic back pain. Those treated with chiropractic care had fewer lost workdays, and although the initial costs were higher, in the long run (2 years), costs were lower for those receiving chiropractic care. In fact, Meade projected that if all the patients in the study had received chiropractic care it would have resulted in a "reduction of some 2,900,000 days in sickness absence during the two years (of the study), saving about 13 million (British pounds) in output (medical) and 2.9 million (British pounds) in social security payments."[58]

In addition to their successes with treating musculoskeletal disorders and dysfunction, most chiropractors have also noted positive health effects from adjustive and manual therapy in areas outside the musculoskeletal system (see Ch. 7). From the time of its origins, chiropractors have viewed their healing art as having wide-ranging health benefits.[61] Philosophically, this is symbolized by the chiropractic holistic health-care viewpoint, which stresses the important relationship between the structure and function of the NMS system and its effects on homeostatic regulation and health maintenance.[62]

Unfortunately, clinical research in the area of manual therapy and somatovisceral disease is minimal. The functional visceral conditions that may respond to chiropractic care, under what circumstances, and to what degree have yet to be studied and clearly identified. Whether the removal of mechanical malfunction of the spine may be helpful in treating functional disorders but not organic disease is debated and unanswered.

Under these circumstances, the profession should be cautious in predicting the reliability of, or guaranteeing an oucome for, therapies that have limited clinical research support. At the same time, the profession should not discount the potential positive health effects noted in clinical practice. Patients without any contraindications to manual therapy and a suspected somatovisceral disorder should not be refused treatment, but they should not be solicited with the implied guarantee of a positive result.

The major objective of almost all adjustive therapy is the alleviation of aberrant joint alignment and function. The specific mechanical and physiologic changes induced to effect a reduction in symptoms and an improvement in joint function and health have not been specifically determined. Several hypotheses exist as to the mechanism by which chiropractic therapy effects the underlying NMS causes of joint dysfunction and somatovisceral disorders. They include concepts that may be broadly divided into mechanical, analgesic, circulatory, and neurobiologic categories. The following discussion touches on some of the proposed mechanisms but is by no means comprehensive.

Mechanical Hypothesis

In the mechanical arena, manual therapy is directed toward reversing or minimizing the soft tissue pathology and mechanical dysfunction associated with disorders or injuries of the NMS system. The soft tissue derangements responsible for mechanical dysfunction may be initiated by trauma, repetitive motion injuries, postural decompensation, developmental anomaly, immobilization, reflex changes, psychosocial factors, and/or aging and degenerative disease. These injuries and disorders often result in soft tissue fibrosis, adaptational shortening, loss of flexibility, and altered joint mechanics.[63–68]

The scope of manual therapies available to treat mechanical joint dysfunction is extensive. The selection and application of each should be based on an understanding of the pathophysiology of the disorder being treated and knowledge of the procedures therapeutic effects.

In the early stages of soft tissue injury and repair, manual therapy is directed toward decreasing pain and inflammation, preventing further injury, and promoting flexible healing. Early appropriate manual therapy and mobilization may minimize the formation of extensive fibrosis and the resulting loss of extensibility.[63,65–73] Excessive immobilization can retard and impair the healing process and can promote further atrophy and degeneration in articular soft tissue and cartilage.[67–81] By promoting an early return to activity, the detrimental effects of immobilization may be minimized. Early activation promotes strong flexible repair and remodeling and breaks the pattern of deconditioning and illness behavior, which can be so detrimental to recovery.[82,83] Gentle distractive adjustments, passive joint mobilization, friction massage, and effleurage are commonly applied manual therapies in this stage.

If the initial injury to the connective tissue is minor, repair may proceed quickly without significant structural change or resulting impairment. If the tissue damage is marked, however, the issuing fibrous repair may result in "a scar, visible or hidden, which has matured to fill the injured area, but lacks the resilience, strength, and durability of the original tissue. Such an asymmetric scar, produced either by injury, degeneration, or surgical trauma, may produce severe disturbances of biomechanical performance."[82] Therefore, when injury or degenerative disease results in contracture, stiffness, joint hypomobility, and chronic pain or impairment, therapies shift toward a more vigorous approach and are directed toward the restoration of mobility and function. They include adjustments, mobilization, therapeutic muscle stretching, connective tissue massage, trigger-point therapy, myofascial release techniques, and the like.[84] In this stage, manual therapies are most effective when coupled with activities and exercises that promote soft tissue remodeling and muscle strength. However, applying spinal exercises without first incorporating an assessment and treatment of joint dysfunction may be detrimental. If joint hypomobility persists, active exercise may stimulate movement at the compensatory hypermobile joint, instead of the hypomobile joints. This may lead to the further breakdown and attenuation of the joint stabilizing structures, further complicating joint instability.

Cavitation

The physical mechanism by which adjustments are speculated to have a mechanical effect on joint pain and immobility is by inducing rapid separation of joint surfaces. Typically, this occurs at the end range of passive joint motion when a quick thrust overcomes the remaining joint fluid tension. The quick separation of the joint is theorized to produce a cavity within the joint, the induction of joint cavitation, and an associated "cracking" sound.

Cavitation is the "formation of vapor and gas bubbles within fluid through the local reduction of pressure." It is a well-established physical phenomena; evidence strongly suggests it also occurs during the application of adjustive therapy.[15,85–89] It has long been known that water confined in a container with rigid walls can be stretched, and if stretched sufficiently, cavitation occurs. The pressure inside the liquid drops below the vapor pressure, bubble formation and collapse occur, and a cracking sound is heard.[90] The case for synovial joint cavitation and cracking is supported by experimental evidence conducted on metacarpophalangeal (MP) joints, the cervical spine, and the thoracic spine.[15,85–89] Unsworth et al.[88] suggested that cracking is not due to bubble formation but rather to the rapid collapse of bubbles caused by fluid flow from the higher pressure periphery to the lower pressure joint center. Meal and Scott,[89] however, have more recently shown that the crack produced in the MP joint and in the cervical spine are actually double cracks separated by several hundredths of a second. Bubble formation is a possible source of the first crack. Herzog[87] demonstrated sound recordings during the application of thoracic adjustments that closely approximated those obtained during the cavitation of MP joints.

Besides the cracking itself, cavitation is considered to be associated with several postadjustive phenomena: transitory increase in passive range of motion; temporarily increased joint space; an approximately 20-minute refractory period, when no further joint cracking can be produced; and radiolucency with subsequent joint separation (Fig. 4.2). The postadjustive increase in joint range of movement has been labeled *paraphysiologic movement* by Sandoz because it represents motion induced only after cavitation[15] (see Fig. 3.17).

The postcavitation refractory period and associated phenomena may be explained by microscopic bubbles of carbon dioxide remaining in solution for approximately 20 minutes. During this period, the bubbles will expand with any subsequent joint separation, maintaining the pressure within the joint. The expanded bubble appears as the radiolucency on a radiograph of

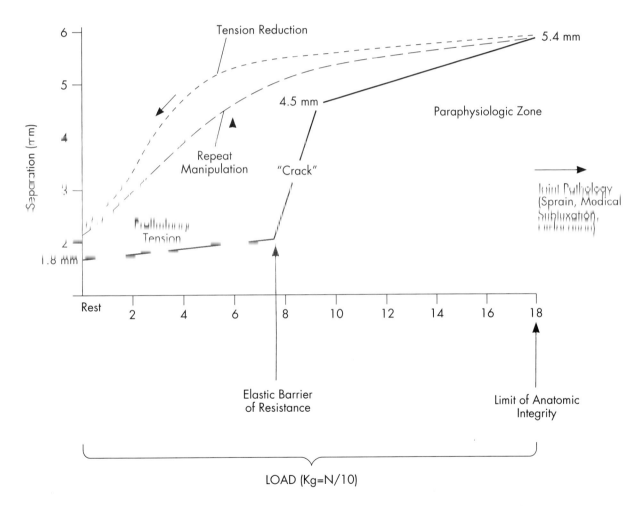

Figure 4.2 Graph representing the effects of joint separation and cavitation: As the joint tension increases with joint surface separation, a quick and dramatic separation occurs and a cracking noise is produced; the resting joint spacing is increased, but further joint separation results in no further cavitation response.

the distracted joint. Because the pressure cannot drop until the gas bubbles are reabsorbed, no further cavitation can occur.[88] Furthermore, the coaptation force contributed by fluid stretching will be absent, causing a decrease in force holding the joint surfaces together, and thus resulting in the increased passive range of motion noted by Sandoz.[15,86] The increased joint space may be explained by the slow viscoelastic flow of excess synovial fluid between the joint surfaces.[88]

Although the presented theory is founded on inferences generated from experiments with MP joints separated in a nonphysiologic direction,[15,85,86,88,89] manipulation of the thoracic and cervical spine did produce very similar sound profiles.[87,89] Therefore, in the absence of contradictory information, it seems reasonable at this time to assume that a similar mechanism is responsible for spinal joint cracking.

The process of cavitation is not assumed to be therapeutic in and of itself, but rather it represents a physical event that signifies joint separation, stretching of periarticular tissue, and stimulation of joint mechanoreceptors and nociceptors. These events, in turn, theoretically alleviate or reduce pain, muscle spasm, joint hypomobility, and articular soft tissue inflexibility.

Joint Fixation (Joint Locking)

Several theories concerning the cause of joint fixation have been advanced. Derangements of the posterior joints, intercapsular adhesions, and intradiscal derangement have been proposed as interarticular sources; segmental muscle spasm, periarticular soft tissue fibrosis, and shortening, as extra-articular sources.

Interarticular block

Entrapment of the interaphophysary meniscus within the posterior spinal joints has been hypothesized as a cause of episodic acute back pain and joint looking.[91–97] The menisci are purportedly drawn into a position between the joint margins by uncoordinated false movements or by sustained occupational or sleeping postures (Fig. 4.3). With resumption of normal postures, pain resulting from impaction of the menisci and/or traction of the articular capsule induces reactive muscle spasm and joint locking. The development of a painful myofascial cycle is initiated as prolonged muscle contraction leads to muscle fatigue, ischemia, and more pain. If spasm and locking persist, the articular cartilage may mold around the capsular meniscus, causing it to become more rigidly incarcerated within the joint[96–98] (Fig. 4.3). To interrupt the cycle of pain, muscle cramping, and joint locking, distractive adjustments have been presented as a viable therapy capable of inducing joint separation, cavitation, and liberation of the entrapped meniscoid[98] (Fig. 4.4).

Bogduk and Engel[99] question the plausibility of meniscus entrapment as a source of acute joint locking. They contend that meniscoid entrapment would require the meniscus to have a firm apex strongly bound to the capsule by connective tissue. Their morphologic studies did not confirm such an anatomic entity. They did imply, however, that a piece of meniscus torn and dislodged from its base could form a loose body in the joint, capable of acting as a source of back pain and amenable to manipulation.

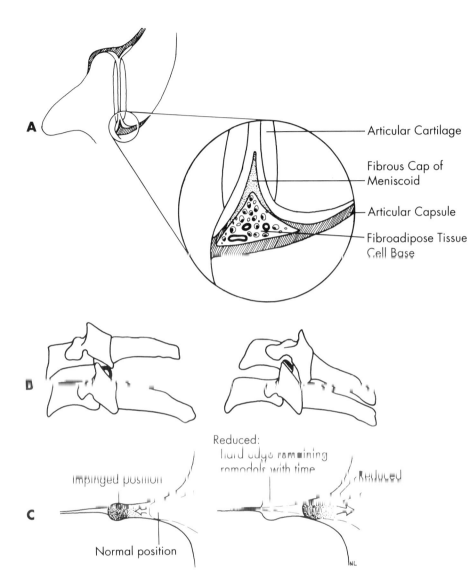

Figure 4.3 Position and postulated incarceration of synovial joint meniscoids. **(A)** Diagrammatic representation of the structural components of a meniscoid in a lumbar facet. (Modified from Dupuis,[186] with permission.) **(B)** Meniscoids entrapment in cervical facet joints restricting extension and flexion movements. **(C)** Entrapment of meniscoids is postulated to produce deformation of the articular cartilage surface: after reduction and over time the articular cartilage will remodel. (Modified from Lewit,[98] with permission.)

Other theories of interarticular soft tissue entrapment suggest that impingement of synovial folds or hyperplastic synovial tissue are additional sources of acute back pain and locking.[100–102] Bony locking of the posterior joints at the end range of spinal motion have also been proposed. It is suggested that the developmental incongruencies and ridges in joint surface anatomy, combined with the complex coupled movements of the spine, may lead to excessive joint gaping at the extremes of movement, which may in turn lead to bony locking as the surfaces reapproximate.[100] In both circumstances, distractive adjustive therapy has the potential to reduce the locking.

Interarticular adhesions

Interarticular adhesions may result from joint injury, inflammation, or immobilization.[67,74,75] Joint injury or irritation leading to chronic inflammation

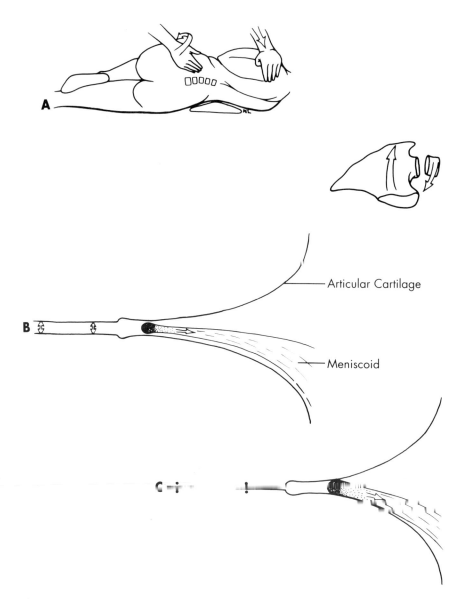

Figure 4.4 Techniques producing joint distraction have the potential to produce cavitation and reduce entrapment of meniscoids. (A) Technique applied to induce flexion, lateral flexion, and rotation in the left lumbar facets. (B) Separation and expulsion of entrapped meniscoid. (C) Return to normal resting position.

and joint effusion may induce synovial tissue hyperplasia, invasion of fibrous connective tissue and consequent interarticular adhesions.[24,74] Additionally, Gillet[103] has suggested that prolonged joint immobilization secondary to periarticular ligamentous shortening may eventually lead to fibrous adhesion formation between joint surfaces. Adjustive therapy is suggested as a procedure that may induce quick distraction and break the intra-articular adhesions.

Interdiscal block

The mechanical derangements of the intervertebral disc (IVD) that may lead to joint dysfunction are postulated to result from pathophysiologic changes associated with aging, degenerative disc disease, and trauma. Farfan[104] has proposed a model of progressive disc derangement based on repetitive rotational stress to the motion segment. He postulates that repetitive torsional loads of sufficient number and duration may, over time, lead to a fatigue injury in the outer annular fibers. The process begins with circumferential distortion and separation in the outer annular fibers followed by progression to radial fissuring and outward migration of nuclear material. The rate of fatigue and injury depend on the duration and magnitude of the force applied. In the individual with disrupted segmental biomechanics, the process is potentially accelerated as an altered axis of movement leads to increased rotational strain on the IVD.

The significance of torsional stress, especially without coupled flexion, on the IVD has been questioned. The sagittal orientation of the lumbar facets, and the protective rotational barrier they provide, bring into question the susceptibility of the lumbar discs to rotational torsion.[105–108] In vitro experimental evidence demonstrates that torsion of the lumbar spine is resisted primarily by the apophyseal joints and that injury to the articular cartilage occurs before significant mechanical stress is transferred to the IVD.[106,108] This suggests that pure rotational damage to the IVD could occur only after significant disruption of the posterior joints. However, the disc does appear to be vulnerable to flexion injuries.[107] Flexion is not inhibited by the articular facets, and distortion and disruption of the posterior annulus may occur with excessive flexion, especially when coupled with positions of lateral bending, loading, and twisting.

Further complicating discal injury are the likely autoimmune reactions triggered by cellular disruption. Naylor[109] has suggested that a discal injury with its associated connective tissue repair and vascularization is sufficient to create an antibody–antigen inflammatory reaction. The net effect is diminished proteoglycan production, reduction of the nucleus polyposus, loss of fluid content, and progression and acceleration of nuclear degeneration. As the nucleus atrophies, the disc becomes more susceptible to loading, and additional tractional forces may be transferred to the annulus.

Interwoven into the natural history of degenerative disc disease may be episodes of acute mechanical back pain and joint locking. Maigne and others[13,110–113] have postulated that incidents of blockage may occur during efforts of trunk flexion as nuclear fragments become lodged in fissures in the posterior annulus (interdiscal block) (Fig. 4.5). Consequently, tension

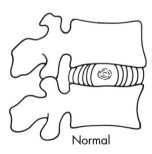

Normal

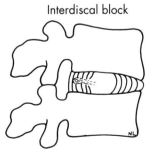

Interdiscal block

Figure 4.5 Fragments of nuclear material migrate in annular defects, creating an interdiscal block.

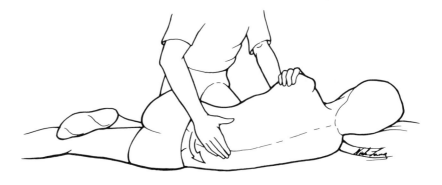

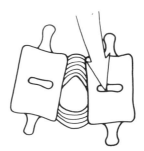

Figure 4.6 Techniques designed to close the side of nuclear migration (open wedge) are performed to force nuclear material toward the center of the disc.

on the posterior annulus and other mobile elements of the involved motion segment are produced, initiating local muscle guarding and joint locking. Cyriax[113] proposes that these lesions may induce tension on the dura mater, inducing lumbago and muscle splinting. Once local pain and muscle spasm are initiated, a self-perpetuating cycle of pain, cramping, and joint locking may result.

Adjustive therapy has been proposed as a viable treatment for interrupting this cycle of acute back pain and joint locking. In addition to the distractive effect on the posterior joints, adjustive therapy is thought to have a potential direct effect on the IVD; either by directing the fragmented nuclear material back toward a more central position or by forcing the nuclear fragment toward a less mechanically and neurologically insulting position. Two separate mechanical concepts have been proposed as models for how this might occur. Gonstead adjustive technique has presented a model using adjustments to close down the side of nuclear migration (slippage) and force the material back toward the center[114] (Fig. 4.6). The second concept, presented by Sandoz,[15] proposes a model where distractive side posture adjustments combine disc distraction with rotation to induce helicoid traction and draw the herniated nuclear material back toward the center (Fig. 4.7).

Clinical trials on the manipulative treatment of lumbar disc herniations are few in number but do indicate a significant improvement for those patients receiving manipulation.[15,115–118] Levernieux[119] noted reduction in

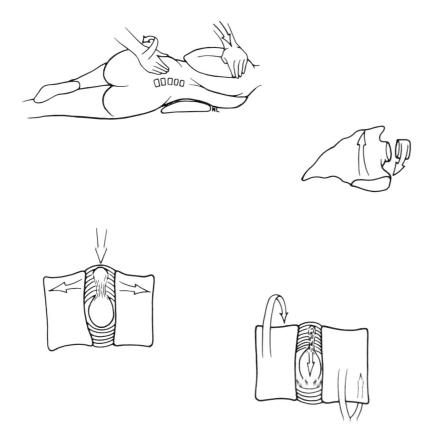

Figure 4.7 Techniques using distraction combined with rotation induce a helicoid traction that is intended to draw nuclear material toward the center of the disc

disc. In relation with axial traction, and Mathis and Yates[18] reported epidurographic reductions in disc herniations with manipulation. In addition, Christman and associates[116] reported a notable improvement in 51 percent of their patients treated with manipulation but no change in disc hernia as measured with myelography. Sandoz[15] concluded that the contradictory findings between these two studies can be accounted for by the fact that epidurography may measure smaller derangements of the disc, whereas myelography reveals only larger protrusions that are less amendable by manipulative care. It is doubtful that manipulation can reduce an external protrusion, but Sandoz[15] has suggested that manipulation may have a role to play in shifting the herniation away from the nerve root, minimizing the mechanical conflict and associated inflammation. In such circumstances, treatment is expected to be more protracted.[15]

The incidence of complications arising from the manipulative treatment of disc herniation patients appears to be low[48,105] This procedure, however, does carry some risk,[49,120–122] and in the absence of clear professional standards, extra caution should be applied in the manipulative treatment of patients with marked disc herniations. To minimize the risk of further annular injury, some have suggested using passive mobilization procedures that emphasize flexion, extension, or lateral flexion instead of side posture rotational adjustments.[120] Disc herniation patients suffering progressive neurologic deficits or midline herniations and the associated cauda equina syndrome should not be considered for manipulation.[105,123]

Muscle spasm

The potential causative role of hypertonic muscles in development of joint dysfunction has been presented by numerous authors.[15,63,103,124–127] The concept that restricted joint movement may result from segmental muscle spasm is supported by the knowledge that muscles not only impart movement but impede movement. Joint movement depends on a balance between its agonist and antagonists. If this balance is lost and antagonistic muscles are unable to elongate, owing to involuntary hypertonicity, then the joint may be restricted in its range and/or quality of movement.

Muscle spasm may be initiated by direct provocation or injury to myofascial structures or indirectly by stimulation or injury to associated articular structures. Direct overstretching and tearing of muscle leads to stimulation of myofascial nociceptors and protective muscle splinting. The intersegmental muscles of the spine may be especially vulnerable to incidents of minor mechanical stress and overstretching. They are not under voluntary control. They act primarily to stabilize and integrate segmental movements in response to global movements of the trunk. As a result, they may be especially vulnerable to unguarded movements and the induction of reactive splinting.

Korr[125] suggests that unguarded and uncoordinated movements may approximate the short segmental muscles of the back and reduce annulospiral receptor activity in the muscle spindle complex and produce muscle spasm. Maigne[124] envisions a similar lesion (articular strain) but speculates that it results from abnormal sustained postures or poorly judged movements that induce minor intersegmental muscle overstretching and cramping. Both speculate that segmental muscle spasm, once initiated in the back, may be hard to arrest. Contracted segmental muscles of the back, unlike the voluntary appendicular muscles, are not easily stretched by the contraction of antagonistic muscle groups. As a result, this condition may not be inhibited by active stretching and therefore may be less likely to be self-limiting.[124]

Myofascial cycle

A central complicating feature of many of the internal and external derangements of the motion segment is the induction of a self-perpetuating myofascial cycle of pain and muscle spasm. The articular soft tissues are richly innervated with mechanoreceptors and nociceptors, and traction or injury to these structures may lead to the initiation of local muscle splinting. With time, the continued muscle contraction leads to further muscle fatigue, ischemia, pain, and maintenance of muscle spasm and joint locking (Fig. 4.8).

High-velocity adjustments are suggested as treatments that may be effective in interrupting this cycle. Several theories exist as to the mechanism by which adjustments relieve muscle spasm. Korr[125] speculates that quick traction and excitation of the Golgi tendon organs (GTO), located in the muscle tendon junction, provide one such mechanism. When stimulated, they purportedly act as brakes to limit excessive joint movement and possible injury by inhibiting motor activity. The concept is that adjustments induce

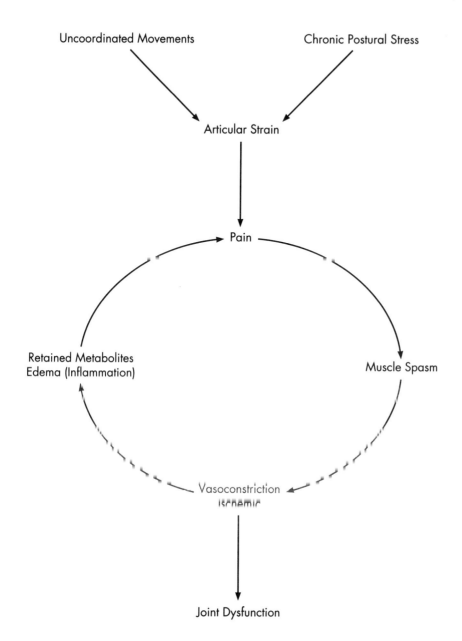

Figure 4.8 The self-perpetuating cycle of myofascial pain and muscle spasm.

a strong stretch on the muscle tendon complex, activate the GTO, and induce reflex muscle relaxation (autogenic inhibition).

Although this model seems reasonable, evidence suggests that the GTO has a less profound effect than initially envisioned. Watts and colleagues[128] found that stimulation of the GTO produces a very meager inhibitory effect on α-motor neuron activity. This information implies that the GTO plays a more minor role in the inhibition of muscle spasm than initially proposed and brings into question its relationship to postadjustive muscle relaxation.

In contrast, stimulation of articular low- and high-threshold mechanoreceptors and nociceptors has demonstrated a notable inhibitory effect on segmental motor activity.[129] Additionally, high-velocity distractive adjustments induce enough force to stimulate these structures and induce a burst of somatic afferent receptor activity.[87,130] Based on this information, it may be prudent to place more emphasis on the potential role of joint and soft tissue mechanoreceptors and nociceptors in the inhibition of muscle spasm and the interruption of painful myofascial cycles and of joint locking.

Periarticular fibrosis and adhesions

As mentioned previously, acute or repetitive trauma may lead to articular soft tissue injury. In the process of fibrotic repair, adhesions and contractures may develop, resulting in joint hypomobility. Distractive adjustments are advanced as procedures capable of effectively treating these derangements by stretching the affected tissue, breaking adhesions, restoring mobility, and normalizing mechanoreceptive and proprioceptive input.[63–66]

It is further postulated that manipulation may sever the adhesive bonds, stretch tissue, and promote mobility without triggering an inflammatory reaction and reoccurrence of fibrosis. However, when articular or nonarticular soft tissue contractures are encountered, incorporation of procedures that minimize inflammation and maintain mobility should be considered. Viscoelastic structures are more amenable to elongation and deformation if they are first warmed and then stretched for sustained periods.[131] Therefore, the application of moist heat, ultrasound, and other warming therapies might be considered before applying sustained manual traction or home-care stretching exercises.

Joint Instability

Although emphasis has been on the adjustive treatment of mechanical disorders leading to joint hypomobility, manipulative therapy also may have a role in the treatment of clinical joint instability.

Clinical joint instability can be defined as a loss of stiffness in the controlling intersegmental soft tissues that leads to a loss of motion segment equilibrium and an increase in abnormal translational and/or angular movements.[132,133] Common proposed causes include acute trauma, repetitive use injuries, and compensation for adjacent motion segment hypomobility.[134] Joint instability may predispose the patient to reoccurring episodes of interarticular blocks and may be seen more frequently in individuals who have some degree of hypermobility that is due to advanced training in athletics, gymnastics, or ballet dancing.[134] Clinical joint instability is not to be confused with gross orthopedic instability resulting from marked degeneration, traumatic fracture, or dislocation.

Adjustive therapy applied in this condition is not intended to restore lost movement but rather to reduce the episodic pain, temporary joint locking, joint subluxation, and muscle spasm that are so commonly encountered in patients with unstable spinal joints. Adjustive therapy delivered in these circumstances is considered to be palliative, not curative. It should not be applied over an extended period, and it should be incorporated with stabilization therapy, appropriate exercise, and life-style modification.[134]

Analgesic Hypothesis

The reduction of pain and disability from spinal manipulation is well recognized and clinically documented.[29,57,58,136–139] The mechanisms by which manipulation inhibits pain, however, are matters of speculation and still under investigation. Proposed hypotheses have suggested that manipulation has the potential to remove the source of mechanical pain and inflammation and/or induce stimulus-produced analgesia.

The case for decreasing pain by removing its mechanical source is empirical and deductive. The pain associated with mechanical disorders of the musculoskeletal system is a product of physical deformation, inflammation, or both.[140] It is reasoned that manual therapy that is effective at reversing or mitigating underlying structural and functional derangements will remove the source of pain, as structures are returned to normal function.

The argument for stimulus-produced analgesia is bolstered by experimental evidence that suggests that chiropractic adjustments induce sufficient force to simultaneously activate both superficial and deep somatic mechanoreceptors, proprioceptors, and nociceptors. The effect of this stimulation is a strong afferent segmental barrage of spinal cord sensory neurons, capable of inhibiting the central transmission of pain[130,141–143] (Fig. 4.9).

Gillette[130] suggests that spinal adjustments may initiate both a short-lived phasic response, triggered by stimulation of superficial and deep mechanoreceptors, and a longer lived tonic response, triggered by noxious-level stimulation of nociceptive receptors. The phasic response is hypothesized to initiate a local gating effect but pain inhibition would terminate with cessation of therapy. The tonic response initiated by noxious levels of mechanical stimulation is more powerful and capable of outlasting the duration of applied therapy.[141]

Adjustments that induce joint cavitation and capsular distraction may be a source of nociceptive stimulation capable of initiating relatively long-lasting pain inhibition. This concept supports the premise that the slight discomfort that may be associated with adjustments is casually associated with a positive therapeutic effect.[29]

The short-term bursts of proprioceptive and nociceptive input associated with adjustments, much like transcutaneous electrical nerve stimulation (TENS) and acupuncture, have also been theorized to increase the levels of neurochemical pain inhibitors.[137] Both a local release of enkephalins, initiated by stimulation of the neurons of substantia gelatinosa, and a systemic increase in plasma and cerebrospinal fluid (CSF) endorphin levels, initiated by simulation of the hypothalamic pituitary axis, have been proposed. Both substances act as endogenous opioid pain inhibitors and may play a role in the analgesic effects of adjustments.

Doctor reassurance and the laying on of hands may also impart a direct analgesic effect, which must be factored into the equation when calculating the effects of adjustments and manual therapy. The contact established during a skilled evaluation of the soft tissues indicates the physician's sense of concern and skill. Paris[146] states that with the addition of a skilled evaluation involving palpation for soft tissue changes and altered joint mechanics, the patient becomes convinced of the clinician's interest, concern, and manual

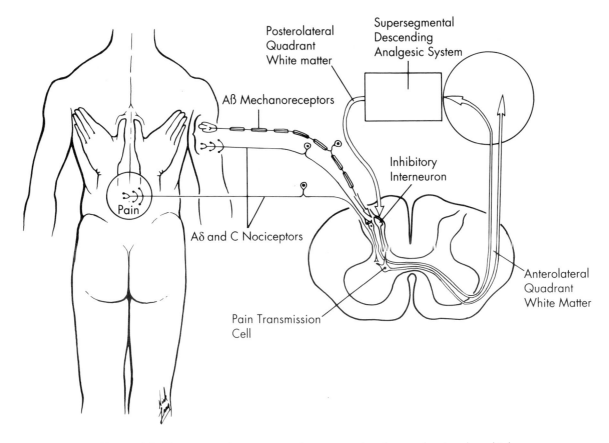

Figure 4.9 Diagrammatic representation suggesting the mechanism by which a high-velocity chiropractic adjustment inhibits the central transmission of pain through activation of mechanoreceptors. 'Modified from Gillette,[145] with permission.)

skills. If the examination is followed by treatment and an adjustive cavitation ("crack"), further positive placebo effects may be registered. The astute clinician accepts and reinforces this phenomena if it influences the patient's recovery. This does not excuse misrepresentation or irresponsible exaggeration of the therapeutic effect.

Neurobiologic Hypothesis

Chiropractic, osteopathy, and manual medicine have envisioned manual therapy affecting not only somatic disorders but also visceral disorders through neurologic means.[12,147–151]

The early paradigm presented in chiropractic stressed a model of altered nerve root function as the basis for secondary somatic or visceral dysfunction. It was theorized that subluxations induce structural alteration of the intervertebral foramina, leading to compression of the contained neurovascular structures and impaired function of the nerve root as electrical transmission and/or axoplasmic flow is impeded (nonimpulsed-based model). The postulated net result of this process (nerve interference) was dysfunc-

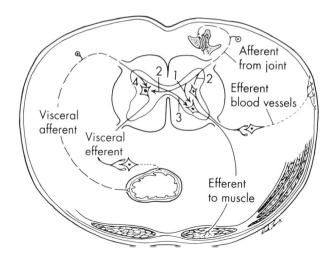

Figure 4.10 Afferent and efferent pathways from and to the viscera and somatic structures that can produce **(1)** somatosomatic, **(2)** somatovisceral, **(3)** viscerovisceral, and **(4)** viscerosomatic reflex phenomena. (Modified from Schmidt,[188] with permission.)

tion or disease in the somatic and visceral structures supplied by the affected nerve root.[12,147–152]

Though the plausibility of uncomplicated subluxations inducing nerve root compression seems unlikely,[151–153] it is plausible that subluxations associated with other pathologic or degenerative changes may predispose or contribute to nerve root compression syndromes.[152,154,155] In such circumstances, adjustive therapy that reduces a position of fixed subluxation and root irritation may have an effect on reducing nerve root traction, compression or inflammation.

Beginning with the work of Homewood,[151] the profession has gradually moved away from reliance on a *nonimpulsed-based* model and toward a more dynamic *impulsed-based* model of subluxation-induced neurodysfunction. As presented earlier (see Ch. 3), the impulsed-based paradigm presents a model where somatic dysfunction and/or joint dysfunction induce persistent nociceptive and altered proprioceptive input. This persistent afferent input triggers a segmental cord response, which in turn induces the development of pathologic somatosomatic or somatovisceral disease reflexes[130,150,156–161] (Fig. 4.10). If these reflexes persist, they are hypothesized to induce altered function in segmentally supplied somatic or visceral structures.

Chiropractic adjustive therapy has the potential for arresting both the local and distant somatic and visceral effects, by normalizing joint mechanics and terminating the altered neurogenic reflexes associated with joint dysfunction. This model has become the focus of more attention and investigation as chiropractors search for an explanation to the wide-ranging physiologic effects that they have clinically observed to be associated with spinal adjustive therapy. This relationship is not consistent, and the frequency of response is undetermined, but the anecdotal and empirical experiences of the profession are significant enough to warrant serious further investigation.

An additional model of subluxation-induced neurodysfunction focuses attention on the potential direct mechanical irritation of the autonomic nervous system. The paradigm for irritation of sympathetic structures is based on the anatomic proximity and vulnerability of the posterior chain ganglion, between T1 and L2, to the soma of the posterior chest wall and costovertebral joints. Altered spinal and costovertebral mechanics are hypothesized to mechanically irritate the sympathetic ganglia and to induce segmental sympathetic hypertonia.[162] The target organs within the segmental distribution then theoretically become susceptible to altered autonomic regulation and function as a result of altered sympathetic function.

In contrast to the sympathetic chain, the parasympathetic system, with its origins from the brain, brain stem, and sacral segments of the spinal cord, does not have anatomic proximity to the spinal joints. Models of mechanically induced dysfunction of the parasympathetic system propose dysfunction in cranial, cervical, and pelvic mechanics as potential sources of entrapment or tethering of the parasympathetic fibers. Altered cervical, cranial, or craniosacral mechanics are theorized to induce traction of dural attachments and the cranial nerves as they exit through the dura and skull foramina. The treatment goal in mechanically induced autonomic dysfunction is to identify the sites of joint dysfunction and implement appropriate manual therapy to balance membranous tension.[163]

From the discussion of spinal dysfunction and its potential neurobiologic effects on health, it must be remembered that spinal dysfunction may be the product of, not the cause of, somatic or visceral dysfunction or disease.[164] Spinal pain and dysfunction may be secondary to a disorder that needs direct treatment. Manual therapy may be a fitting component of appropriate care but would be inadequate as the singular treatment. The patient with caffeine-induced gastritis who develops secondary midback pain and dysfunction (viscerosomatic disorder) (Fig. 4.16) should not receive manual therapy without also being counseled to discontinue ingestion of caffeinated beverages. The spine is a common site of referred pain, and when a patient with a suspected mechanical or traumatic disorder does not respond as anticipated, the possibility of other somatic or visceral disease should be reconsidered.

Neuroimmunology

An interaction exists between the function of the central nervous system and the body's immunity that supports the chiropractic hypothesis that neural dysfunction is stressful to the body locally and globally. Moreover, with the resultant lowered tissue resistance, modifications to the nonspecific and specific immune responses occur, as well as altered trophic function of the involved nerves. Selye[165–167] has demonstrated neuroendocrine–immune connections in animal experiments and clinical investigations.

Physiologic, psychological, psychosomatic, and sociologic components compose the stress response. From studies of overstressed animals, Selye observed nonspecific changes which he labeled the *general adaptive syndrome* (*GAS*). He also observed very specific responses that depended on the stressor and on the part of the animal involved, which he termed *local adaptive syndrome* (*LAS*). Further, he established a stress index comprising major pathologic results of overstress, including enlargement of the adrenal cortex, atrophy of lymphatic tissues, and bleeding ulcers. Selye also felt that long-term stress would lead to diseases of adaptation including cardiovascu-

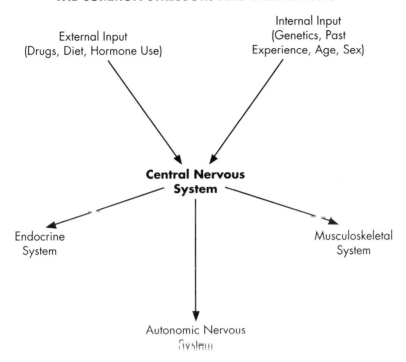

THE COMMON STRESSORS AND THEIR EFFECTS

External Input
(Drugs, Diet, Hormone Use)

Internal Input
(Genetics, Past
Experience, Age, Sex)

**Central Nervous
System**

Endocrine
System

Musculoskeletal
System

Autonomic Nervous
System

Figure 4.11 Internal and external conditioning can affect emotional stimuli, resulting in autonomic, endocrine, or musculoskeletal changes.

lar disease, high blood pressure, connective tissue disease, stomach ulcers, and headaches.

Because all individuals do not develop the same syndrome with the same stressor, Mason suggested that emotional stimuli under the influence of internal (genetics, past experiences, age, sex) or external (drugs, diet, hormone use) conditioning are reflected in the responses of the endocrine, autonomic, and musculoskeletal systems[168] (Fig. 4.11). It is thought that any stressful activity will set the stress mechanism in motion, but whether the effects will be tolerated depends on the influence of the existing conditioning factors. Moreover, even though all parts of the body are exposed equally to stress, it is the weakest link that breaks down first. Therefore, it is the conditioning factors that determine whether the stress will lead to diseases of adaptation or to a physiologic response that allows the body to adapt to stress rather than to succumb to it.[169]

Stein et al. convincingly demonstrated psychosocial and neural influences on the immune system.[170] They showed that the hypothalamus has a direct effect on the humeral immune response, explaining how psychosocial factors can modify host resistance to infection. Moreover, Hess produced sympathetic and parasympathetic responses by stimulating different parts of the hypothalamus.[171] The sympathetic response (ergotropic response) is characteristic of the fight-or-flight mechanism, whereas the parasympathetic response (trophotropic response) produces relaxation that promotes a restorative process. Table 4.9 lists the characteristics and physiologic responses of the ergotropic and trophotropic states.

Table 4.9 Characteristics of the Ergotropic and Trophotropic Response

Ergotropic Responses	Tropotrophic Responses
Primarily sympathetic	Primarily parasympathetic
Excitement, arousal, action	Relaxation
Movement of body and/or parts	Energy conservation
Increased HR, BP, RR	Decreased HR, BP, RR
Increased blood sugar	Increased GI function
Increased muscle tension	Decreased muscle tension
Increased O_2 consumption	Decreased O_2 consumption
Increased CO_2 elimination	Decreased CO_2 elimination
Pupil dilation	Pupil constriction

BP, blood pressure; GI, gastrointestinal; HR, heart rate; RR, respiratory rate.

Leach points out that there is a paucity of studies that directly link vertebral lesions with immunologic competence, though his review of the literature suggests that such a connection is likely.[169] Fidelibus, after conducting a recent review of the literature,[172] concluded that the concepts of neuroimmunomodulation, somatosympathetic reflex, and spinal fixation provide a theoretic basis for using spinal manipulation in the management of certain disorders involving the immune system including asthma, allergic rhinitis, and the common cold. He further postulates that musculoskeletal dysfunction can result in immune dysfunction and that, by removing the musculoskeletal dysfunction, spinal manipulation can affect the immune dysfunction.

Finally, a single high-velocity, low-amplitude thrust in the thoracic spine resulted in an enhanced respiratory burst in polymorphonuclear neutrophils and monocytes drawing a correlation between manipulation and immunoinflammatory processes.[173] In follow-up, Kokjohn et al. hypothesized that the force applied to the thoracic spine by manipulation is sufficient to result in increased plasma levels of substance P, which may prime circulating phagocytic cells for enhanced respiratory burst.[174] However, whether the effect is significant in fighting infection has not been determined, and the exact mechanism whereby manipulation affects phagocytic cells remains speculative, as significant levels of plasma substance P were not determined.

Circulatory Hypothesis

Beneficial vascular responses to adjustive therapy are theorized to result as a product of stimulation of autonomic nervous system or through improved function of the musculoskeletal system.

As discussed previously, joint subluxation/dysfunction has been submitted as a source of altered segmental sympathetic tone. If joint dysfunction can induce a sympathetic response robust enough to induce local or segmental vasoconstriction, then spinal subluxation/dysfunction may be associated with decreased circulation to segmentally supplied tissues. Chiropractic adjustments would then have the potential to improve circulation by restoring joint function and removing the source of sympathetic irritation.

Musculoskeletal integrity and function are additional factors directly impacting the circulatory system. The venous and lymph systems are driven by skeletal muscle movements and changing intrathoracic and intra-abdominal pressures. A healthy respiratory pump depends on a functioning diaphragm and flexible spine and rib cage. Conditions or injuries that lead to the loss of musculoskeletal mobility and strength result in a potential net loss of functional capacity of the musculoskeletal system and its ability to move blood and lymph. Muscle injury or disuse leads to an accompanying loss of vascularization in the affected tissues, and additional blood and lymph flow impedance may occur. Therapy directed at improving mobility and skeletal muscle strength have the potential to improve the functional capacity of the musculoskeletal system and improve circulation.[175]

APPLICATION OF ADJUSTIVE THERAPY

Once a working diagnosis is established, and a decision is reached to employ adjustive therapy, the chiropractor must finally decide what specific adjustive method to apply. The decision is complex and is influenced by factors such as the patient's age, size, flexibility, physical condition, and the acuteness or chronicity of the problem. The ability to make a correct assessment and decision is affected by the physician's knowledge of anatomy, biomechanics, and adjustive mechanics, and by his/her physical attributes and technical skills.

Before adjustments can be applied, the doctor must consider the local anatomy and the geometric plane of the articulation, the nature of the condition to be treated, the patient's health status, and any underlying disease processes. These factors and the mechanical characteristics of the adjustment to be applied will determine the positioning of the patient, the specific contacts, the degree of appropriate preadjustive tension, the magnitude of the applied forces, and the direction of the adjustive thrust (Fig. 4.12).

Each individual joint complex has specific anatomic and biomechanical considerations that affect adjustive therapy. As each spinal region and extremity joint is presented, the unique relationship between regional anatomy, biomechanics, and adjustive mechanics is discussed (Chs. 5 and 6).

Joint Anatomy and Arthrokinematics

Especially important in the performance of adjustive techniques is an awareness of spinal and extremity joint architecture, facet plane orientations, and arthrokinematics. When subluxation/dysfunction is identified, the chiropractic physician must be able to induce joint separation and corrective joint movements without producing joint compression, injury, or distraction at undesired segmental levels. Most adjustive techniques are directed at producing joint distraction either along the articular plane or at right angles (perpendicular) to the articular plane. This cannot be efficiently and effectively accomplished without an understanding of how joints are configured and how they move.

To illustrate this point, consider the application of prone adjustive techniques in the treatment of thoracic flexion and extension dysfunction. In

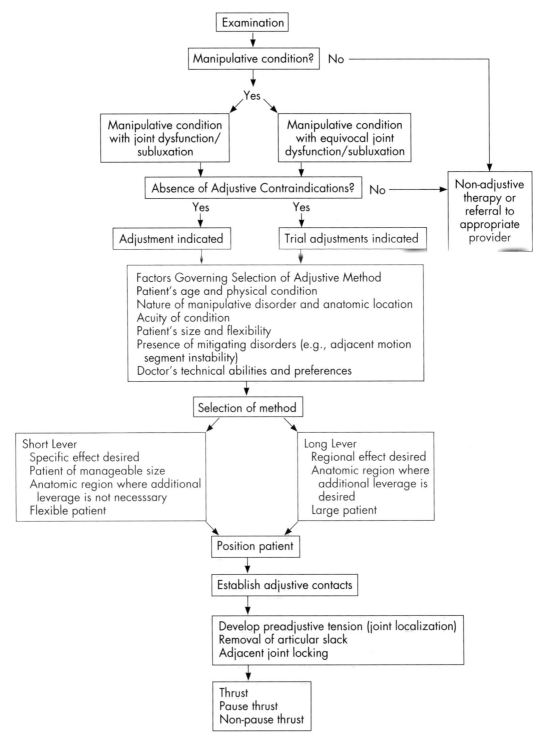

Figure 4.12 Factors to consider before selection and application of an adjustment.

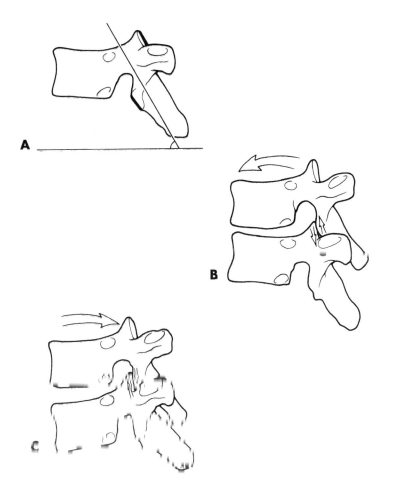

Figure 4.13 The thoracic facets (**A**) lie at a 60-degree angle approaching the coronal plane from the transverse plane; (**B**) separate and glide apart on flexion; and (**C**) approximate with gapping at their superior margins on extension.

the thoracic spine, the articular surfaces are relatively flat. The superior articular processes underlie the inferior articular processes and on average form an angle of approximately 60 degrees to the horizontal. During segmental flexion in the thoracic spine, the posterior joint surfaces separate and glide apart along their joint surfaces. During extension, the posterior joint surfaces approximate and gap at their superior margins at the end range of motion (Fig. 4.13).

When performing prone thoracic adjustments, the doctor typically develops adjustive vectors that either approximate the disc plane or the facet planes. The thrust that parallels the disc plane is perpendicular to the spine and facet facings and will likely induce approximation of the facets in the joint below the contacted vertebrae and perpendicular gapping in the joint superior to the contacted vertebrae (Fig. 4.14). In contrast, a thrust delivered cephalically along facet planes should induce longitudinal distraction in the facet joint inferior to the point of contact and gliding approximation in the joint superior to the point of contact (Fig. 4.15). Therefore, thrusts that parallel the disc plane are intended to induce extension in the joint below the contact and perpendicular gapping above (see Fig. 4.14). Thrusts directed

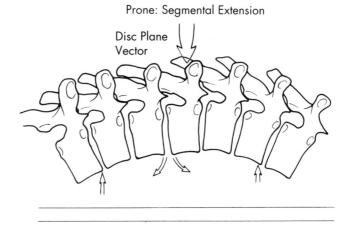

Prone: Segmental Extension

Disc Plane Vector

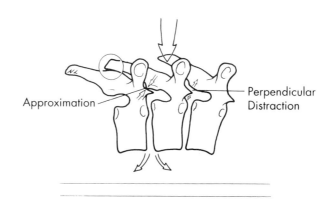

Approximation

Perpendicular Distraction

Figure 4.14 Effects of an adjustive force applied in the disc plane will likely approximate the facets and separate the anterior interbody space below the contact with perpendicular gapping of the facets above the contact, thereby creating extension movement.

cephalically along the facet plane are intended to induce flexion in the joint below the contact and extension above (see Fig. 4.15). These deductions are not possible without knowledge of joint anatomy and arthrokinematics.

Adjustive Mechanics

Each grouping of adjustments has its own mechanical characteristics dependent on adjustive contacts, patient positioning, doctor positioning, and adjustive vectors. Efficient and effective selections cannot be made without an understanding of each adjustment's unique physical attributes.

For example, side posture lumbar adjustments may be used to develop rotational tension and perpendicular facet distraction. In contrast, prone lumbar adjustments maintain a more neutral position of the lumbar spine and therefore minimize the amount of rotational tension. Side posture positions also provide additional leverage and more latitude in the development of and use of the doctor's body weight, providing a possible mechanical advantage. Therefore, if rotational lumbar distraction is desired, a side posture adjustive method should be considered over a prone method. If

Prone: Segmental Flexion

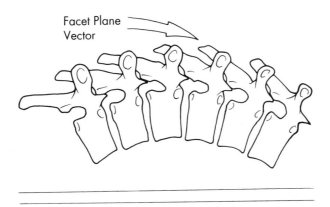

Facet Plane
Vector

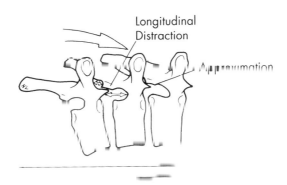

Longitudinal
Distraction

Approximation

Figure 4.15 Effects of an adjustive thrust applied along the facet plane will likely induce the following: longitudinal distraction of the facet joint, approximation on the anterior interbody space below the contact, with a gliding approximation in facet joint above the contact, thereby creating flexion.

lumbar distraction without rotational tension is desired, then a prone lumbar position might be more appropriate. If adjustive mechanical principles are not clear to the practitioner, the adjustive selections may be made by habit or chance, instead of reason.

Adjustive Localization

Adjustive localization refers to the preadjustive procedures designed to localize adjustive forces and joint distraction. They involve the application of physiologic and unphysiologic positions, the removal of articular "slack," and the development of appropriate patient positions, contact points, and adjustive vectors. These factors are critical to the development of appropriate preadjustive tension and adjustive efficiency. Attention to these components is intended to improve adjustive specificity and to further minimize the distractive tension on adjacent joints.

Physiologic and Unphysiologic Movement

Knowledge of the physiologic movements of the spine and extremities is essential to the process of determining how to localize and apply adjustive therapy. Adjustive efficiency and specificity depend on an understanding of the normal ranges of joint movement and how combinations of movement affect ease and range of joint movement. Each spinal region and extremity joint has its own unique range and patterns of movement. Knowing the ranges and patterns of movement allows the doctor to know what combination of movements is necessary to produce the greatest range of movement and what combination is necessary to limit movement.

The spine can flex, extend, laterally flex, and rotate, but in combination, these movements can either act to limit or increase movement. Performance of movement in one plane will limit movement in another plane; flexion of the spine will limit the amount of lumbar rotation, and lumbar rotation will limit the amount of flexion. An additional coupling of motion in a third plane can combine to further restrict or enhance the range of motion. For example, the greatest range of combined lumbar rotation and lateral flexion is achieved if rotation and lateral flexion are executed in opposite directions and coupled with extension instead of flexion.

In this discussion, we refer to combined movements that allow for the greatest total range as *physiologic movement* and to combinations that lead to limited movement as *unphysiologic movement*. Right lateral flexion combined with left rotation and extension is an example of physiologic movement in the lumbar spine. Right lateral flexion combined with right rotation and/or flexion is an example of unphysiologic movement.

Unphysiologic movements bring the joints to positions of locking earlier in their range of motion, limiting their overall range of motion. This strategy is referred to as *joint locking* and is one of the important principles involved in "localizing" the adjustive forces to the affected joint. It is especially valuable when clinical joint instability may be suspected at adjacent joints. By placing adjacent joints in unphysiologic positions, a block of resistance may be created above and/or below the joint to be adjusted. Joints placed in their unphysiologic positions have greater impact between joint surfces, which may decrease the likelihood of paraphysiologic joint movement and gapping at that joint.

The motion segment to be adjusted is placed at the transition point between unphysiologic motion and physiologic motion or between sections placed in unphysiologic locking (Fig. 4.16). The joint to be adjusted must have sufficient slack remaining, so the adjustive thrust may induce gapping or gliding within the joint's physiologic range. If an adjustive thrust is delivered against a joint placed in its close-packed position, there is a greater risk of inducing joint injury.

Removal of Articular Slack

Articular slack refers to the joint play present in all synovial joints and their periarticular soft tissues. Although it is a normal component of joint function, available slack must be removed during or before delivery of an adjustive thrust, if joint cavitation is to occur. Removing articular slack helps

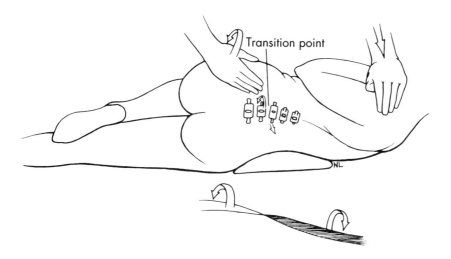

Figure 4.16 The articulation to be adjusted (in this case, L3–L4) is placed in a position between unphysiologic motion above (flexion, left rotation, right lateral flexion) and physiologic motion below (flexion, right rotation, right lateral flexion) or between sections placed in unphysiologic locking.

isolate tension to the specific periarticular soft tissues that may be reducing joint play and impeding joint motion. The removal of articular slack and the development of preadjustive tension also helps to focus the adjustive thrust to the desired level. The energy and force generated by adjustive thrusts may be dissipated into superficial soft tissue and adjacent articular soft tissue if preadjustive tension is not first established. A thrust directed at a joint that has available slack removed will be more focused and will need less force to produce cavitation.[176,177]

The doctor may remove articular slack by passively altering the involved joint or by altering patient positions to move the joint from its neutral position toward its elastic barrier. Joint distraction induced by the doctor may be developed by the gradual transfer of body weight through the adjustive contacts or by diverting tractional forces through the adjustive contacts. The degree of preadjustive tension is gauged by the doctor's sense of joint tension and by the patient's response to pressure. Lighter contacts and less preadjustive tension are necessary when patient discomfort and splinting are encountered.

Joints with limited mobility need less movement to remove articular slack and are often adjusted closer to their neutral positions. Joints with greater flexibility usually necessitate patient positions that move the joint from neutral positions toward the elastic barrier.

Patient Positioning

Appropriate preadjustive joint tension and localization depend critically on patient placement and leverage. Localization of adjustive forces may be enhanced by using patient placement to position a joint at a point of distractive vulnerability. Locking adjacent joints and positioning the joint to be adjusted at the apex of curves established during patient positioning enhances this process and adjustive specificity (Fig. 4.17). Joint localization and joint distraction may be further enhanced if forces are used to either assist or oppose the adjustive thrust. Assisting or opposing forces may be generated either during the adjustive setup and/or during the adjustive

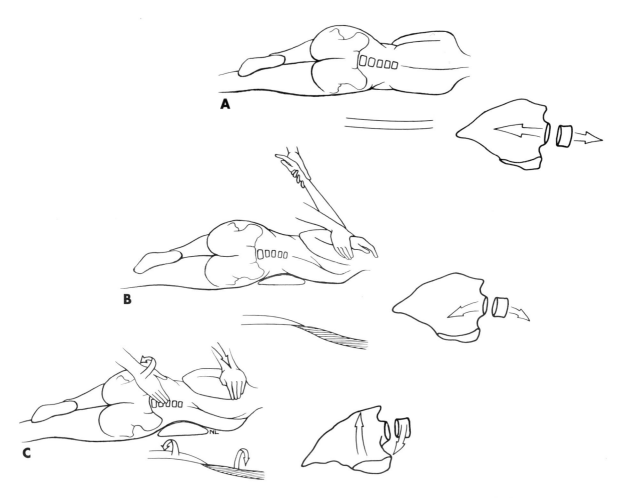

Figure 4.17 Proper patient positioning is necessary to develop appropriate pre-adjustive joint tension. **(A)** Sagittal plane movement (flexion) and separation of the posterior element of the joint. **(B)** Coronal plane movement (lateral flexion) and separation of the joint away from the table. **(C)** Transverse plane movement and development of counterrotational tension.

thrust. Assisted and resisted patient positions refer to the principles involved during the adjustive setup and development of preadjustive tension, not to the generation of assisted or resisted thrusts.

Assisted and resisted positioning

The notion of applying assisted and opposing forces during the performance of manipulation was first described relative to thoracic manipulation by the French orthopedist Robert Maigne.[180] In the chiropractic profession, Sandoz was the first to describe similar terms.[15] Sandoz proposed using the terms *assisted* and *resisted* to describe patient positions that either assist or resist adjustive thrusts. As originally described, assisted and resisted methods were applied only to side posture lumbar adjustments and to those procedures involving a single primary thrust.[15] Both methods are employed to

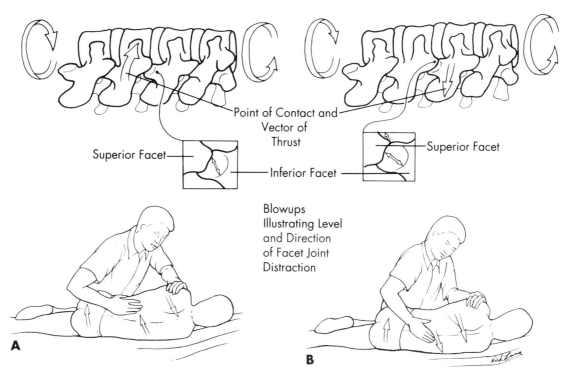

Figure 4.18 **(A)** Resisted patient positioning with mammillary contact established on inferior vertebra. **(B)** Assisted patient positioning with spinous contact established on superior vertebra.

improve the localization of preadjustive tension. Their application is based on the mechanical principle that the point of maximal tension will be developed at the point of opposing counterrotation.

Assisted and resisted methods are distinguished from each other by the positioning of vertebral segments relative to the adjustive thrust. In both circumstances, the trunk and vertebral segments superior to the adjustive contact are prestressed in the direction of desired joint movement. In the assisted method, the contact is established on the superior vertebral segments, and movement of the trunk and the thrust are directed together (Fig. 4.18). Assisted procedures are designed to induce preadjustive tension and positions that assist the adjustive thrust. Resisted procedures employ patient positions in which the segments superior to the adjustive contact are stabilized or moved in a direction opposing the adjustive thrust. In the resisted method, the contact is established on the lower vertebral segment, and the direction of trunk movement and adjustive thrust are in opposing directions (Fig. 4.18).

Sandoz[15] has suggested that resisted positions bring maximal tension to the articulation superior to the established contact (e.g., contact at the L3 mammillary inducing tension at the L2–L3 motion segment) and assisted positions bring maximal tension to the articulation inferior to the established contact (e.g., L2 spinous contact inducing tension at the L2–L3 motion segment). In the assisted method, the point of countertension is inferior to the point of contact because the segments below are stabilized or rotated in a direction opposite the adjustive thrust (Fig. 4.18).

In the resisted approach, the site of countertension is superior to the point of contact because the segments above are stabilized or are rotated in a direction opposite the adjustive thrust (Fig. 4.18). Therefore, either method theoretically can be used to induce cavitation and motion within the same articulation. Although the movement generated is the same, the points of contact and the line of drive differ. With the assisted method, the contact is established on the superior vertebrae of the dysfunctional motion segment; in the resisted method, it is established on the inferior vertebrae. The thrust is oriented in the direction of restriction when using the assisted method and against the direction of restriction when using the resisted method (Fig. 4.18).

Assisted and resisted methods have been most frequently discussed relative to the development of rotational tension of the spine. The same methods and principles, however, may be applied to treat dysfunction in lateral flexion or flexion and extension.

For example, to treat a loss of right lateral bending in the lumbar spine using the assisted method, place the patient on the right side, with a roll placed under the lumbar spine to induce right lateral flexion. Establish a contact on the left mammillary of the superior vertebra with an adjustive vector directed anteriorly and *superiorly* (Fig. 4.19). To treat the same restriction with a resisted method, maintain the same patient positioning, but contact the left mammillary process of the inferior vertebra, and thrust anteriorly and *inferiorly* (Fig. 4.19). Although both techniques are directed at distracting the left facet joints, one is assisting and the other is resisting the direction of bending.

To treat a loss of lumbar flexion with a side posture assisted method, place the patient on either side and induce segmental flexion, contact the superior vertebrae of the involved motion segment, and thrust anteriorly and *superiorly*. Conversely, without changing patient positioning, the same restriction could be treated with a resisted method by simply contacting the lower vertebrae and thrusting anteriorly and *inferiorly* (Fig. 4.20). The same principles described for flexion can easily be applied to treat an extension restriction, the only difference being the prestressing of the patient into segmental extension.

Although the classification scheme of assisted and resisted adjustments is

Figure 4.19 Adjustment for loss of right lateral flexion using the resisted method, by contacting the left mammillary process of the inferior vertebrae, or the assisted method, by contacting the left mammillary process of superior vertebrae.

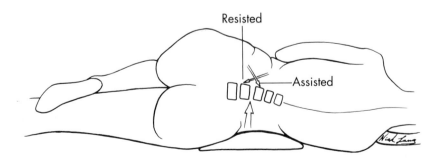

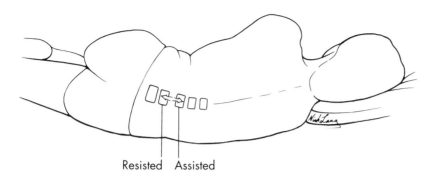

Resisted   Assisted

Figure 4.20 Adjustment for loss of flexion using resisted or assisted methods.

very useful for contrasting different methods, it does create a possible void for those procedures in which both hands establish adjustive contacts and both deliver opposing adjustive thrusts. Counterthrust procedures do not conform to the strict definitions of assisted or resisted methods because these terms are defined relative to the delivery of one thrust, not two. In methods applying counterthrust techniques, both arms thrust; one arm establishes an assisted position and thrust as the other develops a resisted position and thrust. Therefore, based on the previous guidelines, they do not fit either category. However, because these methods typically involve procedures that generate opposing forces across a joint, we propose placing them under the resisted category. To further distinguish them from single thrust-resisted patient positions, they may be further described as resisted counterthrust procedures.

Neutral positioning

Neutral adjustments involve patient positions where the joint is left in a relatively neutral position during the delivery of an adjustive thrust. They are typically used when joint mobility is minimal. Articular slack is removed and preadjustive joint tension is established by the doctor, not by significant alterations in patient positioning.

Principles of patient positioning

If the doctor does not comprehend or apply principles of patient positioning, the risk of developing tension at undesired levels is increased. Although one approach is not necessarily superior to the other, each method has unique attributes that may make it more appropriate in certain circumstances. To make the appropriate distinction and effectively deliver adjustments, the doctor must have a clear understanding of each method's unique mechanical characteristics and differences. For example, a thrust delivered against the left L3 mammillary of a patient lying on the right side with shoulders in neutral may not have the same mechanical effect as in the patient whose shoulders are rotated toward the table into left rotation.

With the patient in the neutral position, the thrust against the left L3 mammillary is typically applied to induce right rotation of L3 relative to L4 (Fig. 4.21). If the same thrust is delivered with the patient's shoulders rotated into left rotation (resisted position), then maximal tension and cavitation may be induced in left rotation at the ipsilateral articulation above

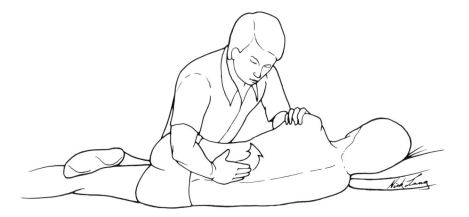

Figure 4.21 Typical adjustment to induce right rotation of L3 relative to L4 using a mammillary contact (neutral position).

(L2–L3). If the physician wishes to induce right rotation at the L3–L4 motion segment with an adjustive technique that involves shoulder counterrotation and a mammillary contact, then the patient should be placed on the opposite side (left) with a mammillary contact established at L4 instead of L3 (Fig. 4.22).

Adjustive Contacts and Vectors

Adjustive contacts specify the placement of the doctor's hands during the delivery of an adjustment. Adjustive vectors describe the direction of the adjustive thrust. Errors in the placement of adjustive contacts or orientation of adjustive vectors may have dramatic effects on adjustive specificity and effectiveness, even if all the appropriate steps have been taken to ensure appropriate patient positioning and preadjustive tension. If the adjustive contacts are established at inappropriate levels, maximal distractive tension and cavitation may not be induced at the intended joint. Similarly, adjustive vectors aimed in inappropriate directions may induce joint compression instead of distraction or cavitation at undesired levels.

For example, if a loss of vertical glide at the T5–T6 motion segment is to be treated with a prone adjustment, a contact should be established at T5 with an adjustive vector directed anteriorly and superiorly. If the contact is

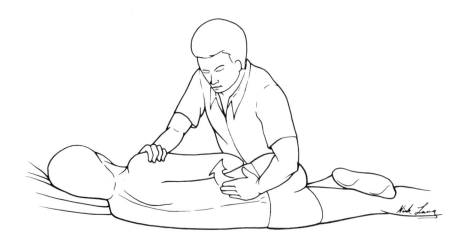

Figure 4.22 If a resisted method is used to induce right rotation of L3 relative to L4, a contact is established on the right mammillary of L4 with the patient lying on the left side instead of the right.

inadvertently established at T6, then distraction may occur at the T6–T7 motion segment instead of T5–T6. If the adjustive thrust is delivered incorrectly and directed too anteriorly, then unnecessary compression is directed to the facet joints and cavitation may occur at the joint above the desired level.

Adjustive Specificity

Application of the principles of patient positioning and joint localization does not ensure that adjustive setups and thrusts will produce movement only at the desired level. The spine is a closed kinetic chain, making it highly unlikely that spinal movements can be induced at one joint at a time. Any adjustive thrust will have some effect on the other components of the three-joint complex and the joints above and below the contacted vertebrae. The goal is not to eliminate all adjacent movement but to stress the skills that increase the probability of producing specific joint cavitation at the desired level, while minimizing movement and tension at adjacent joints. Joint cavitation usually occurs at the end range of passive joint movement, and it may be possible to induce joint cavitation in one joint without cavitating adjacent joints.

DEFINITION OF ADJUSTIVE TECHNIQUE PSYCHOMOTOR SKILLS

There is a wide range of adjustive procedures within the chiropractic profession, some are unique to the profession, and some are practiced by a wide variety of manual therapists. Several of the technique approaches are practiced as a package or system (Appendix 4). They are often the product of clinical practice and usually include multiple procedures of assessment. It is not uncommon for chiropractors to limit their practice to one of these many systems or approaches. We feel that the adherence to one methodologic approach may be a disadvantage. A therapy or technique that works for one patient or problem may not work on a different problem or patient. An integrated approach that incorporates alternative technique approaches may provide effective options. Adjustive technique is a psychomotor skill that requires personal development and modification. Limiting alternatives to one approach may exclude techniques that fit the physical characteristics of the doctor or the patient.

Although some techniques differ dramatically, most thrust techniques share common basic mechanical characteristics and psychomotor skills. To effectively perform adjustive techniques, the chiropractor must have a foundation in these common principles and psychomotor skills.

Patient Position

Patient position (PP) denotes the placement of the patient before the delivery of an adjustment. The standard options are prone, supine, standing, sitting, knee–chest, and side posture. The type of adjusting table used, the position of the table's sectional pieces, and the appropriate use of any additional pillows, rolls, and so on are discussed in this section. When indicated, the positioning of the extremities is described to ensure proper segmental tension. Whenever possible, allow patients to position themselves. Do not rush to move patients around; it is uncomfortable for them and potentially hard on your back.

As previously described, patient positioning is critical to the development of joint preadjustive tension, adjustive specificity, and efficiency. Adjustive specificity and efficiency are products of adjustive leverage, preadjustive tissue resistance, and joint locking. All these factors in turn depend on patient positioning. Increased tissue resistance and locking of adjacent joints are developed by inducing opposing forces and through nonneutral patient positioning. By positioning the joint to be distracted at the apex of secondarily established curves, joint distraction is increased, and the dysfunctional joint is set up as the weak link (Fig. 4.17).

Equipment Varieties and Management

A wide range of specialized adjusting tables and equipment is available to enhance patient comfort and adjustive efficiency (Fig. 4.23). Table options include flat benches, articulated tables, elevation tables, high–low tables, knee–chest tables, manual and automatic distraction tables, and drop tables. Some of the equipment is designed for the application of specific techniques, but most tables may be used with any of the common adjustive methods.

Regardless of the equipment used, some general habits should be developed. Select a table height advantageous to your physical attributes, use clean face paper on the head piece of the adjusting table, and regularly apply a disinfectant to the table. The appropriate table height will vary, depending on the patient's size, your specific physical attributes, and the area being adjusted. The average table height for pelvic, lumbar, and thoracic adjusting is the distance from the floor to the middle or superior aspect of your knee. For supine cervical adjusting, a higher table may be selected to minimize the stress on your back.

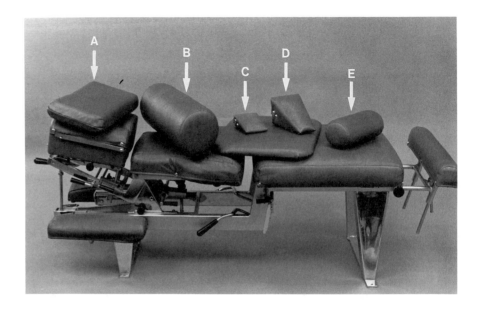

Figure 4.23 Specialized tables and equipment are used to enhance patient comfort and adjusting efficiency. (**A**) Headrest pillow. (**B**) Pelvic or Dutchman's roll. (**C**) Dorsal or pediatric block. (**D**) Pelvic block. (**E**) Sternal roll.

Adjusting bench

An adjusting bench (Fig. 4.24) is a padded, flat table with a face slot. It typically has a brachial cut-out to allow comfortable placement of the patient's shoulders in prone positions (Fig. 4.24A & B). A pelvic bench is very similar to the standard adjusting bench. It is typically wider than the articulated adjusting tables and lacks the brachial cut-out commonly incorporated in other adjusting benches (Fig. 4.24C). A Dutchman's roll or cylindrical cushion is used to achieve the same effects as raising the thoracic and pelvic pieces on an articulated table (Fig. 4.24D).

Articulated and hydraulic tables

An articulated table has movable head, thoracic, pelvic, and foot pieces to properly accommodate the patient in both the prone, side posture, and supine positions (Fig. 4.25A). Elevation tables have the ability to adjust to variable heights for different procedures as well as for different-sized doctors (Fig. 4.25B & C). High–low tables tilt from a vertical to a horizontal position making it easier for a patient to get on and off the table (Fig. 4.25D).

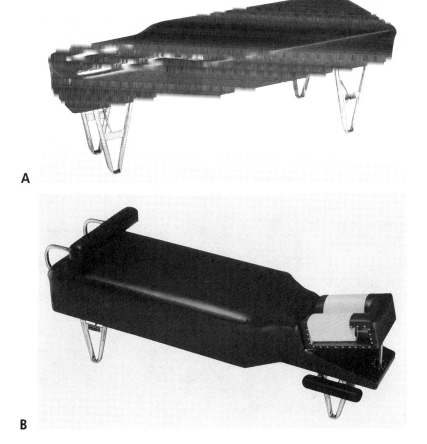

A

B

Figure 4.24 **(A, B)** Typical adjusting benches. (*Figure continues.*)

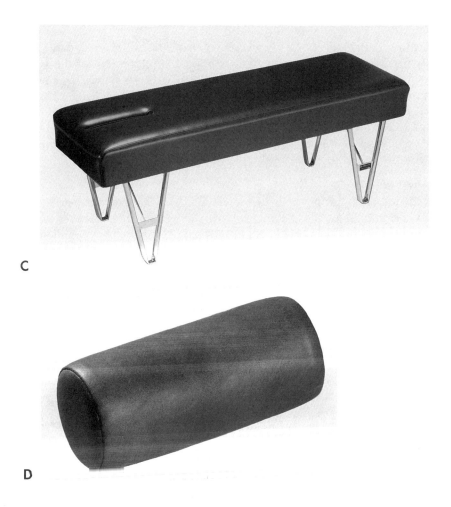

C

Fig. 4.24 (*Continued*). (**C**) Pelvic bench. (**D**) Dutchman's roll. (Photos courtesy of Lloyd Table Company, Lisbon, IA.)

D

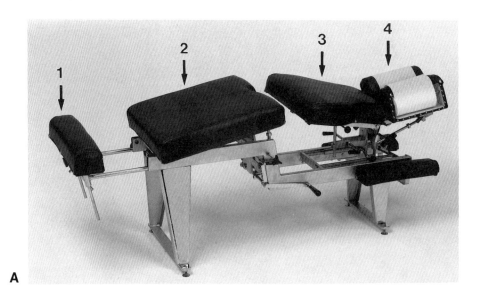

Figure 4.25   Articulated and hydraulic tables. (**A**) Stationary: (1) footrest; (2) pelvic section; (3) thoracic section; (4) headrest. (*Figure continues.*)

A

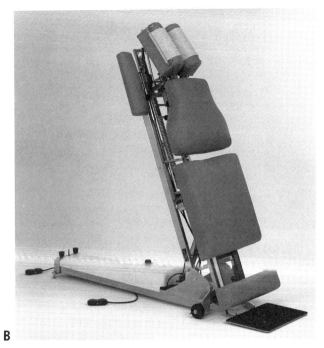

B

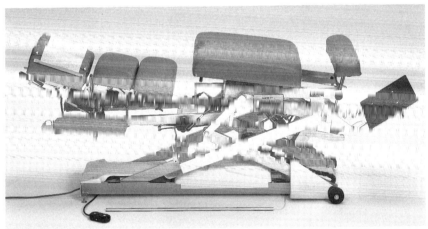

C

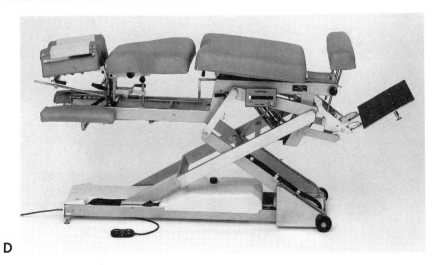

D

Fig. 4.25 (*Continued*). (**B**) Vertical to horizontal tilt. (**C & D**) Elevation to variable heights. (Photos courtesy of Lloyd Table Company, Lisbon, IA.)

To position the patient in the supine position on an articulating table, close and elevate the headrest and lower all other sections to a level position. When performing cervical or upper thoracic adjusting, the headpiece may be lowered. For prone positioning, to achieve a relaxed neutral posture, elevate the footrest, pelvic, and thoracic sections slightly and lower the headrest. Position the patient on the table with the anterior superior iliac spines over the peak formed by the raised pelvic and thoracic sections. The patient's shoulders should not touch the headrest.

Knee–chest table

The knee–chest table (Fig. 4.26) gets its name from the position the patient assumes when on the table. The chest and face are supported by a head or chest piece with the lower trunk unsupported. The patient's knees rest on the base of the table, while the spine remains parallel to the floor.[181] This table is especially useful in treating lower thoracic and lumbar extension restrictions and for those patients with large abdomens for whom the prone position is uncomfortable. Patients beyond the first trimester of pregnancy will be more comfortable and have less anxiety in the knee–chest position than prone when having posterior to anterior thrusts applied to the lower back. Cervical, thoracic, and lumbar techniques can be performed in this position. Take caution when using this position to avoid hyperextension with potential injury to the posterior joints and overstretch of the abdominal wall.

Using an articulated table, one can achieve a similar position either by raising the pelvic piece and allowing the thoracic piece to drop away or by having the patient kneel on a pillow at the head end of the table with the face on the headrest and forearms on the armrests. The kneeling modification should be used only in unusual circumstances.

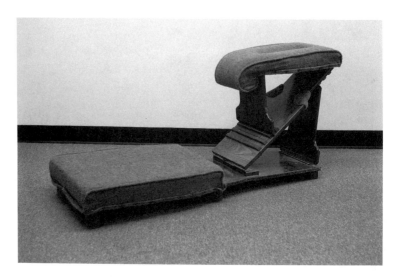

Figure 4.26 Knee–chest table.

Drop tables

Mechanical drop pieces are available on any or all of the sections of an articulated table (Fig. 4.27). Drop mechanisms allow for the elevation of sectional pieces and the subsequent free fall of those sections when sufficient

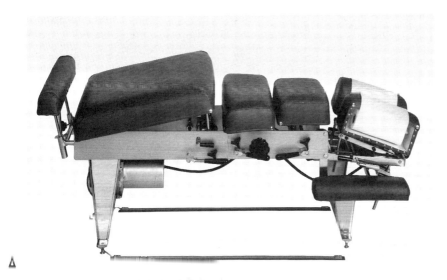

A

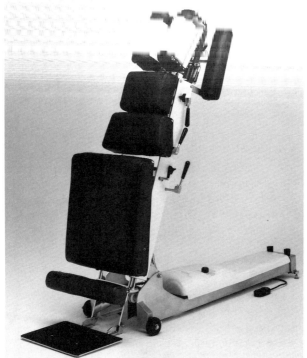

B

Figure 4.27   Mechanical drop pieces on an articulated table. (**A**) Stationary: (1) pelvic section cocking lever; (2) lumbar section cocking lever; (3) thoracic section cocking lever; (4) cervical section cocking lever. (**B**) High-low. (Photos courtesy of Lloyd Table Company, Lisbon, IA.)

adjustive force is applied against the patient. The drop sections elevate a fixed amount (approximately one-half inch), but the degree of resistive tension varies. Before delivering an adjustment, cock and elevate the drop piece and establish the appropriate degree of resistive tension. The amount of tension varies, depending on the size of the patient, the extent of established preadjustive tension, and the force of the adjustive thrust. Do not ascertain the degree of tension established in the drop mechanism by thrusting against the patient. Determine tension by placing the patient on the table and thrusting against the table, not the patient.

Although no supporting clinical data exist, drop-piece mechanisms have been promoted as a technology for increasing adjustive efficiency. One claim suggests that the degree of adjustive muscular effort and force may be reduced because the drop of the table decreases the counterresistance of the table and the patient. The other assertion is that the adjustive thrust is enhanced by the counterreactive force generated across the joint when adjustive thrusts are maintained through the impact of the drop piece. One of the potential disadvantages of the drop mechanism is the noise generated during the dropping action, which makes it difficult to perceive specific joint movement with the thrust.

Distraction tables

The distraction table (Fig. 4.28) offers a form of mechanical assistance for the application of manual therapy by having a fully movable pelvic section. The mobile pelvic piece provides a long-lever action that can place the lumbar spine through the normal individual ranges of motion of flexion, extension, lateral flexion, and rotation as well as the combined movement of circumduction. Some procedures use a manual contact and a manual leverage to create distraction, holding the segment in sustained long-axis traction. Other tables have a motorized pelvic section that can provide a continuous passive movement to the spinal segments and their soft tissues in general. Many of these tables include ankle straps, which should be used for patient safety when the pelvic section is rotated. Take caution not to use excessive flexion with segmental distraction, because this can have a negative effect on the posterior portion of the disc.

Cervical chair

The cervical chair (Fig. 4.29) is a padded chair with a movable backrest. The backrest is adjusted so that the patient's spine remains straight and the area to be adjusted lies just below the doctor's forearm when the elbow is flexed to 90 degrees. The patient should sit with legs comfortably straightened and hands relaxed on the thighs.

Doctor's Position

Doctor's position (DP) denotes the doctor's stance and position in relation to the adjusting table and patient. It is critical to select an appropriate table height to maintain a balanced and relaxed stance. If the table is too high, you are at a mechanical disadvantage, and if the table is too low, unnecessary stress may be applied to your back. Place your center of gravity as close as

Principles of Adjustive Technique 177

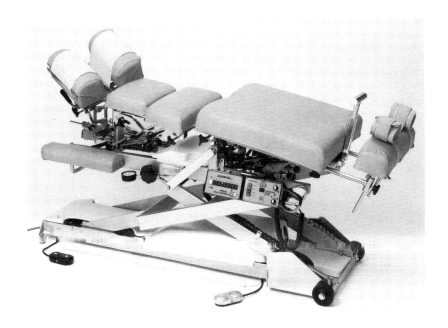

Figure 4.28 Distraction table. (Photo courtesy of Lloyd Table Company, Lisbon, IA.)

possible to the segmental contact point, and whenever appropriate, use body weight to maintain preadjustive joint tension

The productive use of your weight and positioning is essential to your protection and efficient adjusting. Chiropractic is a physical profession, and to avoid fatigue and injury, sound body mechanism must be practiced. Whenever possible, use gravity and body weight to produce preadjustive tension and movement. This helps minimize muscular effort and fatigue. Maintain a neutral spinal posture by bending at the knees, hips, and abducting the thighs when adapting to table height. As much as possible, your legs should bear the workload, thereby protecting your own back.

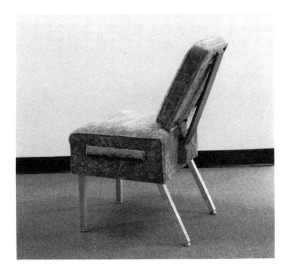

Figure 4.29 Cervical chair.

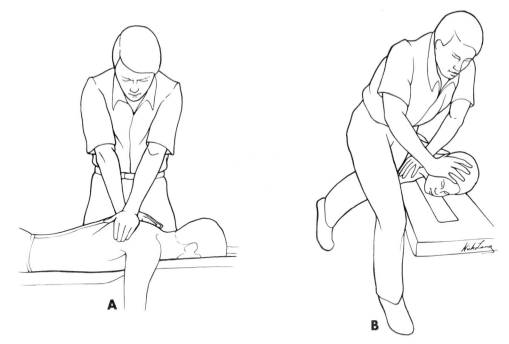

Figure 4.30 Illustration of two common doctor positions; (**A**) the square stance and (**B**) the fencer's stance, or lunge position.

The effective use of body weight can minimize the effort expended in developing preadjustive tension and in delivering an adjustive thrust. By increasing the mass behind the adjustive thrust, force can be increased during the adjustment without increasing the velocity.[176–179] Placing your center of gravity behind the line of drive allows you to transfer appropriate body weight into the adjustive setup and thrust. Using body weight and leg strength saves energy for the adjustive thrust and permits the upper extremities to remain more relaxed. Various named stances have been used to describe adjustive techniques. Figure 4.30 illustrates two of the common stances; other modifications are discussed and illustrated in the regional sections on adjusting.

Contact Point

The contact point (CP) designates which hand is the thrusting hand and the specific area of the hand that will develop the actual patient contact. The contact point may be described anatomically or by a numbering convention developed to represent the common contact points (Fig. 4.31). This text describes the contacts anatomically.

Indifferent Hand

The indifferent hand (IH) specifies which hand is used to stabilize the patient, fixate adjacent joints, or reinforce the contact hand, as well as how the patient is to be contacted and what additional forces are necessary to maintain positioning and stabilization.

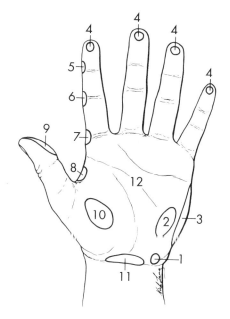

Figure 4.31 Contact points on the hand; (1) pisiform; (2) hypothenar; (3) metacarpal, or knife-edge; (4) digital, used typically with the index and middle fingers; (5) distal interphalangeal (DIP); (6) proximal interphalangeal (PIP); (7) metacarpophalangeal (MP), or index; (8) web; (9) thumb; (10) thenar; (11) calcaneal; (12) palmar.

The indifferent hand is not always passive during the delivery of an adjustment. There are circumstances when the indifferent hand moves from the realm of stabilization into either assisting or counterresisting an adjustment. In the accompanying illustrations, an arrow is used to demonstrate adjustive vectors and a triangle is used to demonstrate stabilization points (Fig. 4.32).

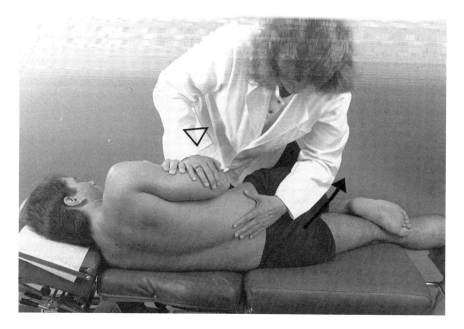

  represents point of stabilization

represents adjustive force and vector

Figure 4.32 Arrows indicate adjustive vectors; a triangle indicates stabilization.

Segmental Contact Point

The segmental contact point (SCP) specifies anatomically where the adjustive contact or contacts are to be established on the patient. The segmental contact point or points are listed and described specifically in this chapter and in Chapters 5 and 6. Where possible, they are illustrated in photographs or drawings. The SCPs are typically bony landmarks located close to the joint to be distracted. Adjustive contacts established at the level of the dysfunctional joint are referred to as *short-lever (direct) adjustments*. Adjustive contacts established at some distance from the level of the dysfunctional joint are referred to as *long-lever (indirect)* adjustments, and adjustments that combine short and long lever contacts are referred to as *semidirect*.

In spinal adjusting, a single thrusting contact is conventionally taken on the superior vertebrae of the dysfunctional motion segment. Methods that incorporate thrusting contacts on the lower vertebra or both vertebrae of the involved motion segment are also effective and in common use (see Figs. 4.33 and 4.39).

Remember that the drawings depicting bony contact points are intended to be illustrative. Segmental contacts focused at specific bony landmarks cannot be established without contacting overlying or adjacent soft tissues, and the site of segmental contact can be only as diminutive as the size of the doctor's contact point (see Fig. 4.33).

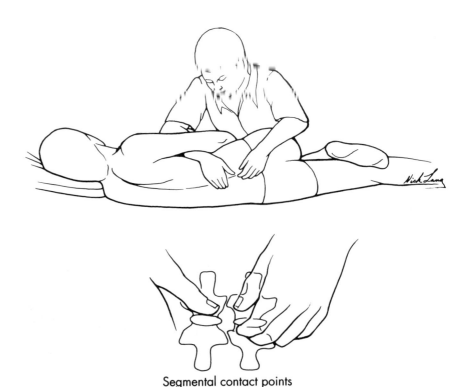

Figure 4.33 Segmental contact points are bony landmarks located close to the joint(s) to be adjusted. In this illustration, segmental contacts are illustrated for a spinous push-pull adjustment.

Segmental contact points

Tissue Pull

A superficial tissue pull is typically taken during the establishment of an adjustive contact. Proper tissue pulls are necessary to ensure that a firm contact is established before a thrust is delivered. If this is not taken into consideration, the contact point may slip during the thrust and dissipate the force or negate the specificity of the adjustment. The indifferent hand may be used to draw the tissue slack as the contact point is established. Tissue pulls are invariably initiated in the direction of the adjustive thrust and as such will not be listed separately.

Vector (Line of Drive)

The vector (V) denotes the direction of the adjustive thrust. The direction of adjustive thrust is usually described in anatomic terms. An adjustive vector delivered in the prone position with a downward and cephalic orientation is described as a posterior to anterior (P/A) and inferior to superior (I/S) vector. Adjustive vectors are illustrated by solid arrows (see Fig. 4.32).

Attention to vector alignment is necessary to ensure anatomically sound, specific, and efficient adjustments. To produce joint distraction and movement without producing injury, one must have knowledge of the functional anatomy and kinematics and match the adjustive vector accordingly. The adjustment must be delivered within the limits of physiologic movement to prevent injury. Knowledge of the articular facet facings and how joint surfaces glide in relation to each other during movement (arthrokinematic movements) is critical to effective adjusting.

A single adjustive thrust and cavitation may not free multiple directions of joint restriction.[182] Therefore, at times, a single articulation may be adjusted in multiple directions, with different adjustive vectors applied for each adjustive thrust.

Thrust

The adjustive thrust can be defined as the application of a controlled directional force, the delivery of which effects (or constitutes) an adjustment. The adjustive vector describes the direction of applied force; the adjustive thrust refers to the production and implementation of that force. The adjustive force is typically generated through a combination of practitioner muscular effort and body weight transfer. The chiropractic adjustive thrust is a ballistic, high-velocity, low-amplitude force designed to induce joint distraction and cavitation without exceeding the limits of anatomic joint motion.

Adjustive thrusts are traditionally divided into two physical forms, distinguished by whether the adjustment is delivered with or without an active recoil.[183] They are often further categorized by whether they are delivered with the joint in a relatively neutral position or toward its end range of motion at the elastic barrier.

Recoil thrust

The recoil thrust involves the application of a high-velocity, low-amplitude ballistic force, characterized by the delivery of an active thrust coupled with a passive recoil. It is produced by inducing rapid elbow extension and

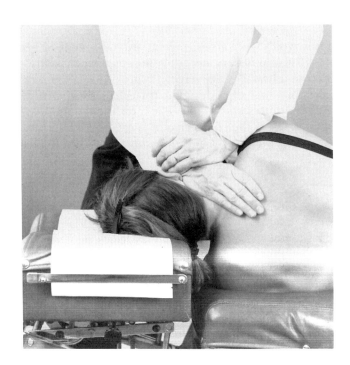

Figure 4.34 The recoil thrust is induced by quickly contracting and immediately relaxing the pectoral muscles and elbow extensors simultaneously.

shoulder adduction followed by passive elbow flexion. The active thrust is induced by simultaneously contacting the pectoral muscles and extensor muscles of the elbows. The recoil is induced by rapid cessation of the thrust and the elastic rebound that results from impact with the patient and the stretch of the doctor's arms[15] (Fig. 4.34). This method typically involves unilateral hand contacts while the other hand reinforces the contact hand. Both arms thrust equally during the delivery of the adjustment; the vector is determined by the orientation of the doctor's episternal notch relative to the contact point. This thrust is most commonly delivered with the joint placed in a neutral position.

Impulse thrust (dynamic thrust)

Impulse thrusts also employ a high-velocity, low-amplitude force but do not involve a recoil. The velocity may be varied, with either a slow or fast termination. This thrust is most commonly delivered at the elastic barrier, but it may also be delivered from a neutral starting position. When delivered from a neutral starting position, articular slack is removed before the delivery of the thrust. Thrusts delivered at the elastic barrier are accomplished by positioning the joint at the end of its passive range of motion. A high-velocity, low-amplitude thrust is then delivered to induce joint cavitation and paraphysiologic movement (Fig. 4.35).

Impulse thrusts may be delivered through one arm or both arms. When one arm is used, the hand of the other arm becomes the indifferent hand and either reinforces the contact or stabilizes the patient at another site. When used for stabilization, the indifferent hand can maintain the patient

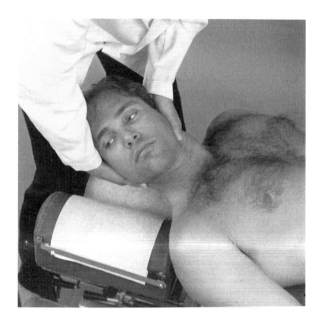

Figure 4.35 An impulse thrust is a high velocity, low amplitude force with no recoil.

in a neutral position or induce positions or forces that assist or resist the adjustive force.

All adjustive thrusts involve relatively high-velocity forces but vary in the degree of associated body weight coupled with the adjustment. Where less mass and total force are desired, the thrust is typically delivered only through the upper extremities. This is commonly the case in the cervical spine and involves adjustments delivered through the wrists, elbows, and shoulders. When more total force is desired, the doctor transfers additional weight from the trunk and/or pelvis into the adjustive thrust. This is accomplished by flexing the trunk and/or knees and hips during the delivery of an adjustment. The adjustive force is generated through the upper extremities and is typically reinforced by a simultaneous contraction of the abdominal muscles and diaphragm. Faye[184] has described this as a process similar to the event that occurs during sneezing or spitting.

In prone thoracic, lumbar, and pelvic adjusting, the thrust is commonly delivered by combining an impulse through the upper extremities with a body drop thrust through the trunk. Prone adjustments may also be delivered primarily through the trunk by locking the doctor's arms and dropping at the trunk and hips.

Lumbar and pelvic side posture adjustments, which commonly demand more total force, invariably involve the transfer of trunk and pelvic weight into the adjustive thrust. This is accomplished by coupling an impulse thrust with a drop of the trunk, pelvis, and lower exremities by flexing the knees and hips.

A common technique variation in side posture lumbar adjusting couples a segmental contact with a reinforcing thrust through the doctor's leg. Instead of the doctor's weight resting against the patient's upper thigh and hip, a contact on the patient's knee is established. The impulse is then

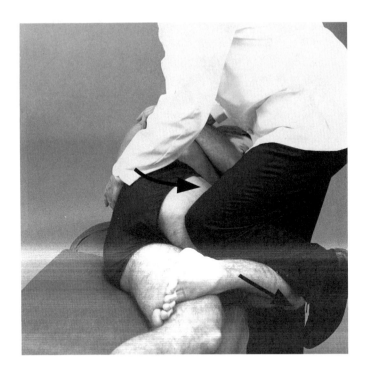

Figure 4.36 Long levers (upper leg) and short levers (spinous process) can be combined to deliver a segmental impulse thrust.

delivered by combining a pulling impulse through the arm with a quick extension of the doctor's knee (Fig. 4.36). In this method, the leg provides the additional leverage and force instead of the doctor's body weight.

Although for didactic purpose it is useful to separate the adjustive thrust into its component parts, it can be misleading and distracting to the student who is trying to perfect the art of adjusting. Instead of focusing on the act as a singular event, the novice often tries to develop a thrust by mentally producing each event separately, resulting in an unfocused, uncoordinated thrust. The experienced thrust, developed through repetitive practice, is a fluid procedure done reflexively or habitually and not as a series of steps.

Assisted and resisted thrusts

Assisted and resisted thrusts are not to be confused with assisted and resisted patient positions. *Assisted and resisted positions* refer to the placement of the patient before the delivery of an adjustment. *Assisted and resisted thrusts* refer to thrusts delivered through both arms.

When both arms are active in producing an adjustive force, the thrust may be equally or unequally distributed and may be delivered in the same direction or opposing directions. When both arms thrust in the same direction, an assisted thrust occurs, and both adjustive forces induce movement in the direction of joint restriction. In spinal adjustments, this approach involves methods that apply additional assisting forces through contacts established on the superior vertebra of the dysfunctional motion segment.

The treatment of a thoracic rotational dysfunction with a sitting thoracic adjustment illustrates this approach. This technique incorporates a segmen-

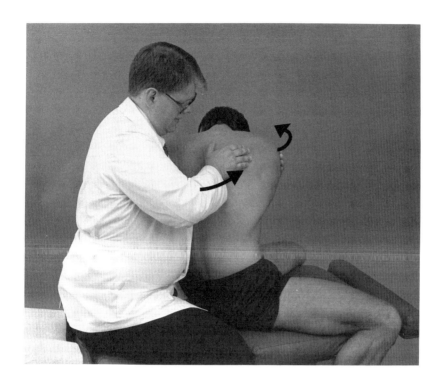

Figure 4.37 An example of an assisted thrust has the patient's trunk rotated in the direction of joint restriction (away from the malposition), with the adjustive force applied to the superior vertebra in the direction of joint restriction.

tal contact on the transverse process of the superior vertebrae of the dysfunctional motion segment with an assisting hand contact on the opposite
forearm (Fig. 4.37). When performing the adjustment, rotate the patient in
the direction of joint restriction (away from the malposition) and induce a
thrust by both the contact hand and the assisting hand.

Thrusts delivered against the direction of joint restriction may also effectively be applied, but they are less common and harder to visualize. This
method is most commonly applied in the lumbar spine and involves a
segmental contact on the inferior vertebra of the dysfunctional motion
segment with an additional contact established inferiorly on the patient's
leg. The vertebral segments above the contact are rotated in the direction
of restriction, opposite the direction of the thrust, and preadjustive tension
is localized to the articulation above the contact. At tension, a thrust is
delivered to the lower contacts, but cavitation and movement are generated
in the direction of restriction at the articulation above the contact.

This method is effectively illustrated by the treatment of a right rotational
restriction at L4–L5 with a side posture spinous pull adjustment (Fig. 4.38).
When applying this method, the doctor places the patient on the left side
and establishes a fingertip contact on the left side of the L5 spinous process.
The patient's right shoulder is stressed posteriorly, creating right posterior
trunk rotation. Simultaneously, the patient's pelvis is drawn anteriorly by
the pressure of the doctor's leg on the patient's right knee, developing
counterrotation. At the point of articular tension, a pulling thrust is delivered through the contact arm as the doctor quickly extends the knee, increas-

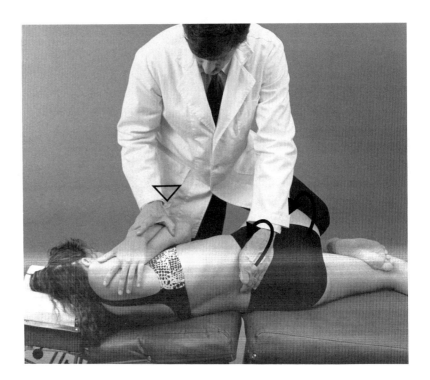

Figure 4.38 An example of a resisted thrust has the patient's trunk rotated in the direction opposite to joint restriction (toward the malposition) with the adjustive force applied to the inferior vertebra in the direction opposite the joint restriction.

ing the pelvic rotation. The resisting thrusts are generated through the vertebral contact along with your leg instead of your other hand.

Counterthrusts

Counterthrust techniques are delivered in opposing directions to maximize the motion across a given joint. In the spine, this procedure is most commonly applied in the treatment of rotational dysfunction. The side posture lumbar spinous push pull technique is an example of a resisted counterthrust technique (Fig. 4.39). During this procedure, the contacts are established on adjacent spinous processes and the superior arm thrusts in the direction of restriction as the inferior arm thrusts in the direction opposite the restriction.

Nonpause thrust

Following the removal of articular slack, a thrust may be delivered with or without a pause. When the thrust is performed without a pause, the slack is removed, and the thrust is delivered by accelerating and thrusting at the point of appropriate tension. An illustrated example is a wave crashing on the beach; removal of slack relates to the wave rolling toward the beach, and the thrust corresponds to the wave breaking against the shoreline. This approach is effective in maintaining adjustive momentum and avoiding patient guarding.

Pause thrust

When thrusts are performed with a pause, the doctor takes a moment to assess the degree of established joint tension and tissue resistance before

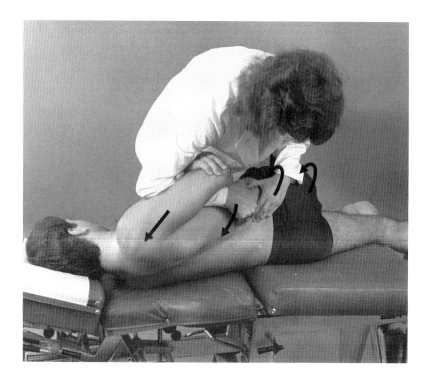

Figure 4.39 A counter thrust is delivered in opposing directions to maximize distraction across a specific joint.

Table 4.10 Basic Rules for Effective Adjustive Technique

1. Select the most efficient and specific technique for the primary problem.
2. Position the patient in a balanced, relaxed, and mechanically efficient position.
3. The doctor should be relaxed and balanced with his or her center of gravity as close to the contact points as possible.
4. The contacts should be taken correctly and specifically.
5. Articular and soft tissue slack should be removed before thrusting.
6. Any minor alterations in position or tension should be made before thrusting.
7. Visualize the structures contacted and the direction of your adjustive vector.
8. Guard against the loss of established preadjustive joint tension. Do not noticeably back off before thrusting.
9. The thrust must be delivered with optimum velocity and appropriate depth.
10. During the thrust, use additional body weight where appropriate (body drop). This is especially important in side posture pelvic and lumbar adjusting, where most of the adjustive force is derived from a body-drop thrust.
11. It is just as important to know when not to adjust as to know when and where to adjust.
12. *Primo est non nocere*—First, do no harm.

thrusting. This allows testing of the setup and evaluation of the patient's responses to tension and pressure. If sufficient articular slack has not been removed or if abnormal binding induces patient discomfort, the doctor may modify the degree of preadjustive tension or the adjustive vector before applying the thrust. Following the pause, the doctor raises off the patient slightly to regain momentum and apply body weight into the thrust. During this process it is critical to maintain the established preadjustive tension through the hands and points of secondary contact. It may be appropriate to back off the point of restriction very slightly, so the thrust can be directed at the point of restriction and not too deeply into the joint's anatomic limits. However, if the doctor loses too much tension, the thrust can become nonfocused and uncomfortable.

Remember that any procedure that has the potential to do good has the potential for harm. Table 4.10 lists some basic rules or principles for the effective and safe use of chiropractic adjustive technique.

REFERENCES

1. Lamm LC, Wegner E: Chiropractic scope of practice: what the law allows. Am J Chiro Med 2(4):155, 1989

2. Department of Statistics: 1985 Survey. J Am Chiro Assoc 23(2):68, 1986

3. Commission of Inquiry Into Chiropractic: Chiropractic in New Zealand. Reprinted by Palmer College of Chiropractic, 1979

4. Vear HJ: Standards of chiropractic practice. J Manipulative Physiol Ther 8(1):33, 1985

5. Nyiendo J, Haldeman S: A prospective study of 2,000 patients attending a chiropractic college teaching clinic. Med Care 25(6):516, 1987

6. Kelner M, Hall O, Coulter I: Chiropractors: Do they help? Fitzhenry & Whiteside Ltd, Toronto, 1980

7. Shekelle PG, Brook RH: A community-based study of the use of chiropractic services. Am J Public Health 81(4):439, 1991

8. ACA Council on Technic: Chiropractic terminology—a report. J Am Chiro Assoc 25(10):46, 1988

9. Bergmann TF: The chiropractic spinal examination. p. 97. In Ferezy JS (ed): The Chiropractic Neurological Examination. Aspen Publishers, Rockville, MD, 1992

10. Vear HJ: Introduction. p. 1. In Vear HJ (ed): Chiropractic Standards of Practice and Quality of Care. Aspen Publishers, Rockville, MD, 1992

11. Bartol KM: A model for the categorization of chiropractic treatment procedures. J Chiro Tech 3(2):78, 1991

12. Palmer DD: Textbook of the Science, Art and Philosophy of Chiropractic. Portland Printing House, Portland, OR, 1910

13. Stephenson RW: The Art of Chiropractic. Palmer School of Chiropractic, 1947.

14. Levine M: The Structural Approach to Chiropractic. Comet Press, New York, 1964, p. 85.

15. Sandoz R: Some physical mechanisms and affects of spinal adjustments. Ann Swiss Chirop Assoc 6:91, 1976

16. Bartol KM: Algorithm for the categorization of chiropractic technic procedures. J Chiro Tech 4(1):8, 1992

17. Bartol KM: The categorization of chiropractic procedures. p. 24. In: Proceedings of the Sixth Annual Conference on Research and Education. Monterey, CA, 1991

18. Osterbauer PJ, Fuhr AW: The current status of activator methods chiropractic technique, theory, and training. J Chiro Tech 2:168, 1990

19. Greenman PE: Principles of soft tissue and articulatory (mobilization with impulse) technique. p. 71. In: Principles of Manual Medicine. Williams & Wilkins, Baltimore, 1989

20. Maigne R: Personal method: the rule of no pain and free movement. p. 137. In: Orthopedic Medicine: A New Approach to Vertebral Manipulations. Bannerstone House. Springfield, IL, 1972

21. Wood KW: Acute torticollis: Chiropractic therapy and management. Chir Tech 3:3, 1991

22. Hammond B: Torticollis. Eur J Chiro 31(3):162, 1983

23. Triano JJ: The subluxation complex: outcome measure of chiropractic diagnosis and treatment. J Chiro Tech 2(3):114, 1990

24. Kirkaldy-Willis WH: The pathology and pathogenesis of low back pain (Ch. 5). The three phases of the spectrum of degenerative disease (Ch. 8). In Kirkaldy-Willis WH (ed): Managing Low Back Pain. 3rd Ed. Churchill Livingstone, New York, 1992

25. Phillips RB, Howe JW, Bustin G et al: Stress x-rays and the low back pain patient. J Manipulative Physiol Ther 13:127, 1990

26. Haas M, Nyiendo J, Peterson C et al: Lumbar motion trends and correlation with low back pain. Part I. A roentgenological evaluation of coupled lumbar motion in lateral bending. J Manipulative Physiol Ther 15:145, 1992

27. Haas M, Nyiendo J: Lumbar motion trends and correlation with low back pain. Part II. A roentgenological evaluation of quantitative segmental motion in lateral bending. J Manipulative Physiol Ther 15:224, 1992

28. Haas M, Peterson D: A roentgenological evaluation of the relationship between segmental mal-alignment and motion in lateral bending. J Manipulative Physiol Ther (in press)

29. Kirkaldy-Willis WH, Cassidy JD: Spinal manipulation in the treatment of low back pain. Can Fam Physician 31:535, 1985

30. Peters RE: The facet syndrome. J Aust Chiro Assoc 13(3):15, 1983

31. Guebert GM: Standards for contraindications to spinal manipulative therapy. In Vear HJ (ed): Chiropractic Standards of Practice and Quality of Care. Aspen Publishers, Baltimore, MD, 1992

32. Gatterman MI: Contraindications and complications of spinal manipulative therapy. J Am Chiro Assoc 15:75, 1981

33. Maigne R: p. 168. In: Orthopedic Medicine: A New Approach to Vertebral Manipulations. Bannerstone House, Springfield, IL, 1972

34. Shekelle PG, Adams AH: The Appropriateness of Spinal Manipulation for Low-Back Pain: Project Overview and Literature Review. RAND Corp, Santa Monica, CA, 1991

35. Ladermann JP: Accidents of spinal manipulations. Ann Swiss Chiro Assoc 7:161, 1981

36. Brewerton DA: Conservative treatment of painful neck. Proc R Soc Med 57:16, 1964

37. Kleynhans AM: Complications of and contraindications to spinal manipulative therapy. p. 359. In Haldeman S (ed): Modern Developments in the Principles and Practice of Chiropractic. Appleton-Century-Crofts, East Norwalk, CT, 1980

38. Schafer RC: Chiropractic Physician's Handbook. Clinical Malpractice: Basic Preventive and Defensive Procedures. National Chiropractic Mutual Insurance, Des Moines

39. Terrett AGJ: Vascular accidents from cervical spinal manipulation: a report of 107 cases. J Aust Chiro Assoc 17:15, 1987

40. Bland JH: Disorders of the Cervical Spine. WB Saunders, Philadelphia, 1987

41. Toole JF, Tucker SH: Influence of head position upon cerebral circulation. Studies on blood flow in cadavers. Arch Neurol 2:616, 1960

42. Hardesty WH, Witcare WB, Toole JF et al: Studies on vertebral artery blood flow in man. Surg Gynecol Obstet 116:662, 1963

43. Farris AA, Poser CM, Wilmore DW, Agnew CH: Radiographic visualization of neck vessels in healthy men. Neurol 13:386, 1963

44. George PE: Identification of high risk pre-stroke patient. J Am Chiro Assoc 15(S):26, 1981

45. Terrett AGJ: Importance and interpretation of tests designed to predict susceptibility to neurocirculatory accidents from manipulation. J Am Chiro Assoc 13(2):2, 1983

46. Ferezy JS: Neural Ischemia and Cervical Spinal Manipulation. The Chiropractic Neurological Examination. Aspen Publishers, Rockville, MD, 1992

47. Darbert O, Freeman DG, Weis AJ: Spinal meningeal hematoma, warfarin therapy and chiropractic adjustment. JAMA 214:2058, 1970

48. Matthews JA, Yates DAH: Reduction of lumbar disc prolapse by manipulation. Br Med J 3:696, 1969

49. Jennet WB: A study of 25 cases of compression of the cauda equina by prolapsed IVD. J Neurol Neurosurg Psychiatry 19:109, 1956

50. Kane RL et al: Manipulating the patient: a comparison of the effectiveness of physician and chiropractor care. Lancet 1:1333, 1974

51. Cherkin DC, MacCornack FA: Health care delivery. Patient evaluations of low back pain care from family physicians and chiropractors. Zoes J Med 150(3):351, 1989

52. Cherkin DC, MacCornack FA, Berg AO: The management of low back pain—a comparison of the beliefs and behaviors of family physicians and chiropractors. West J Med 149:475, 1988

53. American Chiropractic Association: Comparison of Chiropractic and Medical Treatment of Nonoperative Back and Neck injuries 1976–77. American Chiropractic Association, Des Moines, IA, 1978

54. Brunarski DJ: Clinical trials of spinal manipulation: a critical appraisal and review of the literature. J Manipulative Physiol Ther 7(4):243, 1984

55. Nyiendo J: Chiropractic effectiveness. Series No. 1. Oregon Chiropractic Physicians Association Legislative Newsletter April 1991

56. Anderson R et al: A meta-analysis of clinical trials of spinal manipulation. J Manipulative Physiol Ther 15:181, 1992

57. Waagen GN, Haldeman S, Cook G: Short term trial of chiropractic adjustments for the relief of chronic low back pain. Manipulative Med 2:63, 1986

58. Meade TW, Dyer SD, Brown W: Low back pain of mechanical origin: randomised comparison of chiropractic and hospital outpatient treatment. Br Med J 300:1431, 1990

59. Nyiendo J: Disabling low back Oregon workers' compensation claims. Part III: Diagnosing and treatment procedures and associated costs. J Manipulative Physiol Ther 14(5):287, 1991

60. Greenwood JG: Work-related back and neck injury cases in West Virginia. Orthop Rev 14(2):51, 1985

61. Montgomery DP, Nelson JM: Evolution of chiropractic theories of practice and spinal adjustment, 1900–1950. Chiro History 5:71, 1985

62. Strasser A: The chiropractic model of health: a personal perspective. Dig Chiro Econ 13(2):12, 1988

63. Stonebrink RD: Evaluation and Manipulative Management of Common Musculo-Skeletal Disorders. Western States Chiropractic College, Portland, Oregon, 1990

64. Grieve GP: Aetiology in general terms. p. 175. In: Common Vertebral Joint Problems. Churchill Livingstone, Edinburgh, 1988

65. Kirkaldy-Willis WH: The pathology and pathogenesis of low back pain (Ch. 5). In Kirkaldy-Willis WH (ed): Managing Low Back Pain. 3rd Ed. Churchill Livingstone, New York, 1992

66. Cyriax J: Textbook of Orthopedic Medicine. Vol. I: Diagnosis of Soft Tissue Lesions. 8th Ed. Bailliere Tindall, London, 1982

67. Salter RB: The biologic concept of continuous passive motion of synovial joints. The first 18 years of basic research and its clinical application. Clin Orthop 242:12, 1989

68. Salter RB: Motion vs. rest: Why immobilize joints? J Bone Joint Surg [Br] 64:251, 1982

69. Gelberman R, Manske P, Akeson W: Kappa Delta Award paper: flexor tendon repair. J Orthop Res 4:119, 1986

70. Kellet J: Acute soft tissue injuries—a review of the literature. Med Sci Sports Exerc 18(5):489, 1986

71. Fitz-Ritson D: Chiropractic Management and Rehabilitation of Cervical Trauma. J Manipulative Physiol Ther 13(1):17, 1990

72. Waddell G: A new clinical model for the treatment of low-back pain. Spine 12(7):632, 1987

73. Mealy K, Brennan H et al: Early mobilization of acute whiplash injuries. Br Med J 292:656, 1986

74. Akeson W, Amiel D, Woo S: Immobility effects on synovial joints. The pathomechanics of joint contracture. Biorheology 17:95, 1980

75. Van Royen BJ, O'Driscoll SW, Wouter JAD: Comparison of the effects of immobilization and continuous passive motion on surgical wound healing in the rabbit. Plast Reconstr Surg 78:360, 1986

76. Amiel D, Woo S L-Y, Harwood F: The effect of immobilization on collagen turnover in connective tissue: a biomechanical–biochemical correlation. Acta Orthop Scand 53:325, 1982

77. Rubak JM, Poussa M, Ritsila V: Effects of joint motion on the repair of articular cartilage with free periosteal grafts. Acta Orthop Scand 53:187, 1982

78. McDonough AL: Effects of immobilization and exercise on articular cartilage—a review of literature. J Orthop Sports Phys Ther 3:2, 1981

79. Akeson WH, Amiel D, Mechanic GL: Collagen cross-linking alterations in joint contractures: changes in the reducible cross links in periarticular connective tissue collagen after nine weeks of immobilization. Connect Tissue Res 5:15, 1977

80. Woo S L-Y, Matthews JV, Akeson WH: Connective tissue response to immobility. Correlative study of biomechanical and biochemical measurements of normal and immobilized rabbit knees. Arthritis Rheum 18(3):257, 1975

81. Enneking WF, Horowitz M: The intra-articular effects of immobilization of the human knee. J Bone Joint Surg [Am] 54:973, 1972

82. Mayer T, Gatchel R: Functional Restoration for Spinal Disorders: The Sports Medicine Approach. Lea & Febiger, Philadelphia, 1988

83. Fordyce W, Roberts A, Sternbach R: The behavioral management of chronic pain: a response to critics. Pain 22:112, 1985

84. Schafer RC: Basic Chiropractic Procedural Manual. Emphasizing Geriatric Considerations. 4th Ed. American Chiropractic Assoc, Arlington, Virginia, 1984

85. Roston JB, Wheeler Haines R: Cracking in the metacarpophalangeal joint. J Anat 81:165, 1947

86. Sandoz R: The significance of the manipulative crack and of other articular noises. Ann Swiss Chiro Assoc 4:47, 1969

87. Herzog W: Biomechanical studies of spinal manipulative therapy. JCCA 35(3):156, 1991

88. Unsworth A, Dowson D, Wright V: Cracking joints. Ann Rheum Dis 30:348, 1971

89. Meal GM, Scott RA: Analysis of the joint crack by simultaneous recording of sound and tension. J Manipulative Physiol Ther 9(3):189, 1986

90. Harvey EN, McElroy WD, Whiteley AH: On cavity formation in water. J Appl Physics 18:162, 1947

91. Schmorl G, Junghans H: The Human Spine in Health and Disease. 2nd Ed. pp. 221–223. Grune & Stratton, Orlando, FL, 1971

92. Maigne R: Orthopedic Medicine. A New Approach to Vertebral Manipulations. pp. 30, 31. Charles C Thomas, Springfield, IL, 1972

93. Giles LGF, Taylor JR: Innervation of lumbar zygapophyseal joint synovial folds. Acta Orthop Scand 58:43, 1987

94. Giles LGF: Lumbar apophyseal joint arthrography. J Manipulative Physiol Ther 7(1):21, 1984

95. Giles LGF: Lumbo-sacral and cervical zygapophyseal joint inclusions. Manipulative Med 2:89, 1986

96. Kos J, Wolf J: Les menisques intervertebraux et leur role possible dans les blocages vertebraux. Ann Med Phys 15:203, 1972

97. Kos J, Wolf J: [Translation of reference 94 into English.] J Orthop Sports Phys Ther 1:8, 1972

98. Lewit K: Manipulative Therapy in Rehabilitation of the Locomotor System. pp. 17–20. Butterworths, Boston, 1985

99. Bogduk N, Engel R: The menisci of the lumbar zygopophyseal joints. A review of their anatomy and clinical significance. Spine 9:454, 1984

100. Badgley CE: The articular facets in relation to low back pain and sciatic radiation. J Bone Joint Surg 23:481, 1941

101. Hadley LA: Anatomico-Roentgenographic Studies of the Spine. 5th Ed. Charles C Thomas, Springfield, IL, 1964

102. Kraft GL, Levinthal DH: Facet synovial impingement. Surg Gynecol Obstet 93:439, 1951

103. Gillet H: The anatomy and physiology of spinal fixations. J Nat Chiro Assoc 33(12):22, 1963

104. Farfan MF: Torsion and compression. In: Mechanical Disorders of the Low Back. Lea & Febiger, Philadelphia, 1974

105. Cassidy JD, Haymo WT, Kirkaldy-Willis WH: Manipulation (Ch. 16). In Kirkaldy-Willis WH (ed). Managing Low Back Pain. 3rd Ed. Churchill Livingstone, New York, 1992

106. Adams MA, Hutton WC: The role of the apophyseal joints in resisting intervertebral compressive force. J Bone Joint Surg [Br] 62:358, 1980

107. Adams MA, Hutton WC: 1981 Volvo Award in Basic Science. Prolapsed intervertebral disc; A hyperflexion injury. Spine 7(3):184, 1982

108. Adams MA, Hutton WC: The relevance of torsion to the mechanical derangement of the lumbar spine. Spine 6(3):241, 1981

109. Naylor A: Intervertebral disc prolapse and degeneration. The biomechanical and biophysical approach. Spine 1(2):108, 1976

110. Maigne R: Orthopedic Medicine: A New Approach to Vertebral Manipulation. pp. 28–29. Charles C Thomas, Springfield, IL, 1972

111. de Seze S: Les accidents de la deterioration structurale du disque. Semin Hop Paris 1:2267, 1955

112. de Seze S: Les attitudes antalgique dans la sciatique discoradiculaire commune. Semin Hop Paris 1:2291, 1955

113. Cyriax JH: Lumbago, mechanism of dural pain. Lancet, Vol. 1, 427, 1945

114. Herbst R: Gonstead Chiropractic Science and Art. The Chiropractic Methodology of Clarence S. Gonstead, D.C. SCI-CHI Publications, 1968–1980

115. Nwuga VCB: Relative therapeutic efficacy of vertebral manipulation and conventional treatment in back pain management. Am J Phys Med 61:273, 1982

116. Christman OD, Mittnacht A, Snook GA: A study of the results following rotatory manipulation in the lumbar intervertebral-disc syndrome. J Bone Joint Surg [Am] 46:517, 1964

117. Kuo PPF, Loh ZCL: Treatment of lumbar intervertebral disc protrustions by manipulation. Clin Orthop 215:47, 1987

118. Cox JM: Mechanism, diagnosis and treatment of lumbar disc protrusion and prolapse. J Am Chiro Assoc 8:181, 1974

119. Levernieux J: Les Tractions Vertebrales. L'Expansion, Paris, 1960

120. Gatterman MI, Panzer D: Disorders of the lumbar spine. p. 147. In Gatterman MI (ed): Chiropractic Management of Spine Related Disorders. Williams & Wilkins, Baltimore, 1990

121. Richard J: Disc rupture with cauda equina syndrome after chiropractic adjustment. NY State J Med 67:249, 1967

122. Hooper J: Low back pain and manipulation, paraparesis after treatment of low back pain by physical methods. Med J Aust 1:549, 1973

123. Gatterman MI: p. 66. Chiropractic Management of Spine Related Disorders. Williams & Wilkins, Baltimore, 1990

124. Maigne R: Orthopedic Medicine. A New Approach to Vertebral Manipulations. pp. 33, 34. Charles C Thomas, Springfield, IL, 1972

125. Korr IM: Proprioceptors and somatic dysfunction. J Am Osteopath Assoc 74:638, 1975

126. Sandoz RW: Some reflex phenomena associated with spinal derangements and adjustments. Ann Swiss Chiro Assoc 6:60, 1981

127. Grice AS: Muscle tonus change following manipulation. J Can Chiro Assoc 18(4):29, 1974

128. Watts DG, Stouffer EK, Taylor A et al: Analysis of muscle receptor connection by spike-triggered averaging, spindle primary, and tendon organ afferents. J Neurophysiology 80(6):1279, 1976

129. Moore JC: The Golgi tendon organ: a review and update. Am J Occup Ther 38:227, 1984

130. Gillette RG: A speculative argument for the coactivation of diverse somatic receptor populations by forceful chiropractic adjustments. Manipulative Med Dis, 1987

131. White AA, Panjabi MM: Clinical Biomechanics of the Spine. 2nd Ed. pp. 692–694. JB Lippincott, Philadelphia, 1990

132. Muhlemann D: Hypermobility as a common cause for chronic back pain. Ann Swiss Chiro Assoc (in press)

133. Paris SV: Physical signs of instability. Spine 10(3):277, 1985

134. Gatterman MI: p. 47. In: Chiropractic Management of Spine Related Disorders. Williams & Wilkins, Baltimore, 1990

135. Grieve GP: Common Vertebral Joint Problems. 2nd Ed. Churchill Livingstone, Edinburgh, 1988, pp. 407, 412–413

136. Bernard TN, Kirkaldy-Willis WH: Recognizing specific characteristics of nonspecific low back pain. Clin Orthop 217:266, 1987

137. Vernon HT, Dhami MSI et al: Spinal manipulation and beta-endorphin: a controlled study of the effect of a spinal manipulation on plasma beta-endorphin levels in normal males. J Manipulative Physiol Ther 9(2):115, 1986

138. Terrett A, Vernon H: Manipulation and pain tolerance. A conrolled study of the effect of spinal manipulation on paraspinal cutaneous pain tolerance levels. Am J Phys Med 63(5):217, 1984

139. Gitelman R: Spinal manipulation in the relief of pain. In: The Research Status of Spinal Manipulative Therapy. NINDCS monograph no. 15. pp. 277–285. Washington, DC, DHEW publication no. 76-998, 1975

140. Mense S: Slowly conducting afferent fibers from deep tissues. Progress Sensory Physiol 6:140, 1986

141. Roberts WJ, Gillette RG, Kramis RC: Somatosensory input from lumbar paraspinal tissues: anatomical terminations and neuronal responses to mechanical and sympathetic stimuli. Soc Neurosci Abst 15:755, 1989

142. Gillette RG, Kramis RC, Roberts WJ: Spinal neurons likely to mediate low back and referred leg pain. Soc Neurosci Abstr 16:1704, 1990

143. Gillette RG, Kramis RC, Roberts WJ: Convergent input onto spinal neurons likely to mediate low back pain. 3rd IBRO World Congress of Neuroscience Abstracts. 1991

144. Melzack R, Wall PD: Pain mechanisms: a new theory. Science 150:971, 1965

145. Gillette RG: Potential antinociceptive effects of high-level somatic stimulation—chiropractic manipulation therapy may coactivate both tonic and phasic analgesic systems. Some recent neurophysiological evidence. Trans Pacific Consortium Chirop Res 1:A4(1), 1986

146. Paris SV: Spinal manipulative therapy. Clinical Orthopedics and Related Research 179: 1983

147. Palmer BJ: The Science of Chiropractic—Its Principles and Philosophies. Vol. 1. Palmer School of Chiropractic, 1906, Davenport, IA, 1910.

148. Stephenson RW: Chiropractic Textbook. Palmer School of Chiropractic, Davenport, IA, 1948

149. Haldeman S, Hammerich K: The evolution of neurology and the concept of chiropractic. ACA J Chiro 7:S-57, 1973

150. Janse J: History of the Development of Chiropractic Concepts; Chiropractic Terminology. pp. 25–42. In: The Research Status of Spinal Manipulative Therapy. NINCDS monograph no. 15. Washington, DC, DHEW publication no. 76-988, 1975

151. Homewood AE: The Neurodynamics of the Vertebral Subluxation. pp. 11–33. Valkyrie Press, St. Petersburg, FL, 1979

152. Leach RA: Nerve compression hypothesis. p. 49. In: The Chiropractic Theories. A Synopsis of Scientific Research. 2nd Ed. Williams & Wilkins, Baltimore, 1986

153. Crelin Es: A scientific test of the chiropractic theory. Am Sci 61:574, 1973

154. Hadley LA: Anatomico-Roentgenographic Studies of the Spine. pp. 172–183, 422–477. Charles C Thomas, Springfield, IL, 1964

155. Hadley LA: Intervertebral joint subluxation, bony impingement and foramen encroachment with nerve root changes. Am J Roentgenol Rad Ther 65:377, 1951

156. Leach RA: Neurodystrophic hypothesis. p. 153. In: The Chiropractic Theories. A Synopsis of Scientific Research. 2nd Ed. Williams & Wilkins, Baltimore, MD, 1986

157. Coote JH: Somatic sources of afferent input as factors in aberrant autonomic, sensory and motor function. p. 91. In Korr IM (ed): The Neurobiologic Mechanisms in Manipulative Therapy. Plenum, New York, 1978

158. Kiyomi K: Autonomic system reactions caused by excitation of somatic afferents: study of cutaneo-intestinal reflex. p. 219. In Korr IM (ed): The Neurobiologic Mechanisms in Manipulative Therapy. Plenum, New York, 1978

159. Sato A: The Somatosympathetic Reflexes: Their Physiological and Clinical Significance. pp. 163–172. NINCDS monograph no. 15. Washington, DC, DHEW publication no. 76-988, 1975

160. Appenzeller O: Somatoautonomic reflexology—normal and abnormal. p. 179. In Korr IM (ed): The Neurobiologic Mechanisms in Manipulative Therapy. New York, Plenum, 1978

161. Sato A, Swenson R: Sympathetic nervous system response to mechanical stress of the spinal column in rats. J Manipulative Physiol Ther 7(3):141, 1984

162. Kunert W: Functional disorders of internal organs due to vertebral lesions. Ciba Symp 13:85, 1965

163. Greenman PE: Principles of Manual Medicine. pp. 8–10. Williams & Wilkins, Baltimore, 1989

164. Kellgren JH: The anatomical source of back pain. Rheumatol Rehabil 16:3, 1977

165. Selye H: Stress and Disease. McGraw-Hill, New York, 1956

166. Selye H: The Stress of Life. McGraw-Hill, New York, 1956

167. Selye H: Stress Without Distress. JB Lippincott, Philadelphia, 1974

168. Mason JW: A re-evaluation of the concept of non-specificity in stress theory. Psychol Res 8:323, 1971

169. Leach RA: Ch. 12. In: The Chiropractic Theories, a Synopsis of Scientific Research. 2nd Ed. Williams & Wilkins, Baltimore, 1986

170. Stein M, Schiavi RC, Camerino M: Influence of brain and behavior in the immune system. Science 191:435, 1976

171. Hess WR: Functional Organization of the Diencephalon. Grune & Stratton, Orlando, FL, 1957

172. Fidelibus JC: An overview of neuroimmunomodulation and a possible correlation with musculoskeletal system function. J Manipulative Physiol Ther 12:289, 1989

173. Brennan PC, Hondras MA: Priming of neutrophils for enhanced respiratory burst by manipulation of the thoracic spine. p. 160. In: Proceedings of the 1989 International Conference on Spinal Manipulation. Arlington, VA, FCER, 1989

174. Kokjohn K, Kaltinger C, Lohr GE et al: Plasma substance P following spinal manipulation. p. 105. In: Proceedings of the 1990 International Conference on Spinal Manipulation. FCER, Arlington, VA, 1990

175. Greenman PE: Principles of craniosacral (inherent force) technique. p. 113. In: Principles of Manual Medicine. Williams & Wilkins, Baltimore, 1989

176. Haas M: The physics of spinal manipulation. Part III. Some characteristics of adjusting that facilitate joint distractions. J Manipulative Physiol Ther 13(6):305, 1990

177. Haas M: The physics of spinal manipulation. Part IV. A theoretical consideration of the physician impact force and energy requirements to produce synovial joint cavitation. J Manipulative Physiol Ther 13(7):378, 1990

178. Haas M: The physics of spinal manipulation. Part I. The myth of F = ma. J Manipulative Physiol Ther 13(4):204, 1990

179. Haas M: The physics of spinal manipulation. Part II. A theoretical consideration of the adjustive force. J Manipulative Physiol Ther 13(5):253 1990

180. Maigne R: Localization of manipulations of the spine. p. 131. In: Orthopedic Medicine. 3rd Ed. Charles C Thomas, Springfield, IL, 1979

181. Plaugher G, Lopes MA: The knee–chest table: indications and contraindications. J Chiro Tech 2(4):163, 1990

182. Schafer RC: Motion palpation and chiropractic technic. Principles of dynamic chiropractic. 1st Ed. pp. 34, 56. The Motion Palpation Institute, Huntington Beach, CA, 1989

183. Grice AS: Modern Developments in the Principles and Practice of Chiropractic. p. 33. Appleton-Century-Crofts, East Norwalk, CT, 1980

184. Schafer RC, Faye LJ: p. 34. In: Motion Palpation and Chiropractic Technic—Principles of Dynamic Chiropractic. The Motion Palpation Institute, Huntington Beach, CA, 1989

185. Barral J-P, Mercier P: Visceral Manipulation. Eastland Press, Seattle, 1988

186. Dupuis PR: The anatomy of the lumbosacral spine. p. 29. In Kirkaldy-Willis WH (ed): Managing Low Back Pain. Churchill Livingstone, New York, 1988

187. Schmidt RF et al (eds): p. 242. In: Fundamentals of Neurophysiology. Springer-Verlag, New York, 1978

5

The Spine: Anatomy, Biomechanics, Assessment, and Adjustive Techniques

David H. Peterson
Thomas F. Bergmann

STRUCTURE AND FUNCTION OF THE SPINE

The spine is, among its many other functions, the mechanism for maintaining erect posture and for transmitting movements of the head, neck, and trunk. The pelvis helps to form the foundation for posture, and the cervical spine-occipital complex is essentially the postural accommodation unit. The spinal column simultaneously provides stability to a collapsible cylinder, permits movements in all directions with the ability to return to a starting position, supports structures of considerable weight, provides attachments for muscles and ligaments, transmits weight onto the pelvis, and encases and protects the spinal cord while allowing transmission of neural information to and from the periphery. All structures must be interrelated and coordinated.

The functional unit of the spine (motion segment), the smallest component capable of performing the characteristic roles of the spine, is divided into an anterior and posterior portion (Fig. 5-1). The motion segment, then, comprises the two adjacent vertebrae and their associated structures, both intrinsic and extrinsic, forming a complete set of articulations.

The articulations of the vertebral bodies are synchondroses, or cartilaginous joints, connected by the fibrocartilaginous intervertebral discs. In the cervical and lumbar spines, the discs are approximately one-third the thickness of the body of a corresponding vertebrae. In the thoracic spine, this ratio decreases to about one-sixth the thickness. This articulation forms the anterior portion of the vertebral motion unit; its chief function is weight-bearing, although it also provides some shock-absorbing.

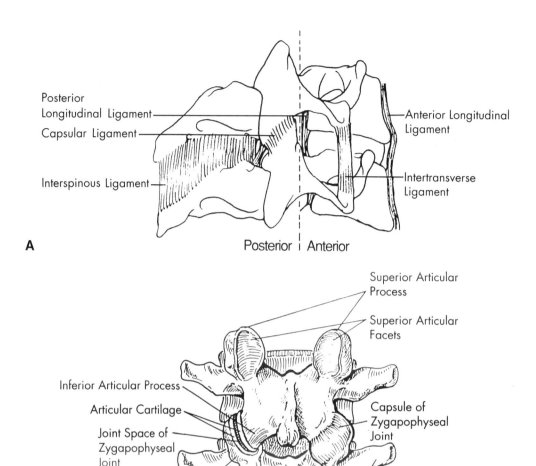

Figure 5.1 Spinal motion segment composed of two vertebrae and contiguous soft tissues: (**A**) intrinsic ligaments; (**B**) view of the posterior joint and joint capsule. (Fig. B from White and Panjabi,[1] with permission.)

Two important ligaments help support the vertebral bodies. These are the anterior longitudinal ligament (ALL) and posterior longitudinal ligament (PLL) (Fig. 5-1). The ALL extends from the inner surface of the occiput to the sacrum. It starts out as a narrow band that widens as it descends. It is thickest in the thoracic spine and thinnest in the cervical spine. The PLL runs from the occiput down the posterior portion of the vertebral bodies. It is a somewhat narrow structure that has lateral extensions and covers part of the intervertebral disc. It is also thickest in the thoracic spine, while equally thin in the cervical and lumbar regions. In the lumbar spine, the

PLL tapers, leaving the posterolateral borders of the disc uncovered and unprotected, with important clinical ramifications. Fibers from the PLL attach to the disc itself.

The articulations between the neural arches of vertebrae are non-axial diarthrodial joints. Each has a joint cavity enclosed within a joint capsule and lined with a synovial membrane (Fig. 5-1). These joints are true synovial joints and form the posterior portion of the vertebral motion unit. They allow a guiding, gliding action for movement. These joints help to determine the amount and direction of motion, which depends on the facings of the articular facets (Fig. 5-2). Furthermore, the facets play a significant role in load-bearing, though this varies between the facets and the disc depending on the position of the spine. Loads will be born more by the facets when the spine is in extension as well as in flexion coupled with rotation.

Support and stability for the posterior joints come from the small segmental ligaments and joint capsule (Fig. 5-1). The ligamentum flavum, a strong and highly elastic structure, connects adjacent lamina. The interspinous and supraspinous ligaments attach from spinous process to spinous process. Occasionally a bursa will be formed between these two ligaments. The intertransverse ligaments are relatively thin and run from transverse process to transverse process.

While each region of the spine has its own unique characteristics, typical vertebrae have common descriptive parts that include a vertebral body, two pedicles, two laminae, four articular processes, two transverse processes, and a spinous process (Fig. 5-3). There are, however, in each region atypical vertebrae, which either lack one of these descriptive features or contain other special peculiarities. The atypical vertebrae are C1, C2, C7, T1, T9, T10, T11, T12, L5 and the sacrum and coccyx. Specific anatomic descriptions and functional characteristics are covered under each specific spinal region.

The intervertebral joint, or motion segment, is made up of three parts, the two posterior joints and the disc forming a three-joint complex in all spinal regions except the upper cervical spine. Changes that affect the posterior joints will also affect the disc and vice versa. The application of rational and effective manipulative treatment depends on an understanding and correlation of the patient's clinical presentation with pathomechanical processes of the spine.

EVALUATION OF SPINAL JOINT FUNCTION

The investigation for spinal function incorporates history taking, physical examination, and where appropriate radiographic, laboratory, and special examinations. The interview and examination should be open-ended, efficient, and directed toward identifying the source and nature of the patient's complaint. This is not to imply that the examination should focus just on the site of complaint. The site of complaint does not necessarily correspond to the source of the dysfunction or pathology. Complaints of pain or aber-

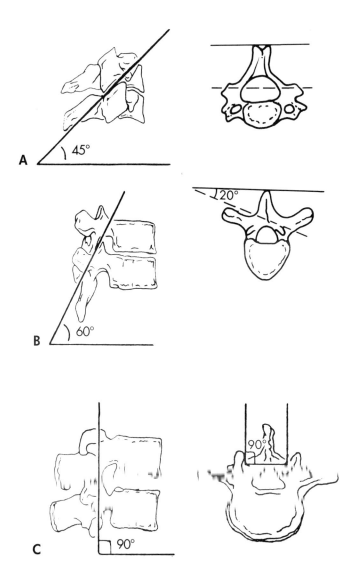

Figure 5.2 Facet planes in each spinal region viewed from the side and above. **(A)** Cervical (C3–7). **(B)** Thoracic. **(C)** Lumbar. (Modified from White and Pan-jabi,[1] with permission.)

rant function may have visceral, not somatic, origin, and disorders within the neuromusculoskeletal (NMS) system may be secondary to somatic disease or dysfunction at distant sites. Consequently, the doctor must develop a method to efficiently scan the spine and the locomotor system for possible sites of disease or dysfunction. Within this context it is impractical to evaluate every

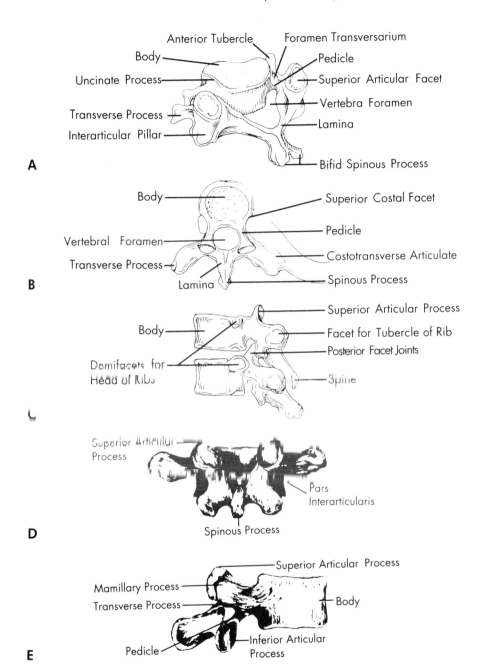

Anterior Tubercle Foramen Transversarium
Body
Uncinate Process
Superior Articular Facet
Pedicle
Transverse Process
Vertebra Foramen
Interarticular Pillar
Lamina
Bifid Spinous Process

A

Body
Superior Costal Facet
Pedicle
Vertebral Foramen
Transverse Process
Costotransverse Articulate
Lamina
Spinous Process

B

Body
Superior Articular Process
Facet for Tubercle of Rib
Posterior Facet Joints
Demifacets for Head of Ribs
Spine

C

Superior Articular Process
Pars Interarticularis
Spinous Process

D

Superior Articular Process
Mamillary Process
Transverse Process
Body
Pedicle
Inferior Articular Process

E

Figure 5.3 The structures that compose the typical (**A**) cervical, (**B,C**) thoracic, and (**D,E**) lumbar vertebrae. (Figs. D and E from Dupuis and Kirkaldy-Willis,[77] with permission.)

joint of the musculoskeletal system during the initial evaluation. The spinal scanning examination should therefore be an abbreviated evaluation designed to quickly scrutinize key areas of spinal joint function. Sites of potential abnormality would then be examined in further detail to isolate the level and nature of spinal joint disorders.

Table 5.1 Physical Scanning Evaluation for Joint Dysfunction

Goal

To serve as a screen for locating possible ares of joint dysfunction in need of a detailed and/or isolation examination.

Components

1. Posture and gait
   a. Evaluates integration of activities of the musculoskeletal system
   b. Evaluates asymmetries in sectional relationships of the spine and extremities
   c. Performed rapidly during initial contact with patient

2. Global range of motion
   a. Active movements of the cervico-thoracic spine in flexion, extension, lateral flexion, and rotation
   b. Active movements of the thoraco-lumbar spine in flexion, extension, lateral flexion, and rotation
   c. Evaluated visually or quantified with instrumentation (inclinometer, goniometer)

3. Motion scan: joint play scan, joint challenging
   a. Usually performed in the seated position; posterior to anterior pressure is applied to the spinal segments while the patient's spine is passively extended, creating a resisted springing quality
   b. A fluid wave, rocking motion should be produced; note any regions of restriction

4. Pain scan: palpable pain and/or skin sensitivity
   a. Evaluates general areas using light palpation or pinwheel
   b. Note location, quality, and intensity of pain produced during the previous activities

Spinal Joint Scan

The scanning examination of the spine is designed to screen for alterations in structure or function indicative of possible joint subluxation and dysfunction. It incorporates the assessment of posture, global range of motion, mobility, and the location of any sites of palpatory pain (Table 5-1).

Posture Scan

The evaluation of static posture incorporates lateral and posterior plumb line assessment. The patient stands with the heels separated approximately 3 inches and the forepart of each foot abducted about 8 to 10 degrees from midline. On the lateral analysis, visible surface landmarks that ideally coincide with the plumb line are the lobe of the ear, shoulder joint, greater trochanter, a point slightly anterior to the middle of the knee joint, and just anterior to the lateral malleolus (Fig. 5-4). On posterior postural examination, the plumb line should pass through the external occipital protuberance, the spinous processes, the gluteal crease, midway between the knees, and midway between the ankles (Fig. 5-4). Look for specific postural faults, including head tilt, head rotation, shoulder unleveling, lateral curves of the spine, pelvic unleveling, and pelvic rotation. Postural faults that are suspected of having a muscular basis should be followed up with evaluations of muscle length, strength, and volume. While there is no single ideal

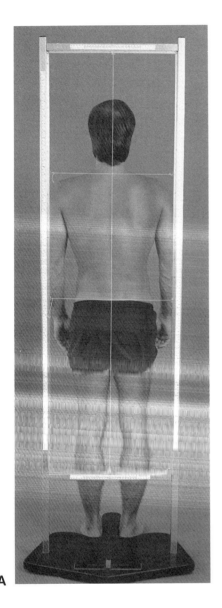 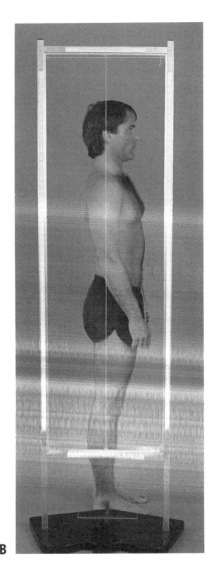

Figure 5.4 **(A)** Posterior and **(B)** lateral plumb line evaluation of posture.

posture for all individuals, the best posture for each person is the one in which the least expenditure of energy occurs because the body segments are balanced in the position of least strain and maximum support.

Global Range of Motion

Evaluate global range of motion of the cervical spine and trunk for both active and passive movements. Evaluate all three cardinal planes of motion and record any reduced, aberrant, asymmetric, or painful movements. During a scanning examination of the spine, estimations of range are typically conducted without the aid of instrumentation; however, inclinometric measurements may be easily incorporated. The specific ranges and methods for evaluating regional mobility of the spine will be discussed later under each separate spinal section. Regional spinal movements that fall within normal ranges do not necessarily exclude segmental joint dysfunction. Segmental joint hypomobility may be masked by hypermobility at adjacent joints.

Pain Scan

The pain scan is designed to screen for sites of possible abnormal bony or soft tissue tenderness. The superficial soft tissues are assessed with light contacts through the palmar surfaces of the fingers (Fig. 5-5A) or by rolling

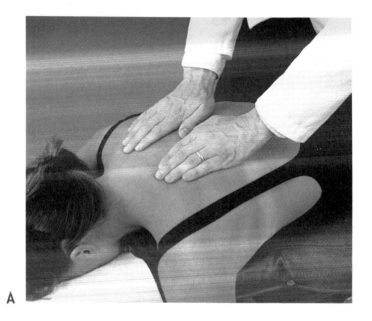

A

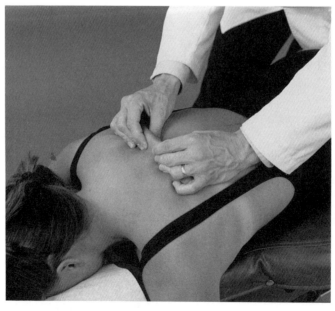

B

Figure 5.5 Evaluation of skin and superficial soft tissue sensitivity and texture with (**A**) light palmar contacts and (**B**) skin rolling technique.

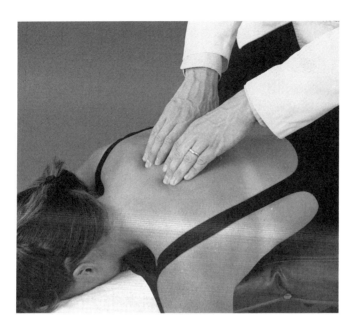

Figure 5.6 Evaluation of the sensitivity, tone, and texture of the deep paraspinal tissues using the palmar surface of the fingertips.

the superficial layer between the fingers and thumbs (Fig. 5-5B). The deeper paraspinal tissues are evaluated with the same palmar contacts but more pressure is applied to explore the deeper layer (Fig. 5-6). Particular attention is directed to identify any tenderness in the soft tissues over the posterior joints.

To identify the soft tissue tenderness, the spinous processes and interspinous spaces are scanned with the fingertips of one or both hands. When employing a single hand contact, the doctor rests the middle finger in the interspinous space and the index and ring finger on each side of the spinous process spanning the interspinous space (Fig. 5-7). The middle finger palpates for interspinous spacing and tenderness, and the index and ring fingers palpate for interspinous alignment and lateral spinous tenderness.

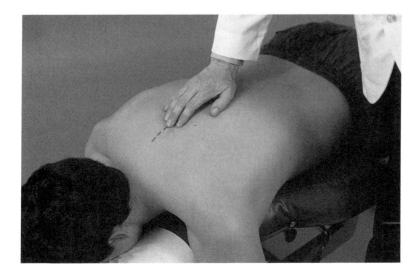

Figure 5.7 Single hand palpation of spinous process alignment and tenderness.

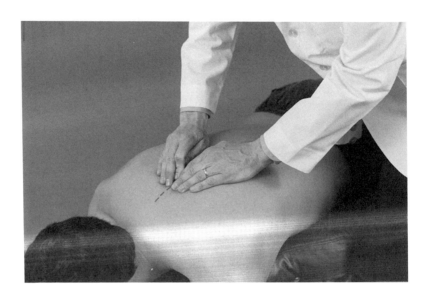

Figure 5.8 Two-hand palpation of spinous process alignment and tenderness.

When the fingers or both hands are applied the fingertips meet in the midline to palpate the interspinous alignment and tenderness (Fig. 5-8).

The lumbar spine and thoracic spine are customarily examined in the prone position. Though the cervical spine may be evaluated in prone or supine positions, it is more commonly evaluated in the supine position using bilateral fingertip contacts.

Motion Scan

Evaluation of spinal mobility incorporates tests to scan regional joint play and passive range of motion. Joint play may be evaluated in sitting or prone positions, while passive range of motion is screened in the sitting position. In both cases the doctor establishes broad contacts against the spinous processes or broad bilateral contacts over the posterior joints. When evaluating joint play, the area evaluated should be positioned as close to the loose-packed position as possible.

When evaluating sitting joint play the doctor sits or stands behind the patient and places the non-palpating arm across the patient's shoulders (Fig. 5-9) or under the patient's flexed arms. The flexed arm position is commonly utilized in the mid to upper thoracic spine and is developed by having the patient interlace his/her fingers behind the neck (Fig. 5-10). In the cervical spine the indifferent hand supports the crown of the patient's head (Fig. 5-11).

With the patient prone, the doctor establishes bilateral contacts on each side of the spine or a reinforced contact over the spinous processes (Fig. 5-12). To scan the spine, slide up or down applying gentle posterior to anterior springing movements. Regions of induced pain or inappropriate movement should be noted for further evaluation.

To screen for sections of possible active and passive movement restriction, place the patient in the sitting position with the arms crossed over the chest. The doctor may either sit behind the patient or stand at the patient's side.

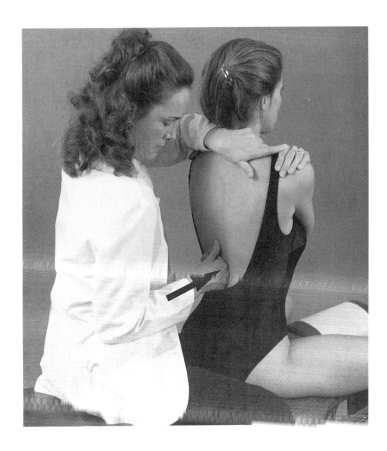

Figure 5.9 Sitting joint play scan of the thoracolumbar region.

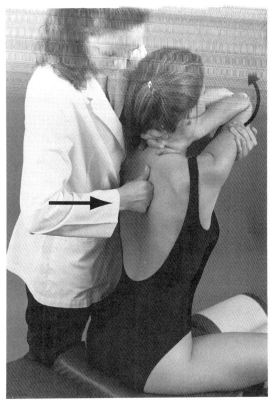

Figure 5.10 Sitting joint play scan of the mid-thoracic region using the flexed arm position.

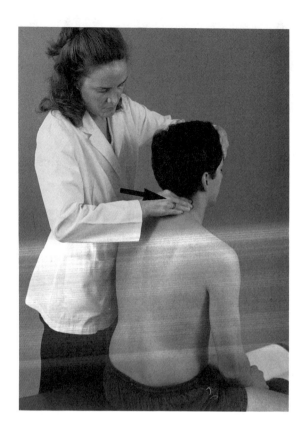

Figure 5.11 Sitting joint play scan of the mid-cervical region.

Trunk movement is controlled by establishing contacts across the patient's shoulder or reaching around to grasp the patient's forearm (Fig. 5-13). Cervical movement is directed by establishing a contact on the crown of the patient's head or forehead (Fig. 5-14). Palpation contacts are established with the fingertips, palm, or thenar surface of the doctor's palpation hand. The contacts should be broadly placed so movement at two to three motion segments may be scanned together.

For lateral flexion and rotation assessment of the lumbar or thoracic regions, contacts are established on the lateral surface of the spinous processes on the side of induced rotation or laterally bending (Fig. 5-13). In the cervical spine the fingertips establish the contacts over the articular pillars (Fig. 5-14). For spinal flexion and extension the contacts are established with fingertip contacts over the interspinous spaces of several adjacent segments (Fig. 5-15). To evaluate movement, guide the patient through the full range of passive motion. During the assessment any regional sites of elicited pain or perceived increased or decreasd resistance should be noted and investigated with more specifically applied methods of segmental motion palpation and end play.

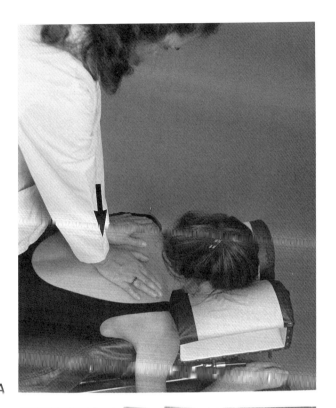

A

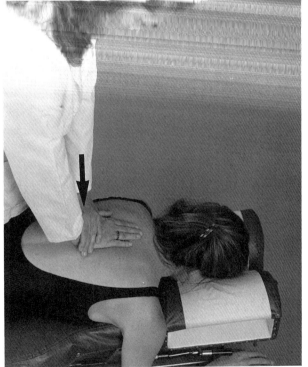

B

Figure 5.12 Prone joint play scan using (**A**) bilateral thenar contacts over the transverse processes and (**B**) reinforced hypothenar contacts over the spinous process.

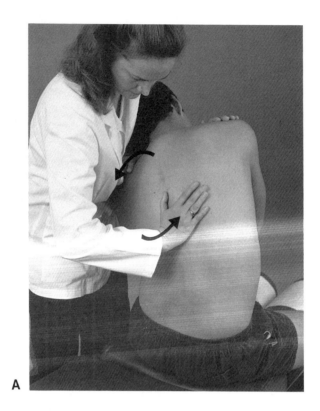

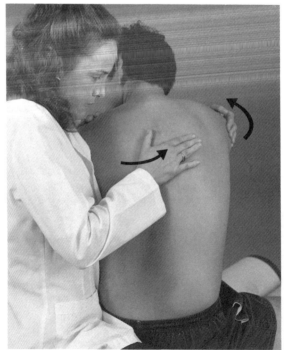

Figure 5.13 (**A**) Evaluation of left lateral flexion movement with doctor standing; (**B**) evaluation of left rotation movement with the doctor seated.

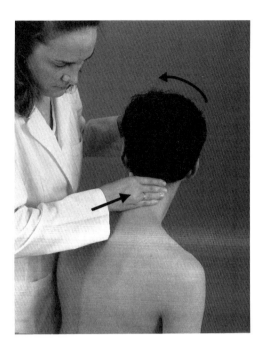

Figure 5.14 Evaluation of cervical rotation with the in-different hand contact on the patient's forehead.

ISOLATION OF JOINT SUBLUXATION/ DYSFUNCTION

As stated previously, the goal of isolation testing is to further separate and define the possible sites of motion segment dysfunction. Many of the procedures used to scan the spine are also applied in the investigation and localization of subluxation and dysfunction (Table 5-2). However, they are applied within a different context to identify more precisely the site and nature of dysfunction/subluxation under question. They incorporate the

Table 5.2 Isolation of Motion Segment Dysfunction (PARTS)

Goal

To identify and define the specific joint dysfunction and specific tissues involved.

P	Location, quality, and intensity of pain or tenderness produced by palpation and pressure over specific structures and soft tissues.
A	Asymmetry of sectional or segmental components identified by static palpation of specific anatomic structures.
R	The decrease or loss of specific movements (active, passive, and accessory) distinguished through motion palpation techniques.
T	Tone, texture, and temperature changes in specific soft tissues identified through palpation.
S	Use of special tests or procedures linked to a technique system.

Neither the scanning (Table 5.1) nor isolation evaluation alone or in combination constitute a complete examination. The doctor of chiropractic must be competent in performing a complete physical evaluation to assess the nature of the patient's condition and determine if the patient is suitable for chiropractic care.

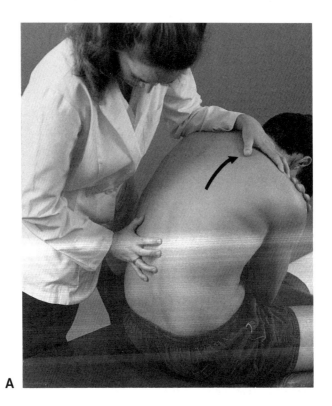

A

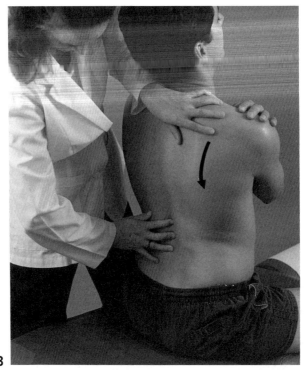

Figure 5.15 Evaluation of upper lumbar (**A**) flexion and (**B**) extension with indifferent hand contact across the posterior aspect of the patient's shoulders.

B

detailed exploration of painful sites; assessment of joint alignment, texture tone, and consistency of associated soft tissues; and the precise evaluation of intersegmental movements and end play. The evaluation of painful tissues often incorporates the application of various directions of applied pressure to determine the directions of painful movement. These procedures are referred to as joint challenging or joint provocation testing.

Evaluation of segmental alignment involves comparing adjacent vertebral segments for symmetry and examining interspinous spaces, spinous processes, cervical articular pillars, thoracic transverse processes, rib angles, and lumbar mammillary processes. Sudden changes in interspinous spacing may identify flexion or extension malposition. Rotational malpositions may be identified by misalignment of adjacent spinous processes and unilateral prominence of the articular pillars, transverse processes, or lumbar mammillary processes. The articular pillars, transverse processes, and mammillary processes are not as distinctly palpable as the spinous processes, but they are less susceptible to congenital or developmental anomaly. Unilateral contraction of segmental muscles produces a sense of fullness and may be mistaken for underlying rotational malposition of the articular pillars, transverse processes, or mammillary processes.

The localization of soft tissue changes also helps in specifying the nature and site of joint disease or derangement. Injured or inflamed joints may be associated with an overlying sense of increased warmth or puffiness. Joint disease or dysfunction is also commonly associated with local soft tissue reactive changes in the segmentally related tissue. This may lead to local or asymmetrical muscle spasm. Long-standing dysfunction may be associated with local areas of induration and contracture. These sites may palpate as areas of deep nodular or rope-like consistency.

Segmental motion palpation and end play tests are essential to identify those segmental movements that are increased, restricted, or painful. Pain elicited at one level and not adjacent levels helps localize the site of possible pathology. Increased resistance identifies a site of possible joint fixation, and increased movement identifies a site of possible joint instability. The identification and segmental location of soft tissue alterations, pain, and end play restriction are critical to identifying not only the level but also the direction of dysfunction. Furthermore, they are often essential to determining the type and directions of the applied adjustive therapy.

Although all of the physical examination procedures discussed are an integral part of joint evaluation, it must not be forgotten that all have limitations. Many are based on the evaluation of symmetry in structure and function, and the degree of variation necessary to produce disease or dysfunction has not been determined. Asymmetry of structure and function is common, and minor abnormalities in alignment and motion may be within the range of normal variation. Furthermore, physical joint examination procedures depend on the skill of the examiner and are susceptible to errors in performance or interpretation. It must also be remembered that the identification of dysfunction does not necessarily identify the cause. All these concerns lead to the necessity to incorporate and contrast all the history and examination findings before a diagnostic conclusion is reached and therapy is applied.

The specific methods applicable to each spinal region will be discussed in detail in each region section.

THE CERVICAL SPINE

The cervical spine has the precarious task of maintaining head posture while allowing for a great deal of mobility. The cervical spine must balance the weight of the head atop a relatively thin and long lever, making it quite vulnerable to traumatic forces. The cervical facets allow movement in all directions; the cervical spine is, therefore, the most movable portion of the vertebral column. The cervical spine has two anatomically and functionally distinct regions, which will be considered individually.

Functional Anatomy of the Upper Cervical Spine

The upper cervical spine is the most complex region of the axial skeleton. It is composed of the atlanto-occipital and atlanto-axial articulations, which serve as a transition from the skull to the rest of the spine. These two functional units are both anatomically and kinematically unique. Neither has an intervertebral disc, and the atlanto-axial articulation incorporates three synovial joints.

The *atlas* has no vertebral body or spinous process (Fig. 5-16). It consists of a bony oval with the two lateral masses connected by the anterior and posterior arches. The lateral masses are formed from enlarged pedicles with concave articular facets superiorly for articulation with the occipital condyles and circular inferior facets for articulation with the axis.

The outstanding feature of the *axis* (C2) is the presence of the odontoid process (dens) (Fig. 5-17). The odontoid is formed by the fusion of the embryologic remnants of the vertebral body of the atlas to the superior aspect of the body of the axis. The spinous process of the axis is large, bifid, and the first palpable midline structure below the occiput. The superior articular surfaces project from the superior aspect of the pedicles to meet the inferior aspects of the atlas lateral masses. Their surfaces are convex and lie in the transverse plane with a slight downward slant laterally. The

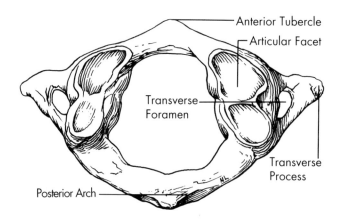

Figure 5.16 The structure of the atlas (C1).

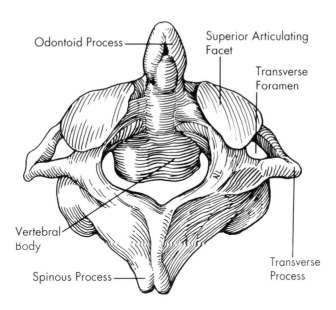

Figure 5.17 The structure of the axis (C2).

atlanto-axial articulation is formed by articular surfaces of the C1–C2 lateral masses. Both articular surfaces are convex, allowing for considerable mobility in rotation. The atlanto-odontal articulation is formed by the anterior arch of the atlas and the odontoid process. The odontoid process is completely surrounded by the anterior arch of the atlas anteriorly, the lateral masses laterally, and the transverse ligament posteriorly (Fig. 5-18). It is a trochoid joint, providing a pivot action.

The atlanto-occipital articulation is a freely movable, synovial, condyloid articulation (Figs. 5-19 and 5-20). The articular surface of the condyles are convex and converge anteriorly, resembling curved wedges that fit into

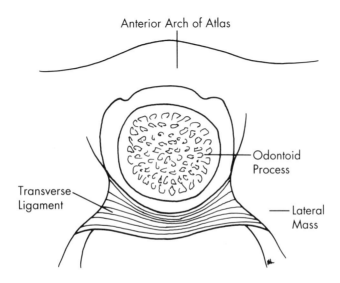

Figure 5.18 The atlanto-odontoid articulation viewed from above.

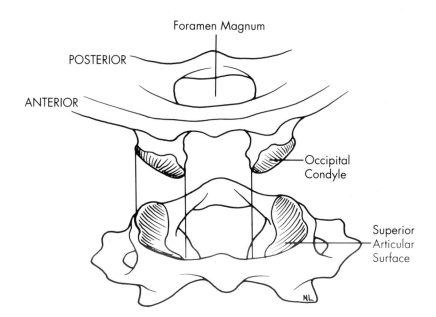

Figure 5.19 The atlanto-odontoid articulation has convex condyles fitting into concave lateral mass.

matching concave surfaces in the lateral masses of the atlas. Individual axes for each condyle exist, demonstrating that there is no single axis for axial rotation.

The muscles that provide the forces necessary for movement, postural support, and primary stability of the upper cervical region include the rectus capitis posterior major, rectus capitis posterior minor, rectus capitis lateralis, rectus capitis anterior, superior oblique, and inferior oblique (Figs. 5-21 and 5-22). All these muscles are supplied with motor fibers from the first cervical nerve and proprioceptive and pain fibers via a communicating branch from the second cervical nerve.

The ligaments that provide added stability of the upper cervical spine include the transverse ligament of the atlas, alar ligaments, posterior longitudinal ligament, posterior atlanto-occipital membrane, anterior atlanto-

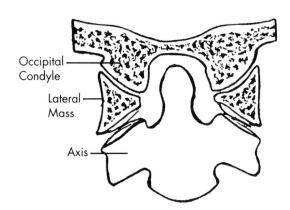

Figure 5.20 A coronal section through the atlanto-occipital and atlanto-axial articulations showing the plane of the facets.

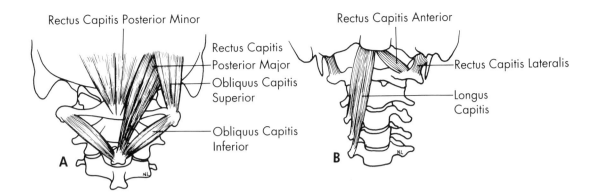

Figure 5.21 The suboccipital muscles: (**A**) posterior view, (**B**) anterior view.

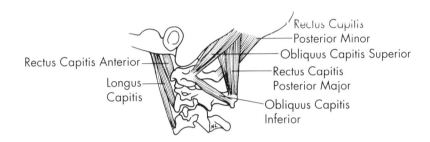

Figure 5.22 Lateral view of the suboccipital muscles.

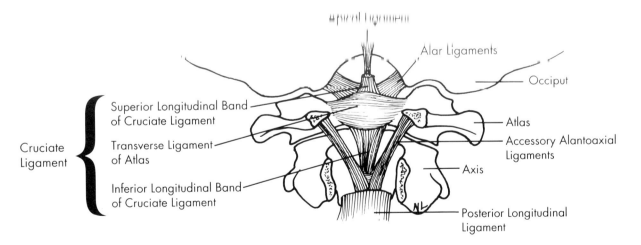

Figure 5.23 Upper cervical spinal ligaments shown with the posterior arch of the atlas and axis removed.

occipital membrane, ligamentum nuchae, and the apical ligament (Fig. 5-23). Because the ligaments of the upper cervical spine can be damaged by trauma, weakened by systemic inflammatory diseases, or be congenitally absent or malformed, testing for their integrity should be done before manipulative therapy is begun.

Table 5.3 Segmental Ranges of Motions for the Upper Cervical Spine

Vertebra	Combined Flexion and Extension	One Side Lateral Flexion[a]	One Side Axial Rotation
C0–C1	25°	5°	5°
C1–C2	20°	5°	40°

[a] Lateral glide or translation (laterolisthesis) occurs with lateral flexion movements of the neck.
(Adapted from White and Panjabi,[1] with permission.)

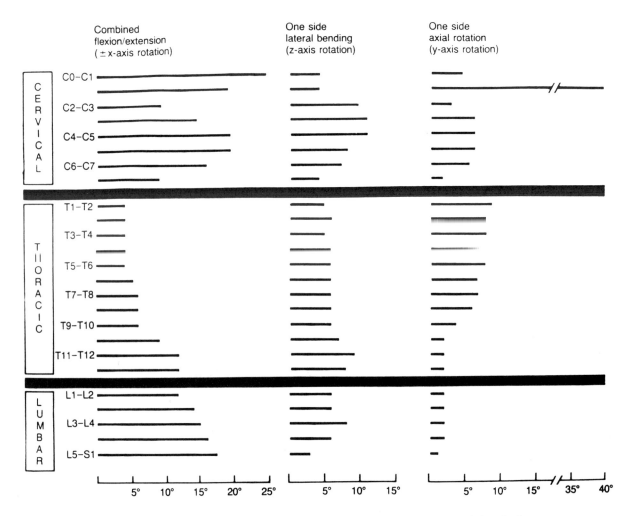

Figure 5.24 Representative values for rotatory ranges of motion at each level of the spine. (From White & Panjabi,[1] with permission.)

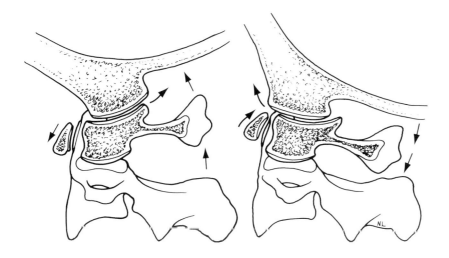

Figure 5.25 Flexion and extension of the occiput on the atlas with concomitant movement of the atlas on the axis.

Range and Pattern of Motion of C0–C1

The principle movement that occurs in the atlanto-occipital articulation is flexion and extension.[1] The combined range is approximtely 25 degrees (Table 5-9) (Fig. 5-24). Flexion and extension movements at C0–C1 are predominantly angular movements in the sagittal plane, without any significant associated coupled motions. During flexion the occipital condyles glide posteriorly and superiorly on the lateral masses of atlas as the occipital bone separates from the posterior arch. During extension, the condyles slide anteriorly on the lateral masses of atlas while the occipital bone approximates the posterior arch of atlas (Fig. 5-25).

Axial rotation at C0–C1 articulation was previously thought to be very limited.[2] However, recent studies have demonstrated a range of 4 to 8 degrees to each side.[1] Rotational movement is limited by the articular anatomy and the connections of the alar ligaments. The movement that does occur is predominantly in the elastic range at the end of total cervical rotation, where it is usually coupled with some small degree of lateral flexion.[3]

Lateral flexion of the atlanto-occipital articulation approximates that of axial rotation. Although the articular design of the atlanto-occipital articulation should allow for greater flexibility in lateral flexion it appears that the attachments of the alar ligament function to limit this motion[1] (Fig. 5-26). Movement occurs primarily in the coronal plane, although it is typically associated with some small degree of coupled rotation in the opposite direction. This leads to rotation of the chin away from the side of lateral flexion. The predominant movements occurring at the articular surface during lateral flexion are coronal plane rotation (roll) and translation (slide). Roll and slide occur in opposite directions because of the convex shape of the occipital condyles and the concave shape of the atlas articular surface. Rotation (roll) occurs in the direction of lateral flexion, and translation (slide) occurs in the direction opposite the lateral flexion (Fig. 5-27).

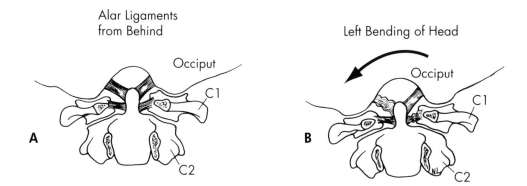

Figure 5.26 The role of the alar ligaments in lateral flexion of the atlanto-occipital articulation: (**A**) posterior view in the neutral position; (**B**) left lateral flexion. Motion is limited by the right upper portion and the left lower portion of the alar ligaments. (Modified from White and Panjabi,[1] with permission.)

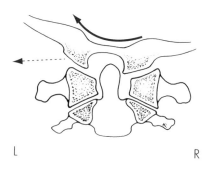

Figure 5.27 Right lateral flexion of the atlanto-occipital articulation demonstrating rolling of the occiput to the right (solid arrow) and sliding to the left (broken arrow).

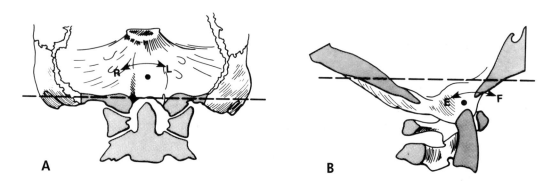

Figure 5.28 The theoretical location of the instantaneous axis of rotation for the atlanto-occipital articulation (dot) in (**A**) lateral flexion (R, L) and (**B**) flexion (F) and extension (E). (From White and Panjabi,[1] with permission.)

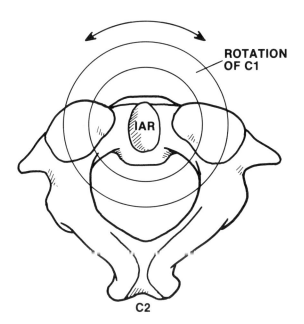

Figure 5.29 The theoretical location of the instantaneous axis of rotation (IAR) for the atlanto-axial articulation in axial rotation. (From White and Panjabi,[1] with permission.)

The instantaneous axes of rotation have not been experimentally determined for the atlanto-occipital articulation. The axes were estimated by Henke "by determining the centers of the arches formed by the outline of the joints in the sagittal and frontal planes"[1] (Fig. 5-28).

Range and Pattern of Motion of C1–C2

The principal movement that occurs at the atlanto-axial joint is axial rotation. Segmental range averages 40 degrees to each side, contributing to over half of the total cervical rotation. The first 25 degrees of cervical rotation occur primarily in the atlanto-axial joint.[3] During rotation the lateral mass and articular surface slide posteriorly on the side of rotation and anteriorly on the side opposite rotation. The motion occurs about a centrally located axis within the odontoid process (Fig. 5-29). An additional subtle vertical displacement of the atlas takes place with rotation owing to the biconvex structure of the articular surfaces (Fig. 5-30).

Flexion and extension movements of the atlas on the axis occur as rocker movements owing to the biconvex facet surfaces. The instantaneous axes of rotation is located in the middle third of the dens. In flexion the posterior joint capsule and posterior arches separate and the atlas articular surface glides forward. In extension the posterior joint capsule and posterior arches approximate and the atlas articular surface glides posterior (Fig. 5-31). Also, the anterior arch of the atlas must ride up the odontoid process during extension and down during flexion. Flexion and extension movements of the atlanto-axial joint are also associated with small translational movements from 2–3 mm in the adult up to 4.5 mm in the child.[1] Any movement greater than these ranges should trigger an evaluation to assess the stability of the C1–C2 articulation and the integrity of the odontoid and transverse ligaments.

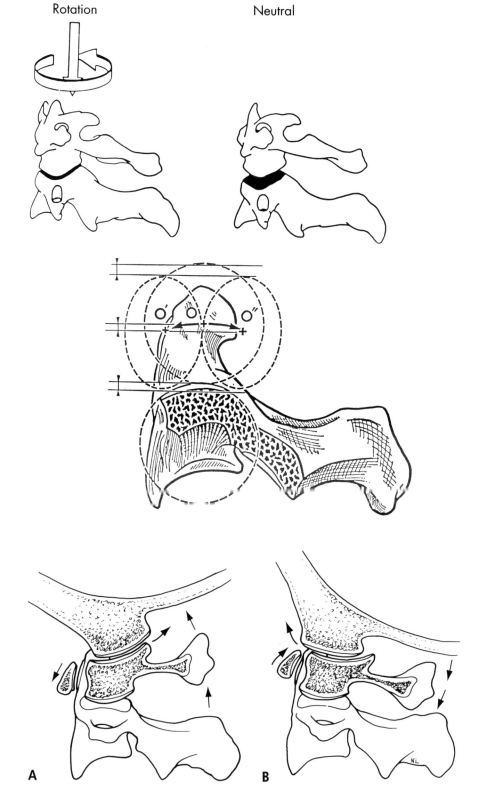

Figure 5.30 Because the articular surfaces are both convex, as the atlas rotates on the axis, a subtle vertical displacement occurs, causing the two segments to approximate one another (∪ = neutral).

Figure 5.31 (A) Flexion and (B) extension of the atlanto-axial articulation with the instantaneous axis of rotation indicated. The anterior curvature of the dens will influence the degree of movement.

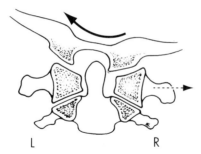

Figure 5.32 Right lateral flexion of the upper cervical spine (solid arrows) with translation of the atlas (broken arrow) toward the right.

Compared with rotation, lateral flexion of the atlanto-axial articulation is limited, averaging approximately 5 degrees to each side.[3] It has been suggested that lateral flexion is coupled with translation, however, this is a controversial subject.[1] The associated translation is purported to occur toward the side of lateral flexion. In other words, right lateral flexion of the cervical spine would be associated with translation of C1 to the right (Fig. 5.32).

Further clouding the issue is the apparent translation that may be visible on an AP open-mouth radiograph with rotational subluxation of the atlas. Rotational movement of the lateral masses about the odontoid process may induce an apparent lateral translation of the atlas on the AP open-mouth owing to projectional widening and narrowing of the lateral masses (Fig. 5.33)

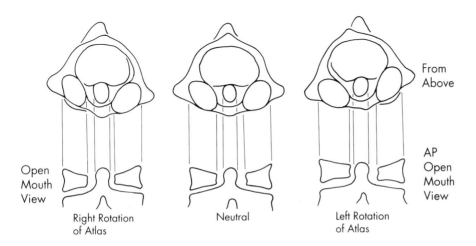

Figure 5.33 Projectional distortion and magnification cause atlas rotation to appear as lateral flexion on an anterior to posterior open-mouth x-ray view.

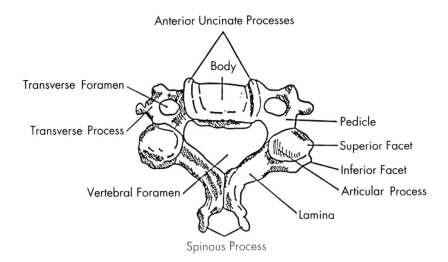

Figure 5.34 Structure of a typical cervical vertebra.

Functional Anatomy of the Lower Cervical Spine (C3–C7)

The typical cervical vertebra (C3–C6) possess the same structural parts as all other true vertebrae, plus some unique and distinctive physical features (Fig. 5-34). The spinous processes are bifid to allow for better ligamentous and muscular attachment. Each transverse process from C6 upwards contains the transverse foramen, allowing for the passage of the vertebral artery. The body of the typical cervical vertebra has anterior and posterior surfaces that are small, oval, and wide transversely. The anterior and posterior surfaces are flat and of equal height. The posterolateral aspect of the superior margin of the vertebral bodies is lipped, forming the uncinate processes, which serve to strengthen and stabilize the region. The uncovertebral articulations (joints of Von Luschka) are pseudojoints that have a synovial membrane with synovial fluid but no joint capsule (Fig. 5-35). They serve as tracts that guide the motion of coupled rotation and lateral flexion. They begin to develop at six years of age and are complete by age eighteen years.

The articular facets are tear-drop shaped with the superior facet facing up and posteriorly while the inferior one faces down and anteriorly placing the joint space at a 45-degree angle midway between the coronal and transverse planes (Fig. 5-36). The disc height to body height ratio is greatest (2 : 5) in the cervical spine, therefore allowing for the greatest possible range of motion (Fig. 5-37).

The short and rounded pedicles of cervical vertebrae are directed posteriorly and laterally. The superior and inferior vertebral notch in each pedicle is the same depth. The laminae are long, narrow, slender, and sloping. The intervertebral foramen in this region are larger than in the lumber or thoracic areas and are triangular in shape.

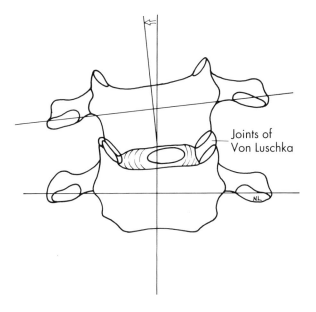

Figure 5.35 The uncinate processes limit pure lateral flexion to only a few degrees while serving as guides to couple lateral flexion with rotation.

Joints of Von Luschka

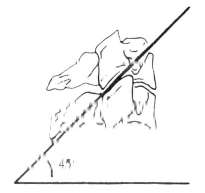

Figure 5.36 The cervical facet planes.

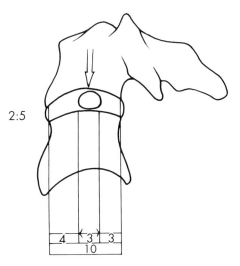

Figure 5.37 The location of the nucleus pulposus and the disc height-to-body ratio in the cervical spine.

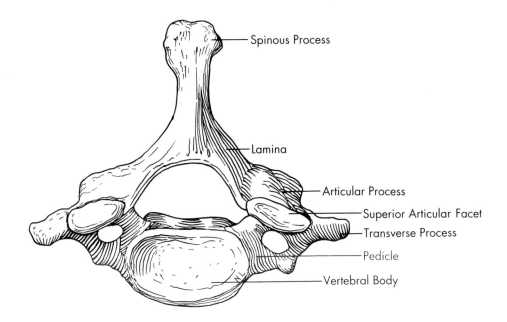

Figure 5.38 The structure of the C7 vertebra (vertebral prominence).

Spinous Process

Lamina

Articular Process

Superior Articular Facet

Transverse Process

Pedicle

Vertebral Body

The C7 vertebra (vertebra prominence) is considered the atypical segment of the lower cervical spine. It demonstrates anatomic characteristics of both the cervical vertebra and thoracic vertebra. It has a spinous process that is quite long and slender, with a tubercle on its end. The inferior articular processes are similar to those in the thoracic spine, while the superior processes match those of the typical cervical vertebra. C7 has no uncinate processes and no transverse foramen. The transverse processes are large, broad, and blunt. The anterior root is shorter and smaller than the remaining cervicals. The transverse processes may become enlarged or develop cervical ribs, with the potential to create thoracic outlet compromise (Fig. 5-30).

Cervical Curve

The cervical spine forms a lordotic curve that develops secondary to the response of upright posture. The function of the cervical curve, and the anterior to posterior curves throughout the spine, is to add resiliency to the spine in response to axial compression forces and to balance the center of gravity of the skull over the spine. The center of gravity for the skull lies anterior to the foramen magnum (Fig. 5-39). The facet and disc planes in large part determine the degree of potential lordosis. Congenital diversity in pillar height and facet angulation, therefore, lead to significant variation in the degree of cervical lordosis present in the population. Additionally, degenerative changes or stress responses in either of these structures may change the "normal" lordosis. With a reduced cervical curve (hypolordosis) more weight has to be born on the vertebral bodies and discs, and musculature effort will increase as the posterior neck muscles work to maintain head

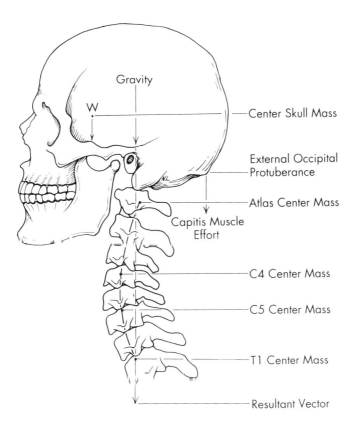

Figure 5.39 The center of gravity for the skull. If the cervical curve changes, the center of gravity will shift.

position and spinal stability. An increased cervical curve (hyperlordosis) increases the compressive load on the facets and posterior elements (Fig. 5-40). There are a number of ideas as to what the normal cervical curve should be and how it should be measured.[2,4–10] There is some agreement that the midpoint is the C5 vertebra (C4-5 interspace). The cervical lordosis apparently extends to the T1-2 motion segment where the transition to the thoracic kyphosis occurs. Measurements for the cervical curve use the C7 level, as this is usually the lowest point that can be seen on a lateral cervical x-ray. Jochumsen[8] proposed classifying the cervical curve by measuring the distance from the anterior body of C5 to a line running from the anterior arch of the atlas to the anterior superior aspect of the body of C7 (Fig. 5-41). Other methods incorporate direct measurement of the curve by forming an angle between a line extending through the center of C1 with a line drawn along the inferior end plate of C7 (Fig. 5-42).

The proposed optimal curve for the cervical spine can be extrapolated from the mechanical principle that states the strongest and most resilient curve is an arc that has a radius of curvature equal to the cord across the arc (Fig. 5-43). The length of the radius, and hence the cord, should equal approximately 7 inches or 17 cm. As the radius increases the curve increases (flattens as in hypolordosis) and vice versa.

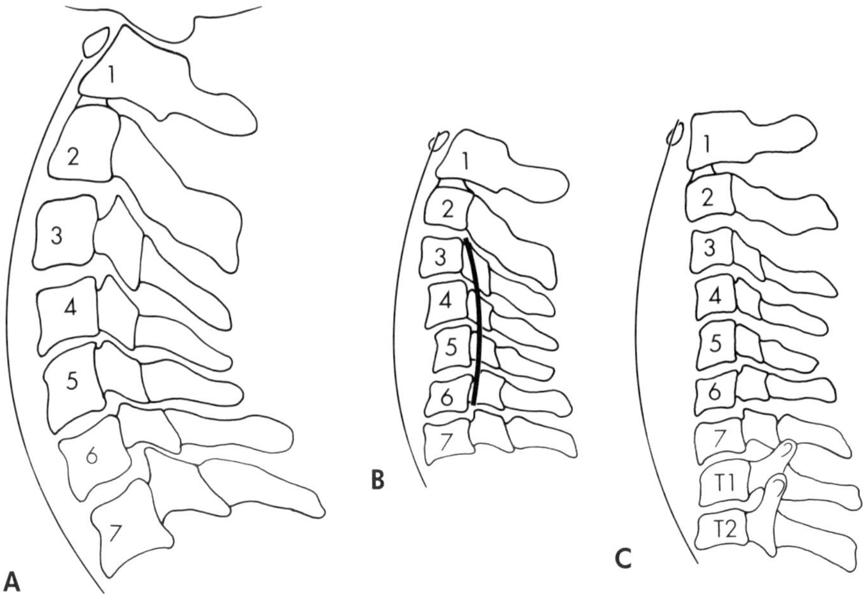

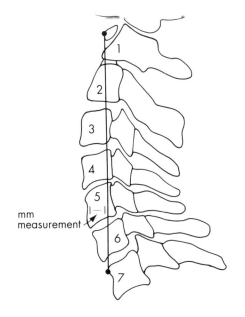

Figure 5.40 The cervical curve extending from C1 to T2: (**A**) normal; (**B**) hypolordosis with a kyphosis involving the middle segments; (**C**) a-lordosis.

A

B

C

Figure 5.41 Jochumsen's measuring procedure for determining the adequacy of the cervical curve.

mm measurement

over 9 mm = hyperlordosis
3 to 8 mm = mean lordosis
1 to 2 mm = hypolordosis
1 to −3 mm = alordosis
under −3 mm = kyphosis

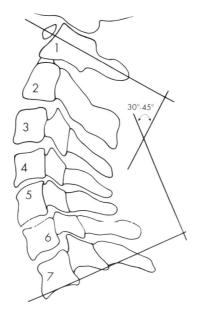

Figure 5.42 The angle of the cervical curve should be about 30 to 45 degrees when measured between lines drawn through C1 and C7.

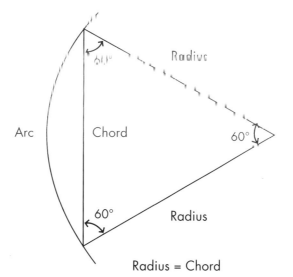

Figure 5.43 Diagram demonstrating the relationship formed when a chord equals the radius of an arc.

Range and Pattern of Motion of the Lower Cervical Spine

The lower cervical spine exhibits its greatest flexibility during flexion and extension movements (Table 5-4) (Fig. 5-24). Lateral flexion exhibits slightly greater movement than rotation. Both rotation and lateral flexion decrease significantly at the thoraco-cervical junction.

Table 5.4 Segmental Ranges of Motion for the Lower Cervical Spine[a]

Vertebra	Combined Flexion and Extension	One Side Lateral Flexion	One Side Axial Rotation
C2–3	5–16 (10)	11–20 (10)	0–10 (3)
C3–4	7–26 (15)	9–15 (11)	3–10 (7)
C4–5	13–29 (20)	0–16 (11)	1–12 (7)
C5–6	13–29 (20)	0–16 (8)	2–12 (7)
C6–7	6–26 (17)	0–17 (7)	2–10 (6)
C7–T1	4–7 (9)	0–17 (4)	0–7 (2)

[a] Given in degrees with average in parentheses.
(Adapted from White and Panjabi,[1] with permission.)

Flexion/Extension

Movement averages approximately 15 degrees of combined flexion/extension per segment and is greatest at the C5–C6 motion segment.[11] Flexion/extension occurs around an axis located in the subjacent vertebra and combines sagittal plane rotation with sagittal plane translation. This pattern of combined segmental angular tipping and gliding develops a stair step effect, which is noted on flexion/extension radiographs (Fig. 5-44).

With flexion the articular joint surfaces slide apart, producing stretching and gapping of the posterior facets and disc and anterior disc approximation and compression. With extension the opposite occurs. The disc is subjected to compression on the concave side and tension on the convex side. The side subjected to tension retracts while the side subjected to compression bulges.[1] The net effect of these two opposing forces is to limit shifting of the nucleus pulposus during movements of flexion and extension and lateral flexion (Fig. 5-45). King et al[12] implanted small metal markers within the lumbar and thoracic intervertebral discs and confirmed the bulging and retraction of the discs during lumbar segmental flexion movements. However, they did note some minor posterior migration of the nucleus that was not identified by previous mathematical models. This phenomena has not been investigated for the cervical spine.

The coupled translation that occurs with flexion and extension has been measured at approximately 2 mm per segment, with an upper range of 2.7 mm.[13] Translational movements do not occur evenly throughout the cervical spine.[11] For every degree of sagittal plane rotation more translation occurs

Figure 5.44 Sagittal plane movement of a cervical motion segment in (**A**) flexion and (**B**) extension locating the instantaneous axis of rotation (IAR) and the stair stepping appearance that occurs with combined tipping and gliding movements.

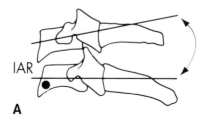

IAR

A

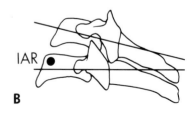

IAR

B

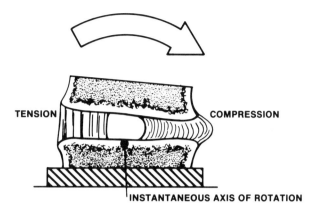

Figure 5.45 Representation of changes in the disc with flexion as well as extension or lateral flexion movements. (From White and Panjabi,[1] with permission.)

in the upper cervical segments than in the lower cervical segments. This leads to a flatter arch of movement in the upper cervical spine (Fig. 5-46). Accounting for radiographic magnification, White and Panjabi[1] have recommended 3.5 mm as the upper end of normal translational movement in the lower cervical segments. Translation beyond 3.5 mm suggests segmental instability.

Lateral Flexion

Lateral flexion averages approximately 10 degrees to each side in the mid cervical segments, with decreasing flexibility in the caudal segments. The instantaneous axis of rotation for lateral flexion has not been determined. Speculation places the axis in the center of the subjacent vertebral body

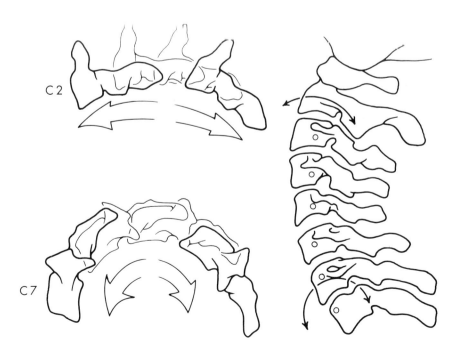

Figure 5.46 With active flexion and extension movements, apparently more translation takes place in the upper segments while more rotation takes place in the lower segments.

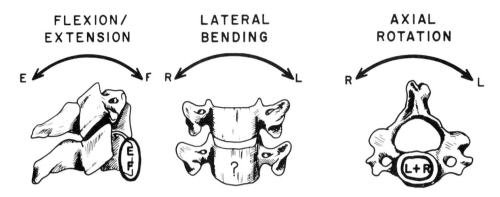

Figure 5.47 The theoretical locations for the instantaneous axis of rotation for each plane of movement in the lower cervical spine. (From White and Panjabi,[1] with permission.)

(Fig. 5-47). Lateral flexion in the lower cervical spine is coupled with rotation in the transverse plane. The coupling is such that lateral flexion and rotation occur to the same side. This leads to posterior vertebral body rotation on the side of lateral flexion, thereby causing the spinous processes to deviate to the convexity of the curve (Fig. 5-48). The degree of coupled axial rotation decreases in a caudal direction.[10] At the second cervical vertebra there are 2 degrees of coupled rotation for every 3 degrees of lateral bending, and at the seventh cervical vertebra there is only 1 degree of coupled rotation for every 7.5 degrees of lateral bending.

During lateral flexion the facets on the side of lateral flexion (concave side) approximate as the inferior facet slides inferiorly and medially because of the coupled rotation. On the opposite side the facets distract and the inferior facet slides superiorly and anteriorly. The intervertebral disc approximates on the side of lateral flexion and distracts on the opposite side (Fig. 5-49).

Rotation

Ranges of motion for segmental axial rotation on average are slightly less than those for lateral flexion, with a similar tendency for decreased movement in the lower cervical segments, especially at the C7–T1 motions segment. The axis of rotation is also somewhat speculative and has been placed by Lysell[10] in the anterior subjacent vertebral body (Fig. 5-47). Rotational movements in the lower cervical spine demonstrate the same coupling as described for lateral flexion. In other words, left or right axial rotation is coupled with lateral flexion to the same side. This leads to a pattern of motion where on the side of cervical rotation (posterior body rotation) the inferior facet glides posteriorly and inferiorly as the contralateral glides anteriorly and superiorly (Fig. 5-50).

Cervical Kinetics

Non-segmental muscles produce integrated global movement of the cervical spine as a result of the head's moving in relation to the trunk. Concentric and eccentric muscle activity is combined, with eccentric activity predominating

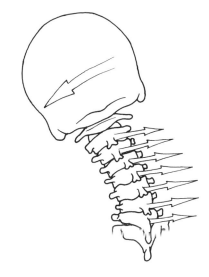

Figure 5.48 Left lateral flexion coupled with physiologic left rotation in the cervical spine.

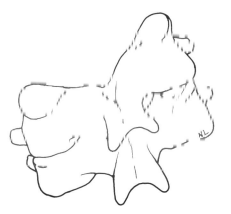

Figure 5.49 Movement of the facet surfaces with left lateral flexion in the lower cervical spine.

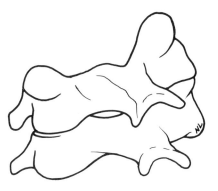

Figure 5.50 The effects of left rotation coupled with left lateral flexion on the articulations in the lower cervical spine.

during flexion/extension and lateral flexion. *Concentric muscle activity* refers to the development of sufficient muscle tension to overcome a resistance, causing the muscle to visibly shorten and the body part to move. However, *eccentric muscle activity* occurs when a given resistance overcomes the muscle tension, causing the muscle to actually lengthen. Relaxation of a muscle against the force of gravity, creating a deceleration of the moving body part, is an example of eccentric muscle activity.[11]

The *segmental (intrinsic) muscles* function to coordinate and integrate segmental motion. The intrinsic muscles act as involuntary integrators of overall movement. Normal movements of the cervical spine are initiated by movements of the head, but with conscious effort movement may be initiated at lower segmental levels. They operate by the same concentric and eccentric principles as the larger non-segmental muscles. Flexion is initiated by anterior cervical muscles and controlled or limited by eccentric activity of the semispinalis, longissimus, and splenius muscle groups. Flexion is further limited by the elastic limits of myofascial tissue, nuchal ligament, joint capsule, PLL, ligamentum flavum, posterior IVD, anterior vertebral bodies, and the chin hitting the chest.

Extension is initiated by posterior cervical muscles controlled or limited by the eccentric activity of the SCM, scaleni, and longus coli muscle groups. Extension is further limited by the elastic limits of the myofascial tissue, anterior IVD, ALL, joint capsule, posterior vertebral bodies, and articular pillars.

Lateral flexion is initiated by ipsilateral contraction and controlled or limited by the contralateral eccentric activity of the splenius capitis, semispinalis cervices, and longus coli muscle groups. Lateral flexion is further limited by the elastic limits of some myofascial tissue, contralateral joint capsule, periarticular ligaments, flavel ligament, IVD, ipsilateral joint capsule, and ipsilateral articular pillars.

Rotation is initiated by concentric contraction of the ipsilateral splenius capitis and cervicis, longissimus cervicis, and contralateral semispinalis muscles. Eccentric muscle contraction occurs simultaneously to guide and break movements and involves action of the contralateral splenius capitis, cervicis, longissimus cervicis, and ipsilateral semispinalis and scaleni muscles. Movement is further limited by capsular and periarticular ligaments and segmental muscles.

Evaluation of the Cervical Spine

Observation

Examination of the cervical spine begins with a visual examination of the alignment and range of motion of the cervical spine in the sagittal, coronal, and transverse planes. Alignment in the coronal plane is evaluated by observing the orientation of the head relative to the trunk and shoulders, the leveling of the mastoid processes, and the symmetry of the cervical soft tissues. Sagittal plane alignment is assessed by observing the status of the cervical curve and orientation of the patient's chin. Tucking or elevation of the chin in the presence of a normal cervical curve may indicate upper cervical dysfunction. Orientation of the head in the transverse plane may

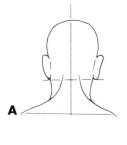

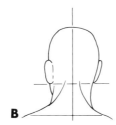

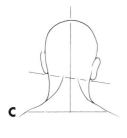

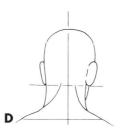

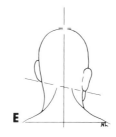

Figuer 5.51 Common cervical postural presentations: (A) normal; (B) occiput fixed in left posterior rotation; (C) occiput fixed in right lateral flexion or atlas in left laterolisthesis; (D) atlas fixed in right posterior or left anterior rotation; (E) axis fixed in right rotation and right lateral flexion. (Modified from Pratt,[17] with permission.)

be assessed by observing the patient from the posterior, noting any turning of the head (Fig. 5-51).

Global range of motion is most effectively evaluated in the sitting position. Take care to observe for recruitment of trunk movement and stabilization of the shoulders if necessary. During flexion the patient should be able to touch the chin to the chest and during extension look straight up at the ceiling. During rotation the patient should be able to approximate the chin to the shoulder and during lateral flexion approximate the ear to within two to three fingers' width of the shoulder (Fig. 5-52). Variations with sex and age are quite common. If range of motion is evaluated in circumstances other than screening evaluations, it should be conducted with the use of inclinometry for more accurate recordings of the ranges (see Fig. 3-11 and Table 5-5).

Static Palpation

Palpation for alignment, tone, texture, and tenderness of the bony and soft tissue structures of the neck is conducted with the patient in the supine or

Table 5.5. Global Ranges of Motion for the Cervical Spine

Motion	Normal Range	Range Without Impairment
Flexion	60°–90°	60°
Extension	75°–90°	75°
Lateral flexion	45°–55°	45°
Rotation	80°–90°	80°

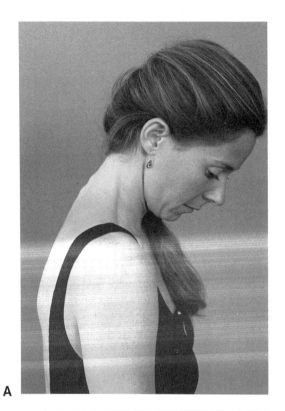

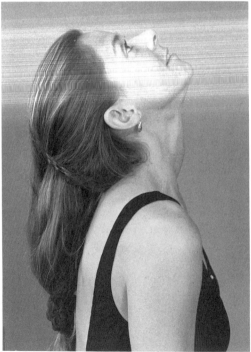

Figure 5.52 Cervical global ranges of motion: (**A**) flexion; (**B**) extension; (*Figure continues.*)

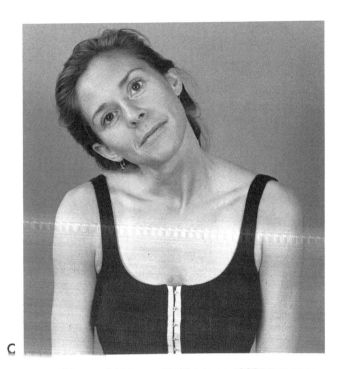

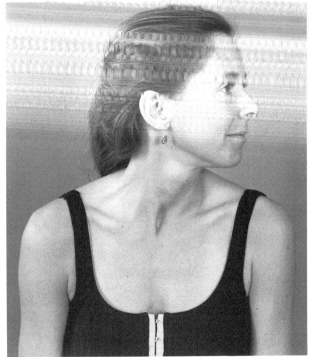

Figure 5.52 (*Continued*). (**C**) right lateral flexion; (**D**) left rotation.

sitting position. During supine evaluation stand or kneel at the head of the table, and during the seated evaluation stand behind the patient.

Upper cervical spine

The suboccipital muscles are evaluated by using the palmar surfaces of the fingertips to make a bilateral comparison of tone, texture, and tenderness (Fig. 5-53). Bony alignment of the atlanto-occipital joint is evaluated by placing the tip of the index finger in the space between the mandibular ramus and the anterior tip of the atlas transverse process and between the inferior tip of the mastoid process and the atlas transverse process (Fig. 5-54).

Spacing between the atlas transverse process and the mandibular ramus and between the atlas transverse process and mastoid processes should be symmetric on both sides. The space between the angle of the jaw and atlas transverse processes may be opened with an extension malposition and closed with a flexion malposition. With lateral flexion subluxations the mastoids may be unlevel, and increased spacing may be noted in the interspace between the atlas transverse process and mastoid process.

Bony alignment of the atlanto-axial joint is evaluated by comparing the relative alignment of the atlas and axis transverse processes. This is accomplished by establishing bilateral contacts with the doctor's index and middle fingers over each articulation (Fig. 5-55). Posterior prominence of the atlas or palpable stair stepping of the atlas and axis transverse processes indicate possible rotational malposition of the atlas. Lateral prominence of the atlas and/or narrowing of the atlas mastoid interspace indicates possible lateral flexion malposition of the atlas.

Asymmetry in suboccipital muscle tone and/or tender and taut suboccipital muscles are further indications of possible upper cervical joint dysfunction. However, the upper cervical spine is at the end of a kinetic chain, and asymmetries in tone and alignment are commonly encountered. They may

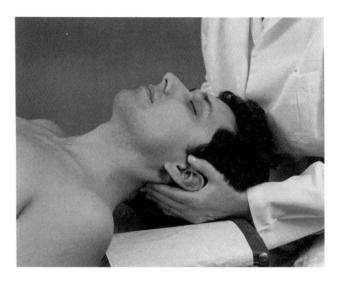

Figure 5.53 Palpation of suboccipital muscle tone and texture.

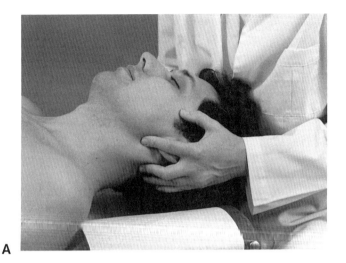

A

B

Figure 5.54 Palpation for (A) flexion, extension, or rotation alignment and (B) lateral flexion alignment of the atlanto-occipital articulation.

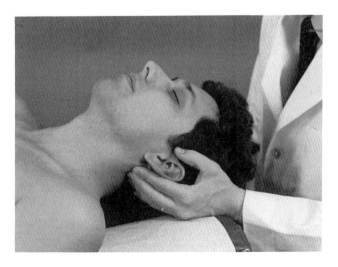

Figure 5.55 Palpation for rotation and lateral flexion alignment of the atlanto-axial articulation.

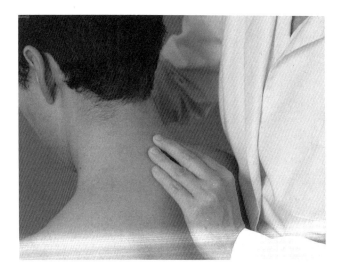

Figure 5.56 Palpation for the alignment of the spinous processes in the lower cervical spine.

be normal variations or sites of compensational adaptation instead of primary joint dysfunction.

Lower cervical spine (C2–C7)

Bony contour, tenderness, and alignment are assessed by palpating the spinous process, interspinous spaces, and posterior articular pillars. In the sitting position the interspinous spaces may be palpated with the middle finger while the index and ring fingers lay along the lateral margins to compare alignment of adjacent spinous processes (Fig. 5-56). The spinous processes are bifid and difficult to palpate in the mid-cervical spine. They

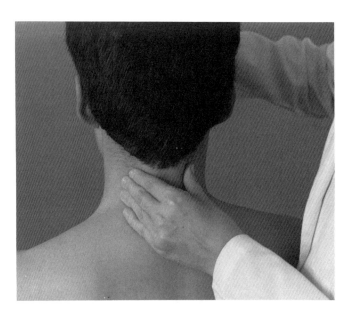

Figure 5.57 Palpation for the alignment of the articular pillars in the mid-cervical spine.

become more accessible if the neck is placed in a slight flexion. The articular pillars are not as accessible to direct palpation but are probably a more reliable landmark for detecting rotational malpositions.

To evaluate the alignment of the articular pillars and tone, texture, and tenderness of the paraspinal soft tissues, establish segmental contacts on each side of the spine. In the sitting position use the thumb and index fingers (Fig. 5-57), and in the supine position the palmar surfaces of the fingers of both hands make a bilateral comparison.

Motion Palpation

Cervical joint play, segmental range of motion, and end play may be evaluated with the patient in either a sitting or supine position. Stand behind the seated patient; stand, kneel, or squat at the head of the table during a supine evaluation.

Joint play

To evaluate joint play and posterior to anterior glide with the patient in the seated position, position the patient's neck in a neutral position and establish segmental contacts bilaterally over posterior joints with the palmar surfaces of the index finger and thumb. With the patient's forehead supported by the indifferent hand, gently spring each individual motion segment in a fluid posterior to anterior gliding motion along the horizontal plane (Fig. 5-58).

In the supine position, assess posterior to anterior glide by contacting

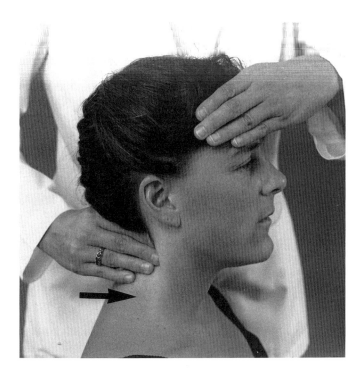

Figure 5.58 Sitting joint play evaluation for posterior to anterior glide in the mid-cervical spine.

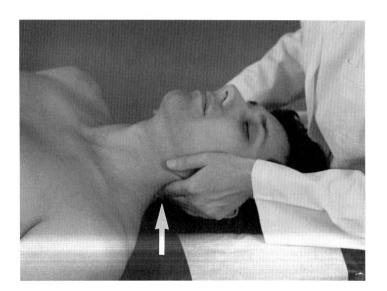

Figure 5.59 Supine joint play evaluation for posterior to anterior glide in the mid-cervical spine.

the posterior joints with the palmar surfaces of the fingertips. The patient's head rests on the table while the fingertips spring posterior to anterior against the articular pillars (Fig. 5-59). Lateral to medial glide may be assessed by contacting the posterolateral surface of adjacent vertebrae with the radial or palmar surface of the doctor's index fingers. Testing is performed by springing toward the midline with one hand as the other hand counter stabilizes (Fig. 5-60).

During posterior to anterior joint play assessment, the doctor should feel a subtle gliding and recoil at each segment tested. The movement should be uniform on each side and pain free; unilateral resistance or a tendency for the spine to rotate out of the sagittal plane may indicate segmental fixation. Lateral to medial glide is less giving than anterior to posterior glide, and a perceptible decrease in movement should be noted when the adjacent vertebra is counter-stabilized. Excessive sponginess and lack of elastic resistance with either procedure indicates possible hypermobility or instability.

Segmental range of motion and end play (C0–C1)

C0–C1 flexion/extension. Atlanto-occipital flexion/extension may be evaluated by placing the tip of the index finger in the space bertween the mandibular ramus and the anterior tip of the atlas transverse process. The doctor's indifferent hand supports the top of the head in the sitting position and cups the patient's contralateral occiput and mastoid in the supine position. The patient's chin is elevated and tucked to instill extension and flexion in the upper cervical spine. The space between the mandibular ramus and atlas transverse process opens during extension and closes during flexion (Fig. 5-61). Fixation in this plane leads to a loss of rolling of the occiput on the atlas and unchanged spacing between the angle of the jaw and the atlas transverse process.

To evaluate end play, apply additional springing over-pressure at the end

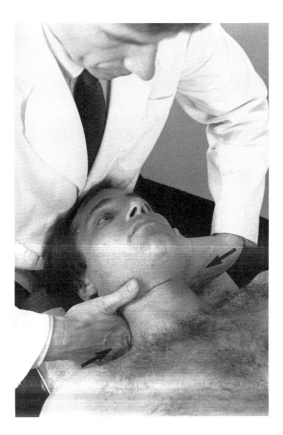

Figure 5.60 Supine joint play evaluation for lateral to medial glide in the mid-cervical spine.

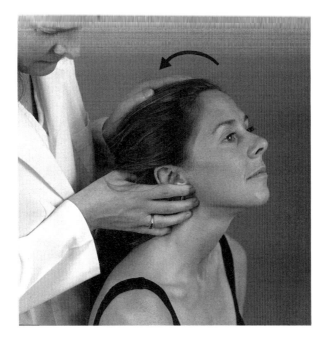

Figure 5.61 Palpation for extension movement of the right atlanto-occipital articulation.

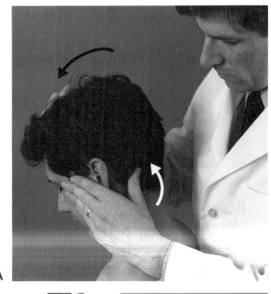

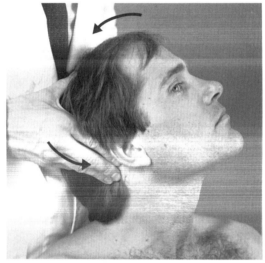

Figure 5.62 End play evaluation of the atlanto-occipital articulation: **(A)** flexion and **(B)** extension.

range of motion. For flexion, the contacts are established under the inferior rim or the occiput with pressure applied upward. For extension, the contacts are established over the mastoid and posterior occiput, with pressure applied forward and downward (Fig. 5-62). Flexion end play has a firmer quality as it is limited by the strong posterior neck muscles.

C0–C1 rotation. The index finger is placed between the mandibular ramus and the anterior tip of the atlas transverse process. The head is passively rotated away from the side of contact. The gap between the mandibular ramus and the atlas transverse process will open on the side opposite rotation and close on the side of rotation. Occipital rotation is limited and occurs at the end of cervical rotation (Fig. 5-63).

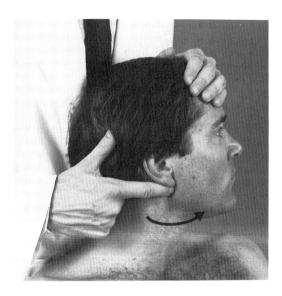

Figure 5.63 Palpation of left rotation and anterior glide of the right atlanto-occipital articulation.

C0–C1 lateral flexion. Lateral flexion is evaluated by placing the index finger between the inferior tip of the mastoid process and the atlas transverse process (Fig. 5-64). The head is laterally flexed away from the side of contact, and the gap between the mastoid and atlas transverse should open on the side opposite the lateral flexion. End play is evaluated on the side of lateral flexion for medial glide and on the contralateral side for superior glide. To evaluate medial glide, the doctor contacts the posterior lateral aspect of the occiput with the lateral surface of the index finger (or fingertips of the index and middle fingers). The patient's head is laterally flexed toward the side of contact while the doctor springs medially at the end range of motion (Fig. 5-65). Superior glide is evaluated by establishing fingertip contacts

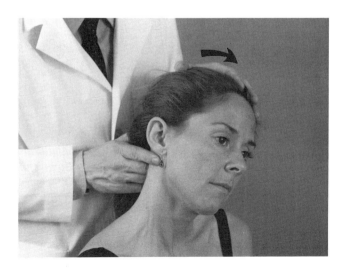

Figure 5.64 Palpation of left lateral flexion and superior glide of the right atlanto-occipital articulation.

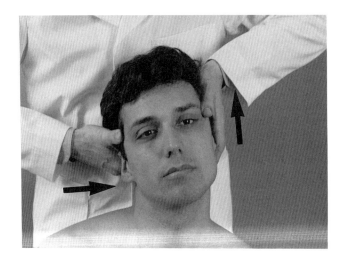

Figure 5.65 Palpation of right lateral flexion end play of the atlanto-occipital articulation. The doctor's right hand applies medial pressure while the left hand distracts superiorly.

under the mastoid process on the opposite side and springing headword at the end range of motion.

Segmental range of motion and end play (C1–C2)

C1–C2 rotation (posterior to anterior glide). To evaluate atlanto-axial rotation, contact the posterolateral aspect of the transverse process of the atlas and axis overlapping the C1–C2 intertransverse space with the palmar surfaces of the middle and index fingers. The contacts are established on the side opposite cervical rotation, while the head is laterally flexed a few degrees toward the contact and passively rotated away from the side of contact (Fig. 5-66). The doctor should palpate anterior rotation of C1 and separation of the C1–C2 intertransverse space on the side opposite rotation (side of

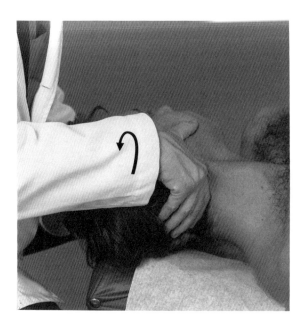

Figure 5.66 Palpation of left rotation and anterior to posterior glide of the right atlanto-axial articulation.

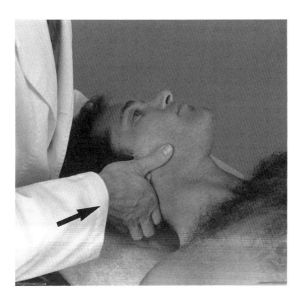

Figure 5.67 Palpation of right to left medial glide of C1.

contact). At the end of passive rotation, evaluate end play by applying forward overpressure against the transverse process of C1. The atlanto-axial articulation lacks a strong interlaminar ligament and has a loss joint capsule allowing for a comparatively flexible end play.

C1–C2 medial glide. Establish an index contact on the lateral surface of the atlas transverse process. The patient's head is laterally flexed toward the side of contact while medial springing pressure is applied against the atlas transverse process from the concave side toward the convex side (Fig. 5-67). Lateral flexion at the atlas is limited; this procedure is designed to assess the small degree of medial glide that should be present, not the active range of lateral flexion.

C1–C2 flexion/extension. Establish bilateral contacts over the C1–C2 articulation. Employ the index and middle fingers on one side and a thumb contact on the other. The patient's head is flexed and extended at the C1–C2 articulation. Palpate for posterior inferior glide of the atlas during extension and anterior superior glide during flexion (Fig. 5-68). At the end of passive motion, evaluate end play by springing anterior and superiorly for flexion and anteriorly and inferiorly for extension. The end play is elastic but firm compared with rotation end play.

Segmental range of motion and end play (C2–C7)

The lower cervical spine may be evaluated with the patient in the sitting or supine position. In the sitting position, the doctor controls movement by contacting the patient's forehead or the crown of the patient's head. In the supine position, passive movement is controlled by cupping the patient's contralateral occiput and mastoid.

Rotation (posterior to anterior glide). Evaluate movement by placing the palmar surface of the index or index and middle fingers over the articular

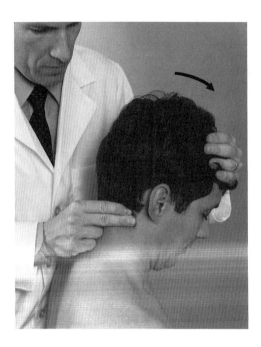

Figure 5.68 Palpation of flexion at the atlanto-axial articulation.

pillars. With the patient in the sitting position, use either an upright (palm up) or reverse (palm down) hand contact method (Fig. 5-69). Establish palpation contacts on the posterior surface of the articular pillars on the side opposite cervical rotation. The patient's head is passively rotated as anterior glide on the side opposite the direction of induced rotation is palpated. The superior pillar should move forward relative to those below, and the soft tissue should elongate under the contact. With full rotation you should note a stair-stepping effect from the lower to upper cervical spine. At the end of passive motion, evaluate end play by springing from the posterior to the anterior, along the facet planes, normally encountering firm, elastic but giving end play.

Rotation (anterior to posterior glide). When evaluating this motion with the patient in the sitting position, stand behind the patient, opposite the side of contact. Establish a soft contact with the ventral surface of the index and middle fingers over the anterolateral surface of the articular pillars. Take care to avoid excessive pressure over the anterior neurovascular structures. The stabilization hand contacts the patient's forehead or top of the patient's head. The patient's head is laterally flexed away and rotated toward the side of contact to induce anterior to posterior gliding and perpendicular gapping of the articulation under the point of contact. In addition to the anterior to posterior palpation vector, an inferior to superior orientation should be maintained so that the palpation vector is at a 90 degree angle to the facet plane (Fig. 5-70). Evaluate end play motion by springing from the anterior to the posterior along the same palpation vector.

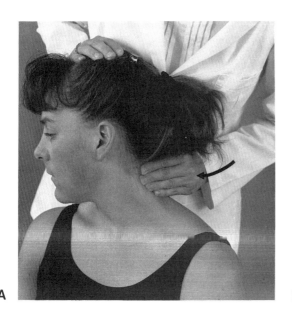
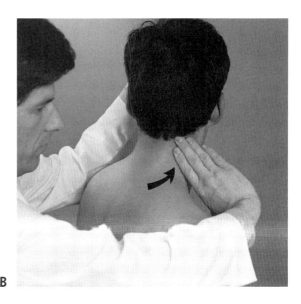
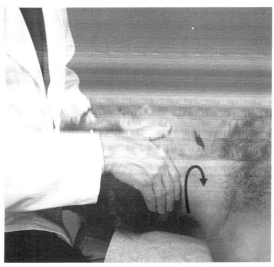

Figure 5.69 Palpation of rotation and posterior to anterior glide at the C3–C4 articulation: (**A**) right rotation with the palm down; (**B**) left rotation with the palm up; (**C**) left rotation in the supine position.

You may also perform this method with the patient in the supine position by establishing a soft anterior lateral pillar contact with the thumb of your hand corresponding to the side of palpation (Fig. 5-71).

C2–C7 lateral flexion. To assess lateral flexion, establish segmental contacts over the articular pillars slightly posterior to the mid-coronal plane. If the contacts are placed too far anterior they can become uncomfortable to the

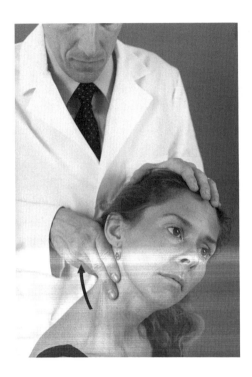

Figure 5.70 Palpation of right rotation and anterior to posterior glide of the right C2–C3 articulation in the seated position.

patient. Segmental contacts may be established unilateral or bilaterally. They may be established with the index and middle fingers of one or both hands or with the fingers and thumb of the same hand. When employing unilateral fingertip contacts, stand to the side opposite the contact and change palpation hands and sides as you evaluate movement to each side (Fig. 5-72). With the patient in the supine position, kneel at the head of the table and employ bilateral fingertip or index contacts (Fig. 5-73).

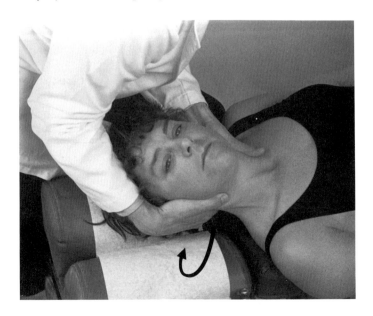

Figure 5.71 Palpation of right rotation and anterior to posterior glide of the right C2–C3 articulation in the supine position.

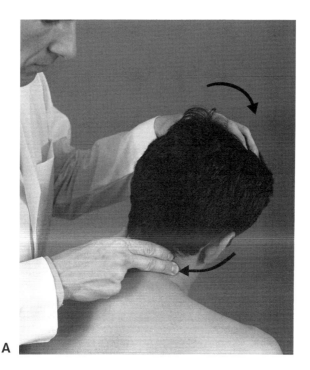

A

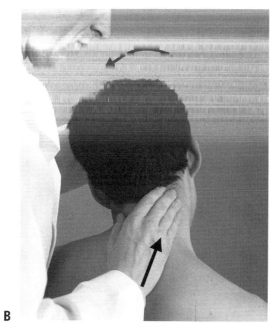

B

Figure 5.72 Palpation of (**A**) right lateral flexion and inferior, medial glide of C5–6 and (**B**) left lateral flexion and superior glide of the right C5–C6 articulation.

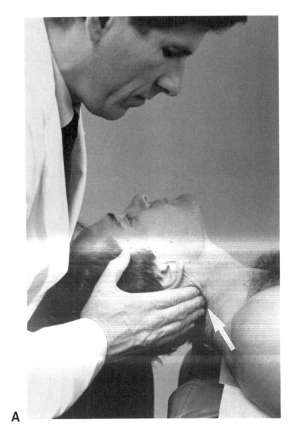

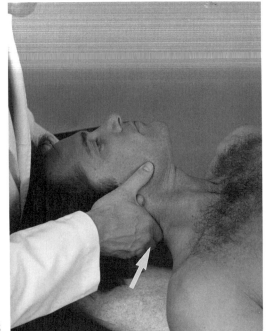

Figure 5.73 Palpation of right lateral flexion and inferior, medial glide in the supine position with (**A**) a fingertip contact and (**B**) an index contact of the right C5–C6 articulation.

During the assessment of lateral flexion, palpate bending and inferior glide of the articular pillar on the side of lateral flexion and superior glide and elongation of the soft tissues on the side opposite the lateral flexion (Fig. 5-72). At the end of passive motion, evaluate end play by applying additional overpressure by pushing toward the midline from the side of lateral flexion (concave toward convex). The vector should incorporate an inferior inclination to avoid compressing the soft tissues. End play may also be evaluated on the side opposite lateral flexion by applying additional headward distraction with the opposing hand as medial pressure is applied from the side of lateral flexion. During the latter, feel for the elastic stretch and elongation of the soft tissue on the convex side of bending. The end play quality for lateral flexion is similar to that of rotation—firm but giving and elastic.

C2–C7 flexion/extension. To evaluate segmental flexion and extension, establish bilateral or unilateral contacts over the posterior articular pillars. Establish the segmental contacts with the fingertips or with the fingertips and thumb of the same hand (Fig. 5-74). During extension, palpate posterior and inferior gliding of the articular pillars. During flexion, palpate anterior/superior gliding of the articular pillars. Evaluate flexion end play by applying additional overpressure in an anterior and superior direction, and evaluate extension by applying additional overpressure in an anterior and inferior direction. The quality of end play for flexion is more resistant owing to strong posterior neck muscles.

ADJUSTMENTS OF THE CERVICAL SPINE

Adjustments of the cervical spine are performed with the patient in sitting, prone, and supine positions. Most are assisted techniques and involve adjustive positions that involve movement of head and motion segments superior to the dysfunctional segment in the direction of joint restriction and adjustment. Therefore, the majority of the adjustments presented (assisted methods) developed tension in the motion segment immediately inferior to the segmental contact. Resisted methods are used less frequently. When applied they are typically used in the treatment of rotational dysfunction and the loss of posterior medial glide and gapping of the involved joint. Resisted cervical or thoracocervical adjustments develop maximal tension in the motion segment superior to the established contact.

The cervical spine is flexible and composed of small structures. It is easy to overpower the neck, so caution must be used in the delivery of cervical adjustments. Adjustive thrusts are delivered through the doctor's upper extremities. Although the majority of the adjustive impulse is predominantly delivered through the contact hand, the indifferent hand often provides additional assistance.

Rotational Dysfunction

Rotational dysfunction of the cervical spine may result from loss of anterior-superior glide of the facets on the side opposite the direction of rotation restriction (side of posterior body rotation) and/or posterior-inferior glide and gapping on the side of rotational restriction (Fig. 5-75). The side and

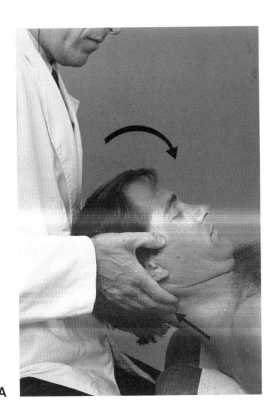

A

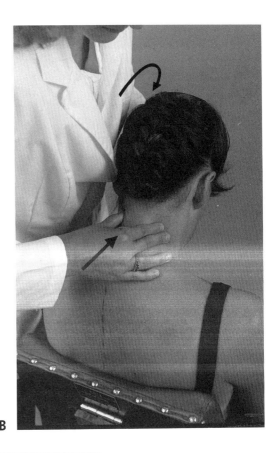

B

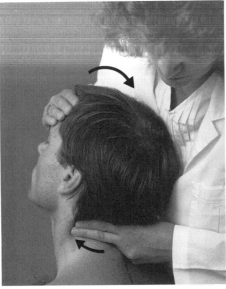

C

Figure 5.74 Palpation of cervical flexion of the C3–C4 articulation in (A) the supine position and (B) the seated position. (C) Palpation of cervical extension of the C3–C4 articulation.

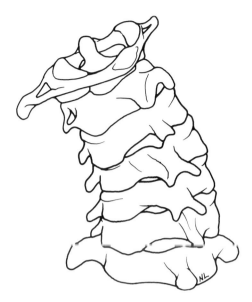

Figure 5.75 Posterior view of the cervical spine illustrating left rotation and characterized by anterior superior glide of the right facet joints and posterior inferior glide of the left facet joints.

site of fixation is assessed by comparing the end play quality of posterior to anterior glide on one side to the anterior to posterior glide on the other.

Dysfunction in anterior glide may be treated with assisted methods by contacting the posterior pillar of the superior vertebrae on the side of posterior body rotation (side opposite the rotation restriction). In the lower cervical spine the adjustive thrust would be directed anteriorly and superiorly (Fig. 5-76). In the case of the atlanto-axial joint the contact is established on the posterior lateral mass, and the thrust is directed horizontally (see Fig. 5-85B).

Restrictions in posterior glide and gapping may be treated with either assisted or resisted methods. In both techniques the cervical spine is laterally flexed away from the side of contact to lock the contralateral joints and distract the joint to be adjusted. With assisted methods, the contacts are established on the ipsilateral anterolateral pillar of the superior vertebrae on the side of rotational restriction (side opposite the posterior body rotation). The adjustive thrust is directed in a posterior direction (Fig. 5-77). When applying resisted methods the contacts are established on the spinous process of the inferior vertebra on the side opposite the rotation restriction (inferior vertebra on the side of posterior body rotation). The adjustive thrust is directed medially through the spinous contact, resisted by the counter rotational positioning of the patient's head (Fig. 5-78). The methods described are designed to isolate the adjustive forces to the side of fixation and reduce tension to contralateral joints that may not be fixated.

Lateral Flexion Dysfunction

Lateral flexion dysfunction of the cervical spine may result from a loss of inferior medial glide on the side of lateral flexion dysfunction (open wedge) and/or a loss of contralateral superior glide on the side opposite lateral

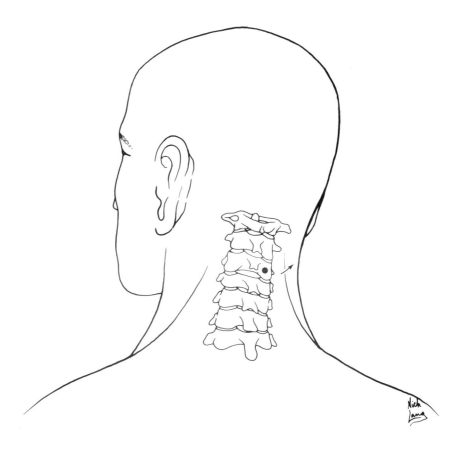

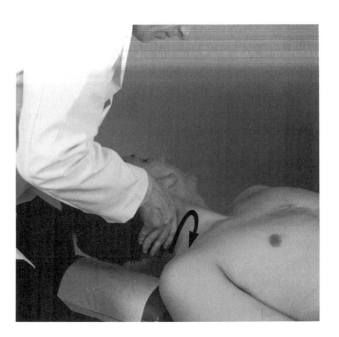

Figure 5.76 Index contact applied to the right C3 articular pillar (dot) with adjustive force directed anteriorly and superiorly (arrow) to induce left rotation and anterosuperior glide of the right C3–C4 articulation.

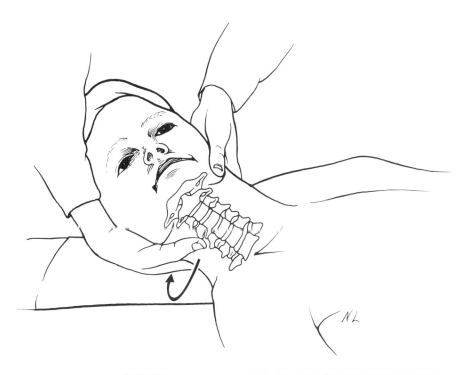

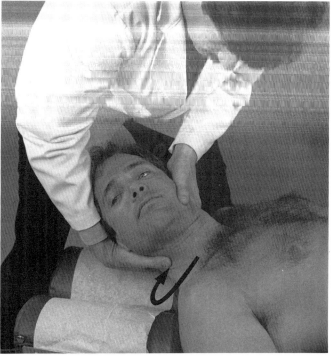

Figure 5.77 Assisted method. Thumb contact established over the right anterolateral pillar of C4 with adjustive force directed posterior (arrow) to induce right rotation and posterior glide in the right C4–C5 articulation.

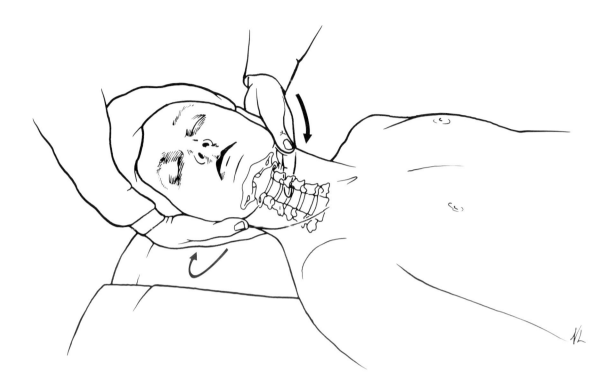

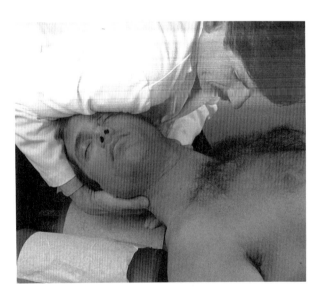

Figure 5.78 Resisted method. Index contact established on the left spinous process of C4 with adjustive force directed medially (arrows) to induce gapping and relative right rotation in the right C4–C5 articulation.

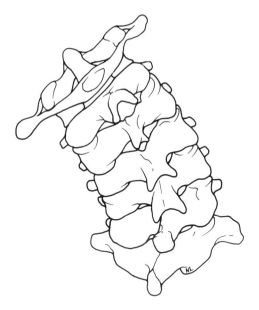

Figure 5.79 Posterior view of the cervical spine illustrating left lateral flexion and superior glide of the right facet joints and inferior glide of the left facet joints.

flexion restriction (closed wedge) (Fig. 5-79). The exception is the atlanto-axial articulation, which has horizontal facet planes and very limited lateral flexion. Determination of sites and direction of restriction are assessed by end feel evaluation.

Lateral flexion dysfunction is typically treated with assisted methods. In the lower cervical spine, ipsilateral inferior glide is induced by contacting the articular pillar or the spinous process of the superior vertebra on the side of lateral flexion restriction and applying adjustive thrusts medially and inferiorly along the facet planes (Fig. 5-80A). Contralateral superior glide is induced using the same techniques but may be enhanced if the indifferent hand applies a simultaneous assisting thrust in a headward direction on the side opposite the lateral flexion restriction. Techniques directed at inducing unilateral long axis distraction of the posterior joints may also be applied to treat restriction in superior glide (Fig. 5-80B). Lateral flexion restrictions in the atlanto-occipital joint are distinctive because of the unique anatomy. They may involve decreased medial and inferior glide on the side of lateral flexion and/or decreased lateral and superior glide on the side opposite the lateral flexion restriction. To induce medial inferior glide the doctor contacts the patient on the side of lateral flexion restriction and thrusts medially (see Fig. 5-83B). To treat restriction in superior glide, specific methods directed at contacting the side of dysfunction and inducing long axis distraction may be applied (Fig. 5-81).

Flexion/Extension Dysfunction

Flexion restrictions (extension malpositions) involve a loss of anterior superior facet gliding and may be treated with methods specifically designed to treat this restriction (Fig. 5-82). These methods are typically applied in a

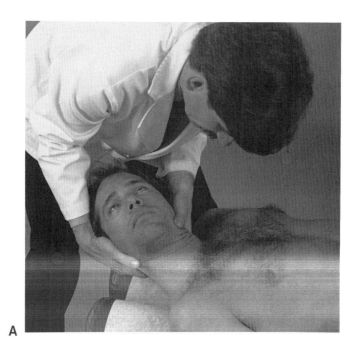

A

Figure 5.80 **(A)** Index contact applied to the left posterolateral articular pillar of C3 with adjustive force directed medially and inferiorly (arrow) to induce left lateral flexion and inferior glide of the left C3–C4 articulation and superior glide of the right C3–C4 articulation. **(B)** Adjustment applied to induce long axis distraction in the left C2–C3 articulation.

B

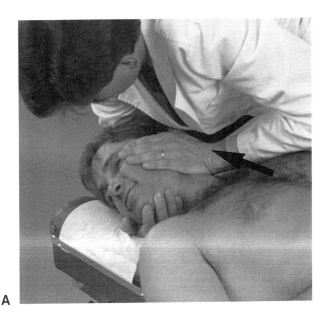

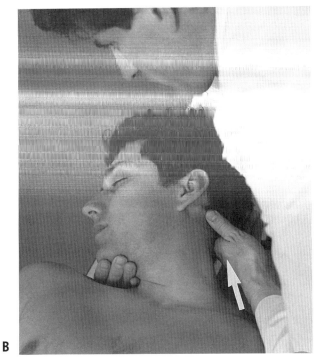

Figure 5.81 (**A**) Hypothenar contact applied to the left inferior aspect of the occiput to flex and/or distract the left atlanto-occipital articulation. (**B**) Thumb contact applied to the left inferior aspect of the occiput to flex and/or distract the left atlanto-occipital articulation.

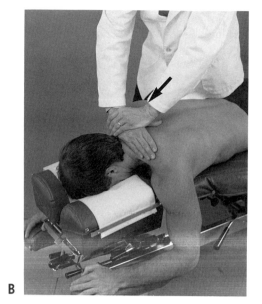

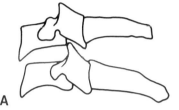

A   B

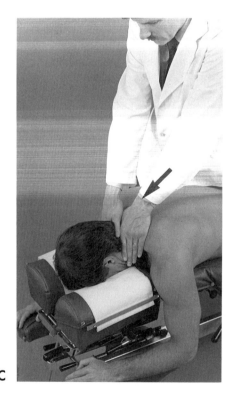

Figure 5.82 (**A**) Lateral view of the cervical spine demonstrating flexion and antero-superior gliding of the posterior joints. (**B**) Adjustment applied to mid-cervical spine to induce flexion. (**C**) Adjustment applied to mid-cervical spine to induce extension. (**D**) Lateral view of the cervical spine demonstrating extension and inferior gliding of the posterior joints.

C   D

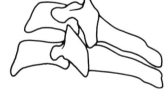

prone position. Additionally, many of the previous methods described for treating lateral flexion restrictions (loss of superior glide) and rotational restrictions (anterior glide) induce movements that may effectively treat components of flexion dysfunction. Adjustments that induce long axis distraction may also alleviate restrictions in flexion by inducing joint gapping (Fig. 5-80B).

Cervical extension induces motion that stretches the capsule and its periarticular tissue in directions not specifically addressed with rotation or lateral flexion adjustments (Fig. 5-82C&D). Therefore, extension restrictions (flexion malpositions) are more effectively addressed by adjustive techniques and vectors directed specifically for this dysfunction. Extension adjustments may be directed to reduce unilateral or bilateral segmental joint fixations. When treating bilateral joint restrictions, place the patient in the prone position with contacts established in the midline over the spinous process or both articular pillars (Fig. 5-105A). When treating unilateral dysfunction, place the patient in the supine or prone position and establish the contact on the side of restriction over the posterior aspect of the cervical articular pillar (Fig. 5-85C).

To induce segmental extension prestress the joint into extension and deliver a thrust anteriorly to induce posterior inferior gliding and anterior capsular gapping. When applying extension adjustments, use extreme caution to avoid excessive extension and joint compression. The thrust must be shallow and gentle.

Atlanto-occipital restrictions in flexion (extension malposition) are treated with methods directed at inducing posterior superior glide or long axis distraction of the occipital condyle (Figs. 5-81, 5-86, 5-91). Restrictions in extension (flexion malposition) are treated with methods directed at inducing anterior inferior glide of the occipital condyle (Figs. 5-105A and 5-99). The thrust is directed mainly in the sagittal plane, with limited cervical rotation and some segmental lateral flexion to isolate the joint.

Abbreviations used in illustrating technique

The following abbreviations are used throughout the chapter.

IND,	indications	→ Arrows on photographs indicate direction of force.
PP,	patient's position	
DP,	doctor's position	
SCP,	segmental contact point on patient	▲ Triangles on photographs indicate stabilization.
CP,	contact point	
IH,	indifferent hand	
VEC,	vector	
P,	procedure	

Supine Upper Cervical Adjustments

Occipital lift (Fig. 5-81)

IND: Restricted flexion C0–C1. Extension malposition C0–C1. Loss of long axis distraction C0–C1.

PP: The patient lies supine with the doctor supporting the patient's head off the end of the table and turned away from the side of dysfunction.

DP: Stand at the head of the table facing cephalad on the side of adjustive contact, in a low fencer stance with weight shifted toward superior leg.

CP: Hypothenar of your caudal hand with fingers pointing vertically and resting on the skull (Fig. 5-81A). You may employ an optional thumb contact (Fig. 5-81B).

SCP: Inferior edge of the occiput, medial to the mastoid.

IH: Your indifferent hand and fingers wrap around the patient's chin while your forearm supports the patient's head.

VEC: Inferior to superior.

P: Establish the contacts and rotate the patient's head away from the side of adjustive contact. Apply pre-adjustive long axis distraction by leaning your bodyweight headward. At tension deliver a shallow, vertically directed thrust superiorly through the contact hand and body.

Hypothenar occiput (Fig. 5-83)

IND: Restricted rotation, lateral flexion, or extension, C0–C1. Rotation, lateral flexion or flexion malpositions, C0–C1.

PP: The patient lies supine with the head off the end of the table, supported by doctor and turned away from the side of dysfunction.

DP: The doctor stands at the head of table on the side of the adjustive contact angled 45 to 90 degrees to the patient.

CP: Hypothernar of the hand corresponding to the side of segmental contact (e.g., the doctor's right hand establishes the contact when contacting the right occiput). The contact hand is arched to cup over the patient's ear with fingers resting on the angle of the jaw. Index or thenar contacts may be employed as alternatives to the hypothenar contact.

SCP: Posterior supramastoid groove, just posterior to the ear.

IH: Doctor's indifferent hand supports and cradles the patient's head with fingers running along the base of the occiput.

VEC: Posterior to anterior, superior to inferior and laterally to medial to induce extension. Lateral to medial and superior to inferior to induce lateral flexion.

P: The doctor establishes the contacts and laterally flexes the head toward the side of contact while rotating it away. The degree of associated occipital extension or lateral flexion is dependent on the dysfunction being treated. After joint tension is established an impulse thrust is generated through the doctor's shoulder along the desired vector. Care should be taken to minimize rotational tension to the upper cervical spine.

Extension, C0–C1 (Fig. 5-83A). When inducing extension or ipsilateral anterior inferior glide laterally flex the occiput toward the side of contact and prestress into extension.

Lateral flexion, C0–C1 (Fig. 5-83B). When inducing lateral flexion or ipsilateral medial glide and contralateral superior glide, limit extension of the occiput and induce lateral flexion toward the side of adjustive contact.

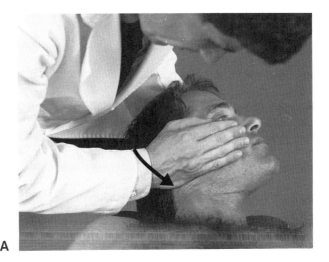

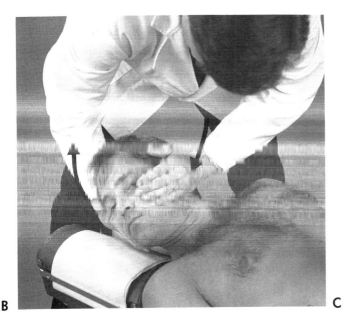

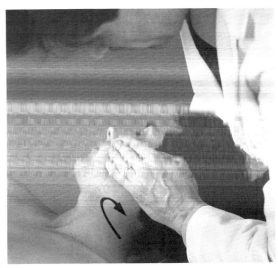

Figure 5.83 (**A**) Hypothenar contact applied to the right inferior aspect of the occiput to extend the atlanto-occipital articulation. (**B**) Hypothenar contact applied to the left lateral aspect of the occiput to left laterally flex the atlanto-occipital articulation. (**C**) Hypothenar contact applied to the left posterolateral aspect of the occiput to right rotate the left atlanto-occipital articulation.

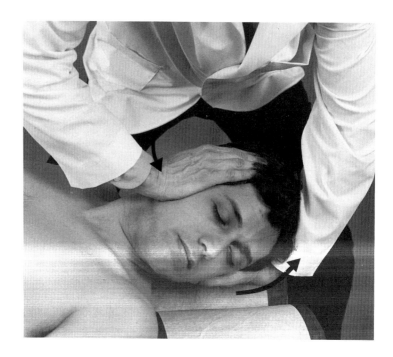

Figure 5.84 Hypothenar (calcaneal) contact above the right zygomatic arch to right laterally flex the atlanto-occipital articulation.

Rotation, C0–C1 (Fig. 5-83C). When inducing occipital rotation or ipsilateral anterior glide, rotate the patient's head away from the side of adjustive contact. **Avoid full rotational tension when treating rotational restrictions in the upper cervical spine. This position may produce unnecessary tension on the vertebral artery.** Rotational movement between the occiput and the atlas is very limited, and it is not necessary to develop full cervical rotation to develop tension at the C0–C1 articulation. The incorporation of slight lateral flexion toward the side of contact aids in developing earlier rotational tension.

Calcaneal zygomatic (Fig. 5-84)

IND: Lateral flexion restrictions, lateral flexion malpositions, C0–C1.

  PP: The patient lies supine with the head rotated away from the side of contact and lateral flexion restriction.

  DP: Stand at the side of the table behind the patient's head in a square stance.

  CP: A calcaneal contact (heel of the hand) of the caudal hand, fingers pointing toward the vertex of the skull.

SCP: The zygomatic arch

  IH: Your cephalad hand cups the down side ear with the palm while your fingers wrap around occiput and upper cervical vertebra.

VEC: Lateral to medial

   P: As your indifferent hand exerts superior traction separating the down side articulations and approximating the up side articulations, deliver an impulse thrust through both arms, creating a "scooping" action lateral to medial.

Index atlas (Fig. 5-85)

IND: Restricted rotation, lateral flexion, or extension of C1–C2. Rotation, lateral flexion, or flexion malposition of C1–C2.

PP: The patient lies supine.

DP: Stand at the head of table on the side of the adjustive contact, angled 45° to 90° to the patient.

CP: Proximal ventro-lateral surface of the index finger of your hand corresponding to the side of segmental contact. Your thumb rests on the patient's cheek while the remaining fingers support the contact and cup the base of the occiput.

SCP: Lateral aspect of the transverse process of the atlas for inducing lateral flexion (medial glide). Posterolateral aspect of the transverse process of the atlas for inducing rotation. Posterior surface of the lateral mass for inducing extension.

IH: Your indifferent hand cradles the patient's head and supports the contralateral occiput.

VEC: Posterior to anterior with clockwise or counter clockwise rotation to induce rotation. Posterior to anterior to induce ipsilateral extension. Medial to lateral to induce lateral flexion.

P: Rotates the patient's head away from the side of dysfunction and establish the contact. The degree of additional rotation, extension, or lateral flexion depends on the dysfunction being treated. After joint tension is established generate an impulse thrust through your shoulder along the desired vector.

Rotation (Fig. 5-85A). When treating rotational dysfunction and inducing ipsilateral anterior glide, rotate the patient's head away from and slightly laterally flexed toward the side of adjustive contact. At tension deliver a rotational impulse thrust through the wrist and forearms. **Avoid full rotational tension with extension when treating rotation restrictions in the upper cervical spine. This position may produce unnecessary tension on the vertebral artery.** Rotational tension may be achieved earlier in the arc of motion by inducing slight lateral flexion toward the side of contact.

Lateral flexion (Fig. 5-85B). When treating restrictions in lateral flexion and inducing ipsilateral medial glide, contact the lateral surface of the atlas transverse, minimize rotation of the cervical spine and thrust lateral to medial by adducting the shoulder.

Extension (Fig. 5-85C). When treating extension restrictions the doctor minimizes the rotation of the cervical spine while pre-stressing the joint into extension. The contact is established over the posterior lateral mass and a thrust is delivered anteriorly by inducing shoulder flexion.

Sitting Upper Cervical Adjustments

Occipital lift (Fig. 5-86)

IND: Restricted flexion and/or lateral flexion, loss of long axis distraction, C0–C1. Extension and/or lateral flexion malpositions, C0–C1.

PP: The patient sits in a cervical chair with the head turned away from the side of contact and resting against your chest.

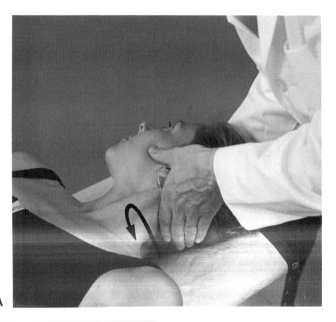

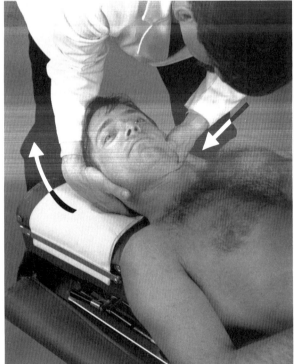

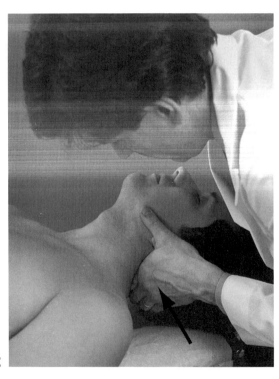

Figure 5.85 (**A**) Index contact applied to the left atlas transverse process to right rotate the left C1–C2 articulation. (**B**) Index contact applied to the left atlas transverse process to left laterally flex and/or laterally glide left to right the C1–C2 articulation. (**C**) Index contact applied to the posterior aspect of the left atlas transverse process to extend the left C1–C2 articulation.

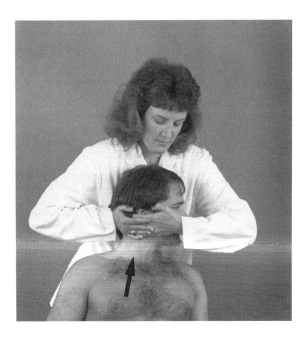

Figure 5.86 Middle finger contact applied to the right lateral and inferior aspect of the occiput to distract in the long axis and/or laterally flex the right atlanto-occipital articulation.

DI: Stand behind the patient slightly toward the side of cervical rotation.

CP: Proximal palmar surface of the middle finger of the hand corresponding to the side of head rotation (e.g., your left hand establishes the contact on the right occiput when the patient's head is rotated to the left).

SCP: Inferior border of occiput and lateral border of the mastoid process on the side of dysfunction.

IH: The indifferent hand reinforces the contact hand and stabilizes the patient's head against your chest.

VEC: Inferior to superior for flexion or long axis distraction. Lateral to medial for lateral flexion dysfunction.

P: Place the patient in the sitting position and rotate the patient's head away from the side of contact. Reach around the patient's face to contact the dysfunctional joint (a pillow may be used to cushion the patient's head against your chest). Develop pre-adjustive joint tension by tractioning vertically with arms and legs.

   To induce long axis distraction and/or occipital flexion, thrust headward with a lifting impulse generated through the arms and legs.

   To induce lateral flexion, accentuate bending of the patient's head away from you and thrust lateral to medial through the contact arms while maintaining long axis distraction.

Index occiput (Fig. 5-87)

IND: Restricted rotation, lateral flexion, or extension, C0–C1. Rotation, lateral flexion, or flexion malpositions of C0–C1.

PP: The patient sits relaxed in a cervical chair.

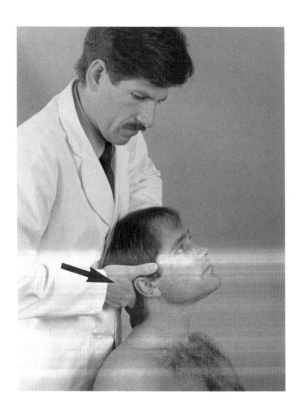

Figure 5.87 Index contact applied to the right posterior and inferior aspect of the occiput to extend the right atlanto-occipital articulation.

DP: Stand behind the patient toward the side of segmental contact.

CP: Ventro-lateral surface of the index finger of the hand corresponding to the side of segmental contact. The palm is turned up with wrist straight. The forearm is approximately 45 degrees to the patient, with the remaining fingers cupping the lower occiput.

SCP: Supramastoid groove on the side of lesion.

IH: The indifferent hand cups the patient's head and supports the contra-lateral occiput.

VEC: Posterior to anterior, superior to inferior, and lateral to medial to induce extension. Lateral to medial, superior to inferior, and posterior to anterior to induce lateral flexion.

P: Establish stabilization and segmental contact points, keeping contact arm angled approximately 45 degrees to the patient's shoulders. Laterally flex the patient's head toward the side of contact with slight rotation away. The degree of comparative extension and lateral flexion depends on the direction of C0–C1 restricted movement. When inducing extension and ipsilateral anterior glide direct the adjustive vector more anteriorly, and when inducing lateral flexion and ipsilateral medial glide, direct the thrust more medially. Take care to minimize rotational tension to the upper cervical spine.

Index atlas—sitting (Figs. 5-88 and 5-89)

IND: Restricted rotation, lateral flexion, or extension of C1–C2. Rotation, lateral flexion, or flexion malposition of C1–C2.

PP: The patient sits relaxed in a cervical chair.

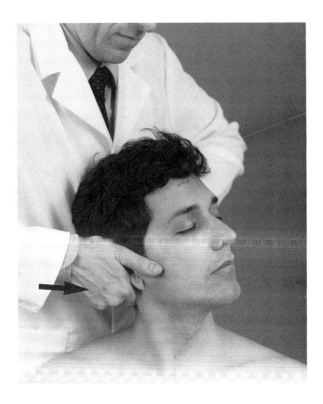

Figure 5.88 Index contact applied to the posterior aspect of the atlas to left rotate and glide posterior to anterior the right C1–C2 articulation.

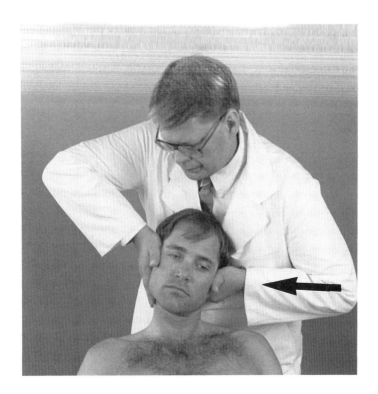

Figure 5.89 Index contact applied to the left atlas transverse process to left laterally flex the C1–C2 articulation.

DP: Stand behind the patient, toward side of segmental contact.

CP: Proximal ventral surface of the index finger of the hand corresponding to the side of segmental contact. The palm is turned up with the wrist straight. The forearm is approximately 90 degrees to the patient with the remaining fingers cupping the lower occiput.

SCP: Lateral aspect of the transverse process of the atlas for inducing lateral flexion (medial glide). Posterolateral aspect of transverse process of the atlas for inducing rotation. Posterior surface of the lateral mass for inducing extension.

IH: The indifferent hand supports and cradles the patient's head by cupping the patient's ear and inferior occipital rim.

VEC: Posterior to anterior with clockwise or counter clockwise rotation to induce rotation. Posterior to anterior to induce extension. Medial to lateral to induce lateral flexion.

P: Rotate the patient's head away from the side of dysfunction and establish the contacts. The degree of additional rotation, extension, or lateral flexion depends on the dysfunction being treated. After joint tension is established generate an impulse thrust through your shoulder along the desired vector.

Rotation (Fig. 5-88). When treating rotational dysfunction and inducing ipsilateral anterior glide, rotate the patient's head away from and slightly laterally flexed toward the side of adjustive contact. At tension deliver a rotational impulse thrust through the wrist and forearms. **Avoid full rotational tension with extension when treating rotation restrictions in the upper cervical spine. These positions may produce unnecessary tension on the vertebral artery.** Rotational tension may be achieved earlier in the arc of motion by inducing slight lateral flexion toward the side of contact.

Lateral flexion (Fig. 5-89). When treating lateral flexion dysfunction and inducing ipsilateral medial glide, minimize rotation of the cervical spine and thrust lateral to medial by adducting the shoulder.

Extension. When treating extension restrictions minimize rotation of the cervical spine while pre-stressing the joint into extension. Establish the contact over the posterior lateral mass and thrust anteriorly by inducing shoulder flexion.

Digit atlas (rotary break) (Fig. 5-90)

IND: Restricted rotation, C1–C2. Rotational malposition, C1–C2.

PP: The patient sits relaxed in a cervical chair.

DP: Stand facing the patient on the side opposite the segmental contact.

CP: Palmar surface of the middle finger of the hand corresponding to the side of segmental contact. The thenar of the contact hand rests on the cheek of the patient.

SCP: Posterolateral aspect of atlas transverse.

IH: With fingers running vertically, the indifferent hand stabilizes the patient's head by supporting the contralateral occiput and temporal region.

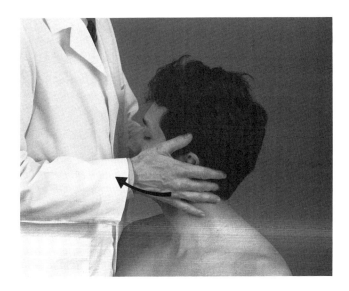

Figure 5.90 Middle finger contact applied to the posterior aspect of the left atlas transverse process to right rotate and glide posterior to anterior the left C1–C2 articulation.

VEC: Posterior to anterior with clockwise or counter clockwise rotation.

P: Rotate the patient's head away from and slightly laterally flexed toward the side of adjustive contact. Induce rotation and ipsilateral anterior glide by developing a pulling impulse thrust through the contact hand by quickly extending the shoulder. (The same concerns discussed previously for minimizing extension and rotational tension in the upper cervical spine apply here also.)

Prone Upper Cervical Adjustments

Thenar occiput distraction (Fig. 5-91)

IND: Restricted flexion, C0–C1. Loss of long axis distraction C0–C1. Extension malposition, C0–C1.

PP: The patient lies prone with the head placed in slight flexion.

DP: Stand on either side of the patient in a fencer stance caudal to the contact, facing cephalad.

CP: Thenar eminence of both hands.

SCP: Establish the contacts bilaterally on the inferior aspect of the occiput, medial to the mastoid.

VEC: Inferior to superior, posterior to anterior.

PRO: Center your body over the patient in low fencer position caudal to the contacts and tractions headward. Tension may be developed through both contacts or centered to one side. After joint tension is reached deliver a cephalically directed thrust through the arms and trunk. The impulse may be directed to one or both articulations. This adjustment may be effectively performed on a drop table or performed as a mobilization procedure.

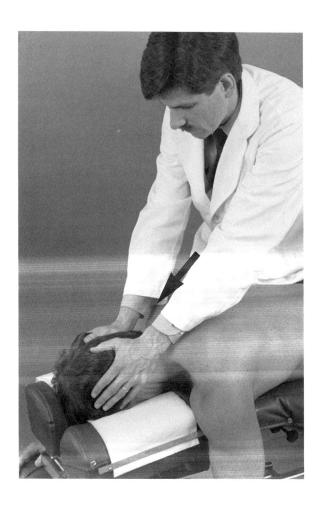

Figure 5.91 Bilateral thenar contacts applied to the posterior and inferior aspect of the occiput to flex the atlanto-occipital articulation.

Thenar occiput extension (Fig. 5-92)

IND: Restricted extension, flexion malposition, C0–C1.

  PP: The patient lies prone, with the head placed in slight extension.

  DP: Stand on either side of the patient in a fencer stance facing cephalically centered over the contacts.

  CP: Thenar eminence of both hands.

SCP: Establish the contacts bilaterally on the posterior occiput, at or above the level of the superior nuchal line.

VEC: Posterior to anterior.

   P: Center your body over the patient and deliver an impulse thrust anteriorly. Tension may be developed through both contacts or centered to one side. This adjustment may be effectively performed on a drop table or performed as a mobilization procedure.

Supine Cervical Adjustments

Index pillar (modified rotary break) (Fig. 5-93)

IND: Restricted rotation, lateral flexion, or extension, C2–C7. Rotation, lateral flexion, or flexion malpositions of C2–C7.

  PP: The patient lies supine.

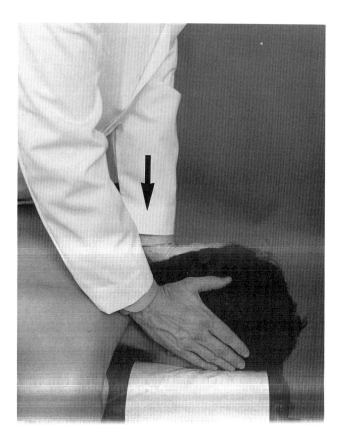

Figure 5.92 Bilateral thenar ~~contacts applied to the pos~~terior aspect of the occiput to extend the atlanto-occipital articulation.

HP: Stand at the head of the table on the side of the adjustive contact angled 45 to 90 degrees to the patient.

CP: Ventro-lateral surface of the index finger of the hand corresponding to the side of segmental contact. The thumb or thenar rests on the patient's cheek as the remaining fingers reinforce the contact. Use the proximal surface of the index finger in upper cervical segments and the distal surface in the lower cervical segments.

SCP: Posterolateral articular pillar of superior vertebrae.

IH: Your indifferent hand cradles the patient's head and supports the contralateral occiput and upper cervical spine.

VEC: Posterior to anterior with slight inferior to superior inclination and clockwise or counter clockwise rotation to induce rotation. Posterior to anterior to induce extension. Medial to lateral and superior to inferior to induce lateral flexion.

P: Rotate the patient's head away from the side of dysfunction and establish the adjustive contact. The degree of additional rotation, extension, or lateral flexion depends on the dysfunction being treated. After joint tension is established, generate an impulse thrust through your shoulder along the desired vector.

Rotation (Fig. 5-93A). Establish the adjustive contact on the superior articular pillar, rotate the patient's head away, laterally flexing it toward the side of contact. Lateral flexion is incorporated in the positioning of this

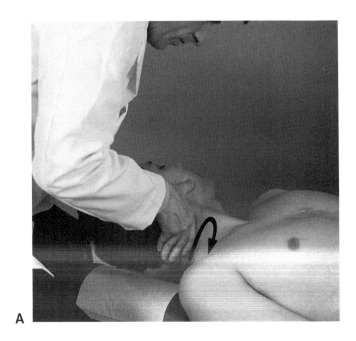

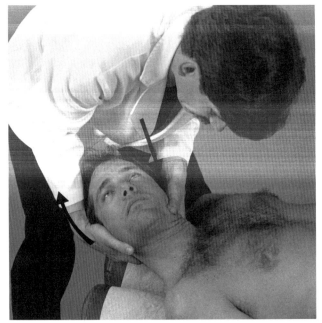

Figure 5.93 (**A**) Index contact applied to the posterior aspect of the right C2 articular pillar to left rotate and glide the right C2–C3 articulation posterior to anterior. (**B**) Index contact applied to the lateral aspect of the C3 articular pillar to left laterally flex the C3–C4 articulation, gliding the left side inferiorly and the right side superiorly.

adjustment to induce unphysiologic movement and locking at the joints above the contact. However, the degree of lateral flexion must not be excessive or it leads to compression and locking of the joint to be distracted. The lower the cervical dysfunction, the more flexion and lateral flexion is necessary to isolate the involved segment. Deliver the thrust through the wrists and forearms in a clockwise or counter clockwise direction along the planes of the facet joint. This method is applied to induce posterior to anterior rotation and ipsilateral distraction in the articulation inferior to the contact.

Lateral flexion (Fig. 5-93B). To induce lateral flexion, laterally flex the head toward the side of contact while minimizing rotation. To induce ipsilateral inferior glide, thrust medially and inferiorly through the contact hand by adducting the shoulder. Contralateral superior glide is also induced with this thrust and may be enhanced if the indifferent hand distracts vertically during the impulse.

Extension. To induce segmental extension pre-stress the involved joint into extension, contact the posterior pillar, and thrust anteriorly and slightly medially through the shoulder.

Index/spinous (Fig. 5-94)

IND: Restricted rotation and/or lateral flexion of C2–T3. Rotation and/or lateral flexion malpositions of C2–T3.

PP: The patient lies supine.

DP: Stand at the head of table on the side of the adjustive contact, angled 45 to 90 degrees to the patient.

CP: Ventro-lateral surface of the index finger of the hand corresponding to the side of segmental contact with the remaining fingers reinforcing the contact.

SCP: Lateral surface of the spinous process (Fig. 5-94A).

IH: Your indifferent hand cradles the patient's head and supports the contralateral occiput and upper cervical spine. Support and control of the patient's head may be enhanced by placing the arm of your contact hand against the patient's forehead and gripping it between the arm and forearm.

VEC: Lateral to medial and superior to inferior.

P: Rotate the patient's head slightly away from you and establish a contact on the lateral surface of the spinous process. The degree of additional rotation or lateral flexion depends on the dysfunction being treated. After joint tension is established, generate an impulse thrust through your shoulder along the desired vector.

Lateral flexion (Fig. 5-94B). Establish the adjustive contact on the superior vertebra on the side of lateral flexion restriction (side of open wedge). Laterally flex the patient's head toward the side of adjustive contact and deliver an impulse thrust medially and inferiorly through the segmental contact. The indifferent hand may remain stationary or deliver a simultaneous distractive thrust cephalically. Thrusts delivered primarily with the contact arm are likely to maximize forces to the side of contact. Distraction of the contralateral facet joint is enhanced by increasing the distractive force through the indifferent hand.

Rotation. Rotational dysfunction may be treated with resisted patient positions or neutral patient positions depending on the side of desired distraction.

The resisted adjustive approach is designed to induce rotation and distrac-

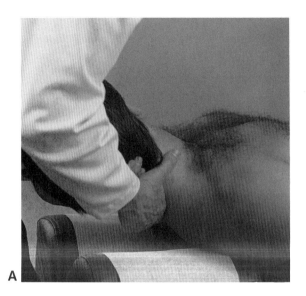

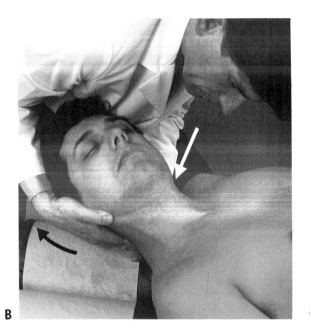

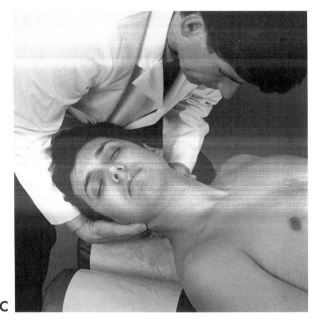

Figure 5.94 **(A)** Index contact applied to the lateral aspect of the C6 spinous process to left rotate the C6–C7 articulation. **(B)** Index contact applied to the left lateral aspect of the C6 spinous process to left laterally flex the C6–C7 articulation. **(C)** Resisted method. Index contact applied to the left lateral aspect of the C4 spinous process to right rotate the C3–C4 articulation, gliding the left side posterior to anterior and right side anterior to posterior.

tion in the facet joint contralateral and superior to the side of adjustive contact. When a resisted method is employed the adjustive contact is established on the lateral surface of the inferior vertebra on the side opposite the rotation restriction. Pre-adjustive tension is developed by rotating the neck in the direction of restriction as counter pressure is applied against the spinous process. Lateral flexion is also induced toward the side of contact to distract the contralateral facet joints and block the ipsilateral facet joints (Fig. 5-94C). To deliver the impulse, counter thrust with both hands. The contact hand thrusts medially by inducing adduction of the shoulder. The indifferent hand induces counter rotation by supinating the forearm.

To induce rotational distraction and medial glide of the facet joint ipsilateral and inferior to the side of contact employ a more neutral patient position. Establish the contact on the superior spinous process on the side of rotational restriction, decrease the degree of lateral flexion, and rotate the patient's head away from the side of contact. The head should be rotated only far enough to rest it in your indifferent hand. By limiting cervical rotation you limit movement to the upper cervical spine and avoid inducing counter opposing rotation in the lower cervical and upper thoracic segments. At tension an impulse thrust is delivered primarily through the contact hand by inducing adduction of the shoulder.

Thumb pillar posterior (Fig. 5-95)

IND: Rotational restrictions and malpositions of C2–C7.

PP: The patient lies supine.

DP: Stand at the head of the table on the side of the adjustive contact, angled approximately 90 degrees to the patient.

CP: Palmar surface of the thumb of the hand corresponding to the side of segmental contact. The palm is turned down with fingers resting on the patient's cheek.

SCP: Posterolateral pillar of the superior vertebra.

IH: Your indifferent hand cradles the patient's head and supports the contralateral occiput and upper cervical spine.

VEC: Posterior to anterior with slight inferior to superior inclination and clockwise or counter clockwise rotation.

PRO: After the contact is established, the patient's head is rotated away and laterally flexed toward the side of contact. Lateral flexion is incorporated in the positioning of this adjustment to induce locking of the joints above the contact. However, the degree of lateral flexion must not be excessive or it leads to compression and locking of the joint to be distracted. The degree of lateral flexion necessary to isolate the lower cervical segments increases in a caudal direction. At tension direct an impulse thrust anteriorly by inducing rotation through your shoulder. This method is applied to induce posterior to anterior rotation and ipsilateral distraction in the articulation inferior to the contact.

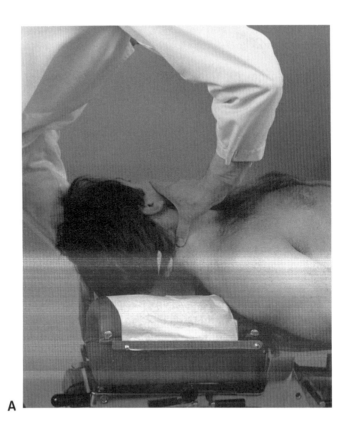

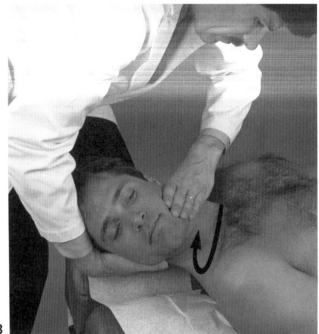

Figure 5.95 Thumb pillar posterior technique: (**A**) thumb contact applied to the posterior aspect of the right C3 articular pillar, and (**B**) the procedure shown from the other side to right rotate and glide the left C3–C4 articulation posterior to anterior.

Thumb pillar anterior (Fig. 5-96)

IND: Restricted rotation or combined restricted rotation and opposite side lateral flexion, C2–C7. Rotation and lateral flexion malpositions, C2–C7.

PP: The patient lies supine.

DP: Stand at the head of the table opposite the side of the adjustive contact, angled approximately 45 degrees to the patient.

CP: Palmar surface of the thumb of the hand corresponding to the side of segmental contact. The palm is turned up with fingers and palm of the contact hand supporting the occiput and upper cervical spine.

SCP: Anterolateral pillar of superior vertebra (Fig. 5-96A).

IH: Your indifferent hand cups over the ear supporting the contralateral occiput (Fig. 5-96B). Support of the patient's head may be improved by placing the arm of your contact hand against the patient's forehead and gripping it between the arm and forearm (Fig. 5-96C).

VEC: Anterior to posterior with slight inferior to superior inclination, inducing clockwise or counter clockwise rotation.

PRO: After the contacts are established, rotate the patient's head toward and laterally flexed away from the side of adjustive contact. At tension direct an impulse thrust posteriorly by inducing adduction of your shoulder and supination of the forearm. This adjustment is applied to induce anterior to posterior rotation and ipsilateral joint gapping (perpendicular gapping) at the articulation below the contact (Fig. 5-96D).

This adjustment may be combined with the index spinous adjustment to induce a resisted adjustive effect. In this scenario the indifferent hand contacts the spinous of the lower vertebrae on the contralateral side. At tension both hands thrust toward the midline to induce counter rotation and perpendicular facet joint gapping (Fig. 5-96E).

Hypothenar pillar (Fig. 5-97)

IND: Restrictions in rotation, lateral flexion, and/or long axis distraction, C2–C7. Malpositions in rotation and lateral flexion and decreased interosseous spacing, C2–C7.

PP: The patient lies supine, head rotated with side of contact up.

DP: Stand at the side of the table behind the patient's head.

CP: Pisiform-hypothenar contact of the caudad hand with the wrist in full extension.

SCP: Articular pillar of the superior vertebra; posterior aspect for rotational dysfunction, lateral aspect for lateral flexion dysfunction, and inferior aspect for long axis dysfunction.

IH: The cephalad hand grasps the patient's chin allowing the head to rest on your forearm.

VEC: Posterior to anterior for rotation; lateral to medial for lateral flexion; inferior to superior for long axis.

P: The indifferent hand provides cephalad traction. At tension, deliver an impulse thrust along the facet plane or perpendicular to the facet plane depending on the restriction treated. Take care not to induce extension.

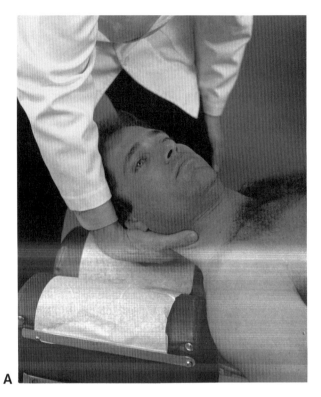

A

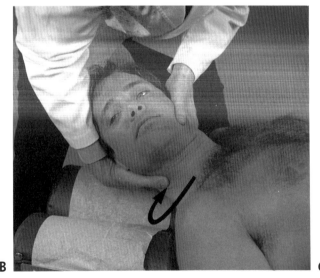

B

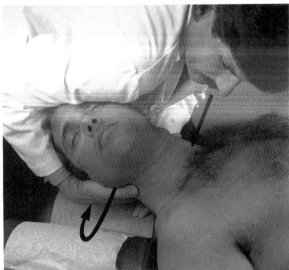

C

Figure 5.96 Thumb pillar anterior technique: (**A**) thumb contact applied to the anterior and lateral aspect of the right C2 articular pillar; (**B**) the procedure shown to right rotate and glide anterior to posterior the right C2–C3 articulation, and (**C**) a counter thrust technique with contacts applied to the anterolateral aspect of the right C2 articular pillar and the left lateral aspect of the C3 spinous process. Note support for contacts with the doctor's shoulder.

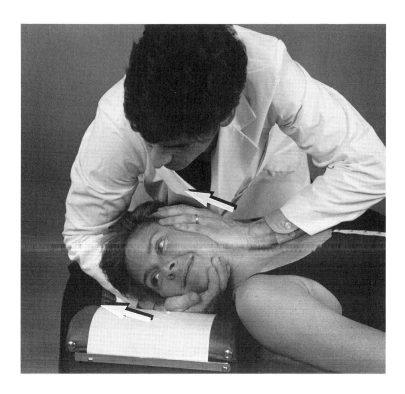

Figure 5.97 Hypothenar contact applied to the left inferior and lateral aspect of the C2 articular pillar to distract in the long axis the left C2–C3 articulation.

Sitting Cervical Adjustments

Digit pillar rotatory break (Fig. 5-98)

IND: Rotational restriction and malpositions, C2–C7.

PP: The patient sits relaxed in a cervical chair.

DP: Stand facing the patient on the side opposite the segmental contact.

CP: Palmar surface of the middle finger of the hand corresponding to the side of segmental contact with the palm resting on the patient's cheek.

SCP: Articular pillar of superior vertebrae.

IH: With fingers running vertically the indifferent hand stabilizes the patient's head by supporting the contralateral occiput and temporal region.

VEC: Posterior to anterior with slight inferior to superior inclination and clockwise or counter clockwise rotation.

P: Rotate the patient's head away from the side of contact and laterally flex it slightly toward the side of contact. At tension, direct a pulling impulse thrust anteriorly along the facet planes by inducing shoulder extension. Take care not to extend or induce excessive lateral flexion when treating rotational dysfunction.

Index pillar—sitting (Fig. 5-99)

IND: Restricted rotation, lateral flexion, or extension of C2–C7. Rotation, lateral flexion, or flexion malpositions, C2–C7.

PP: The patient sits relaxed in a cervical chair.

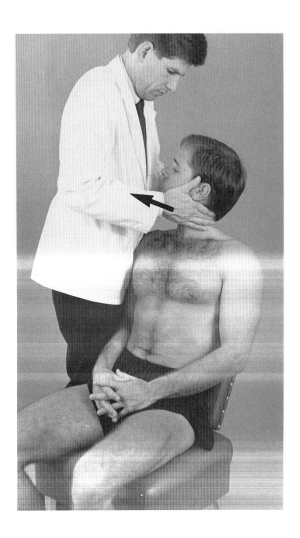

Figure 5.98 Digital contact applied to the left C4 articular pillar to right rotate the left C4–C5 articulation.

DP: Stand behind the patient, toward the side of segmental contact.

CP: Index finger of hand corresponding to the side of segmental contact. The palm is turned up with the thumb and thenar resting on the patient's cheek. In the upper cervical spine establish the contact toward the proximal surface of the index finger and toward the distal surface in the lower cervical.

SCP: Articular pillar of superior vertebrae.

IH: With finger pointing down, the hand and fingers stabilize the opposing occiput and cheek.

VEC: Posterior to anterior with slight inferior to superior inclination and clockwise or counter clockwise to induce rotation (Fig. 5-99A). Posterior to anterior to induce extension. Lateral to medial to induce lateral flexion (Fig. 5-99B).

P: Place the patient in a cervical chair, establish segmental contact points and rotate the patient's head away from and slightly laterally flex it toward the side of adjustive contact. To induce rotation, lateral

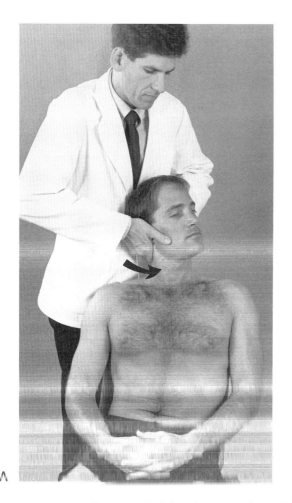 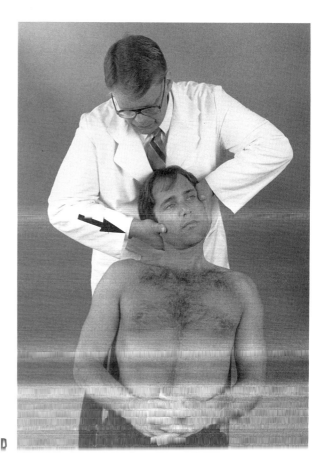

A   B

Figure 5.99 (**A**) Index or reinforced digital contact applied to the right articular pillar to left rotate the C3–C4 articulation, gliding the right side posterior to anterior. (**B**) Index contact applied to the right lateral aspect of the C3 articular pillar to right laterally flex the C3–C4 articulation, gliding the left side inferiorly and the right side superiorly.

flexion, or extension apply the same adjustive vectors presented for the supine index pillar adjustment.

This adjustment is a modification of the Gonstead style cervical chair adjustment. It is not intended to be a duplication.

Index spinous—sitting (Fig. 5-100)

IND: Restricted rotation and/or lateral flexion of C2–T3. Rotational and/or lateral flexion malpositions, C2–T3.

 PP: The patient sits relaxed in a cervical chair.

DP: Stand behind the patient, toward the side of segmental contact.

CP: Index finger of hand corresponding to the side of segmental contact. The palm is turned up with the thumb resting on the patient's cheek.

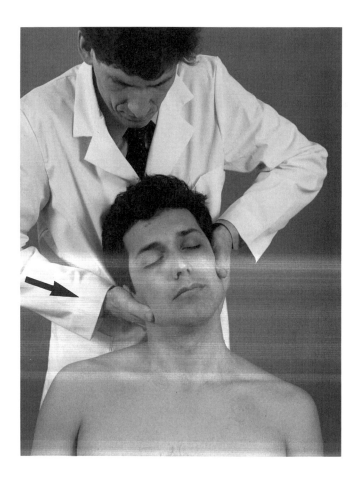

Figure 5.100 Index contact applied to the right lateral aspect of the C4 spinous process to right laterally flex and/or right rotate the C4–C5 articulation.

SCP: Lateral aspect of the spinous process.

IH: With fingers pointing down, the hand and fingers stabilize the opposing occiput and cheek.

VEC: Lateral to medial for rotational restriction. Lateral to medial and superior to inferior for lateral flexion restriction.

P: Place the patient in a cervical chair, establish segmental contact points, and rotate the patient's head away from and slightly laterally flex it toward the side of adjustive contact. To induce rotation and ipsilateral medial glide, thrust medially while minimizing cervical rotation away.

For lateral flexion dysfunction the head is laterally flexed toward the side of adjustive contact. At tension an impulse thrust is delivered medially and inferiorly by inducing adduction of the shoulder. This vector may induce both ipsilateral inferior glide and contralateral superior glide.

This adjustment is a modification of the Gonstead style cervical chair adjustment. It is not intended to be a duplication.

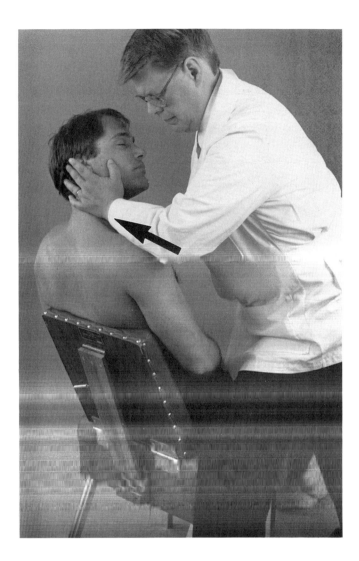

Figure 5.101 Hypothenar contact applied to the anterior and lateral aspect of the right C4 articular pillar to right rotate and glide the right C4–C5 articulation anterior to posterior.

Hypothenar pillar (Fig. 5-101)

IND: Restricted rotation or combined restricted rotation and opposite side lateral flexion of C2–C7. Rotation and lateral flexion malpositions, C2–C7.

PP: The patient sits relaxed in a cervical chair.

DP: Stand in front of the patient toward the side of contact.

CP: Hypothenar of hand corresponding to the side of adjustive contact. The fingers of the contact hand extend obliquely vertically to provide stabilizing support to the patient's head.

SCP: Anterolateral pillar of superior vertebrae.

IH: With fingers running vertically the indifferent hand stabilizes the contralateral upper cervical spine and occiput.

VEC: Anterior to posterior and slightly inferior to superior.

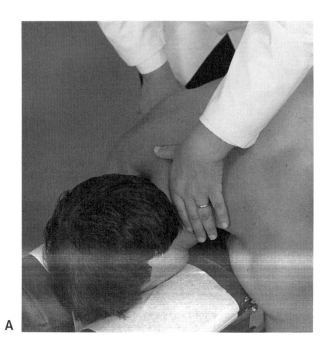

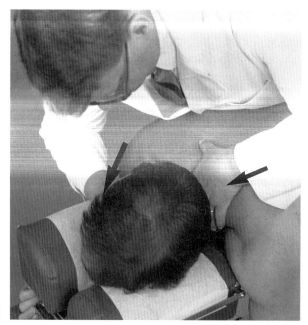

Figure 5.102 Index pillar—prone technique: (A) index contact established over the posterior aspect of the left C5 articular process; (B) procedure shown to left laterally flex and right rotate the left C5–C6 articulation.

P: Stand in a fencer stance on the side of adjustive contact and establish a broad fleshy hypothenar contact over the anterolateral articular pillar. Rotate the patient's head toward and laterally flex it away from the side of adjustive contact. At tension direct an impulse thrust perpendicularly to the facet plane by thrusting posteriorly and superiorly through your shoulder. Slight vertical traction is maintained through both hands during the delivery of the adjustment. This adjustment is applied to induce anterior to posterior rotation and ipsilateral joint gapping (perpendicular gapping) at the articulation below the contact.

Prone Lower Cervicals

Index pillar—prone (Fig. 5-102)

IND: Restricted rotation or lateral flexion of C2–C7. Malpositions in rotation and/or lateral flexion, C2–C7.

PP: The patient lies in the prone position with the headrest lowered to induce slight thoraco-cervical flexion.

DP: Stand in a fencer stance on either side of table facing cephalad.

CP: Index finger (lateral aspect of the metacarpophalangeal joint of the index finger) of the hand corresponding to the side of the adjustive contact. The wrist is held in ulnar deviation with the fingers pointing to the floor and the thumb resting on the posterior cervical soft tissues.

SCP: Posterior aspect of the articular pillar of the superior vertebra (Fig. 5-102A).

IH: A thumb-web contact is established at the inferior rim of the occiput while the palm and fingers contact the cheek and side of the face.

VEC: Posterior to anterior and slightly inferior to superior for rotation restrictions. Posterior to anterior and superior to inferior for lateral flexion restrictions.

P: As your indifferent hand tractions the head cephalad, laterally flexes and slightly rotates to tension, deliver an impulse thrust incorporating elbow extension, shoulder abduction, and wrist radial deviation.

Rotation. To induce rotation contact the posterior pillar on the side opposite the rotational restriction and rotate the head in the direction of joint restriction. At tension thrust anteriorly, medially, and superiorly.

Lateral flexion. To induce lateral flexion, contact the articular pillar on the side of lateral flexion restriction (open wedge side) and laterally flex the neck toward the side of contact. At tension thrust medially, anteriorly, and inferiorly (Fig. 5-102B).

Index pillar thumb spinous (Fig. 5-103)

IND: Restricted lateral flexion of C2–C7. Malpositions in lateral flexion, C2–C7.

PP: The patient lies in the prone position with the headrest lowered to induce slight thoraco-cervical flexion.

DP: Stand in a fencer stance on the side of adjustive contact facing caudad.

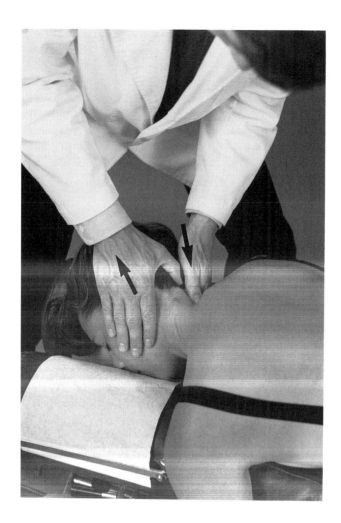

Figure 5.103 Index contact applied to right posterior aspect of the C5 articular pillar with thumb contact applied to the right side of the C5 spinous process to right laterally flex the C5–C6 articulation, gliding the right side inferiorly and the left side superiorly.

CP: Proximal lateral surface of the index finger and distal palmar surface of the thumb. The wrist is held in ulnar deviation with the fingers pointing toward the floor.

SCP: Posterior aspect of the articular pillar and lateral surface of the spinous process.

IH: The palm of the indifferent hand cups the ear with the fingers pointing caudally and resting on the cheek and jaw.

VEC: Lateral to medial, posterior to anterior, and superior to inferior.

P: Place the patient in a prone position, stand at the head of the table facing caudally, and laterally flex the patient's head toward the side of adjustive contact. Pre-adjustive tension is developed by applying medial and inferior pressure through the contact hand while applying cephalic tension through the indifferent hand. At tension deliver an impulse thrust through the contact hand reinforced by a distractive thrust with the indifferent hand.

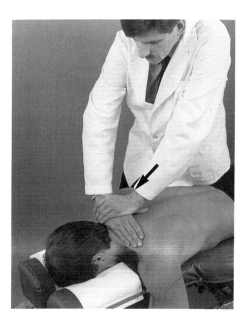

Figure 5.104 Hypothenar contact applied to the posterior and inferior aspect of the C6 spinous process to flex the C6–C7 articulation.

Hypothenar spinous (Fig. 5-104)

IND: Flexion or extension restrictions or malpositions of C2–C7.

  PP: The patient lies prone. The headpiece is slightly lowered for flexion restrictions (extension malpositions).

  DP: Stand in a fencer stance facing cephalad, with the center of gravity positioned caudal to the contact for flexion restrictions and over the contact for extension restrictions

  CP: Mid-hypothenar (knifedge) of cephalad hand.

  SCP: Spinous process of superior segment for flexion restriction (extension malposition). Interspinous space of dysfunctional motion segment for extension restriction (flexion malposition).

  IH: The indifferent hand reinforces the contact hand with fingers pointing vertically.

VEC: Posterior to anterior and inferior to superior for flexion restrictions; posterior to anterior for extension restrictions.

   P: When treating flexion dysfunction position the patient's cervical spine into flexion and center your body over the patient slightly caudal to the contact. After joint tension is reached deliver a cephalically directed impulse thrust through the arms and trunk.

        When treating extension dysfunction position the patient's cervical spine in a neutral or slightly extended position and center your body over the contact. Extension is induced by delivering an impulse thrust anteriorly through the arms and trunk. When performing this adjustment observe extra caution to avoid excessive depth and hyperextension of the neck.

        Both of these adjustments can be performed on a drop table. A drop mechanism that allows for downward and forward movement may provide a mechanical advantage over a straight downward drop by minimizing the compression and providing axial distraction.

Bilateral index pillar (Fig. 5-105)

IND: Restricted flexion or extension of C2–C7. Loss of superior or inferior glide, C2–C7. Flexion or extension malpositions, C2–C7.

PP: The patient lies with the neck in slight flexion for flexion restrictions (extension malpositions) and extension for extension restrictions (flexion malpositions).

DP: Stand in a fencer stance facing cephalad with the center of gravity caudal to the contact for flexion restrictions and over the contact for extension restrictions.

CP: Proximal index of both hands with thumbs crossing in the midline.

SCP: Posterolateral pillars.

VEC: Posterior to anterior and inferior to superior for flexion dysfunction, posterior to anterior for extension restrictions.

P: When treating flexion dysfunction center your body over the patient in a fencer position caudal to the contact. After joint tension is reached deliver a cephalically directed impulse thrust through the arms and trunk. When treating extension dysfunction orient your center of gravity over the site of contact and induce extension by

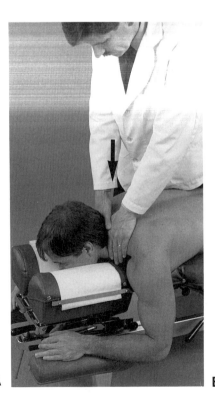
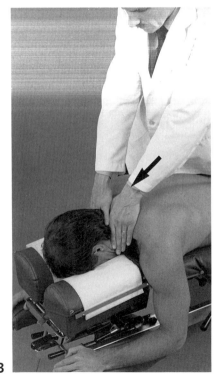

Figure 5.105 Bilateral index contacts established over the posterior aspect of the C4 articular pillars to (**A**) extend or (**B**) flex the C4–C5 articulation.

A   B

delivering an impulse thrust posterior to anterior. When performing these adjustments observe extra caution to avoid excessive depth and hyperextension of the neck. Both of these adjustments can be performed on a drop table.

THE THORACIC SPINE

In the thoracic spine, protection and function of the thoracic viscera take precedence over intersegmental spinal mobility. While the limiting anatomic structures make the thoracic spine the least mobile part of the spinal column, the small movements that do occur within the functional units are still significant. While few people have what could be considered a normal thoracic spine, most clinical attention has been focused around the cervical and lumbar regions. The thoracic region is, however, an area that must be considered important because of the possible mechanical changes to the functional unit that may result in effects to the elements of the autonomic nervous system. Furthermore, the addition of the articulations for the ribs makes the thoracic region an exceptional structure. Finally, this region seems to be prone to chronic postural problems affecting sections of the thoracic spine (scoliosis) and the supporting soft tissues (myofascial pain syndromes).

Functional Anatomy

The body of the typical thoracic vertebra (T2 to T8) is heart shaped with both the anterior to posterior and side to side dimensions of equal length. The anterior surface of the body is convex from side to side while the posterior surface is deeply concave. Both the superior and inferior surfaces of the body are flat with a ring around the margin for attachment of the intervertebral disc. The pedicles of thoracic vertebrae are short and have inferior vertebral notches deeper and larger than in any other part of the spine. The laminae are short, broad, thick, and overlapping. The spinous processes are long and slender, with a triangular shape in cross-section. They point obliquely downward, overlapping in the mid-thoracic spine, limiting extension movement. The transverse processes arise from behind the superior articular processes. They are thick, strong, and relatively long with a concave facet on the anterior side. The intervertebral foramen in this region are essentially circular in shape and fairly small when compared with other areas of the spine (Fig. 5-106).

The articular facets form an angle of approximately 60 degrees to the coronal plane and 20 degrees to the sagittal plane (Fig. 5-107). The inferior articular process arises from the laminae to face inferior, medial, and anterior. The superior articular process arises from near the lamina-pedicle junction to face superior, lateral, and posterior. The inferior articular process lies posterior to the superior articular process of the vertebra below.

The intervertebral discs are comparatively shallow in the thoracic spine. The disc height to body height ratio is 1:5, making it the smallest ratio in the spine (Fig. 5-108). This low ratio contributes to the decreased flexibility of the thoracic spine. The nucleus is also more centrally located within the annulus of the thoracic discs than it is in either of the other two spinal

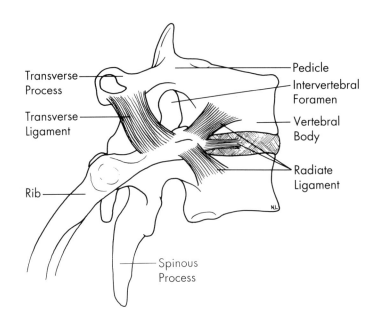

Figure 5.106 Typical thoracic motion segment; note structural difference of anterior and posterior body heights.

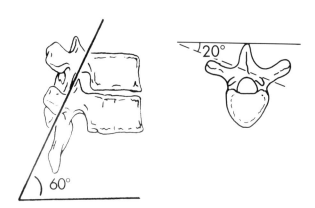

Figure 5.107 The thoracic facet planes.

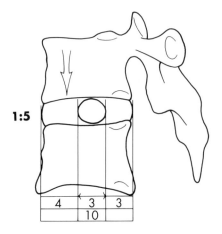

Figure 5.108 The location of the nucleus and the disc height-to-body ratio in the thoracic spine.

regions. One special feature of thoracic vertebrae is the presence of costover-tebral and costotransverse joints, which form the articulations for the ribs (Fig. 5-106). The costovertebral joints (demi-facets) are located on either side of the vertebral body to form an articulation with the heads of the ribs. The costotransverse joints are located on the anterior aspects of the transverse processes to articulate with the tubercles of the ribs.

The thoracic atypical vertebra include T1, T9, T10, T11, and T12. The vertebral body of T1 resembles that of C7 and possesses a whole facet for articulation with the first rib. The T9 vertebra may have no demifacets below, or it may have two demifacets on either side (in which case, the T10 vertebra will have demifacets only at the superior aspect). T10 has one full rib facet located partly on the body of the vertebra and partly on the tubercle. The T11 segment has complete costal facets, but no facets on the transverse processes for the rib tubercle. This vertebra also begins to take on character-istics of a lumbar vertebra. The spinous process is short and almost com-pletely horizontal. T12 has complete facets on the vertebra for articulation with the ribs but otherwise resembles a lumbar vertebra. The inferior articu-lating surfaces of T12 are convex and are directed laterally and anteriorly in the sagittal plane like those in the lumbar spine. The transverse processes are replaced by superior, inferior, and lateral tubercles (Fig. 5-109).

Thoracic Curve

The thoracic spine forms a kyphotic curve of less than 55 degrees [14] with an accepted range of 20 to 50 degrees[15,16] and an average of 45 degrees[2] (Fig. 5-110). It is a structural curve present from birth and maintained by the wedge shaped vertebral bodies that are approximately 2 mm higher posteriorly. The thoracic curve begins at T1–T2 and extends down to T12 with the T6–7 disc space as the apex.[17]

The thoracic curve can be influenced by the postural stress produced by an habitual position of forward shoulders or round upper back that occurs in a sedentary lifestyle. A stretch weakness of the middle and lower trapezius muscles results in a condition of chronic muscle strain.[18] As the thoracic kyphosis increases, it crowds the thoracic viscera, interfering with normal physiologic functioning.

Juvenile kyphosis (Scheuermann's Disease) and osteoporosis also result in an increased thoracic kyphosis. In juvenile kyphosis the wedge shape of the vertebral body is exaggerated, but the etiology remains inconclusive. Theories of the pathogenesis include aspetic necrosis, end plate fracture, infection, endocrine abnormalities, trabecular deficiencies, vitamin defi-ciencies, fluoride toxicity, and mechanical factors.[19] Osteoporosis reduces the number and size of trabeculae in the vertebral body, diminishing the axial loading stretch and resulting in compression fractures, which accentu-ate the kyphotic curve. Dietary deficiencies, malabsorption syndromes, ste-roid use, and endocrine disorders have been implicated in the etiology of osteoporosis.[20]

A change in the primary thoracic curve is likely to produce a change in the secondary curves in the cervical and lumbar spine. The lumbar curve tends to increase, while the cervical curve decreases or shifts forward, creat-ing a cervical "poking" posture.

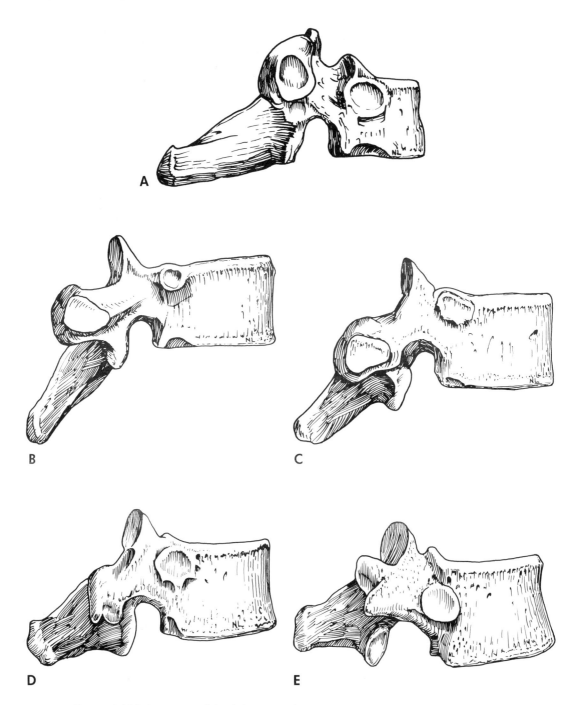

Figure 5.109 Structure of the (**A**) T1 vertebra, (**B**) T9 vertebra, (**C**) T10 vertebra, (**D**) T11 vertebra, and (**E**) T12 vertebra.

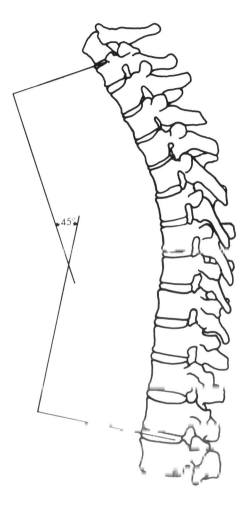

Figure 5.110 Measurement of the thoracic curve.

Range and Patterns of Motion

Of the three cardinal planes of movement, the sagittal plane movement of flexion and extension is the most restricted. Rotation and lateral flexion demonstrate nearly equal movement, with each exhibiting nearly twice as much movement as flexion and extension (Table 5-6) (Fig. 5-24).

Movement in the upper thoracic spine is generally less than the lower. The exception is rotation, which decreases dramatically in the lower thoracic segments as the facet facings become more sagittal.[1] The instantaneous axis of movement for the thoracic spine, like other spinal regions, remains somewhat tentative. Panjabii et al.,[21] using fresh cadaveric specimens, have determined the likely sites for flexion/extension, lateral flexion, and rotation (Fig. 5-111).

Table 5.6 Average Ranges of Motion for the Thoracic Spine

Vertebra	Combined Flexion and Extension	One Side Lateral Flexion	One Side Axial Rotation
T1–T2	4	5	9
T2–T3	4	6	8
T3–T4	4	5	8
T4–T5	4	6	8
T5–T6	4	6	8
T6–T7	5	6	7
T7–T8	6	6	7
T8–T9	6	6	9
T9–T10	6	6	4
T10–T11	9	7	2
T11–T12	12	9	2
T12–L1	12	8	2

(Adapted from White and Panjabi,[1] with permission.)

Flexion and Extension

Combined flexion and extension in the thoracic spine averages approximately 6 degrees per motion segment, demonstrating a cephalocaudal increase in flexibility. Movement averages 4 degrees in the upper thoracic spine, 6 degrees in the mid-thoracic spine, and 12 degrees in the lower two thoracic segments.[1] Extension is more limited than flexion because of the impaction of the articular processes and spinous processes.

Thoracic flexion and extension combine sagittal plane rotation with slight sagittal plane translation. The degree of combined translation is minimal and uniform throughout the thoracic spine.[1] During flexion the articular

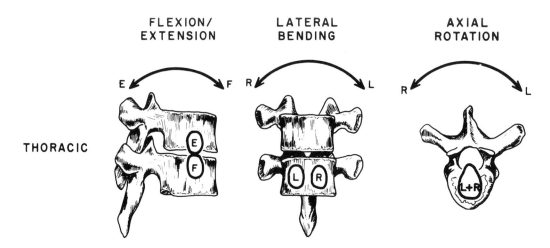

Figure 5.111 Instantaneous axis of rotation for (**A**) flexion and extension, (**B**) lateral flexion, and (**C**) axial rotation in a thoracic segment. (From White and Panjabi,[1] with permission.)

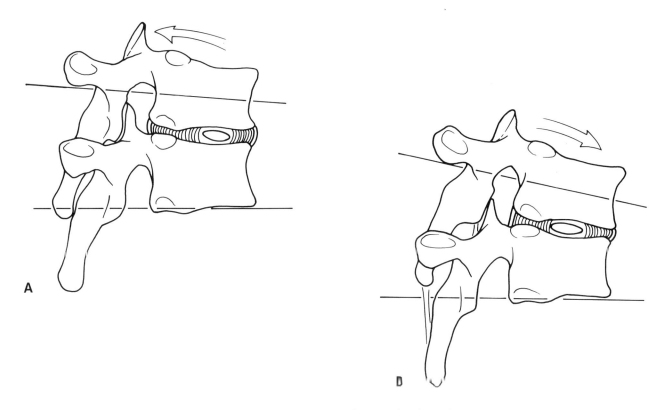

Figure 5.112 (**A**) Extension and (**B**) flexion of a thoracic segment.

facet glide apart as the IVD opens posteriorly. During extension the facet joints and posterior disc approximate (Fig. 5-112).

Lateral Flexion

Lateral flexion averages approximately 6 degrees to each side, with the lower two segments averaging 7 to 9 degrees. Lateral flexion is coupled with axial rotation throughout the thoracic spine. This is especially apparent in the upper thoracic spine where the pattern duplicates that of the cervical spine. The coupling is such that lateral flexion and rotation occur to the same side (i.e., body rotation to the concavity, and spinous deviation to the convexity)[1,22] (Fig. 5-113). In the middle and lower thoracic spine the coupling is less distinct and may occur in either direction (Fig. 5-114).

It is often assumed, however, that the lower thoracic segments have a tendency to follow the coupling pattern of the lumbar spine. The lumbar pattern is opposite to that of the cervical and upper thoracic segments and incorporates lateral flexion with coupled axial rotation in the opposite direction[23,24] (Fig. 5-114). White and Panjabi[1] pointed out, however, that coupling patterns still remain controversial and one must guard against any strong conclusions.

During lateral flexion the IVD and facet joints approximate on the side of lateral flexion and separate on the side opposite the lateral flexion (Fig. 5-113). In the upper thoracic spine the inferior articular facets also glide

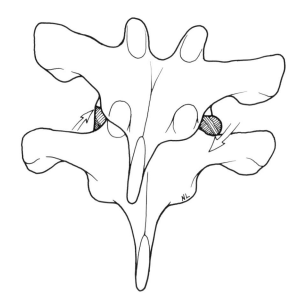

Figure 5.113 Lateral flexion of an upper thoracic segment showing coupling movement in rotation and lateral flexion to the same side as in the cervical spine.

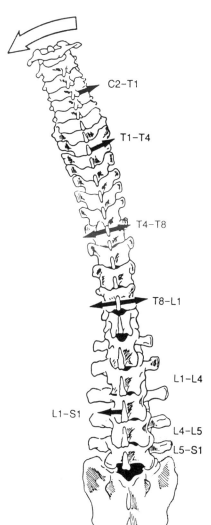

Figure 5.114 Coupled relationship of lateral flexion and axial rotation throughout the spine. The cervical and upper thoracic regions have lateral flexion coupled with ipsilateral rotation while the lumbar spine and lower thoracic regions have lateral flexion coupled with contralateral rotation. (From White and Panjabi,[1] with permission.)

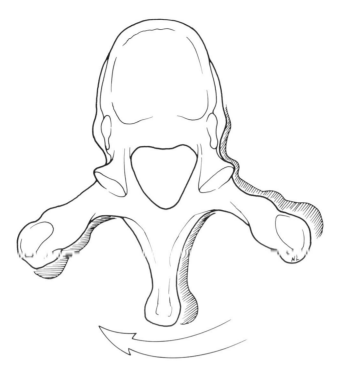

Figure 5.115 Horizontal view illustrating right rotation of the superior (light) vertebra relative to the inferior (dark) vertebra.

medially relative to the superior articular facet on the side of lateral flexion and laterally on the side opposite the lateral flexion. This is due to the strong coupled axial rotation present in the upper thoracic spine.

Rotation

Segmental axial rotation averages 8 to 9 degrees in the upper thoracic spine (Fig. 5-115). Rotational motion decreases slightly in the middle thoracic spine and drops off dramatically to approximately 2 degrees in the lower two or three thoracic segments.[1] The marked decrease in rotational mobility in the lower segments no doubt reflects the transition from coronal plane facets to sagittal plane facets.

Rotational movements in the thoracic spine are also coupled with lateral flexion. In the upper thoracic spine rotation is coupled with same side lateral flexion. This leads to medial and inferior gliding of the inferior facet relative to the superior facet on the side of trunk rotation, and lateral and superior gliding of the inferior facet on the side opposite trunk rotation (Fig. 5-113). The coupling is not as marked in the lower segments as it is in the upper segments.[2] This may occur because the facets of the lower thoracic spine become more sagittal in their orientation.

Kinetics of the Thoracic Spine

The same principles of concentric and eccentric muscle activity discussed for the cervical spine apply to the trunk. Non-segmental muscles, which effect the entire thoracic spine but can also act segmentally, include the erector spinae, rectus abdominis, quadratus lumborum, and abdominal obliques. The segmental muscles that influence each thoracic motion segment include multifidi, interspinalis, intertransversarii (small in the thoracics), and rotatores.

Flexion is initiated by concentric activity of the rectus abdominis and controlled or limited by eccentric activity of the erector spinae. Flexion is further limited by the elastic limits of the myofascial tissue, ligamentum flavum, interspinous ligament, supraspinous ligament, PLL, capsular ligaments, posterior IVD; and bony impact of the vertebral bodies.

Extension is initiated by concentric activity of the erector spinae and controlled or limited by eccentric activity of the rectus abdominis. Extension is mainly limited by the bony impact of the spinous and articular processes, but the anterior longitudinal ligament, anterior IVD, and elastic limits of myofascial tissue also contribute.

Lateral flexion is initiated by concentric activity of ipsilateral erector spinae and quadratus lumborum and controlled or limited by contralateral eccentric activity of the same muscles. Further limiting of lateral flexion movement occurs through impact of the articular facets, contralateral capsular, ligamentum flavum, intertransverse ligament and elastic limits of contralateral segmental and non-segmental muscles.

Rotation is initiated by concentric activity of ipsilateral erector spinae, multifidus and rotatores and controlled or limited by concentric and eccentric activity of the abdominal obliques and erector spinae. Rotation is further limited by the articular capsules, interspinous ligament, supraspinous ligament, ligamentum flavum, bony impact of the articular facets, and the elastic limits of bilateral segmental and non-segmental muscles.

FUNCTIONAL ANATOMY AND BIOMECHANICS OF THE RIB CAGE

Ribs 2 through 9 articulate posteriorly with the transverse process, the superior vertebral body of the same vertebra, and the inferior aspect of the vertebral body of the vertebra above. Ribs 1, 10, 11 and 12 articulate with the transverse process and the vertebral body of the same vertebra only. The articulations that are formed between the vertebral and costovertebral bodies and the transverse and costotransverse processes are each tightly secured by ligaments (Fig. 5-116). Both of these articulations are true synovial joints. The costotransverse articulation is surrounded by a joint capsule with further strength from the costotransverse ligaments. The costovertebral articulations have a single capsular ligament surrounding the two demifacet articulations, which is further strengthened by the radiate ligament.

These synovial joints are prone to the same pathologic conditions that affect other synovial joints, including the subluxation and dysfunction complex. Furthermore, the ribs play an integral part in the normal activity of the thoracic functional unit and should be a significant consideration in evaluation for thoracic dysfunction.

Anteriorly, the first seven ribs connect to the sternum directly, while the eighth, ninth, and tenth ribs attach indirectly via the costocartilage (Fig. 5-117). The eleventh and twelfth ribs are free floating with no anterior

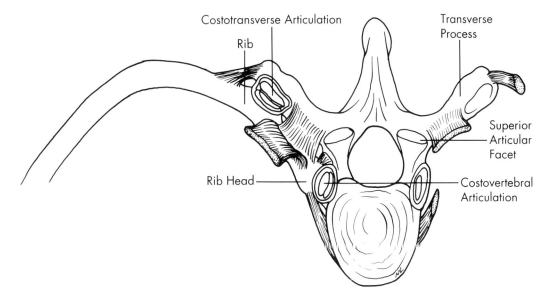

Figure 5.116 Axial view of a thoracic vertebra with rib attachments.

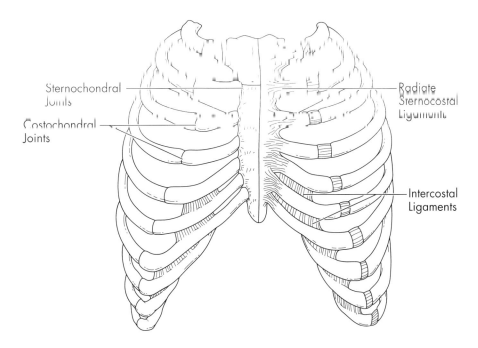

Figure 5.117 Anterior attachments of the ribs to the sternum: 2–7 directly, 8–10 via costocartilage.

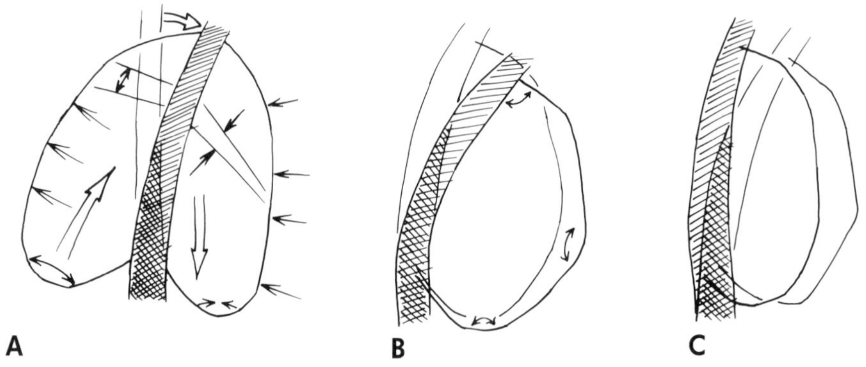

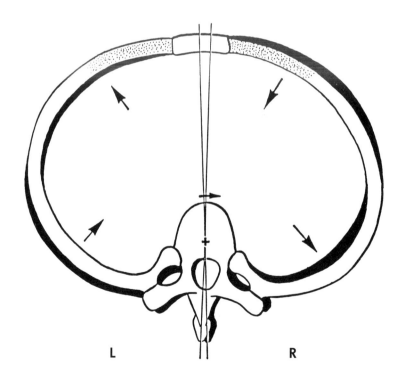

Figure 5.118 The effects of (**A**) lateral flexion, (**B**) flexion, and (**C**) extension on the shape of the rib cage.

attachment. The anterior articulations move mainly because of the elastic quality of the costocartilage. Calcification and subsequent decreases in movement can occur with age.

Movements of the Rib Cage With Spinal Movements

The ribs influence movement of the individual thoracic vertebra and the rib cage influences the movement of the entire thoracic spine. With flexion and extension, the ribs move correspondingly with the thoracic spine, resulting in the posterior intercostal spaces opening up with flexion and closing with extension. The entire rib cage must flatten superiorly and inferiorly, increasing the sternal angle, for flexion of the thoracic spine

Figure 5.119 The effects of right rotation of a thoracic vertebra on its associate rib, leading to accentuation of the concavity of the rib on the side of vertebral rotation and flattening of the concavity of the rib on the opposite side. (From Kapandji,[79] with permission.)

L   R

to take place. The converse is true for extension (Fig. 5-118). A similar relationship occurs with lateral flexion as the rib cage is depressed on the side of lateral flexion. Furthermore, the lateral intercostal spaces open on the convex and close on the concave side. With thoracic rotation the rib angle is accentuated on the side of posterior trunk rotation, while flattening of the rib angle occurs on the side of anterior trunk rotation (Fig. 5-119).

Movement of the Rib Cage With Respiration

Individually and collectively the ribs undergo two main types of motion during respiration. These movements are commonly referred to as "bucket handle" and "pump handle" movements.

Bucket handle movement increases the transverse diameter of the rib cage by elevating the rib and its costochondral arch (Fig. 5-120). Bucket handle movement is greater in the lower thoracic spine where the relatively flat tubercular facets of the ribs and corresponding articular facets of the transverse processes allow the rib to ride up and down against the transverse process. The lower ribs may therefore roll around an axis connecting the costovertebral and sternochondral joints. This allows for elevation and depression of the ribs with respiration and a movement that simulates the rolling movement of a bucket handle when it is elevated on its hinges.[25]

Pump handle movement increases the anterioposterior diameter of the rib cage. It occurs more in the upper rib cage than the lower and results from the elevation of the anterior aspect of the rib cage with the upward and forward movement of the sternum. In contrast to the lower ribs, the tubercular facets of the upper ribs are situated in the pump-shaped sockets on the transverse processes. Therefore the rib is free to move only along the costovertebral and costotransverse joints. With inspiration the rib head rolls downward, elevating the anterior end of the rib like the handle on a pump[24] (Fig. 5-120).

Kinetics of Respiration

During quiet respiration thoracic mobility is minimal as the diaphragm is the main muscle of respiration. The intercostal muscles are slightly active to supply tension, and the qudratus lumborum fixes the twelfth rib to provide a stable attachment. However, during forced respiration the external intercostal muscles become active to elevate the ribs and receive secondary help as needed from the scaleni, pectoralis minor, serratus anterior, and iliocostalis cervicis, which will show a rhythmic increase and decrease of activity during forced inspiration and expiration respectively.

Expiration is usually a passive process resulting from the elastic tension produced in the ribs, costocartilage, and pulmonary parenchyma. Forced expiration is produced by the internal intercostal muscles, which receive secondary help from the abdominal muscles, iliocostalis lumborum, longissimus, and quadratus lumborum. The activity of the expiratory muscles are also used to perform the valsalva maneuver, increasing intraabdominal pressure.

Because of the influences of the iliocostalis cervicis, longissimus cervicis, scalenes, and serratus posterior and superior muscles, the upper ribs tend

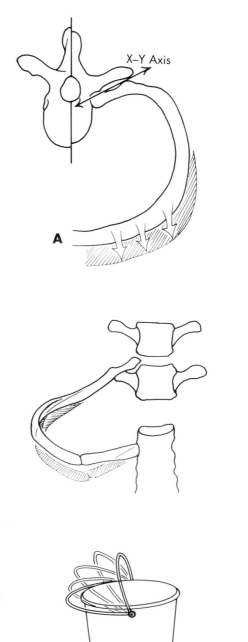

X–Y Axis

A

B

C

Figure 5.120 Movements of the ribs. Pump handle movement in (A) an axial view with rib rotating around the XY axis elevating the rib in front and (B) a lateral view demonstrating elevation of the rib and anterior to posterior expansion of the rib cage. (C) Bucket handle movement illustrating transverse expansion of the rib cage.

to be pulled and fixated superiorly. Similarly, because of the effects of the longissimus thoracis, iliocostalis lumborum, quadratus lumborum, and serratus posterior and inferior muscles, the lower ribs tend to be pulled and fixated inferiorly. However, the iliocostalis thoracis muscle may produce the opposite movement in each area, depressing the upper ribs and raising the lower ribs.

FUNCTIONAL ANATOMY AND CHARACTERISTICS OF THE TRANSITIONAL AREAS

The thoracocervical (C6–T3) and thoracolumbar (T10–L1) segments form a transition between the thoracic spine and the cervical and lumbar regions. Hence some characteristics or activities are shared from both regions and some are unique to each region.

The Thoracocervical Junction (C6–T3)

The notable structural changes in this segment include spinous processes that become more elongated, point caudal, and lose the bifid characteristic of the cervical spine. Furthermore, there are no uncinate processes or transverse foramen. There are the development of costotransverse and costovertebral articulations as well as an increased slope to the articular facets, creating a 60 degree angle toward the coronal plane and a 20 degree turn toward the sagittal plane. Because of the distal attachment of the cervical muscles including the splenius, longissimus, and semispinalis cervicis as well as the semispinalis capitis muscles, cervical spine movements will involve the upper thoracic spine. The presence of ribs in this area provide stability but also decrease motion. Movements in all directions are decreased between C6 and T3, but the coupled movements in this area are

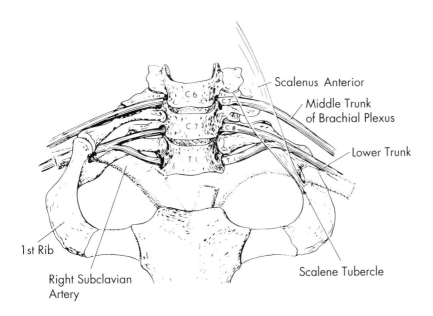

Figure 5.121 The cervico-thoracic junction and its relationship to the neurovascular bundle. (From Grieve,[59] with permission.)

the same as for the typical cervical region (i.e., lateral flexion is coupled with rotation to the same side).

The significance of this area is twofold. First, this area is structurally and functionally related to the neurovascular structures of the upper extremities, as this area forms the thoracic outlet (Fig. 5-121). Secondly, the thoracocervical junction has been deemed a difficult area to apply manipulative therapy. This reputation has been established because of the necessary structural characteristics for a transition from the most mobile area of the spine to the area that is least mobile, as well as the external characteristics of distribution of body fat (dowager hump) and the presence of the shoulder and scapular muscles. However, an understanding of the functional anatomy and biomechanics in this area combined with the appropriate techniques will make the thoracocervical junction no more difficult to adjust than any other area.

The Thoracolumbar Junction (T10–L1)

The thoracolumbar transition area is similar to the thoracocervical junction in that it must serve to join an area of greater mobility with one of lesser mobility, as well as to change from a primary (kyphotic) curve to a secondary (lordotic) curve. The most significant structural characteristic in this area is the change from the coronal facet plane in the thoracic spine to the sagittal plane facets in the lumbr spine (Fig. 5-122). This transition, though typically thought to occur at the T12–L1 segment, has been shown to occur at any of the segments between T10 and L1. Davis[26] reported the change was found to occur most commonly at the T11–T12 level (Table 5-7).

Of further clinical importance is the distribution of the lateral branches of the posterior primary rami of the spinal roots of T12, L1, and L2. These nerves form the cluneal nerves and innervate the skin and superficial structures of the upper posterolateral buttock, posterior iliac crest, and groin area (Fig. 5-123). Dysfunction within the lower thoracic segments

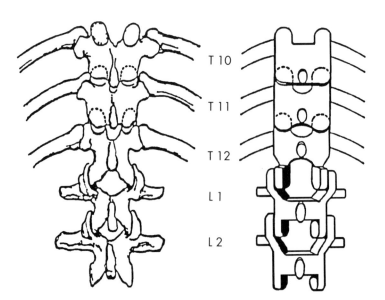

T 10

T 11

T 12

L 1

L 2

Figure 5.122 The thoraco-lumbar transition is characterized by a change in facet planes from coronal to sagittal.

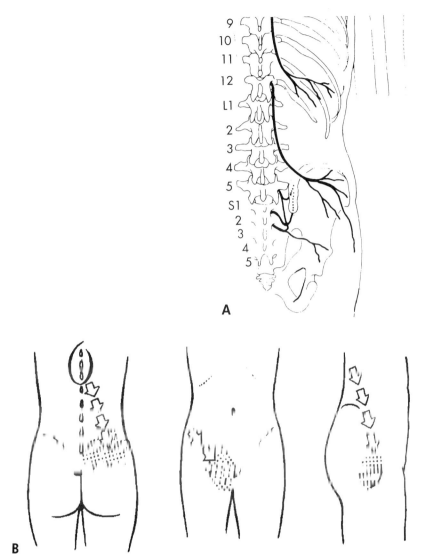

Figure 5.120 (A) The course of the cluneal nerves and (B) possible distribution of pain findings and sensory changes. (Fig. A from Grieve,[59] and Fig. B from Basmajian,[78] with permission.)

Table 5.7 Frequency of Level Demonstrating Transition from Coronal Facets to Sagittal Facets

Segment	Percent
T10–T11:	7.46
T11–T12:	68.66
T12–L1:	23.88
Total:	100.00

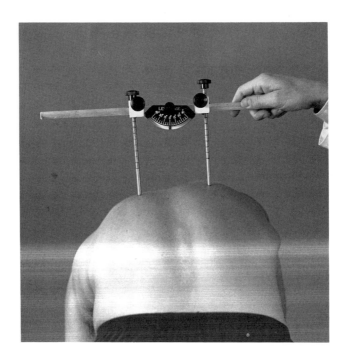

Figure 5.124 Scoliometer demonstrating a right thoracic rib hump.

may refer pain into these regions and be mistaken for disorders of the lumbosacral or sacroiliac regions, which also commonly refer pain to these zones. Maigne[27] believes this syndrome can account for up to 60 percent of chronic and acute backache, generally considered the result of lumbar or sacral joint changes.

EVALUATION OF THE THORACIC SPINE

Observation

Before palpation is begun a visual examination should be made to observe for any deviations in posture or symmetry. Observations should be made with the patient in the sitting, standing, and recumbent positions. Postural syndromes that may predispose the patient to spinal dysfunction and pain are common in the thoracic spine and should not be overlooked. Idiopathic scoliosis has its greatest expression in the thoracic spine, and any noted curvatures should be assessed for flexibility (Fig. 5-124).

Alignment in the coronal plane is evaluated by observing the orientation of the spinous processes, symmetry of paraspinal soft tissues, and contours of the rib cage. The alignment of the shoulders and angles of the scapula should be observed and compared relative to the iliac crests. Sagittal plane alignment is assessed by observing the status of the thoracic curve and noting the position of the gravity line. Orientation of the trunk in the transverse plane is noted by looking at the shoulders and vertebral borders of the scapula for any winging (Fig. 5-125).

Global motion of the thoracic spine is typically not separated from lumbar movements. Both are measured and recorded as movements of the entire

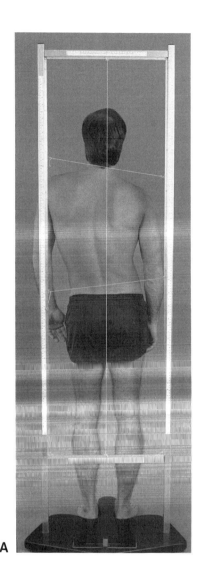

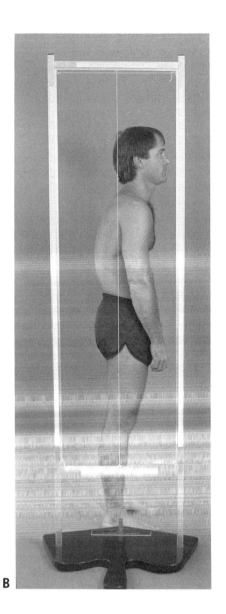

Figure 5-125. Postural evaluation. (A) Posterior plumb line demonstrating shoulder and pelvic unleveling to opposite side creating a "C" shape scoliosis. (B) Lateral plumb line demonstrating a round back deformity with an anterior shift in the upper body.

trunk. However, when desired, regional movements of the thoracic spine may be easily assessed with the inclinometric measuring methods previously described in Chapter 3 (Fig. 3-10). Table 5-8 presents the average global ranges of motion for the thoracic spine.

Static Palpation

Static palpation of the spine and posterior chest wall is commonly performed with the patient in the prone position. During the evaluation, stand to the side of the patient and accommodate to the patient by bending at the knees, hips, and waist. Palpation typically begins with an assessment of superficial

Table 5.8 Global Ranges of Motion for the Thoracic Spine

Flexion	25°–45°
Extension	25°–45°
One Side Lateral Flexion	20°–40°
One Side Rotation	30°–45°

temperature and sensitivity, followed by the assessment of consistency and mobility of the dermal layer and muscular layer. Palpation of bony landmarks incorporates a scanning assessment of contour, tenderness, and alignment of the spinous processes, transverse processes, rib angles, interspinous spaces, and intercostal spaces. In addition, the alignment of the scapula and its borders and angles are customarily included in the evaluation of the thoracic spine.

Potential tenderness and alignment of the spinous processes, interspinous spaces, and transverse processes are assessed with unilateral or bilateral fingertip contacts (Fig. 5-126). Paraspinal muscle tone is evaluated by applying bilateral contacts with the palmar surfaces of the fingers or thumbs to explore for areas of tenderness and altered muscle tone and texture (Fig. 5-127).

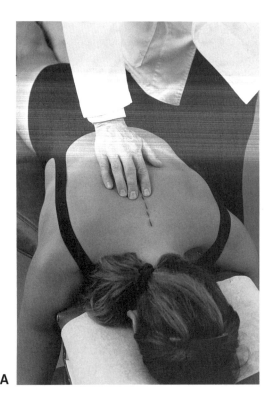

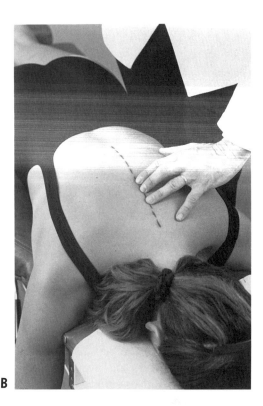

Figure 5.126 Palpation of (A) rotational alignment and sensitivity of thoracic spinous processes and (B) interspinous spaces and sensitivity.

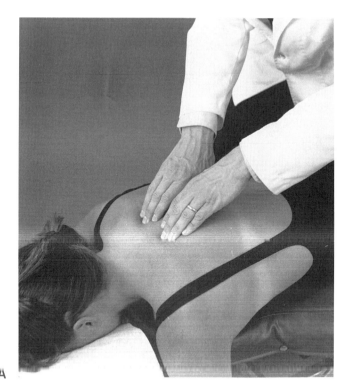

A

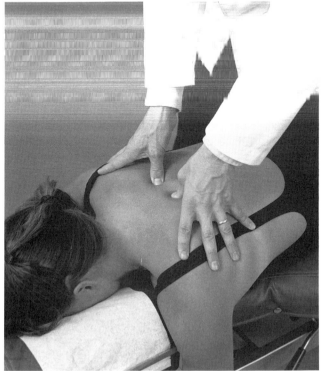

B

Figure 5.127 Palpation of transverse process alignment and sensitivity using (**A**) fingertip contacts and (**B**) thumb contacts.

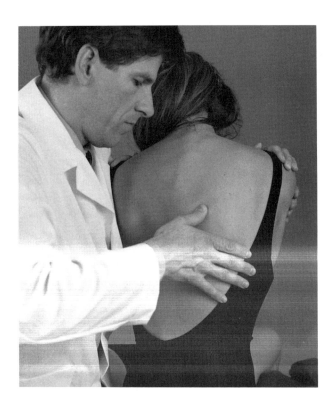

Figure 5.128 Palpation of the right T6 rib angle.

Rib alignment and tenderness is assessed by palpating along the rib angles with the fingertips or thumb. Palpation may be conducted with the patient in the sitting or prone position. The sitting evaluation has the advantage of being able to induce trunk rotation to accentuate the ribs for palpation. When assessing rib alignment in the sitting position, the patient is asked to cross the arms across the chest and flex slightly forward. The doctor then sits or stands beside the patient and rotates the patient forward on the side to be palpated (Fig. 5-128).

The rib angles should be uniform in prominence and non-tender. A tender or distinctly palpable lump that stands out in relation to the adjacent ribs may indicate rib dysfunction. Take care to differentiate a prominent rib from a myofascial trigger point (the former will be bony and immobile; the latter softer and more mobile). The pain associated with costotransverse dysfunction is often accentuated with respiration and may radiate to the anterior chest wall. Dysfunction of the costosternal junction may also be present with or without posterior dysfunction. Evaluate the anterior chest wall for myofascial or joint dysfunction when the patient complaints of pain of the posterior or anterior chest wall.

Motion Palpation

Joint Play

The thoracic spine should be scanned for sites of painful or abnormal joint play with the patient sitting or prone. Areas of elicited abnormality should be further assessed with posterior to anterior and counter rotational

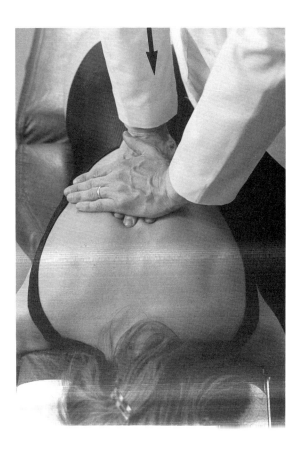

Figure 5.129 Prone mid-tho-racic joint play evaluation using bilateral fingertip con-tacts over the transverse pro-cesses and applying a poste-rior to anterior vector of force

joint play procedures. With the patient in the prone position, posterior to anterior glide is assessed by establishing contacts over the spinous process or bilaterally over the transverse processes. Posterior to anterior pressure is gradually applied and a springing motion is created. During posterior to anterior joint play assessment, each joint tested should be challenged with vectors that run perpendicular to the joint plane (Fig. 5-129) and vectors that are inclined headward along the facet plane (Fig. 5-130). Perpendicular vectors challenge extension movements of the articulation, and superiorly directed vectors assess gliding movements of the facet joints that would contribute to movements of flexion, lateral flexion, and rotation. During posterior to anterior joint play assessment, a subtle gliding and recoil should be felt at each segment tested.

To further isolate the specific level of pain and possible dysfunction, counter rotational joint play and provocation testing may be applied. To perform this procedure, place thumbs on opposing sides of adjacent spinous processes and apply springing pressure toward the midline with the superior spinous while counter stabilizing the inferior spinous (Fig. 5-131). This procedure is less giving than anterior to posterior glide and a perceptible decrease in movement is encountered when pressure is applied to the adjacent vertebra. Pain and/or altered resistance to movement is a positive response. Pain elicited at one level and not at adjacent levels helps localize

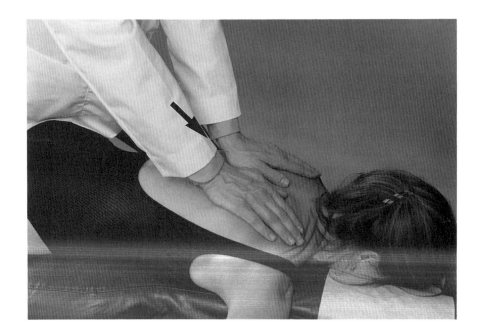

Figure 5.130 Prone mid-thoracic joint play evaluation using bilateral thenar contacts over the transverse processes and applying a posterior to anterior and inferior to superior (facet plane vector) vector of force.

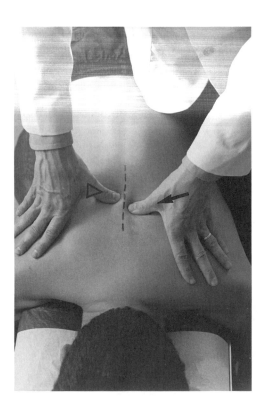

Figure 5.131 Counter rotational joint play evaluation for left rotational movement of T7 relative to T8; a stabilizing contact is established on the right side of the T8 spinous process while the left side of the T7 spinous process is stressed from left to right.

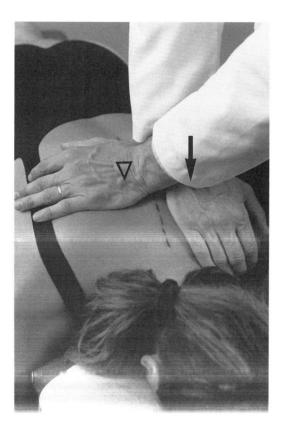

Figure 5.132 Counter rotational joint play evaluation for left rotational movement of T5 relative to T6; a stabilizing contact is established over the right T6 transverse process while the left transverse process of the T5 is stressed posterior to anterior.

the site of possible dysfunction. Decreased resistance identifies a site of possible joint fixation and increased movement a site of possible joint instability. If desired, this procedure may be performed with the contacts located over the transverse processes instead of the spinous processes. With transverse process contacts springing movements are applied in an anterior superior direction against the superior transverse process while counter stabilizing the joint below through contact on the transverse process below (Fig. 5-132).

Thoracic Segmental Motion Palpation and End Play

Movement is typically evaluated with the patient in the sitting position with arms flexed and folded across the chest so the hands can grasp the opposing shoulders. The doctor's position may be sitting behind or standing beside the patient; the standing position is usually preferred when evaluating the upper thoracic segments. Movement is controlled through contacts on the patient's shoulders for the middle and lower thoracic segments or the crown of the patient's head when evaluating the upper thoracic segments (Fig. 5-133). Indifferent hand contacts on the patient's head are to be avoided in patients with cervical complaints.

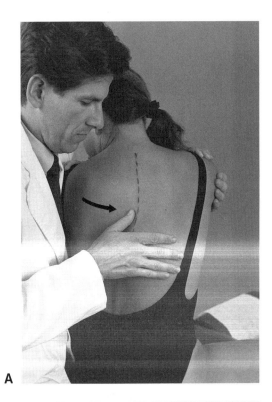

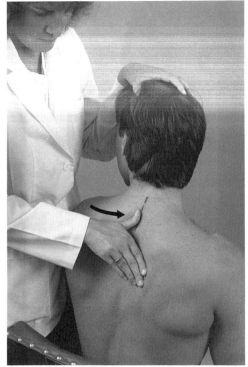

Figure 5.133 Palpation of left rotational movement at the (**A**) T7–T8 level and (**B**) the T2–T3 level using a thumb contact across the left interspinous space.

Rotation

The segmental contact is established against the lateral surface of the adjacent spinous process on the side of induced rotation. The palpating thumb is placed so that the pad spans the interspinous space. The support hand reaches around the front of the patient and grasps the opposite flexed arm or shoulder and rotates the patient's trunk toward the side of contact (Fig. 5-133). During normal rotation, the superior spinous process should be palpated, rotating away from the spinous below. Movement should occur in the direction of trunk rotation. If separation is not noted and adjacent spinous processes move together, segmental restriction should be suspected.

To assess end play, additional overpressure is applied through the contact and indifferent hands at the end of passive motion. Firm elastic but giving motion should be encountered. Contacts may be established against the superior spinous process on the side of induced rotation (Fig. 5-133) or over the transverse process and posterior joint on the side opposite the induced rotation (Fig. 5-134). Comparing the quality of end play between these two contacts may be helpful in determining the side of joint restriction.

Lateral flexion

To assess lateral flexion, a segmental contact against the lateral surface of adjacent spinous processes is established on the side of induced lateral flexion. The doctor either sits or stands behind the patient toward the side of induced lateral flexion. If a sitting position is selected, movement is

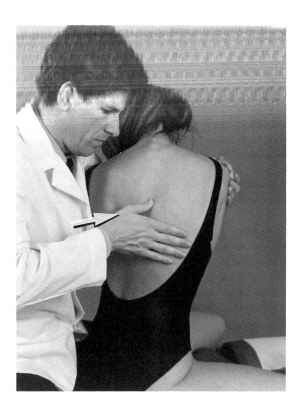

Figure 5.134 Palpation of left rotational end play with anterior superior glide of the right T7–T8 articulation.

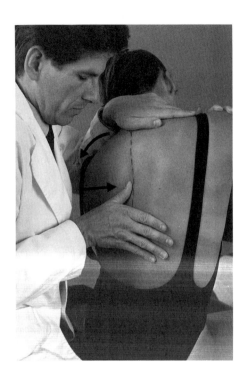

Figure 5.135 Palpation of left lateral flexion movement at T6–T7 using a thumb contact across the left T6–T7 interspace, with the doctor seated.

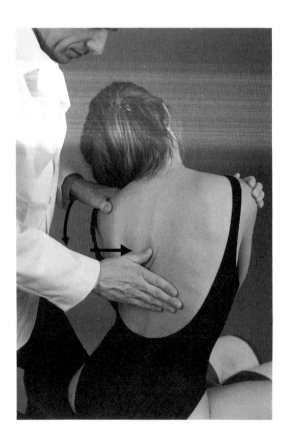

Figure 5.136 Palpation of left lateral flexion at the T6–T7 level with the doctor standing.

guided by placing the forearm across the patient's shoulders (Fig. 5-135). In the standing position, movement is directed by placing the doctor's hand on the patient's shoulder on the side of induced lateral flexion (Fig. 5-136). In the lower thoracic spine, slight patient flexion is produced to accentuate the spinous process and reduce coupled rotation.

Movement is induced by asking the patient to bend to the side as downward pressure is applied through the indifferent arm. As bending is being actively produced, medial pressure is applied through the contact hand to help accentuate the bending at the site of palpation. The indifferent arm and contact arm work together to isolate the site of lateral flexion by adjusting the amount of applied downward pressure and tilting of the patient. During this movement the spinous should be felt to shift toward the opposite side (convex side) while the spine bends smoothly around the contact point. End play is evaluated by shifting the contact to the superior spinous process on the side of induced lateral flexion and applying additional overpressure at the end range of motion.

Flexion and extension

The segmental contacts are established over the interspinous spaces with the doctor's fingertips or thumb. When evaluating flexion and extension in the upper thoracic spine, movement is guided by placing the indifferent hand on the crown of the patient's head. When evaluating flexion in the middle to lower thoracic segments, the forearm is placed across the patient's shoulders (Fig. 5-137). To evaluate extension, the indifferent forearm is placed across the patient's shoulders or the patient interlaces fingers behind the neck while the patient's flexed arms are lifted. The latter method is commonly applied in the upper thoracic spine or when assessing extension end play (Fig. 5-138). To assess motion, actively or passively flex and extend the spine. Take care to place the apex of bending at the level of palpation. During flexion the interspinous spaces should open symmetrically and during extension they should approximate

Flexion end play is assessed by hooking the inferior aspect of the superior spinous between the thumb and flexed finger and springing in the anterior and superior direction with the contact hand while downward pressure is applied through the contact on the patient's shoulders. Extension end play is evaluated by pushing anteriorly after full extension has been reached. Extension end play is inhibited by the impact of the spinous processes and has a more rigid quality than flexion, lateral flexion, or rotation. In the upper thoracics, a side posture position may be used for all the above palpation methods (Figs. 5-139–5-142).

Rib Motion Palpation

Ribs 3 through 12

The evaluation of rib mobility incorporates an assessment of bucket handle movement and costotransverse end play. End play is assessed by placing the patient in the sitting position and inducing slight flexion, lateral flexion, and rotation of the patient away from the side of palpation. The palpation contact is established with the doctor's thumb or fingertips over the rib angle just lateral to costotransverse articulation. The doctor reaches around

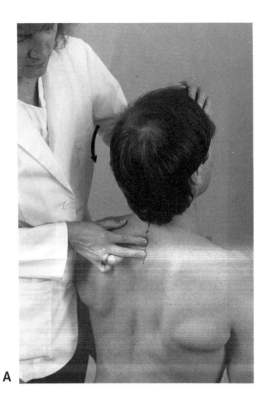

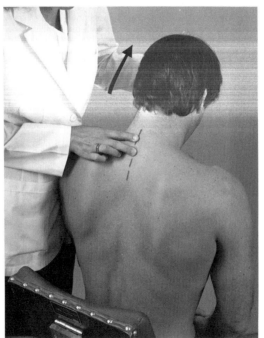

Figure 5.137 Palpation of (A) extension movement and (B) flexion movement in the upper thoracic spine using fingertip contacts in the inter-spinous spaces.

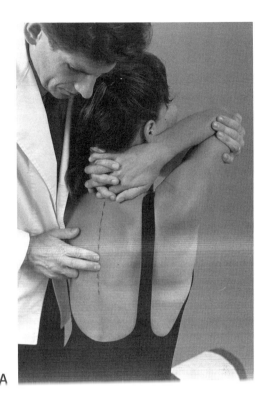

A

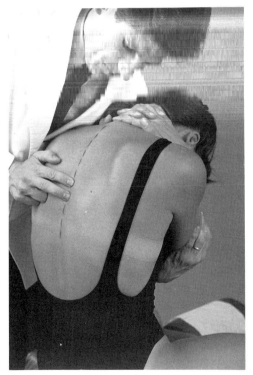

B

Figure 5.138 Palpation of (**A**) extension movement and (**B**) flexion movement in the middle thoracic spine using fingertip contacts in the interspinous spaces.

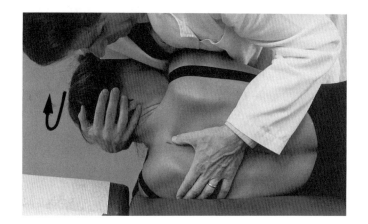

Figure 5.139 Palpation of right rotational movement of T1 relative to T2 using a thumb contact across the right interspinous space in the side posture position.

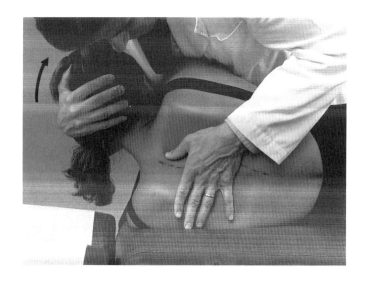

Figure 5.140 Palpation of right lateral flexion movement of T1 relative to T2 using a thumb contact across the right interspinous space in the side posture position.

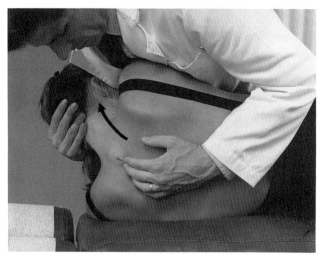

Figure 5.141 Palpation of flexion movement of T1 relative to T2 using a fingertip contact in the interspinous space in the side posture position.

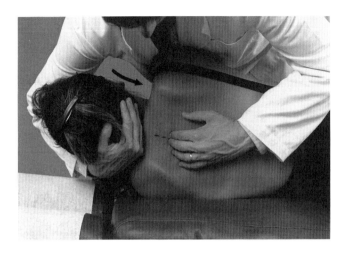

Figure 5.142 Palpation of extension movement of T2 relative to T3 using a fingertip contact in the interspinous space in the side posture position.

with the non-palpating hand to grasp the patient's shoulder and induce rotation. The patient is rotated and the rib is stressed posterior to anterior at the end of rotation (Fig. 5-143). A rib that remains distinctly prominent and provides firm resistance relative to adjacent segments indicates rib dysfunction.

To assess bucket handle motion the doctor places his/her fingertips in the intercostal spaces at the mid-axillary line. The doctor's indifferent arm

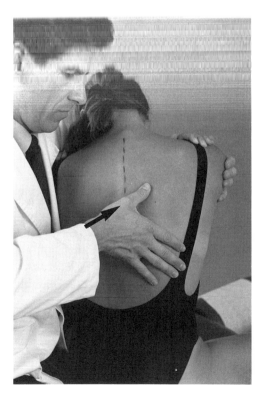

Figure 5.143 Palpation of posterior to anterior end play of the right T7 rib articulation using a thumb contact over the right T7 rib angle.

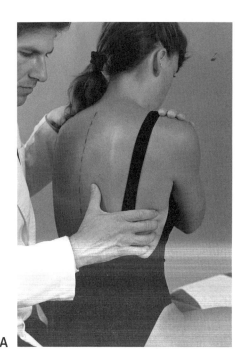

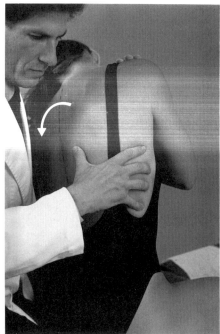

Figure 5.144 Palpation for bucket handle rib movement: (**A**) Starting position with fingers in the intercostal spaces in the midaxillary line, and (**B**) left lateral flexion movement to evaluate opening of the right intercostal spaces.

is placed across the patient's shoulders and the patient is laterally flexed toward and away from the side of contact (Fig. 5-144). The intercostal spaces should open with lateral flexion away and close with lateral flexion toward the contacts. Absence of symmetrical opening and closing may indicate dysfunction at the costotransverse joint or stiffness in the intercostal soft tissues.

Respiratory movements of the upper and lower ribs may also be evaluated by having the patient lie in the prone and supine positions as the respiration movement of the rib cage and intercostal spaces are palpated (Fig. 5-145).

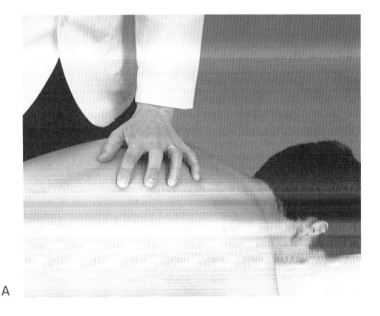

A

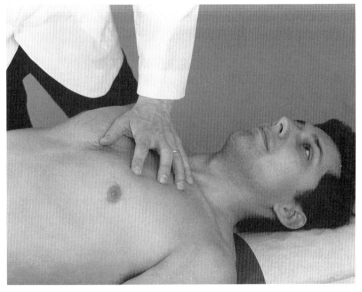

B

Figure 5.145 Palpation of respiratory movements of the rib cage in the (A) prone position and (B) supine position.

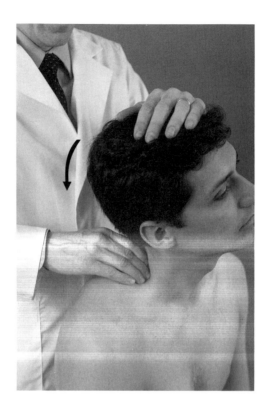

Figure 5.146 Palpation of the first rib using a fingertip contact over the superior aspect of the angle of the right first rib.

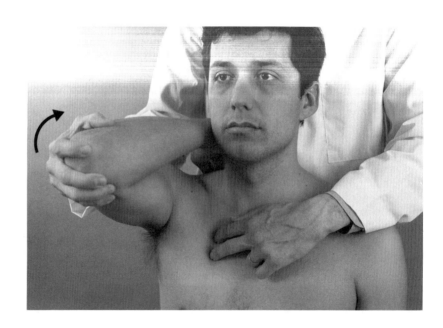

Figure 5.147 Palpation of right anterior rib mobility using a fingertip contact in the right anterior intercostal spaces.

Ribs 1 and 2. To evaluate mobility of the upper two ribs while the patient is in the sitting position, the doctor contacts the posterosuperior portion of the first or second rib with the fingertips. The indifferent hand grasps the crown of the patient's head, rotates it away from the side being palpated, and laterally flexes and extends it toward the side being palpated (Fig. 5-146). During this motion, the rib should fall away from the palpating finger and seem to disappear. Dysfunction should be suspected if the rib remains prominent and immobile during the passive movements of the head.

Anterior rib dysfunction. To evaluate movement of the costosternal joints and anterior intercostal spaces, place the patient in the sitting position and stand behind the patient while contacting the intercostal spaces just lateral to the sternum. Take care to avoid contact with the breasts in female patients. Flex the patient's elbow and shoulder on the side of palpation and grasp the elbow (Fig. 5-147). Move the patient's flexed arm into further flexion and palpate for opening of the intercostal spaces (i.e., the superior rib should move cranially in relation to the inferior rib).

ADJUSTMENTS OF THE THORACIC SPINE

Prone Adjustments

Prone thoracic adjustments are characteristically direct short level methods incorporating specific vertebral contacts (Fig. 5-148). They have the advantage of providing effective and specific access to points of contact while allowing for positions that maximize the incorporation of the doctor's body weight in directing and delivering adjustive thrusts. Although they are commonly delivered with the patient in a relatively neutral position, it is possible to modify prone positioning to induce positions that assist in the development of pre-adjustive tension. Elevation of the thoracolumbar section of an articulating table or dutchman roll may be used to develop segmental flexion, and the thoracolumbar section may be lowered to induce extension. Lateral flexion may be induced by bending the patient to the side or by side bending a flexion table. Rotation of the trunk is not practical on most adjusting tables, though some rotation may be induced with rotation of the pelvic section of flexion tables.

After the patient is appropriately positioned and the contacts are established but before thrusting, the doctor usually removes any remaining articular slack by transferring additional body weight into the contact. At tension the adjustive thrust may be generated solely through the arms but more frequently incorporates a combined body drop and arm thrust.

Knee Chest Adjustments

Knee chest adjustments are similar to prone thoracic adjustments (Fig. 5-149). In most cases the only difference is the modification in positioning the patient must undergo on the knee chest table. Knee chest adjustments may be applied to any region of the thoracic spine and for many of the same circumstances as prone thoracic adjustments. However, they are most

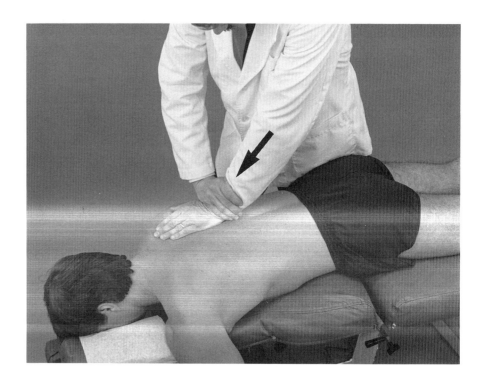

Figure 5.148 Prone unilateral hypothenar transverse adjustment.

effectively applied in the treatment of lower thoracic extension restrictions (flexion malpositions). The knee chest table does not restrict thoracolumbar extension and therefore allows the doctor to maximize movement into extension. This may be especially valuable in the large patient or in circumstances in which the doctor does not have access to an articulating table. While it does provide for maximal extension it also makes the patient vulnerable to hyperextension. Consequently the doctor must be skilled in this procedure and apply it only with shallow, gentle, non-recoil thrusts.

Sitting Adjustments

Sitting thoracic adjustments afford the doctor the opportunity to induce rotation and/or lateral flexion in the development of pre-adjustive tension (Fig. 5-150). They are typically applied as assisted adjustments with the adjustive contact established on the superior vertebra. The indifferent hand contacts the anterior forearm to assist in the development of appropriate trunk rotation. At tension both hands thrust to induce motion in the direction of restriction to induce distraction at the motion segment below the contacted vertebra. They are most commonly applied for rotational restrictions in the middle to lower thoracic spine but may be applied for lateral flexion restrictions or combined rotation and lateral flexion restrictions.

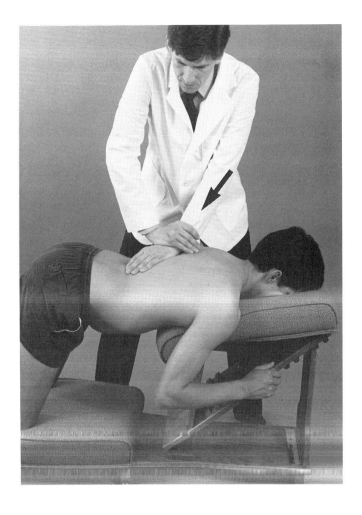

Figure 5.149 Knee chest hypothenar spinous adjustment.

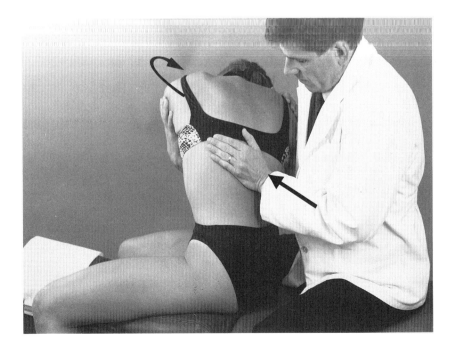

Figure 5.150 Sitting thoracic hypothenar transverse adjustment.

Supine Adjustments

The effectiveness of supine adjustive techniques is a controversial topic within chiropractic. A number of chiropractic colleges do not instruct their students in supine techniques, and a significant percentage of practicing chiropractors also object to their application. The basis for this position appears to be related to the contention that supine techniques are less specific and therefore less effective. Unfortunately this contention has led to a lack of investigation and understanding of the appropriate application of supine techniques. The authors feel supine techniques should not be dismissed out of hand. They can be effective if applied in the proper circumstances, and they should be considered for incorporation in the management of thoracic dysfunction.

One of the major distinctions between prone and supine adjustive techniques is the activity of the posterior spinal contact. In the supine techniques, the posterior contact is customarily passive, and in the prone techniques the contact hand is always involved in delivering an adjustive impulse. In the supine techniques, the posterior contact is a fulcrum point applied to help localize the site of pre-adjustive tension and distraction.

The adjustive impulse in supine technique is generated by thrusting with the weight of the doctor's torso, through the patient, toward the posterior contact (Fig. 5-151). Supine adjustive techniques also involve a strong component of axial traction in the development of pre-adjustive tension and in the delivery of an adjustive impulse. Long axis traction is effective in aiding in the distraction of the posterior joints and is necessary to avoid unnecessary compression to the patient's rib cage. Traction is developed by incorporating an inferior to superior orientation in the adjustive vector. This force is

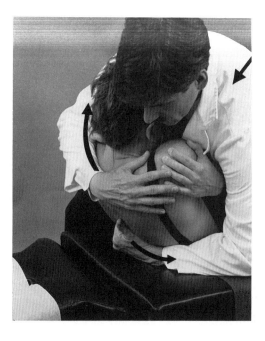

Figure 5.151 Supine thoracic adjustment using a clenched fist for the posterior contact.

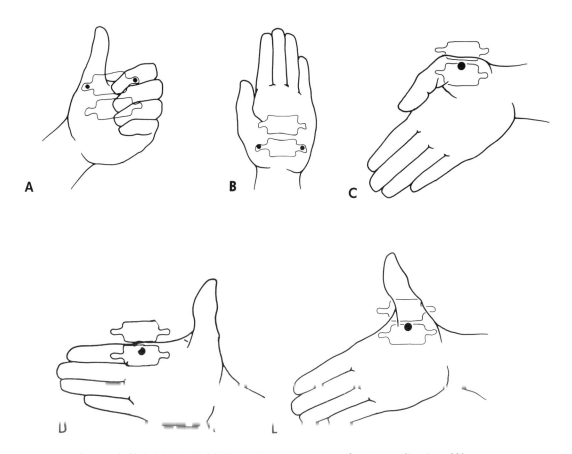

Figure 5-152 Optional hand positions for spinal column adjusting. **(A)** Clenched fist where the thenar and index contacts are established over the transverse processes of the superior or inferior vertebra for treatment of flexion restrictions and the inferior vertebra for treatment of extension restrictions. **(B)** Open palm where the thenar and hypothenar contacts are established over the transverse processes of the superior or inferior vertebra for treatment of flexion restrictions and the inferior vertebra for treatment of extension restrictions. **(C)** Open palm where the thenar contact is established against the inferior tip of the spinous process of the superior vertebra for treatment of flexion restrictions. **(D)** Open palm where the index contact is established against the inferior tip of the spinous process of the superior vertebra for treatment of flexion restrictions. **(E)** Open palm where the thenar contact is unilaterally established against the transverse process of the superior or inferior vertebra for treatment of rotational or lateral flexion dysfunction, this illustrates the contact for a right rotational restriction in the joint above the contact.

generated by the doctor using the upper body weight to traction headward by pushing off the back foot.

The positions of the posterior hand vary depending on the area of application and the dysfunction treated. The optional hand positions (Fig. 5-152) and the appropriate application of each are discussed under each specific adjustment. When applying a bilateral transverse contact, the spinous processes rest in the midline of the doctor's cupped hand or clenched fist as

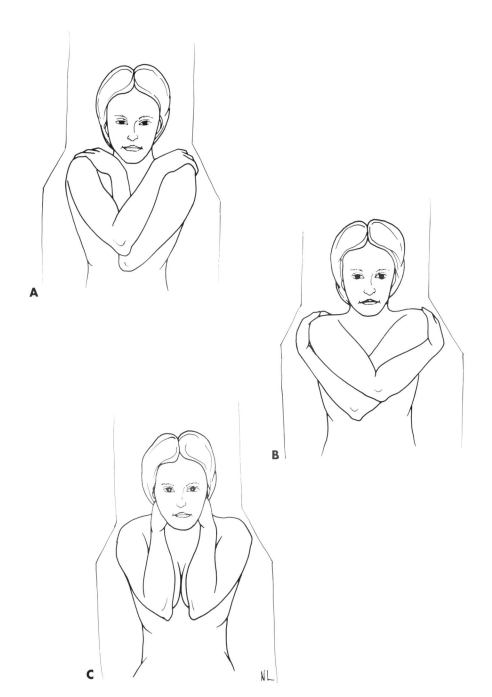

Figure 5.153 Optional patient arm positions in the supine thoracic adjustment: (**A**) right arm crossed over left; (**B**) crossed arm position to separate the scapula; (**C**) pump handle position.

the thenar and phalanxes contact each transverse process. Care must be taken to insure the contacts are established medial to the rib angles and equally balanced. When developing contacts in the lower thoracics it is important to place the hand in a more vertical position to bridge the distance between the table and the patient.

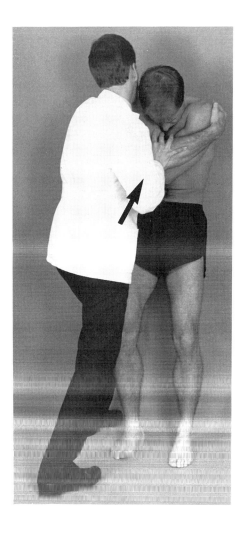

Figure 5-154 The standing thoracic adjustment.

Supine adjustive techniques also allow for a variety of optional patient arm placements (Fig. 5-153). The positioning of the patient's arms is mainly a matter of doctor discretion. However, when crossing the patient's arms across the chest it is important to consider both patient and doctor comfort. To reduce the stress to the patient's anterior chest or breasts, a small sternal role may be placed between the patient's crossed arms. To lessen the pressure against the doctor's upper abdomen or chest a rectangular pillow may be placed between the patient's crossed arms and the doctor. When utilizing crossed arm positions in large patients it is important to cross the arms in a manner that decreases the anterior to posterior diameter of the patient's thorax. Positions that cross the opposing forearm underneath the other (Fig. 5-153B) tend to decrease the distance from the patient's forearms to the table and have the possible advantage of being able to separate the scapula. Positions that interlace crossed arms (Fig. 5-153A) tend to increase the distance from the patient's forearms to the table and have the possible advantage of stabilizing the shoulder girdle.

Standing Adjustments

Standing thoracic adjustments employ the same mechanical principles as supine thoracic adjustments (Fig. 5-154). Most significantly, they provide positions that allow the doctor to develop maximal long axis traction when desired. This is accomplished by tractioning upward through the contacts as the patient's body weight is allowed to drop inferior. The superiorly directed adjustive force opposes the inferiorly directed pull of the patient's weight and develops distraction along the vertical axis of the spine. These positions may be difficult to perform in acute patients who can not withstand weightbearing.

Rotational Adjustments

Rotational dysfunction of the thoracic spine may result from decreased mobility in the posterior joints of the involved motion segment on one side or both sides. Fixation in the joint on the side of rotational restriction (side opposite posterior body rotation) leads to a loss of medial and inferior glide and gapping of the inferior facet relative to the superior facet of the vertebra below (Fig. 5-155). Fixation in the joint on the side opposite the rotational restriction (side of posterior body rotation) leads to a loss of lateral and superior glide of the inferior facet relative to the superior facet (Fig. 5-155). The side and site of fixation is assessed by comparing the end play quality of each side.

Rotational dysfunction leading to a loss of lateral and superior facetal glide may be treated with prone, supine, or sitting adjustive methods. In prone methods the patient is commonly treated with neutral patient postures. The contacts are established on the transverse process of the superior vertebra on the side of posterior body rotation (side opposite the rotation restriction) and the adjustive thrust is delivered anteriorly and superiorly to distract the joint below the contact (Fig. 5-156).

In the upper thoracic spine, resisted patient posture may be applied to induce medial glide and gapping on the side of rotational restriction. With resisted methods, the doctor contacts the inferior vertebra of the dysfunctional motion segment. When applying transverse process contacts, the contacts are established on the side of rotational restriction and when applying contacts on the spinous processes the contacts are established on the side opposite the rotational restriction. The cervical spine is slightly laterally flexed away and rotated toward the side of restriction to induce motion in the direction of restriction as the inferior vertebral contact applies counter pressure (Fig. 5-157). At tension the adjustive thrust is delivered anteriorly and inferiorly with the contact hand to distract the joint above the contact. For example, if the doctor is treating a restriction in left rotation at the T1–T2 motion segment with a resisted approach, the contact is established on the left transverse process of T2 or the right lateral surface of the T2 spinous. The superior segments and head are counter rotated into left rotation, and maximal tension should be generated in the motion segment ipsilateral and superior to the point of adjustive contact (T2) (Fig. 5-157).

When applying sitting, supine, or standing positions to effect rotation

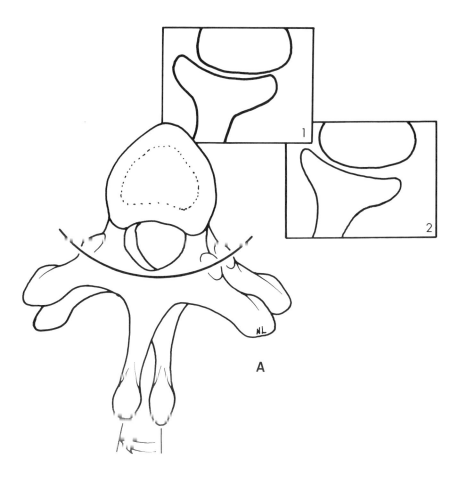

A

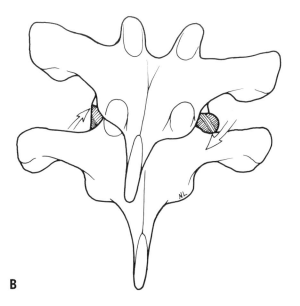

B

Figure 5.155 (**A**) Transverse view of right rotation at T5–T6 showing lateral glide of the left T5 inferior articular surface relative to the T6 articular surface in box 1 and medial glide with end play gapping of the right T5 articular surface relative to T6 in box 2. (**B**) Coronal view illustrating the coupled right lateral flexion associated with right rotation at T5–T6 with superior glide of the left T5 articular surface relative to T6 and inferior glide of the right T5 articular surface relative to T6.

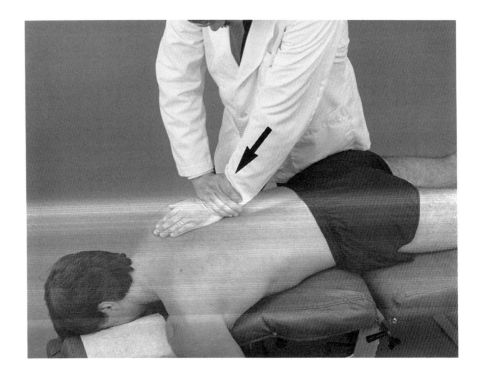

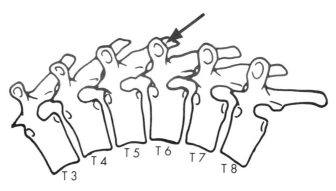

Figure 5.156 Hypothenar transverse contact applied to left transverse process of T6 to induce left rotation and/or left lateral flexion of the right T6–T7 articulation.

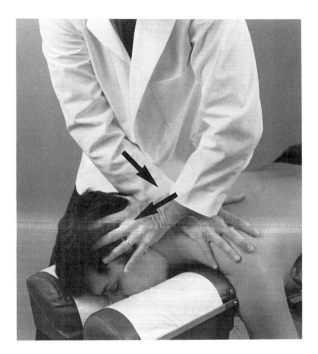

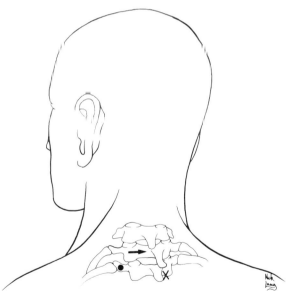

Figure 5.157 Resisted method: hypothenar contact applied to the left transverse process of T2 (dot) or right spinous process of T2 (X) resisted by counter rotation and lateral flexion of the segments above. Depicted is a procedure for treatment of a left rotation restriction at T1–T2 with distraction of the left T1–T2 articulation. Arrows indicate the direction of adjustive and distractive forces.

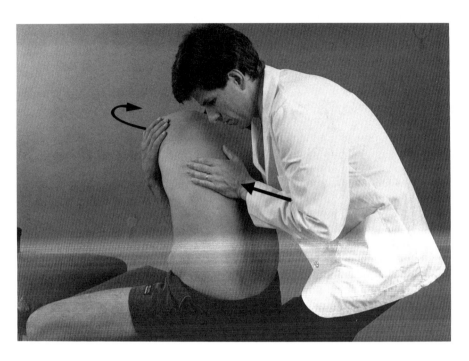

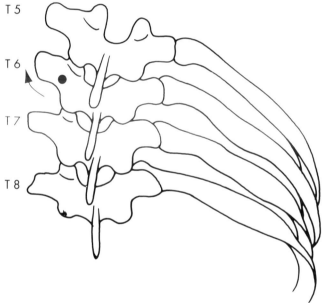

Figure 5.158 Unilateral hypothenar contact applied to the left T6 transverse process (dot) to induce right rotation and/or right lateral flexion with superior glide in the left T6–T7 articulation.

and superior glide it is customary to use assisted methods to aid in the development of trunk rotation. In all assisted methods the adjustive contact is established on the superior vertebra and the thrust is directed to induce distraction in the joint below the contact (Fig. 5-158). In the supine position this necessitates that the doctor maintain the patient in a position of segmental flexion to insure that superior distraction is applied to the joint (Fig. 5-159).

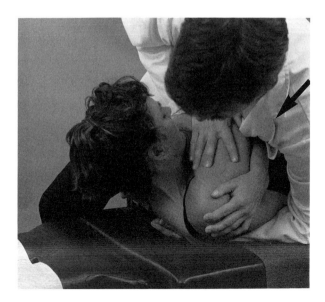

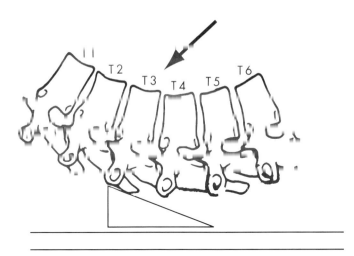

Figure 5.159 Unilateral thenar contact applied in the
right transverse process of
T3 to induce left rotation
and/or left lateral flexion
with superior glide of the
right T3–T4 articulation.
Wedge illustrates the placement of hand and thenar,
and arrow illustrates the direction of adjustive vector
through the doctor's trunk.

Rotational restrictions in the mid and lower thoracic segments leading to restrictions in medial and inferior glide and gapping are commonly treated with neutral or resisted methods. The neutral method is applied in the prone position with the doctor establishing contacts on the side of rotational restriction (side opposite posterior body rotation). The contacts may be established on the spinous process of the superior vertebra or the transverse process of the inferior vertebra. When contacting the spinous process the adjustive thrust is delivered anteriorly and medially to induce rotation in the joint below the contact and distraction in the articulation above (Fig. 5-160). With a transverse process contact, the thrust is delivered anteriorly and inferiorly to induce gapping in the joint above the contact (Fig. 5-161). When applying transverse contacts for rotational dysfunction it is probably more effective to use bilateral contacts on adjacent vertebral segments as

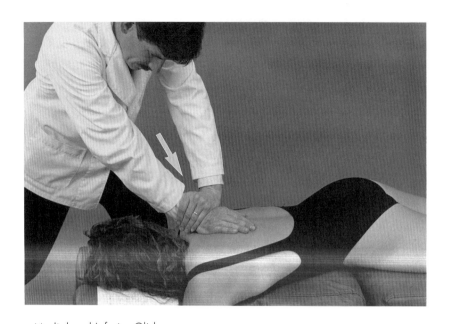

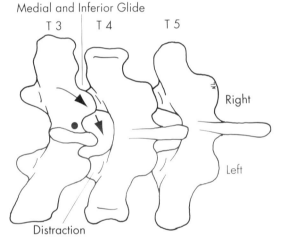

Figure 5.160 Unilateral hypothenar contact applied to the right lateral surface of the T3 spinous process (dot) to induce right rotation and/or right lateral flexion in the T3–T4 articulation. The forces of this adjustment (arrows) are applied to induce inferior medial glide in the right T3–T4 articulation and distraction in the right T2–T3 articulation above the contact.

compared to unilateral contacts (Fig. 5-162). With bilateral contacts the doctor has the option of making one hand a passive counter stabilizer or of counter thrusting through both hands. This should help isolate the adjustive forces to the site of fixation and reduce tension to adjacent joints, which may not be fixated.

Restrictions in rotation and decreased medial glide and gapping may also be treated in the supine position with resisted adjustive methods. In supine methods the doctor establishes a thenar contact on the inferior vertebra of the involved motion segment on the side of fixation and rotates the patient's shoulders toward the side of contact (Fig. 5-163). The contact provides a block to movement and a fulcrum point to localize rotational tension to the joint above the contact. The adjustive thrust is directed posteriorly through the doctor's trunk to induce rotation and gapping in the direction of trunk rotation at the segment above the contact.

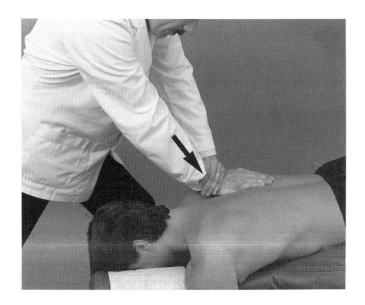

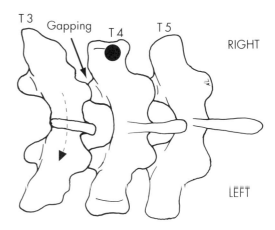

Figure 5.161 Unilateral hypothenar contact applied to the right transverse process of T4 (dot) to induce gapping in the right T3–T4 articulation and right rotation of T3 relative to T4. The adjustive force (solid arrow) is directed posterior to anterior and inferior. Broken arrow illustrates movement of T3 relative to T4.

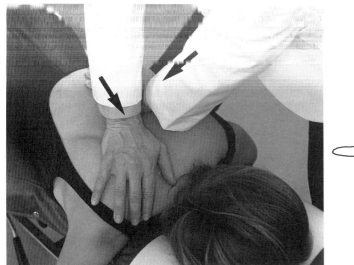

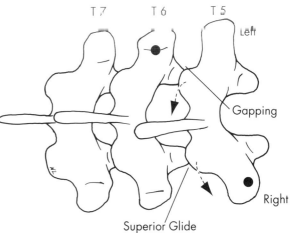

Figure 5.162 Bilateral contacts applied to the T5–T6 motion segment to induce left rotation. The left hypothenar contact is established over the left transverse process of T6 (dot) to induce gapping at the left T5–T6 articulation, and the right thenar contact is established over the right transverse process of T5 to induce superior glide of the right T5–T6 articulation. Solid arrows indicate direction of adjustive force and broken arrows direction of motion of T5 relative to T6.

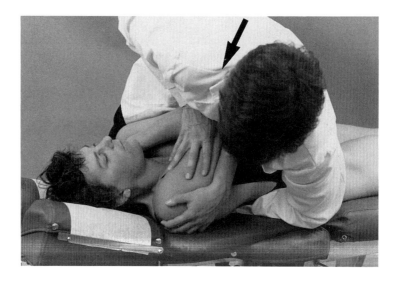

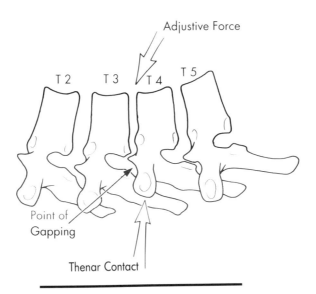

Figure 5.163 Unilateral hypothenar contact applied to the right transverse process of T4 to induce right rotation and gapping in the right T3–T4 articulation.

Lateral Flexion Adjustments

Lateral flexion dysfunction in the thoracic spine may result from a loss of inferior glide of the facet on the side of lateral flexion dysfunction (open wedge side) and/or contralateral superior glide on the side opposite the lateral flexion restriction (closed wedge side) (Fig. 5-164).

Lateral flexion dysfunction may be treated with prone, supine, standing, side posture, or sitting methods. In prone or sitting positions, the contacts are established on the transverse processes or spinous processes. When treating lateral flexion restrictions resulting in decreased superior glide, the doctor establishes a unilateral transverse process contact on the superior vertebra on the side opposite the lateral flexion restriction (close wedge

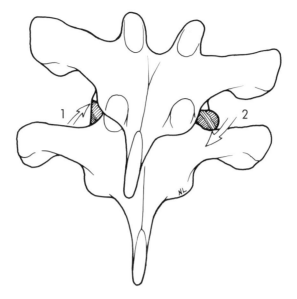

Figure 5.164 Coronal view of right lateral flexion showing (**1**) superior glide of the left T5 articular surface and (**2**) inferior glide of the right T5 articular surface relative to T6.

side) and thrusts anteriorly and superiorly to distract the joint below the contact (Fig. 5-156). When employing spinous contacts in the prone or side posture position the doctor establishes the contacts on the side of open wedging (side of lateral flexion restriction) (Figs. 5-160 and 5-165). The thrust is delivered anteriorly and medially toward the midline to induce inferior glide and closure of the facets and disc on the side of lateral flexion restriction.

Lateral flexion dysfunction may also be treated in the prone position with bilateral transverse contacts. Bilateral contacts may increase the doctor's mechanical advantage and help in the development of tension and movement in both facet joints. When applying this method the contacts are established on each side of the superior vertebra. The contact hand on the side of lateral flexion restriction (open wedge) drives anteriorly and inferiorly to induce inferior glide while the other drives anteriorly and superiorly to induce superior glide (Fig. 5-166).

In prone upper thoracic spine adjusting, the doctor may choose to employ a resisted method. With resisted methods the contact is established on the lower thoracic segment, and pre-adjustive tension is developed by tractioning the cervical segments away from the side of contact (Fig. 5-157). At tension an adjustive thrust is directed anteriorly and inferiorly with the contact hand as counter tension is directed through the indifferent contact. This method is designed to separate and distract the joint above the segmental contact point.

If lateral flexion dysfunction is treated in the sitting, standing, or supine positions, assisted patient positions are commonly employed. The contacts are established on the transverse process of the superior vertebra on the side opposite the lateral flexion restriction (closed wedge side) and the patient is laterally flexed in the direction of restriction. In the sitting position,

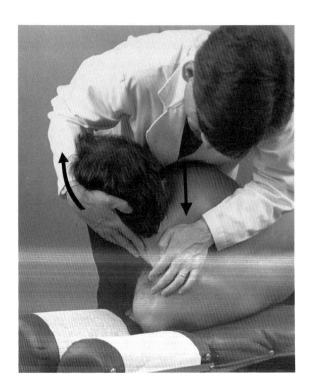

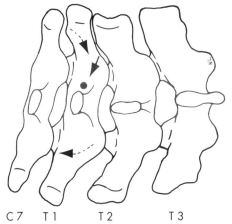

Figure 5.165 Unilateral hypothenar contact applied to the right lateral surface of the T1 spinous process (dot) to induce right lateral flexion with inferior glide of the right T1–T2 articulation and superior glide of the left T1–T2 articulation. Solid arrow indicates the direction of adjustive force, and broken arrow the direction of vertebral movement.

C 7   T 1   T 2   T 3

the thrust is directed anteriorly and superiorly (Fig. 5-158); in the supine and standing positions the thrust is directed through the trunk posteriorly and superiorly. In the supine and standing positions the patient must be maintained in a flexed position to assist in the distraction and superior glide of the involved joint (Fig. 5-159).

Flexion and Extension Adjustments

Flexion and extension dysfunction may be treated with prone, knee chest, supine, or standing patient positions. Flexion restrictions produce a loss of separation and distraction in the posterior joints while extension restrictions

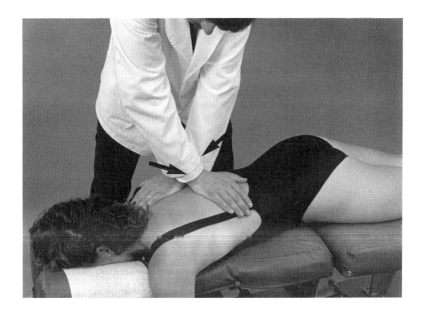

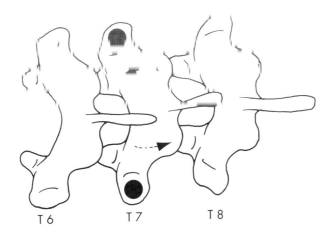

Figure 5.166 Bilateral thenar contacts applied to the transverse processes of T7 (dots) to induce left lateral flexion with superior glide of the left T7–T8 articulation and inferior glide of the right T7–T8 articulation.

T 6   T 7   T 8

produce a loss of inferior glide and approximation in the posterior joints (Fig. 5-167). To induce flexion in the prone and knee chest positions the doctor commonly establishes contacts against the spinous process or transverse process of the superior vertebra and directs the adjustive vector anteriorly and superiorly to induce separation of the joint below the contact (Fig. 5-168). In the upper or lower thoracic spine, where superior vertebral contacts may be hard to maintain, the doctor may contact the inferior vertebra of the involved motion segment. With this method the doctor faces

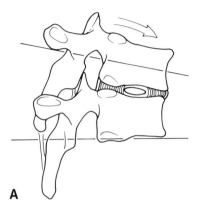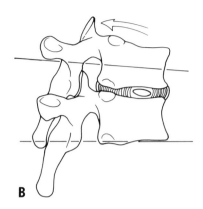

Figure 5.167 Sagittal view of the middle thoracic segments in (**A**) flexion with separation and superior glide of the inferior facet relative to the superior facet below and (**B**) extension with approximation and inferior glide of the inferior facet relative to the superior facet below.

caudally and the adjustive thrust is directed anteriorly and inferiorly to induce separation superior to the contact (a modification for flexion using bilateral knife-edge contacts is shown in Fig. 5-169).

Supine or standing adjustive postures may be especially effective in the treatment of flexion restrictions. Both methods induce long axis traction, which is helpful in the induction of joint separation. The adjustive contacts are established on either the superior or inferior vertebra of the involved motion segment while the patient is maintained in a position of segmental flexion. Superior vertebral contacts are designed to distract the motion segment inferior to the level of the contact hand (Fig. 5-170). Inferior vertebral contacts are designed to distract the motion segment superior to the level of contact. With superior vertebral contacts the doctor tractions headward against the contact to distract the contacted vertebra away from the vertebra below. With inferior vertebral contacts the doctor directs the tissue pull caudally to block movement of the inferior vertebra and induce

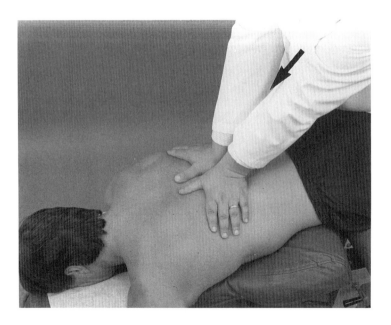

Figure 5.168 Bilateral thenar contacts applied to induce flexion of T7–T8 and superior glide of the T7 facets relative to T8.

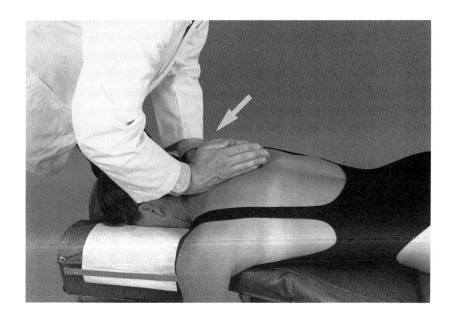

Figure 5.169 Bilateral knife-edge contacts applied to the T3 transverse processes to extend the T3–T4 articulation.

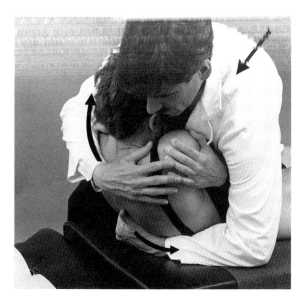

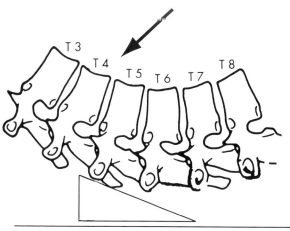

Figure 5.170 Bilateral contacts established on the transverse processes of T5 to induce flexion at the T5–T6 motion segment.

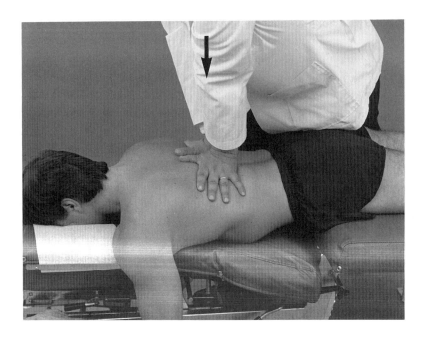

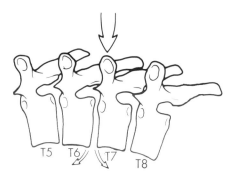

Figure 5.171 Bilateral thenar contacts applied over
the T7 transverse processes
to induce extension at
T7–T8.

separation at the motion segment above the contact. To develop pre-
adjustive tension, the doctor applies headward and posterior pressure
through the patient's trunk. At tension the adjustive thrust is delivered
posteriorly and superiorly through the doctor's torso toward the site of
contact (Fig. 5-170).

To induce extension in the prone or knee chest positions, the doctor
establishes contacts over the transverse process of the superior vertebra.
The doctor's center of gravity is commonly positioned over the contacts
with the adjustive vector directed anteriorly to induce extension at the joint
below the contacts (Fig. 5-171). In the upper or lower thoracics the doctor
may face caudally and direct the vector slightly inferiorly to assist in the
development of tension and extension.

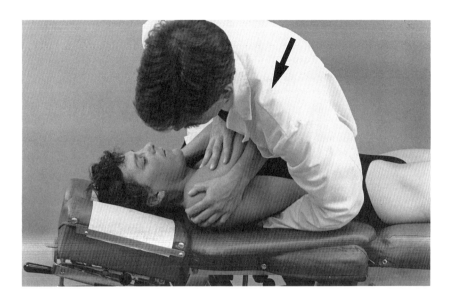

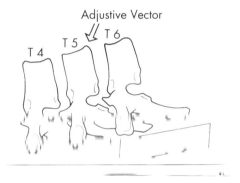

Adjustive Vector

Figure 5.172 Bilateral contacts applied to the left transverse processes of T6 to in
duce distraction of the T5-T6
Block indicates placement
of hand under T6.

In the supine or standing patient positions, the contact is established on the inferior vertebra. The joint to be adjusted is bent into extension over the top of the posterior contact and the doctor thrusts posteriorly using body weight to induce distraction in the joint above the contact (Fig. 5-172). This adjustment should also incorporate long axis distraction to help decompress the joint. Straight posterior to anterior thrusts unnecessarily compress the rib cage and are to be avoided.

ADJUSTMENTS OF THE RIBS

Prone Rib Adjustments

Prone rib adjustments are usually direct short lever or combine short and long lever methods incorporating specific but broader contacts. They are delivered with the patient in a relatively neutral position; the doctor's body weight is used in the development of pre-adjustive tension. Broader contacts are used so that the thrust does not focus the force of the adjustment over a small area of the rib. The rib is more fragile than the vertebral contact points and is therefore more easily fractured.

Sitting Rib Adjustments

Sitting rib adjustments, like sitting thoracic adjustments, afford the doctor the opportunity to induce rotation and/or lateral flexion in the development of pre-adjustive tension. The adjustive contacts are established on the rib angle just lateral to the transverse process and are applied as assisted adjustments. The indifferent hand contacts the anterior forearm to assist in the development of appropriate trunk rotation. At tension, the contact hand induces distraction at the costotransverse articulation vertebra.

Supine Rib Adjustments

Supine rib adjustments can be effective if applied in the proper circumstances; they should be considered for incorporation in the management of dysfunction of the costotransverse and costovertebral articulations. The adjustive impulse in supine rib techniques is generated by thrusting with the weight of the doctor's torso, through the patient, toward the posterior contact. The positions of the contact hand vary depending on the area of application, though a thenar contact is commonly used as it is fleshy enough not to cause pain and broad enough to distribute the force along the rib. The positioning of the patient's arms is mainly a matter of doctor discretion and patient comfort.

Gapping and/or Translational Adjustments

Gapping (joint separation, perpendicular distraction) and/or translation (joint surface gliding) may be produced using the prone, sitting, or supine patient positions. A loss of separation and distraction in the costotransverse articulations produce pain and a loss of pump handle and bucket handle movements. To induce gapping in the prone position, the doctor establishes a contact over the posterior aspect of the rib angle just lateral to the transverse process. The adjustive vector is directed posterior to anterior and medial to lateral to induce separation of the costotransverse joint. An inferior to superior vector is added when the doctor assumes a fencer's stance facing cephalad, and a superior to inferior vector is added when the doctor assumes a fencer's stance facing caudad. Translational movement is induced with a thrust using a vector of posterior to anterior and lateral to medial.

The supine position may also be used to induce separation and/or translation at the costotransverse articulations while producing pump handle movement. The adjustive contacts are established on the posterior aspect of the rib angle just lateral to the transverse process with the patient maintained in a position of flexion. To develop pre-adjustive tension, the doctor applies headward and posterior pressure through the patient's trunk. At tension the adjustive thrust is delivered posteriorly and superiorly through the doctor's torso toward the site of contact.

With the sitting position, a gapping joint separation is produced using an assisted method. A contact is established over the posterior aspect of the rib angle and the patient is rotated forward on the side of contact. The thrust is applied in a posterior to anterior and medial to lateral direction.

Bucket Handle Adjustments

The side posture position is most effectively used for inducing bucket handle movements. The patient lies over a roll to develop preadjustive tension and a contact is applied in the intercostal space against the superior or inferior aspect of the rib in the midaxillary line. With the doctor facing cephalad the contacted rib will be elevated. With the doctor facing caudal the rib will be depressed.

Prone Thoracocervical Adjustments

Thumb spinous (Fig. 5-173)

IND: Restricted rotation and/or lateral flexion, C6–T3. Rotation, lateral flexion, or combined rotation and lateral flexion malpositions, C6–T3.

 PP: The patient lies prone with the headpiece lowered below horizontal to produce slight flexion in the thoracocervical spine.

 DP: Stand in a low fencer stance on either side of the patient facing cephalad. The forward leg approximates the level of the patient's head and your body weight is centered over the midline of the patient.

 CP: Distal palmar surface of the thumb. The thumb is partially abducted and locked with the fingers resting on the patient's trapezius. When standing on the side of adjustive contact your caudal hand establishes the contact (Fig. 5-173A). A fleshy hypothenar contact may be substituted for the thumb contact (Fig. 5-173B). When standing on the side opposite the adjustive contact the cephalic hand establishes the contact.

SCP: Lateral surface of the spinous process

 IH: The indifferent hand supports the upper cervical spine as the fingers contact the inferior occiput

VEC: Lateral to medial with slight posterior to anterior angulation to maintain the segmental contact.

  P: Lightly establish contacts and develop pre-adjustive tension. Deliver an impulse thrust through the contact and the indifferent hands. The impulse generated through the indifferent hand is shallow; take care not to excessively rotate or laterally flex the cervical spine.

Rotation. Thoracocervical rotational dysfunction may be treated with neutral or resisted patient positions.

When applying neutral positions establish the contact on the superior spinous process on the side of rotational restriction (side of spinous rotation) (Fig. 5-173A). Rotate and laterally flex the patient's head toward the side of contact. Cervical rotation is minimized to insure neutral positioning of the thoraco-cervical spine. The thrust is delivered primarily through the contact hand while the indifferent hand produces only modest cephalic distraction.

When employing a resisted method establish the contact on the inferior spinous process on the side opposite the rotational restriction (side opposite the spinous rotation) (Fig. 5-173B). Develop pre-adjustive tension by rotating the patient's head away from and laterally flexing it toward the side of

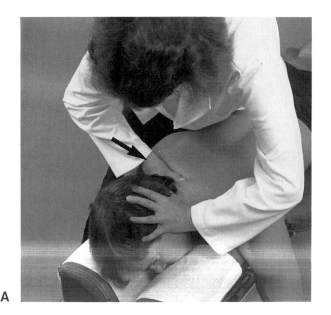

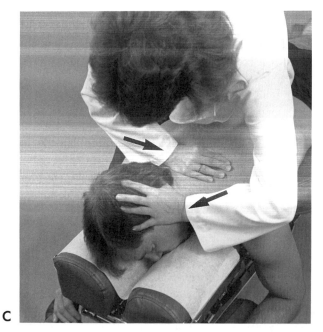

Figure 5.173 **(A)** Neutral method with thumb contact applied to the right lateral aspect of the T2 spinous process to induce right rotation and medial glide of the right T2–T3 articulation. **(B)** Resisted method with a hypothenar contact applied to the right lateral surface of the T3 spinous process to induce left rotation and gapping of the left T2–T3 articulation. **(C)** Hypothenar contact applied to the right lateral surface of the T2 spinous process to induce right lateral flexion with superior glide of the left T2–T3 articulation.

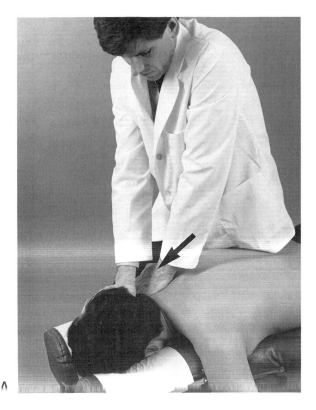
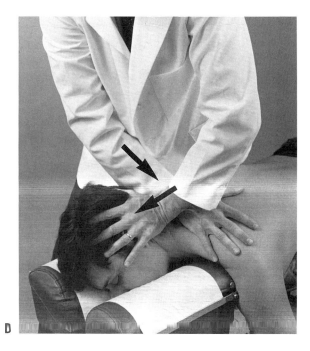

Figure 5.174 **(A)** Neutral position with hypothenar contact applied to the right T1 transverse process to induce left lateral flexion and/or right rotation with superior glide of the right T1–T2 articulation. **(B)** Resisted method with hypothenar contact applied to the left T2 transverse process to induce left rotation and/or right lateral flexion with gapping in the left T1–T2 articulation.

adjustive contact. At tension deliver an impulse counter thrust toward the midline through both hands.

Lateral flexion. When addressing lateral flexion dysfunction, assisted patient positions are usually employed. The contact is established on the superior vertebra on the side of lateral flexion restriction (side of open wedge) (Fig. 5-173C). Pre-adjustive tension is developed by laterally flexing the patient's head toward the side of contact while inducing minimal rotation away. At tension an impulse thrust is generated medially through the contact hand while the stabilization hand applies a thrust cephalically.

Hypothenar transverse (combination move and modified combination move) (Fig. 5-174)

IND: Restricted rotation and/or lateral flexion of C7–T4. Rotation, lateral flexion, or combined rotation and lateral flexion malpositions, C7–T4.

PP: The patient lies prone with the headpiece lowered below horizontal to produce slight flexion in the thoraco-cervical spine.

DP: Stand in a fencer stance on either side of the patient facing cephalad. Your forward leg approximates the level of the patient's head and your upper body weight should be centered over the contact.

CP: Hypothenar (pisiform) of arched hand. When standing on the side of adjustive contact (combination move) the caudal hand establishes the vertebral contact (Fig. 5-174A). When standing on the side opposite the adjustive contact (modified combination move) the cephalic hand establishes the vertebral contact (Fig. 5-174B).

SCP: Transverse process.

IH: The indifferent hand supports the upper cervical spine as the fingers contact the inferior occiput.

VEC: Posterior to anterior and inferior to superior with same side contacts (Fig. 5-174A). Posterior to anterior and superior to inferior with opposite side contacts (Fig. 5-174B).

P: Lightly establish the contacts, gently rotate and traction the patient's head away from the side of contact. At tension deliver an impulse thrust through the contact and indifferent hands. The impulse imparted through the indifferent hand is shallow; take care not to excessively rotate or lateral flex the cervical spine. The impulse is typically assisted by a body drop thrust.

Rotation. Rotational dysfunction may be treated with neutral or resisted patient positions.

With neutral patient positions the doctor typically stands on the side of adjustive contact (Fig. 5-174A). Establish the segmental contact on the superior vertebra of the dysfunctional motion segment on the side of posterior body rotation (side opposite the rotational restriction). Develop preadjustive tension by leaning anteriorly and superiorly with the weight of your torso as the indifferent hand induces lateral flexion and rotation away from the contact. Deliver the thrust anteriorly and superiorly to distract the joint below the contact.

With resisted methods the doctor typically stands on the side opposite the adjustive contact and establishes a contact on the inferior vertebra on the side opposite the posterior body rotation (Fig. 5-174B). Develop preadjustive tension by rotating the patient's head in the direction of restriction as you apply counter pressure against the transverse process contact. At tension both arms counter thrust to induce distraction of the articulation ipsilateral and superior to the contact.

Lateral flexion. Lateral flexion dysfunction may be treated with assisted or resisted methods. In both methods axial rotation is minimized and lateral flexion and gliding distraction is stressed. In the assisted method the doctor typically stands on the side of adjustive contact, establishes a contact on the superior vertebra, and thrusts anteriorly and superiorly (Fig. 5-174A).

In the resisted method the doctor typically stands on the side opposite the adjustive contact, establishes a contact on the inferior vertebra, and thrusts anteriorly and inferiorly in a direction that opposes the thrust generated with the indifferent hand (Fig. 5-174B).

Bilateral thenar transverse (Fig. 5-175)

IND: Restricted flexion or extension of T1–T4. Flexion or extension mal-positions, T1–T4.

PP: The patient lies prone with the headpiece lowered below horizontal for flexion restrictions and neutral for extension restrictions.

DP: Stand at the head of the table facing caudad.

CP: Bilateral thenar contacts running parallel to the spine. (Bilateral knife-edge contacts can also be used.)

SCP: Transverse processes of superior vertebra.

VEC: Posterior to anterior and superior to inferior for extension restrictions (Fig. 5-175A). Posterior to anterior and superior to inferior for flexion restrictions (Fig. 5-175B).

P: Establish hypothenar contacts and develop joint tension by transfer-ring additional body weight into the contacts. For flexion restrictions remove superficial tissue slack by developing an inferior to superior tissue pull. For extension restrictions, a superior to inferior tissue pull is applied. At tension deliver an impulse thrust with a combined thrust through the arms and body.

Hypothenar spinous occiput (Fig. 5-176)

IND: Flexion restrictions or extension malpositions of C7–T4.

PP: The patient lies prone with the headpiece lowered below horizontal to induce thorco-cervical flexion.

DP: Stand in a fencer stance on either side of patient facing headword.

CP: Mid hypothenar of cephalic hand.

SCP: Inferior tip of spinous.

IH: The palm of the indifferent hand cups the base of the occiput while the wrist reinforces the dorsal surface of the contact hand.

VEC: Posterior to anterior and inferior to superior.

P: Establish the adjustive contact by sliding the hypothenar superiorly onto the inferior tip of the spinous. Establish an occipital contact with the indifferent hand and apply cephalic traction. At tension deliver an impulse thrust through the arms, trunk, and body. This adjustment has inferior to superior vector, making it necessary to orient your center of gravity inferior to the established contact points.

Sitting Thoraco-Cervical

Thumb spinous—sitting (Fig. 5-177)

IND: Restricted rotation and/or lateral flexion of C6–T3. Rotation, lateral flexion, or combined rotation and lateral flexion malpositions, C6–T3.

PP: The patient sits, relaxed in a cervical chair.

DP: Stand behind the patient slightly toward the side of spinous contact.

CP: Thumb of contact hand with palm rotated down.

SCP: Lateral surface of the spinous process.

IH: The contralateral hand contacts the top of the patient's head while the forearm supports the lateral head and face.

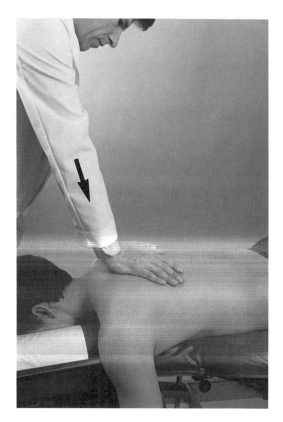

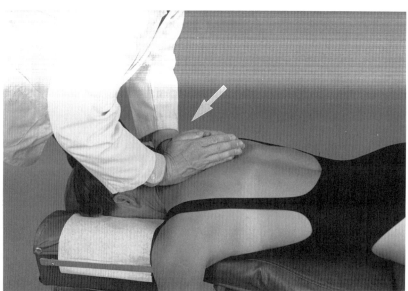

Figure 5.175 Bilateral (A) thenar and (B) knife-edge contacts applied to the T3 transverse processes to extend the T3–T4 articulation.

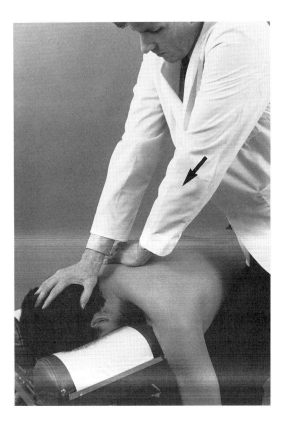

Figure 5.176 Hypothenar contact applied to the spinous process of T2 to induce flexion of the T2–T3 articulation.

VEC: Lateral to medial.
P. Establish the contacts and circumduct the patient's head toward the side of spinous contact. At tension deliver an impulse thrust lateral to medial through the contact hand.

Rotation. Rotational dysfunction may be treated with either assisted or resisted methods.

When treating rotational restrictions with an assisted method contact the superior spinous on the side of rotational restriction (side opposite body rotation) and rotate the patient's head in the direction of restriction (Fig. 5-177A). Generate the adjustive thrust by thrusting toward the midline primarily with the contact arm.

When employing a resisted method contact the inferior spinous process on the side opposite the rotational restricition (side of body rotation of superior segment). Rotate the head and segments above in the direction of restriction. At tension deliver an impulse thrust by thrusting toward the midline through both arms. The greater proportion of the adjustive force is delivered by the contact arm.

Lateral flexion. When treating lateral flexion dysfunction establish the contact on the superior vertebra on the side of lateral flexion restriction (side of open wedge). The patient's neck is laterally flexed in the direction of

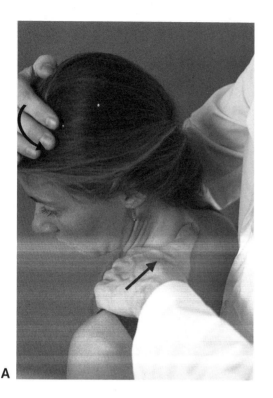
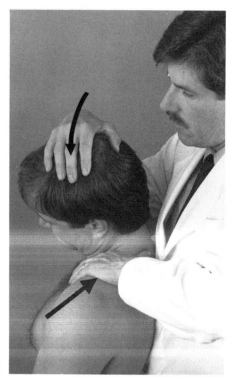

A   **B**

Figure 5.177 **(A)** Assisted method with a thumb contact applied to the left side of the spinous process of T1 to induce left rotation of T1–T2 and medial glide of the left T1–T2 articulation. **(B)** A thumb contact applied to the left side of the spinous process of T1 to induce left lateral flexion of T1–T2 and superior glide of the right T1–T2 articulation and inferior glide of the left T1–T2 articulation.

restriction. At tension direct an impulse thrust toward the midline through the contact arm. The contact thrust is reinforced by a shallow distractive force delivered with the indifferent hand (Fig. 5-177B).

Side Posture Thoraco-Cervical Adjustments

Thumb spinous—side posture (Fig. 5-178)

IND: Restricted rotation and/or lateral flexion of C6–T3. Rotation, lateral flexion, or combined rotation and lateral flexion malpositions, C6–T3.

  PP: Place the patient in side posture with the spine in a neutral position and the patient's head supported in your cephalic hand.

  DP: Stand in front of the patient in a square stance.

  CP: Thumb or thenar of caudal hand.

SCP: Lateral surface of the spinous process.

  IH: The cephalic hand and forearm cradle the patient's cervical spine and head.

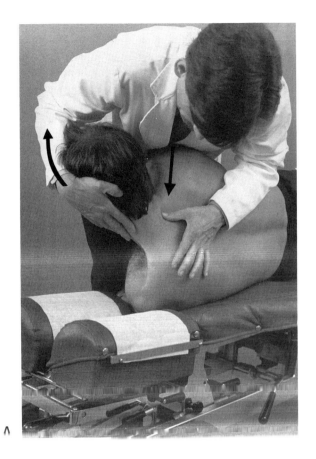

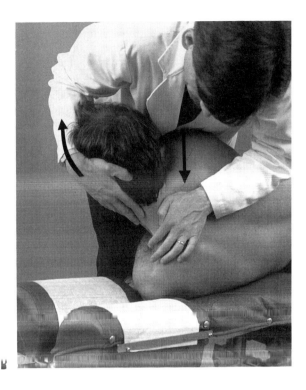

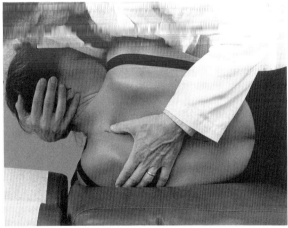

Figure 5.178 (**A**) Thumb or (**B**) thenar contact applied to the right lateral aspect of the C7 spinous process to induce right lateral flexion and superior glide of the left C7–T1 articulation and inferior glide of the right C7–T1 articulation. (**C**) Thumb contact applied to the right lateral aspect of the T1 spinous process to induce right rotation of the T1–T2 motion segment.

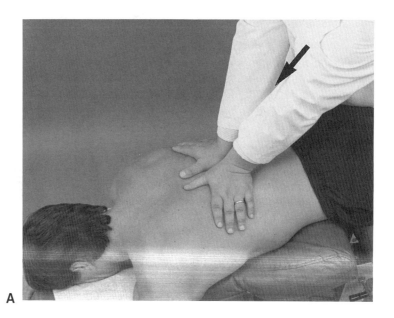

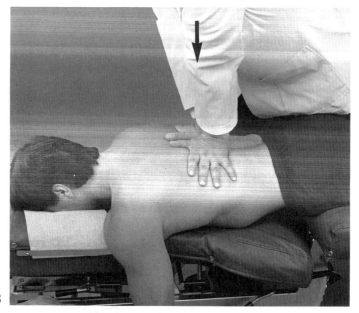

Figure 5.179 Bilateral thenar contacts applied to the T8 transverse processes to induce (**A**) flexion and (**B**) extension of the T8–T9 articulation. (*Figure continues.*)

VEC: Lateral to medial.

   P: Stand in front of the patient and lean over to establish the indifferent and segmental contacts. The contacts must be soft and fleshy or they become uncomfortable to the patient. At tension, deliver an impulse thrust lateral to medial through the contact hand.

Lateral flexion. When treating lateral flexion dysfunction establish the contact on the superior vertebra on the side of lateral flexion restriction (side of open wedge). The patient's neck is laterally flexed in the direction of

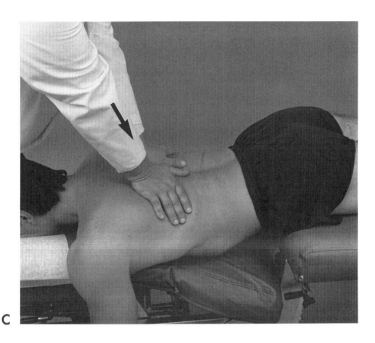

C

Figure 5.179 (*Continued*).
(**C**) Alternate method to create extension facing caudal.

restriction (assisted method). At tension direct an impulse thrust toward the midline through the contact arm. The contact thrust is reinforced by a shallow distractive force delivered with the indifferent hand (A,B).

Rotation. Rotational dysfunction is also treated with assisted methods. Contact the spinous on the side of deviation (side of rotational restriction) and rotate and the patient's head in the direction of restriction. At tension an impulse thrust is directed toward the midline. The contact thrust is reinforced by a shallow rotational pull through the indifferent hand.

Prone Thoracic Adjustments

Bilateral thenar transverse (Fig. 5-179)

IND: Restricted flexion, extension, lateral flexion, or rotation of T4–T12. Flexion, extension, lateral flexion, or rotation malpositions, T4–T12.

 PP: The patient lies prone. To provide added flexion a small roll may be placed under the patient's chest. To provide added extension the thoracic piece may be lowered anteriorly.

 DP: Fencer stance on either side of patient facing headward.

 CP: Bilateral thenar contacts parallel to the spine with fingers fanned and running medial to lateral.

SCP: Transverse processes.

VEC: Posterior to anterior and inferior to superior to induce flexion, lateral flexion, or rotation (Fig. 5-179A). Posterior to anterior to induce extension or rotation. (Fig. 5-179B).

  P: Establish bilateral thenar contacts and develop joint tension by transferring additional body weight into the contacts while tractioning the superficial tissue in the direction of the adjustive vector. When employing a vector that is predominantly posterior to anterior the doctor may use either an inferior to superior or superior to inferior tissue pull. The choice is dependent on the region adjusted and the doctor's preference. At tension an impulse thrust is delivered through the arms, trunk and body. Caution must be observed during the delivery of the thrust to avoid excessive force to the rib cage. This is especially true when delivering straight posterior to anterior thrusts.

Flexion. To induce flexion establish the contacts on the superior vertebra and deliver the thrust anteriorly and superiorly through both contacts (Fig. 5-179A).

Extension. To induce extension establish the contacts on the superior vertebra and deliver the thrust anteriorly through both contacts (Fig. 5-179B,C).

Lateral flexion. To induce lateral flexion establish bilateral contacts on the superior vertebra but deliver the adjustive thrust unilaterally. The thrust

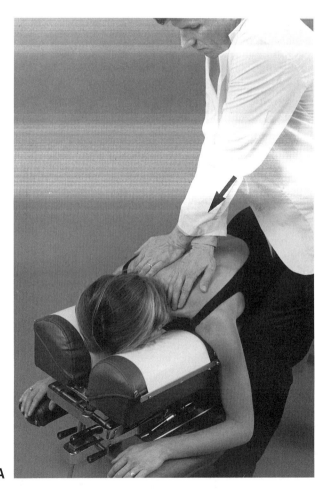

Figure 5.180 Crossed bilateral hypothenar (pisiform) contacts applied to **(A)** the transverse processes of T6 to induce flexion at T6–T7; (*Figure continues.*)

A

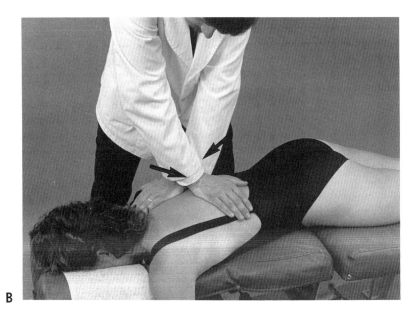

B

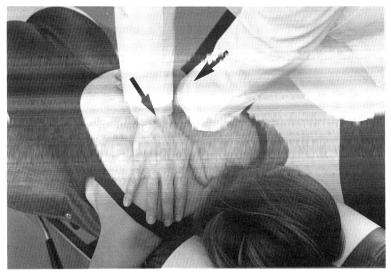

C

Figure 5.180 (*Continued*). (**B**) the right T6 transverse process and left T7 transverse process to induce left rotation with opposite glide of the right T6–T7 and gapping of the left T6–T7 articulation. (**C**) The transverse processes of T6 to induce left lateral flexion with superior glide at the right T6–T7 articulation and inferior glide at the left T6–T7 articulation.

is delivered anteriorly and superiorly through the contact established on the side opposite the lateral flexion restriction (side of closed wedge). This produces ipsilateral gliding distraction in the facet joint inferior to the thrusting hand.

Rotation. To induce rotation establish contacts on the superior or inferior vertebra depending on the side of desired facet distraction (see discussion). With superior vertebra contacts deliver the thrust anteriorly and superiorly on the side of posterior body rotation (side opposite the rotation restriction). With an inferior vertebra contact deliver the thrust anteriorly on the side opposite the posterior body rotation (side of rotational restriction). Inferior vertebra contacts are designed to induce gapping of the posterior joints above the site of contact. Inferior vertebra contacts have not been traditionally employed in this manner (Fig. 5-161).

Bilateral hypothenar transverse (crossed bilateral) (Fig. 5-180)

IND: Restricted flexion, extension, lateral flexion, and/or rotation of T4–T12. Flexion, extension, lateral flexion, and/or rotation malpositions, T4–T12.

PP: The patient lies prone. To provide added flexion a small roll may be placed under the patient's chest.

DP: Stand in a fencer, modified fencer, or square stance depending on the restriction treated. Stand on either side of the patient.

CP: Bilateral hypothenar (pisiform) contacts.

SCP: Transverse processes.

VEC: Posterior to anterior and inferior to superior with the caudal hand and posterior to anterior and superior to inferior with the cephalic hand (see discussion below).

P: Remove superficial tissue slack and establish contacts on the transverse processes. At tension deliver an impulse thrust through the arms, trunk and body.

Flexion. To induce flexion, stand in a fencer stance facing cephalad and establish contacts on the superior vertebra with the hands on edge and fingers running parallel to the spine. At tension deliver an impulse thrust anteriorly and superiorly through both contacts (Fig. 5-180A).

Extension. To induce extension establish the contacts on the superior vertebra and deliver the thrust anteriorly through both contacts.

Rotation. When treating rotational dysfunction stand in a modified fencer or square stance. Establish bilateral hypothenar contacts; hands are arched and arms cross to contact both sides of the spine. The caudal hand contacts the superior vertebra on the side of posterior body rotation (side opposite the rotational restriction). The cephalic hand contacts the contralateral side (Fig. 5-180B). The cephalic hand (hand reaching across the spine) may develop a broad stabilizing contact or a more precise contact on the contralateral inferior vertebra. A thenar contact may be substituted for the hypothenar contact on the crossed hand contact.

Develop pre-adjustive tension by leaning anteriorly into the contacts and tractioning the hands apart. At tension deliver an impulse thrust anteriorly and superiorly with the caudal hand while the cephalic hand stabilizes the contralateral structures or counter thrusts anteriorly and inferiorly on the contralateral inferior vertebra (Fig. 5-180B). The superior vertebral contact is directed at inducing gliding distraction while the inferior vertebral contact is directed at inducing gapping distraction.

Lateral flexion. When inducing lateral flexion establish the segmental contacts bilaterally on the transverse process of the same vertebra. Deliver the thrust through both hands. One hand thrusts anteriorly and superiorly while the other thrusts anteriorly and inferiorly (Fig. 5-180C).

This adjustment may also be used to induce rotation and lateral flexion in the same directions. In this situation contralateral contacts are taken on adjacent vertebra and the thrust is delivered as described for the treatment of rotational dysfunction.

Unilateral hypothenar spinous (Fig. 5-181)

IND: Restricted flexion, lateral flexion, and/or rotation of T4–T12. Extension, rotation, and/or lateral flexion malpositions, T4–T12.

PP: The patient lies prone. To provide added flexion a small roll may be placed under the patient's chest. To provide added extension the thoracic piece may be lowered anteriorly.

DP: Stand in a fencer, modified fencer, or square stance depending on the dysfunction treated.

CP: Mid hypothenar.

SCP: Spinous process.

IH: Supports contact hand on dorsal surface with fingers wrapped around the wrist.

VEC: Posterior to anterior and inferior to superior for flexion restrictions. Lateral to medial, superior to inferior, and posterior to anterior for rotation and/or lateral flexion restrictions.

P: Remove superficial tissue slack and establish a fleshy hypothenar contact against the spinous process. Develop pre-adjustive tension by transferring additional body weight into the contact. At tension deliver an impulse thrust through the arms, trunk, and body.

Flexion. Stand in a fencer stance facing cephalically on either side of the patient. Establish the adjustive contact by sliding the hypothenar contact superiorly onto the inferior tip of the superior spinous process (Fig. 5-181A) with your center of gravity oriented inferior to the level of adjustive contact. At tension thrust anteriorly and superiorly.

Lateral flexion and/or rotation. Stand in a fencer stance or square stance on the side of adjustive contact. Establish the adjustive contact by sliding medially onto the lateral surface of the superior spinous process on the side of rotation and/or lateral flexion restriction (side of spinous rotation). The contact must be fleshy or it may be painful to the patient. While developing the contact a slight clockwise or counter clockwise torquing movement is applied to traction the tissue. This leaves your fingers oriented at an angle of approximately 45 degrees to the long axis of the spine (Fig. 5-181B).

If you wish to induce lateral flexion coupled with same side rotation the cephalic hand is used as the contact. Stand in a square stance or modified fencer stance and face caudally (Fig. 5-181B). This adjustment is commonly applied in the treatment of coupled restrictions in rotation and lateral flexion to the same side (PRS or PLS Palmer Gonstead listings, LPI or RPI National listings).

If you wish to induce lateral flexion coupled with opposite side rotation (PRI or PLS, LPI or RPI) the caudal hand establishes the contact and you stand in a square stance or modified fencer stance facing cephalically (Fig. 5-181C). At tension deliver an adjustive thrust anteriorly, medially, and superiorly.

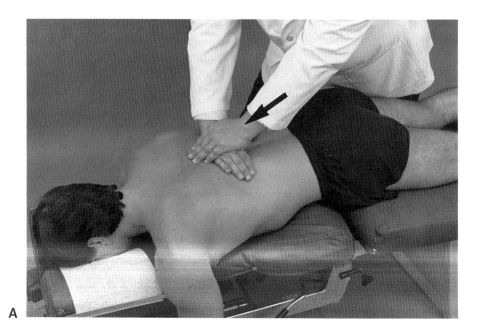

A

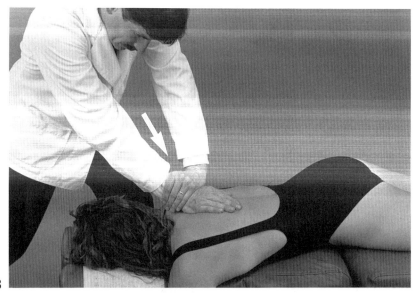

Figure 5.181 Reinforced hypothenar contact applied to (**A**) the inferior aspect of the spinous process of T7 to induce flexion at T7–T8; (**B**) the right lateral surface of the T3 spinous process to induce right lateral flexion and/or right rotation of the T3–T4 articulation with inferior and medial glide of the right T3–T4 articulation. (*Figure continues.*)

B

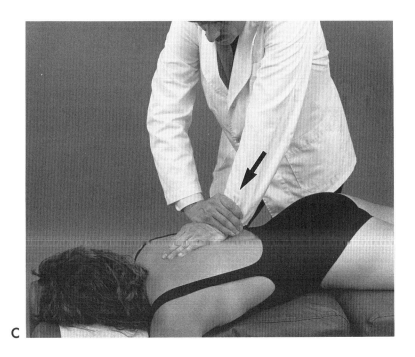

Figure 5.181 (*Continued*) (C) The right lateral surface of the T8 spinous process to induce left lateral flexion and/or right rotation of the T8–T9 articulation with superior and medial glide of the right T8–T9 articulation.

Unilateral hypothenar transverse (Fig. 5-182)

IND: Restricted lateral flexion and/or rotation of T4–T12. Rotation and/or lateral flexion malpositions, T4–T12.

PP: The patient lies prone. To provide added flexion a small roll may be placed under the patient's chest.

DP: Fencer stance in square stance on side of adjustive contact.

CH: Hypothenar (pisiform) of caudal hand with hand arched and fingers running parallel to the spine.

SCP: Transverse process.

IH: Supports contact hand on dorsal surface with fingers wrapped around the doctor's wrist.

VEC: Posterior to anterior coupled with an inferior to superior or superior to inferior vector depending on the dysfunction treated and the vertebra contacted.

P: Remove superficial tissue slack and establish transverse process contacts. Develop pre-adjustive tension by transferring additional body weight into the contacts. At tension deliver an impulse thrust through the arms, trunk, and body.

Lateral flexion. When treating lateral flexion dysfunction establish the contact on the superior vertebra. When contacting the transverse process on the side opposite the lateral flexion restriction (closed disc wedge side) stand in a fencer stance facing cephalically. Establish the contact with the caudal hand and deliver the adjustive thrust anteriorly and superiorly (Fig. 5-182A). When contacting the side of lateral flexion restriction (open disc wedge side) stand in a square or fencer stance and establish the contact with the cephalic hand. Deliver the thrust anteriorly and inferiorly (Fig. 5-182B).

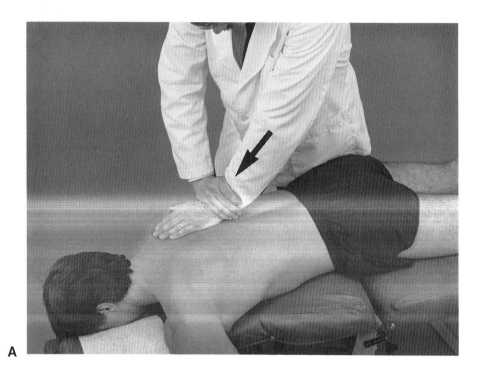

Figure 5.182 Hypothenar contact applied to the right T5 transverse process to induce (**A**) left rotation and/ or left lateral flexion at the T5–T6 articulation with superior glide of the right T5–T6 articulation; (*Figure continues.*)

A

Rotation. When treating rotational dysfunction you may establish contacts on the superior or inferior vertebra of the dysfunctional motion segment. When contacting the superior vertebra establish the contact on the side opposite the rotational restriction (side of posterior body rotation) (Fig. 5-182A). When contacting the inferior vertebra establish the contact on the side of rotational restriction (side opposite posterior body rotation) (Fig. 5-182C). Deliver the thrust anteriorly and superiorly with the superior vertebral contact (Fig. 5-182A) and anteriorly and inferiorly with an inferior vertebra contact (Fig. 5-182C). The side of contact depends on the side of desired distraction and cavitation.

The superior vertebra contact will induce headward distraction and tension in the facet joint inferior to the contact. The inferior vertebral contact should induce more tension and gapping in the joint superior to the contact. The method employing an inferior vertebral contact is not commonly applied.

Hypothenar spinous transverse (Fig. 5-183)

IND: Restricted rotation and or lateral flexion, T4–T12. Rotation and/or lateral flexion malpositions, T4–T12.

 PP: The patient lies prone.

 DP: Modified fencer stance or square stance on side of spinous contact.

 CP: Hypothenar (pisiform) (Fig. 5-183A) or thumb (Fig. 5-183B) contact of the cephalic hand and thenar contact of the caudal hand.

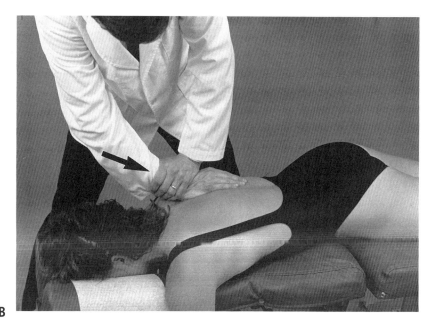

Figure 5.182 (*Continued*). **(B)** right lateral flexion at T5–T6 articulation and inferior glide of the right T5–T6 articulation; **(C)** right rotation at T4–T5 and gapping in the right T4–T5 articulation. (Contact is on right T5 transverse process.)

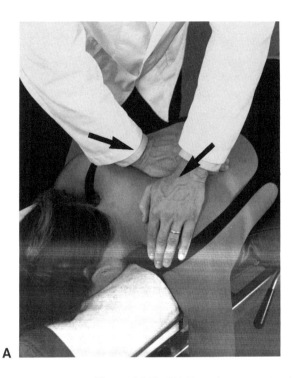

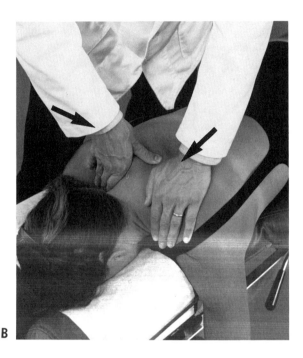

A

B

Figure 5.183 **(A)** Hypothenar or **(B)** thumb contact applied to the right lateral surface of the T4 spinous process and a thenar contact applied to the right T4 transverse process to induce right rotation and/or right lateral flexion at the T4–T5 articulation with inferior and medial glide of the right T4–T5 articulation and superior glide of the left T4–T5 articulation.

SCP: Lateral surface of the spinous process and transverse process of the corresponding vertebra.

VEC: Posterior to anterior, lateral to medial, and superior to inferior with hand contacting the spinous. Posterior to anterior and inferior to superior with transverse process contact.

P: Remove superficial tissue slack by sliding the thumb or hypothenar against the lateral surface of the spinous while sliding the thenar superiorly onto the ipsilateral transverse process. Develop pre-adjustive tension by transferring additional body weight into the contacts. At tension, deliver an impulse thrust through both arms, trunk, and body.

This method combines unilateral spinous and transverse process contacts and has the advantage of developing tension and leverage on both sides of the spine simultaneously. The impulse delivered on the side of spinous contact induces approximation (inferior and medial glide) in the inferior ipsilateral motion segment. The thrust delivered on the side of transverse contact induces distraction (superior glide) in the inferior and ipsilateral motion segment.

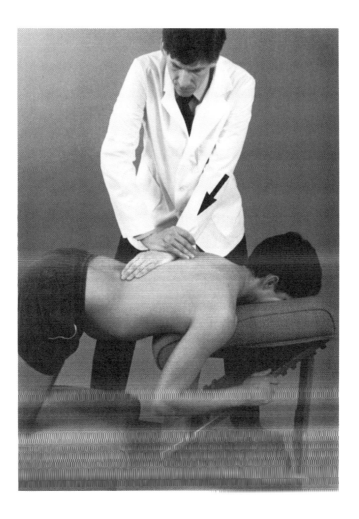

Figure 5.184 Hypothenar contact applied to the left lateral surface of the T8 spinous process to induce extension, left rotation, and/or left lateral flexion with inferior and medial glide of the T7 to T9 articulation using the knee chest position.

Thoracic Knee Chest Adjustments

Hypothenar spinous (Fig. 5-184)

IND: Restricted extension, lateral flexion, and/or rotation of T4–T12. Flexion, rotation, and/or lateral flexion malpositions, T4–T12.

 PP: Position the patient in the knee chest position with the chest support placed so the patient's thoracic spine is level with or slightly lower than the lumbar spine. The patient's femurs should be angled between 95 and 110 degrees.

 DP: Stand at the side of the table in a square stance typically on the side of the contact. You may also stand in a fencer stance facing caudally.

 CP: Hypothenar.

SCP: Lateral surface of the spinous process.

 IH: Supports contact hand on the dorsal surface with fingers wrapped around the wrist.

VEC: Posterior to anterior for extension restriction or flexion malposition; lateral to medial, superior to inferior, and posterior to anterior for rotation and/or lateral flexion restrictions or malpositions.

P: The indifferent hand first raises the patient's abdomen to make the spinous processes more prominent and available for establishing the contacts. Instruct the patient to allow the torso to drop, and at tension, deliver an impulse thrust. The patient is vulnerable to hyperextension in this position and the thrust must be shallow and non-recoiling.

Hypothenar transverse (Fig. 5-185)

IND: Restricted lateral flexion and/or rotation of T4–T12. Rotation and/or lateral flexion malpositions, T4–T12.

PP: Position the patient in the knee chest position with the chest support placed so the patient's thoracic spine is level with or slightly lower than the lumbar spine. The patient's femurs should be angled between 95 and 110 degrees.

DP: Stand at the side of the table in a square stance typically on the side of the contact. You may also stand in a fencer stance facing caudally.

CP: Hypothenar (pisiform).

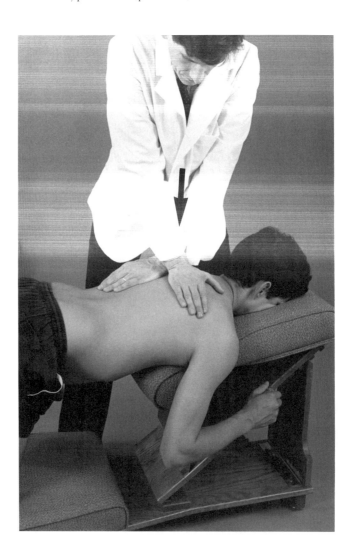

Figure 5.185 Bilateral hypothenar contacts applied to the T5 transverse processes to induce extension at the T5–T6 articulation.

SCP: Transverse process.

  IH: Supports contact hand on the dorsal surface with fingers wrapped around the wrist. The indifferent hand may be placed on opposite side to stabilize or impart an assisting impulse.

VEC: Posterior to anterior for extension restriction or flexion malposition; lateral to medial, superior to inferior, and posterior to anterior for rotation and/or lateral flexion restrictions or malpositions.

   P: The indifferent hand first raises the patient's abdomen to make the transverse process more prominent and available for establishing the contacts. Instruct the patient to allow the torso to drop and at tension, deliver an impulse thrust. The patient is vulnerable to hyperextension in this position and the thrust must be shallow and non-recoiling. If the indifferent hand delivers an assisting thrust it is directed posterior to anterior.

Supine Thoracic Adjustments

Supine thoracic opposite side contact (Fig. 5-186)

IND: Restricted flexion, extension, rotation, and/or lateral flexion, T3–T12. Flexion, extension, rotation, and/or lateral flexion malpositions, T3–T12.

  PP: The patient is requested to sit or lie supine with arms crossed and hands grasping opposing shoulders.

  DP: Stand in a modified fencer stance and reach around the patient to establish the posterior contact.

  CP: The cupped hand, clenched fist, index or thenar of the doctor's contact hand (Fig. 5-159)

 SCP: Bilateral transverse process, unilateral transverse process or interspinous space depending on the dysfunction treated.

  IH: Use the buttress or hand in combination the patient's crossed arms to cradle the patient's neck and upper back (Fig. 5-186A,B).

VEC: Anterior to posterior and inferior to superior to produce flexion or lateral flexion. Anterior to posterior for extension or rotation.

   P: When starting in the supine position first roll the patient toward you to place the posterior spinal contact (Fig. 5-186A). Slide superiorly to establish a superior vertebral contact and inferiorly to establish an inferior vertebral contact. After the spinal contact is established return the patient to the supine position and initiate the indifferent hand contacts (Fig. 5-186C,D,E). During this process it is important that the patient is rolled onto the contact hand with minimal pressure. Undue pressure exerted against the anterior contacts can lead to painful compression against your posterior contact.

     Develop pre-adjustive tension by adding progressive compression and traction through your trunk and anterior contacts. At tension deliver a short amplitude, moderate velocity body drop thrust, generated primarily through your trunk and lower extremities. When applying supine adjustive techniques, it is important to avoid straight compression to the trunk and rib cage. Therefore, all supine adjustments should incorporate some degree of long axis traction. This is

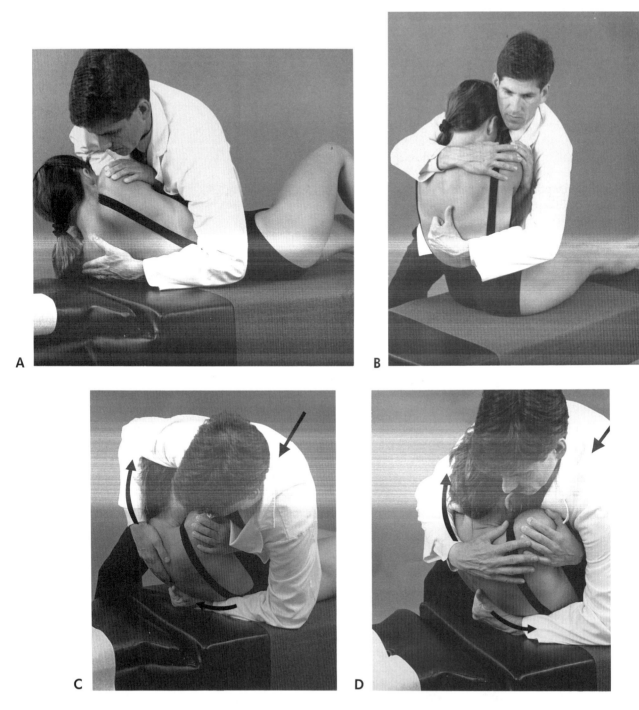

Figure 5.186 Supine thoracic adjustment using an opposite side contact with the patient in a crossed arm position: **(A)** starting in the supine position; **(B)** starting in the seated position; **(C)** assisted method using clenched fist applied to the transverse process of T7 to induce flexion at the T7–T8 articulation (small arrow indicates direction of tissue pull); **(D)** resisted method using clenched fist applied to the transverse process of T8 to induce flexion at the T7–T8 articulation (small arrow indicates direction of tissue pull). (*Figure continues.*)

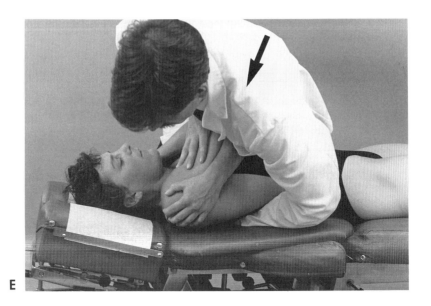

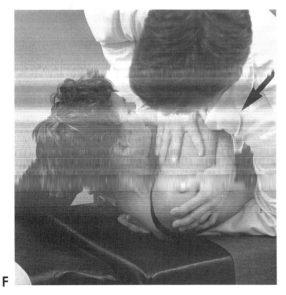

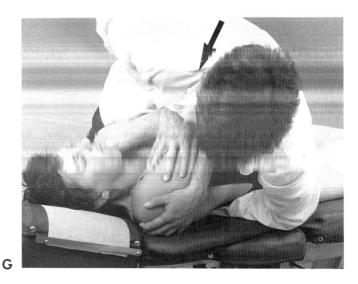

Figure 5.186 (*Continued*). (**E**) Clenched fist contact applied to the T8 transverse process to induce extension at the T7–T8 motion segment. (**F**) Hypothenar contact established on the right T3 transverse process to induce left rotation and superior glide of the right T3–T4 articulation. (**G**) Hypothenar contact applied to the right T4 transverse process to induce right rotation and gapping of the right T3–T4 articulation.

accomplished by applying headward traction during the development of tension.

Supine thoracic adjustments are also commonly started with the patient in a sitting position. This is particularly helpful when adjusting the lower thoracics, adjusting big patients or in situations where rolling the patient onto the contact is too painful (Fig. 5-186B).

Flexion. When treating flexion restrictions (extension malpositions) the patient is maintained in a position of segmental flexion (Fig. 5-186C,D). Place the adjustive contacts bilaterally on the transverse processes or in the midline against the spinous process. Establish the transverse contacts with your cupped hand or clenched fist. The spinous contact is established with your index finger or thenar eminence.

When employing an assisted method, establish the contact on the transverse process or spinous process of the superior vertebra of the dysfunctional motion segment (Fig. 5-186C). At tension deliver the thrust posteriorly and superiorly through the trunk, legs, and posterior contact.

When employing a resisted method, establish the contact on the transverse process or spinous process of the inferior vertebra (Fig. 5-186D). Apply downward counter pressure through the contact to oppose the adjustive thrust, which is directed posteriorly and superiorly through the trunk and legs.

Extension. When treating extension restrictions (flexion malpositions) establish the contact bilaterally on the transverse processes of the inferior vertebra of the dysfunctional motion segment. Develop pre-adjustive tension by inducing segmental extension and deliver the adjustive thrust posteriorly while maintaining headward traction (Fig. 5-186E).

Rotation. To effect rotation you may establish unilateral thenar contacts on either the superior or inferior vertebra of the involved motion segment.

When employing a superior vertebral contact (assisted method) establish the contact on the transverse process on the side opposite the rotation restriction (side of posterior body rotation). Maintain the patient in a flexed position and direct the thrust posteriorly and superiorly (Fig. 5-186F). The thrust through the torso is assisted by a shallow cephalic thrust with the posterior vertebral contact.

When employing an inferior vertebral contact (resisted method) establish the contact on the transverse side of the rotational restriction (side opposite posterior body rotation). For example, when treating a right rotation restriction at T3–T4 (left body rotation) the contact would be established on the right T6 transverse process. During the development of pre-adjustive tension the patient is rolled further toward the side of the posterior contact (Fig. 5-186G). The adjustive thrust is directed posteriorly. The side of selected contact depends on the side of desired distraction and cavitation. The superior vertebra contact (left T3 TP) is directed to induce headward distraction in the facet joint ipsilateral (left) and inferior to the contact. The inferior vertebral contact (right T4 contact) is directed to induce gapping in the facet joint ipsilateral (right) and superior to the contact.

Lateral flexion. Lateral flexion dysfunction is typically treated by establishing unilateral contacts on the side opposite the lateral flexion restriction (side of closed disc wedge).

When employing assisted patient positions, contact the superior vertebra, induce flexion and lateral flexion away, and thrust posteriorly and superiorly through the trunk, legs, and posterior contact.

When employing resisted methods contact the inferior vertebra, laterally flex the patient away, and apply downward counter pressure to oppose the adjustive thrust. This method may be applied to treat combined restrictions in rotation and opposite side lateral flexion.

Supine thoracic same side contact (Fig. 5-187)

IND: Restricted flexion, extension, rotation, and/or lateral flexion, T3–T12. Flexion, extension, rotation, and/or lateral flexion malpositions, T3–T12.

PP: Ask the patient to sit or lie supine with arms crossed and hands grasping opposing shoulders.

DP: Stand in a fencer stance on the side of adjustive contact.

CP: The cupped hand, clenched fist, or thenar of the contact hand.

SCP: Bilateral transverse process, unilateral transverse process, or interspinous space depending on the restriction treated.

IH: You can use the indifferent hand to contact the patient's crossed arms or cradle the patient's neck and upper back.

VEC: Anterior to posterior and inferior to superior to produce flexion or lateral flexion. Anterior to posterior for extension or rotation.

P: Stand on the side of the established contact and instruct the patient to cross the arms. Roll the patient away from you and establish the posterior contact. Then roll the patient back into position and contact the patient's crossed arms or cradle the patient's neck and shoulders (Fig. 5-187A,B). Progressive compression to tighten soft tissue slack is followed by a moderate velocity, short amplitude body drop thrust.

The specific considerations for flexion, extension, and rotational restrictions are the same as previously mentioned in the adjustments described in Fig. 5-186C–G.

Other than personal preference, this method is commonly applied in the treatment of larger patients, or if less contact is desired between the doctor and patient.

Supine thoracic pump handle (Fig. 5-188)

IND: Restricted flexion, extension, rotation, and/or lateral flexion, T3–T12. Flexion, extension, rotation, and/or lateral flexion malpositions, T3–T12.

PP: The patient may begin in either the sitting or supine position with elbows flexed and fingers interlocked or overlapping behind neck.

DP: Stand in a fencer stance on either side of the patient.

CP: The cupped hand, clenched first, or thenar of your contact hand.

SCP: Bilateral transverse process, unilateral transverse process, or interspinous space depending on the dysfunction treated.

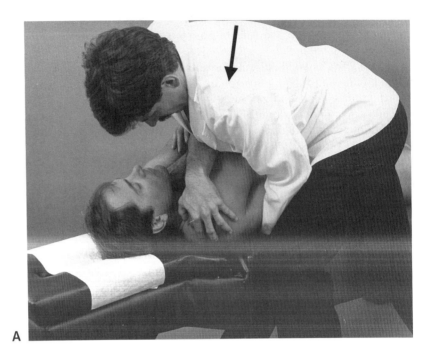

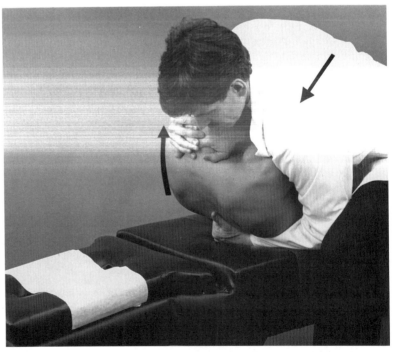

Figure 5.187 Supine thoracic adjustment using a same side contact. (**A**) Contact applied to a mid-thoracic segment to induce extension using a crossed arm position. (**B**) Contact applied to a mid-thoracic segment to induce extension using a pump handle position. (*Figure continues.*)

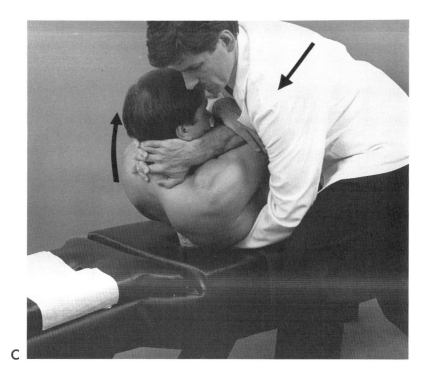

Figure 5.187 (*Continued*). (**C**) Contact applied to a mid-thoracic segment to induce flexion using a pump handle position with a cradling indifferent hand contact.

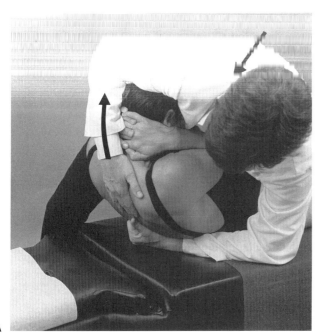

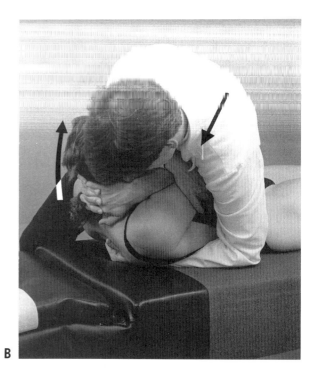

Figure 5.188 Supine thoracic adjustment using an opposite side contact with the patient in a pump handle position to induce flexion in (**A**) a mid-thoracic segment and (**B**) a lower thoracic segment with the doctor cradling the patient.

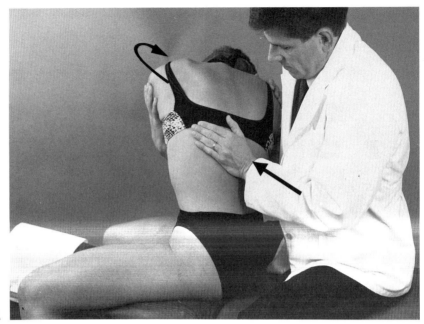

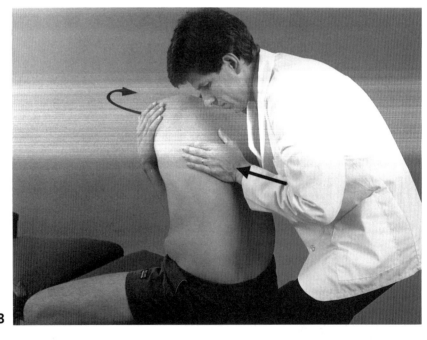

Figure 5.189 Sitting thoracic adjustment, assisted method, with a hypothenar contact applied to the **(A)** left T10 transverse process to induce right lateral flexion with superior glide of the left T10–T11 articulation; **(B)** left T6 transverse process to induce right rotation with lateral and superior glide of the left T6–T7 articulation. (*Figure continues.*)

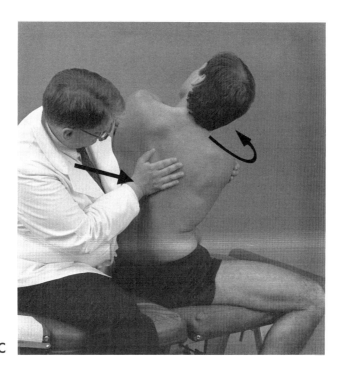

Figure 5.189 (*Continued*). (**C**) Left lateral surface of the T6 spinous to induce left rotation and right lateral flexion with distraction of the left T6–T7 articulation.

IH: Either cradle the patient's neck and upper back with the indifferent hand and arm (Fig. 5-188A) or support the patient by leaning across the patient's forearm with the forearm and upper abdomen (Fig. 5-188B).

VEC: Anterior to posterior and inferior to superior to produce flexion or lateral flexion. Anterior to posterior for extension or rotation.

P: Stand on either side of the patient and establish the posterior contacts. Your indifferent hand and forearm contact the patient's forearms or reach around to cradle the patient's neck and upper back. The development of pre-adjustive tension and the delivery of the adjustive thrust are identical to those previously described. The specific considerations for flexion, extension, and rotational dysfunction are the same as previously mentioned in supine adjustments. This method is especially helpful in inducing flexed patient postures.

Sitting Thoracic Adjustments

Hypothenar transverse—sitting thoracic (Fig. 5-189)

IND: Restricted rotation and/or lateral flexion, T3–T12. Rotation and/or lateral flexion malpositions, T3–T12.

PP: The patient sits with legs straddling the adjusting bench. The arms are crossed with the hands grasping the opposing shoulders.

DP: Sit or stand behind the patient.

CP: Hypothenar or thenar of hand corresponding to the side of contact.

SCP: Transverse or spinous process of superior vertebra.

IH: Your indifferent hand and arm reach around the patient to contact the opposing forearm.

VEC: Posterior to anterior and lateral to medial to produce rotation. Inferior to superior, lateral to medial, and posterior to anterior to produce lateral flexion.

P: Ask the patient to sit and cross the arms. Position yourself behind the patient in either a seated (Fig. 5-189A), straddling, or standing position (Fig. 5-189B). Pre-adjustive tension is typically developed by flexing, laterally flexing, and rotating the patient in the direction of joint restriction (assisted method). Once tension is established deliver an impulse thrust through the contact hand assisted by a pulling and twisting thrust generated through your indifferent arm and trunk. The direction of induced lateral flexion and the point of adjustive contact depends on the dysfunction being treated.

Lateral flexion. Treat lateral flexion dysfunction by contacting the transverse process of the superior vertebra on the side opposite the lateral flexion restriction (closed disc wedge side) (Fig. 5-189A). Develop pre-adjustive

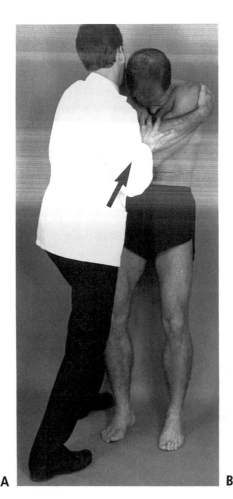
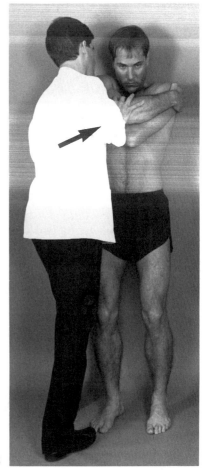

Figure 5.190 Standing thoracic adjustment for a midthoracic segment (**A**) against a wall to induce flexion; (**B**) against a wall to induce extension.

A   **B**

tension by flexing, laterally flexing, and rotating the patient away from the side of contact. At tension, deliver an adjustive thrust superiorly, laterally, and anteriorly.

Rotation. When treating rotational dysfunction you may establish contacts on the spinous process or transverse process.

When utilizing a transverse process contact, establish the contact on the superior vertebra on the side opposite the rotation restriction (side of posterior body rotation). Develop pre-adjustive tension by flexing, rotating, and laterally flexing the patient away from the side of contact (Fig. 5-189B). At tension deliver an adjustive thrust anteriorly, laterally, and superiorly. This method is applied to induce maximal distraction in the facet joint ipsilateral and inferior to the point of contact. It is also applied to treat restrictions in rotation and same side lateral flexion (e.g., right or left rotation restriction coupled with the corresponding right or left lateral flexion restriction).

To employ a spinous process contact, slide medially and establish a fleshy mid-hypothenar contact on the lateral surface of the spinous process on the side of rotational restriction (side of spinous rotation). Develop pre-adjustive tension by flexing, rotating, and laterally flexing the patient away from the side of contact (Fig. 5-189C). At tension deliver an adjustive thrust medially to induce rotation. This contact should induce maximal distraction in the facet joint ipsilateral and inferior to the side of spinous contact, therefore inducing distraction in the facet joints on the side opposite the transverse process contact. This method is also commonly applied when treating combined restrictions in rotation and opposite side lateral flexion (e.g., right or left rotation restriction coupled with the opposing right or left lateral flexion restriction).

Standing Thoracic Adjustments

Standing Thoracic (Fig. 5-190)

IND: Restricted flexion, extension, rotation, and/or lateral flexion, T3–T12. Flexion, extension, rotation, and/or lateral flexion malpositions, T3–T12.

PP: The patient stands leaning against a wall with feet shoulder-width apart and away from the wall. Arms are crossed, with hands grasping opposite shoulders.

DP: Stand on either side of the patient in a fencer stance with your medial leg posterior and body angled about 45 degrees to the patient.

CP: The cupped hand, fist, or open palm of your outside hand reaches behind the patient to contact the patient posteriorly. Your hand must be cushioned from the wall by utilizing a padded wall board or placing a pad between your hand and the wall.

IH: The indifferent hand contacts the patient's crossed arms.

VEC: Inferior to superior and anterior to posterior for flexion and lateral flexion restriction. Anterior to posterior with slight inferior to superior vector for extension and rotation restrictions.

P: Stand to the desired side of the patient, rotate the patient away, and establish the posterior contact. Slide superiorly to establish a superior vertebral contact and inferiorly to establish a inferior vertebral contact. Develop pre-adjustive tension by leaning into the patient while applying vertical traction. As tension is developed it is critical to produce long axis traction by pushing cephalically through your legs and arms. At tension deliver an impulse thrust through your trunk and lower extremities.

Flexion. When treating flexion restrictions (extension malpositions) the superior vertebra of the dysfunctional motion segment is typically contacted. Maintain the patient in a position of flexion and deliver the thrust posteriorly and superiorly (Fig. 5-190A).

Extension. With extension restrictions (flexion malpositions) contact the inferior vertebra, extend the motion segment, and deliver the thrust posteriorly (Fig. 5-190B).

Lateral flexion. Lateral flexion dysfunction is typically treated by establishing unilateral contacts on the side opposite the lateral flexion restriction (side of closed disc wedge).

When employing assisted patient positions contact the superior vertebra, induce flexion and lateral flexion away, then thrust posteriorly and superiorly through the trunk, legs, and posterior contact.

When employing resisted methods contact the inferior vertebra, laterally flex the patient away, and apply downward counter pressure to oppose the adjustive thrust. This method may be applied to treat combined rotation and opposite side lateral flexion dysfunction.

Rotation. When treating rotation dysfunction, adjustive contacts may be established on the superior or inferior vertebra of the dysfunctional motion segment.

When employing a superior vertebral contact (assisted method) establish the contact on the side opposite the rotation restriction (side of posterior body rotation). Position the patient in flexion and deliver a thrust posteriorly and superiorly.

When employing an inferior vertebra contact (resisted method) establish the contact on the side of rotational restriction (side opposite the posterior body rotation) and deliver a thrust posteriorly.

This adjustment may also be used for rib flexion or extension restrictions by moving the contact laterally to the angle of the involved rib.

Standing thoracic long axis distraction (Fig. 5-191)

IND: Restricted flexion, long axis distraction, T3–T12. Extension malpositions, T3–T12.

PP: The patient stands with feet at least 10 inches apart (more if the patient is taller than the doctor), hands interlaced behind the neck and elbows together.

DP: Stand behind the patient in a fencer stance, placing the forward leg between the patient's legs.

CP: A true segmental contact is not established on the back but the sternal angle of the doctor is placed over the region to be distracted.

SCP: Over the spinous processes of the dysfunctional region.

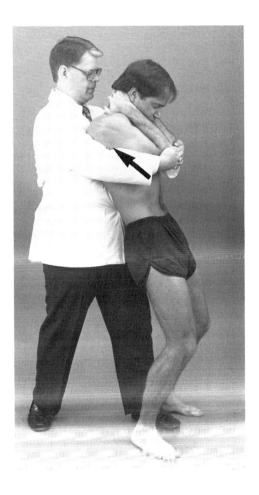

Figure 5.191 Standing thoracic adjustment for a mid-thoracic segment with the doctor standing behind to induce flexion and long axis distraction.

VEC: Anterior to posterior and inferior to superior.
  P: Grasp the patient's forearms, stressing the patient's thoracic spine into flexion. At tension, pull posteriorly and superiorly through the patient's arms. A sternal block can be used to make the contact more specific.

Supine Rib Adjustments

Supine rib/thenar costal (Fig. 5-192)

IND: Rib dysfunction, R2–R12.
  PP: The patient lies supine with arms crossed and hands grasping opposing shoulders. Patient arm placement is at the doctor's discretion. However, the patient's arm closest to the doctor is typically placed across the chest first with the opposite arm crossed over the top. When treating lower rib fixations the patient typically begins in the seated position.
  DP: Stand in a modified fencer stance on either side of the patient.
  CP: Thenar eminence.

SCP: Rib angle.
  IH: Use the indifferent hand to contact the patient's crossed arms or cradle the patient's neck and upper back.
VEC: Anterior to posterior and inferior to superior.
   P: Stand in a low fencer stance on either side of the patient. Access for the contact is achieved by rolling the patient toward you when employing an opposite side contact (Fig. 5-192A).

When treating flexion (superior) malpositions, the superior margin of the rib angle is contacted and downward pressure is applied (Fig. 5-192A). When treating extension (inferior) malpositions, the contact is established on the inferior margin of the rib angle and upward pressure is applied (Fig. 5-192C). Flexion malpositions are purportedly more common in the upper thoracics and extension malpositions more common in the lower thoracics. However, because of the pull of the iliocostalis thoracis muscle, the opposite is quite possible.

At tension direct a moderate velocity thrust through your trunk posteriorly and superiorly. When treating flexion malpositions the vector is angled slightly superior to the contact as the contact hand applies downward pressure (Fig. 5-192B). When treating extension malpositions the vector is directed toward the contact as the contact hand exerts upward pressure (Fig. 5-192D).

In the treatment of lower rib dysfunction the patient is typically started

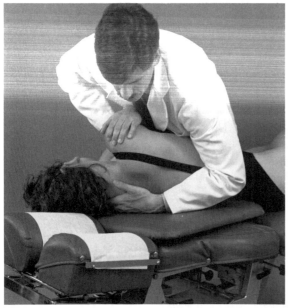
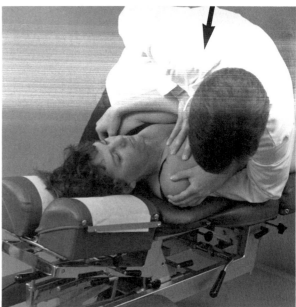

A   **B**

Figure 5.192 Supine rib adjustment using (**A**) a hypothenar contact over the superior margin of the right third rib starting in the supine position; (**B**) vector to induce anterior glide at the right third costotransverse and costovertebral articulations. (*Figure continues.*)

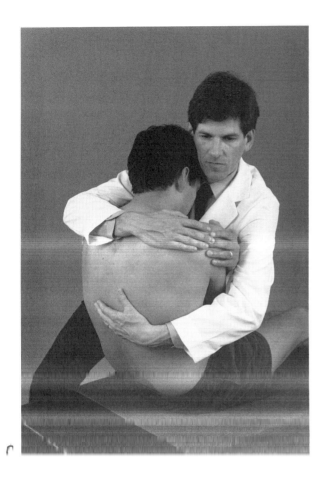

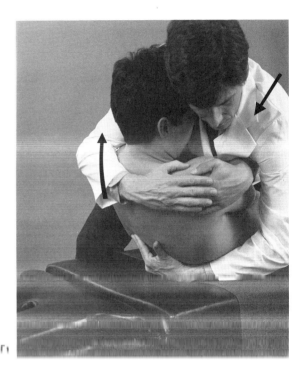

Figure 5-192 (continued). (C) Using a hypothenar contact from the inferior margin of the right eighth rib starting in the seated position; and **(D)** vector to induce anterior glide at the right eighth costotransverse and costovertebral articulations.

in the sitting position (Fig. 5-192B). The patient is maintained in some degree of thoracolumbar flexion and the contact hand is held in a more bridging contact to establish tension in the lower thoracic spine (Fig. 5-192D).

Index costal–supine (Fig. 5-193)

IND: Dysfunction of the first rib.

  PP: The patient lies supine.

  DP: Stand at the head of the table, facing caudad.

  CP: Index contact of the hand corresponding to the side of contact.

SCP: Angle of first rib.

  IH: The indifferent hand cups the patient's ear with the palm while the index and middle fingers lie on either side of the SCM.

VEC: Superior to inferior and lateral to medial.

  P: To facilitate taking the contact, the IH raises the patient's head to

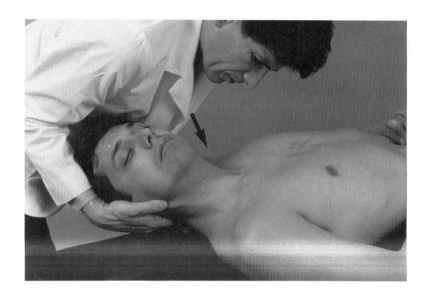

Figure 5.193 Index contact established over the superior aspect of the angle of the left first rib to induce inferior and medial glide at the left T1 costotransverse articulation.

about a 45-degree angle and then extends the head backward over the index contact on the first rib. The head is then rotated about 20 degrees away from the contact and slightly laterally flexed over the contact. At tension, an impulse thrust is delivered toward the opposite fifth intercostal space in the mid-clavicular line.

Prone Rib Adjustments

Hypothenar costal—upper ribs (Fig. 5-194)

IND: Rib dysfunction, R1–R4.

PP: The patient lies prone with the headpiece lowered below horizontal to produce slight flexion in the thoraco-cervical spine. (The patient's head rests on the anterolateral cheek).

DP: Stand in a fencer stance on either side of the patient facing cephalad. The superior leg approximates the level of the patient's head and your upper body weight is centered over the contact.

CP: Hypothenar of arched hand. When standing on the same side of adjustive contact (combination move) the hypothenar of your caudal hand establishes the contact (Fig. 5-194A). When standing on the side opposite the adjustive contact (modified combination move) the hypothenar of your cephalic hand establishes the contact (Fig. 5-194B).

SCP: Rib angle.

IH: The indifferent hand supports the upper cervical spine as the fingers contact the inferior occiput.

VEC: Posterior to anterior and superior to inferior or inferior to superior.

P: Place the patient in the prone position and establish the adjustive contacts. Develop pre-adjustive tension by transferring body weight into the contact while rotating and laterally flexing the patient's head

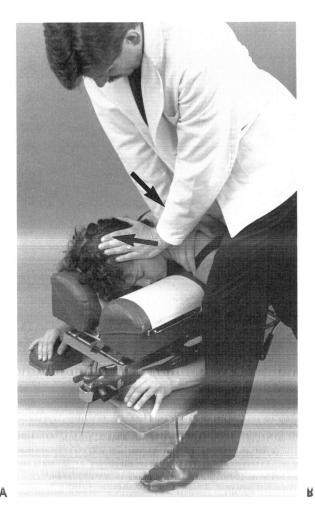

A

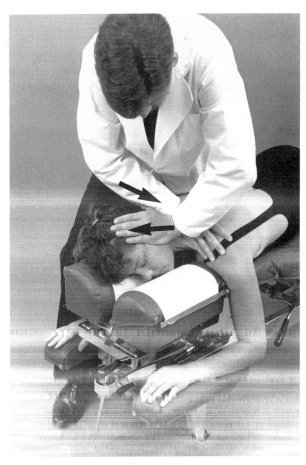

B

Figure 5.194 Hypothenar contact established on the superior margin of the angle of the left first rib applied to distract the left costotransverse and costovertebral articulations of the first rib. **(A)** Doctor stands on the same side as the contact. **(B)** Doctor stands on the opposite side of the contact.

away from the contact. At tension deliver an impulse thrust through the contact and indifferent arms. The impulse delivered through the contact hand is typically assisted by a body drop thrust. The impulse imparted through the indifferent hand is shallow and care should be taken not to excessively rotate or laterally flex the cervical spine.

To maximize distractive tension in the soft tissues or intercostal tissues superior to the contact, apply caudal pressure against the rib angle and deliver the impulse anteriorly and inferiorly (Fig. 5-194A,B).

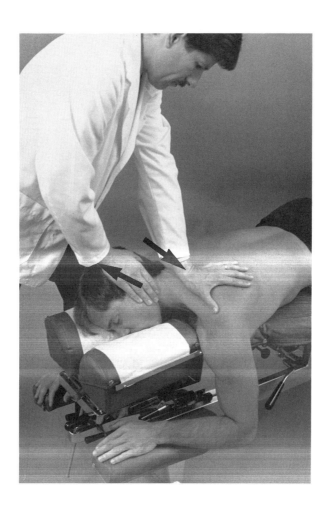

Figure 5.195 Hypothenar contact established over the left angle of the second rib to induce distraction of the left second costotransverse and costovertebral articulations.

Modified hypothenar costal (Fig. 5-195)

IND: Rib dysfunction, R1–R2.

PP: The patient lies prone with the headpiece lowered below horizontal to produce slight flexion in the thoraco-cervical spine. (The patient's head rests on the anterolateral aspect of the cheek).

DP: Stand in a fencer stance at the head of the adjustive bench facing caudad.

CP: Hypothenar of hand corresponding to the side of contact. The arm is straight with the elbow locked.

SCP: Posterosuperior angle of the first or second rib.

IH: Indifferent hand cups the patient's ipsilateral ear while the fingers rest against the lateral face.

VEC: Posterior to anterior and superior to inferior.

P: After establishing the contacts, the patient's head is laterally flexed and rotated away from the contact. At tension an impulse thrust is delivered through the contact hand while a simultaneous counter distraction force is delivered through the indifferent hand. The adjustive force is delivered primarily with a body drop thrust.

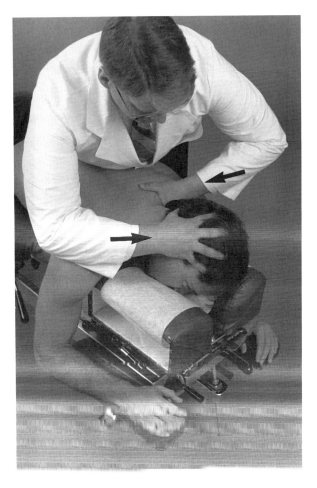

Figure 5.196 Index contact established over the superior aspect of the angle of the left first rib to induce inferior and medial glide at the left costotransverse articulation.

Index costal—prone (Fig. 5-196)

IND: Rib dysfunction, R1.

  PP: The patient lies prone. (The patient's head rests on the anterolateral aspect of the cheek).

  DP: Stand in a low fencer stance facing cephalad on side of rib dysfunction, slightly headward of the adjustive contact.

  CP: Index finger of hand corresponding to the side of contact. The wrist is straight and locked with arm approximately 45 degrees to vertical plane.

SCP: Posterosuperior angle of the first rib.

  IH: Indifferent hand cups the patient's contralateral inferior occiput and lateral skull.

VEC: Superior to inferior, lateral to medial, and posterior to anterior.

  P: After establishing the contacts, laterally flex and rotate the patient's head toward the contact (e.g., with the contact established on the patient's left first rib, the patient's head is left laterally flexed and right rotated). At tension, deliver an impulse thrust through the contact hand while a simultaneous counter distraction force is delivered through the indifferent hand.

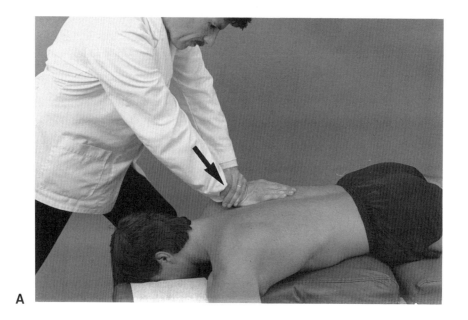

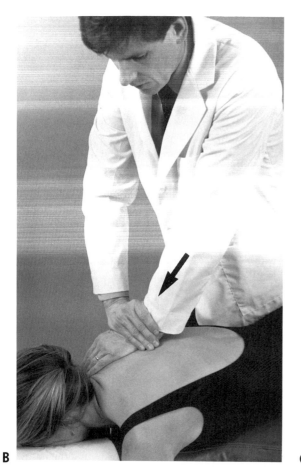

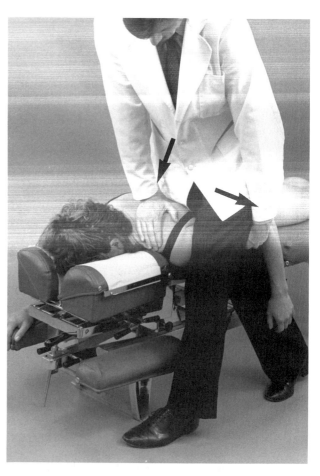

Figure 5.197 Hypothenar contact applied to the **(A)** superior margin of the right fourth rib angle to induce distraction and inferior glide of the right fourth rib costotransverse articulation; **(B)** inferior margin of the right fourth rib angle to induce distraction and superior glide of the right fourth costotransverse articulation, and **(C)** inferior margin of the left third rib angle assisted by left shoulder traction to induce distraction and superior glide of the left third costotransverse articulation.

Hypothenar costal (Fig. 5-197)

IND: Rib dysfunction, R3–R10.

  PP: The patient lies prone, ideally on a table with a brachial cutaway to induce scapular abduction.

  DP: The doctor stands in a fencer stance on the side of adjustive contact.

  CP: Hypothenar of the caudal hand.

SCP: Rib angle.

  IH: Indifferent hand supports the contact hand or develops a broad stabilizing contact on the contralateral rib cage.

VEC: Posterior to anterior and inferior to superior or superior to inferior.

   P: Place the patient in the prone position and establish the adjustive contacts. Develop pre-adjustive tension by transferring body weight into the contact. At tension, deliver an impulse thrust through the contact arm assisted by a body drop thrust. When treating flexion (superior) malpositions, slide laterally and inferiorly onto the superior margin of the rib angle and thrusts anteriorly and inferiorly (Fig. 5-197A). When treating extension (inferior) malpositions slide laterally and superiorly onto the inferior margin or the rib angle and thrusts anteriorly and superiorly (Fig. 5-197B).

     In the upper thoracic spine you may induce additional distraction of the costotransverse joint by abducting and tractioning the patient's ipsilateral shoulder. Straddle the patient's abducted arm and grip it with the indifferent hand and thighs (Fig. 5-197C). Pre-adjustive tension is developed by exerting lateral traction to the patient's shoulder as you transfer additional body weight into the adjustive contact. At tension deliver a high velocity body thrust by dropping and rotating the trunk headward.

Ilial hypothenar costal (Fig. 5-198)

IND: Rib dysfunction, R7–R12.

  PP: The patient lies prone. To provide added flexion a small roll may be placed under the patient's upper abdomen.

  DP: Stand in a square stance (Fig. 5-198A) or a modified fencer stance (Fig. 5-198B) on the side opposite the adjustive contact.

  CP: Hypothenar of cephalic hand.

SCP: Rib angle.

  IH: Fingers of inferior hand reach around to grasp the anterior ilium (ASIS) on the side of adjustive contact.

VEC: Posterior to anterior, inferior to superior, and lateral to medial.

   P: Establish contacts on the rib angle and anterior ilium and induce pre-adjustive tension by lifting and tractioning inferiorly against the ilium as the weight of your trunk is transferred anteriorly and superiorly against the contact. The counter distractive tension induced through the ilium is not marked, and the patient's pelvis should not be rotated off the table more than one to two inches. Deliver the thrust with an impulse and body drop thrust through the contact hand. A thumb-thenar contact can be placed in the intercostal space laterally to influence bucket handle movements.

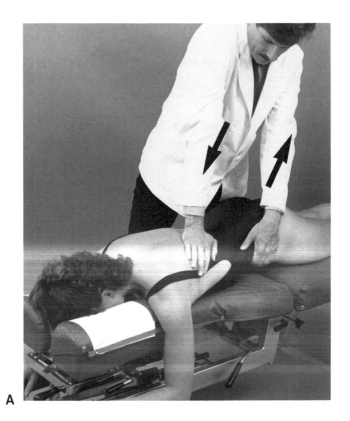

A

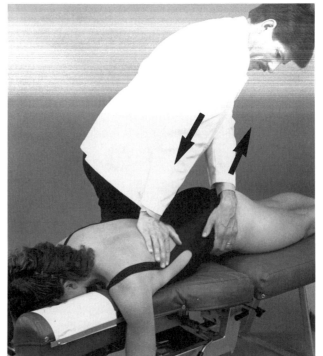

B

Figure 5.198 Hypothenar contact applied to the inferior margin of the left ninth rib angle to induce distraction and superior glide of the left ninth costotransverse articulation. (**A**) Doctor in a square stance. (**B**) Doctor facing caudal.

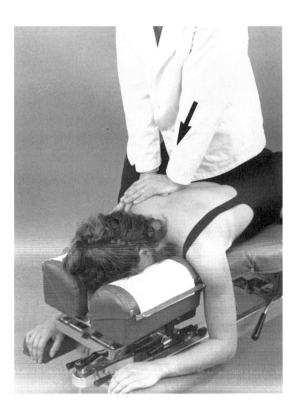

Figure 5.199 Covered thumb contact applied to the right fifth rib angle to induce distraction of the right fifth costotransverse articulation.

Covered thumb (Fig. 5-199)

IND: Rib dysfunction, R3–R12.
  PP: The patient lies in the prone position.
  DP: Stand on the side of contact facing cephalad for inferior to superior vector or caudad for superior to inferior vector.
  CP: The cephalad hand's thumb-thenar contact follows rib contour.
 SCP: Angle of the rib just lateral to the transverse process.
  IH: Place the caudad hand's pisiform-hypothenar contact over contact hands thumbnail with the fingers wrapped around the wrist.
 VEC: Posterior to anterior and either superior to inferior or inferior to superior.
   P: Your body weight is used to take the joints to tension. Deliver a straight arm body drop. Use multiple shallow thrusts on full expiration, each progressively deeper.

Side Posture Rib Adjustments

Web costal—side posture (Fig. 5-200)

IND: Rib dysfunction, R2–R10 (bucket handle dysfunction, intercostal distraction).
  PP: The patient lies with the dysfunctional side up and arm abducted over the head. A Dutchman's roll may be used to induce lateral flexion.
  DP: Stand behind the patient in a fencer stance inferior to the contact.

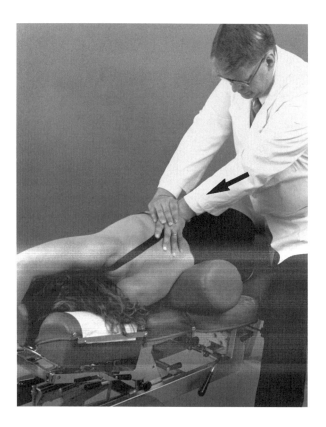

Figure 5.200 Web contact applied to the inferior margin of the right seventh rib in the midaxillary line to induce separation in the intercostal space between the seventh and eighth ribs.

CP: Web contact of the outside hand.
SCP: Inferior margin of the superior rib at the midaxillary line.
IH: The indifferent hand supports the contact hand on the dorsal surface with fingers wrapped around the wrist.
VEC: Inferior to superior and lateral to medial.
P: Establish the adjustive contact by sliding the web of the contact hand onto the superior rib of the dysfunctional intercostal space. Develop pre-adjustive tension by leaning headward. At tension deliver a shallow impulse thrust superiorly and medially to separate the intercostal space. Observe caution to avoid excessive medial pressure to the rib cage. This procedure may be used to mobilize the intercostal space by applying a slow stretch instead of an adjustive thrust.

Sitting Rib Adjustments

Index costal (Fig. 5-201)

IND: Rib dysfunction, R1.
PP: The patient sits relaxed in a cervical chair.
DP: Stand behind the patient toward the side of rib dysfunction.
CP: Index finger of the hand corresponding to the side of dysfunction. The wrist is locked with the arm angled approximately 45 degrees to the horizontal plane.
SCP: Posterosuperior angle of the first rib.

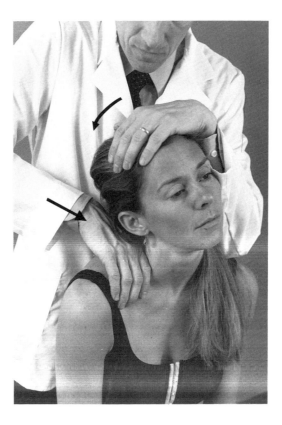

Figure 5.201 Index contact along the superior margin of the right first rib to induce distraction and interior glide in the right first costotransverse articulation.

IH: The indifferent hand grips the top of the patient's head while the forearm rests against the patient's contralateral skull.

VEC: Superior to inferior, lateral to medial, and posterior to anterior.

  P: Lightly establish the contacts and circumduct the patient's head toward the side of rib dysfunction. At tension deliver an impulse through the shoulder of the contact hand while simultaneously delivering a shallow distraction force through the indifferent hand.

Hypothenar costal (Fig. 5-202)

IND: Rib dysfunction, R4–R12.

  PP: The patient sits with legs straddling the adjusting bench. The arms are crossed with the hands grasping the opposing shoulders.

  DP: Sit or stand behind the patient.

  CP: Hypothenar or thenar of hand corresponding to the side of contact.

SCP: Rib angle.

  IH: Indifferent hand and arm reach around the patient to contact the opposing forearm.

VEC: Posterior to anterior and lateral to medial.

  P: Pre-adjustive tension is typically developed by flexing, laterally flexing, and rotating the patient away from the side of contact. Once tension is established, deliver an impulse thrust through the contact hand, assisted by a pulling and twisting thrust generated through the indifferent arm and trunk.

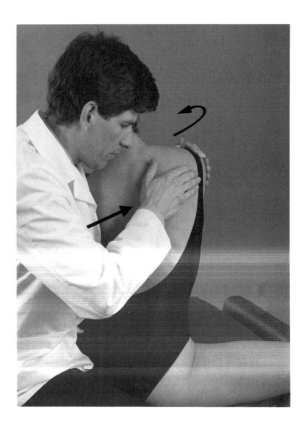

Figure 5.202 Hypothenar contact applied to the right sixth rib angle to induce distraction in the right fifth costotransverse articulation.

Supine Costosternal Adjustments

Covered thumb costal (Fig. 5-203)

IND: Anterior rib dysfunction, R2–R6.
  PP: The patient lies supine with both arms resting on the table.
DP: Stand on the side opposite the adjustive contact.
CP: Thumb of caudal hand.
SCP: Anterior rib just lateral to costosternal junction.
  IH: Palm of superior hand covering the thumb and dorsum of the contact hand.
VEC: Medial to lateral and slightly posterior to anterior.
  P: Slide laterally onto contact with thumb and reinforce the contact with the indifferent hand. Deliver a shallow and gentle impulse thrust, emphasizing a lateral vector to avoid compression of the rib cage.

Sitting Costosternal Adjustments

Hypothenar costal (Fig. 5-204)

IND: Anterior rib dysfunction, R2–R6.
  PP: The patient sits with legs straddling the adjusting bench and arms relaxed in lap.
DP: Sit behind the patient.
CP: Hypothenar of the hand corresponding to the side of adjustive contact.

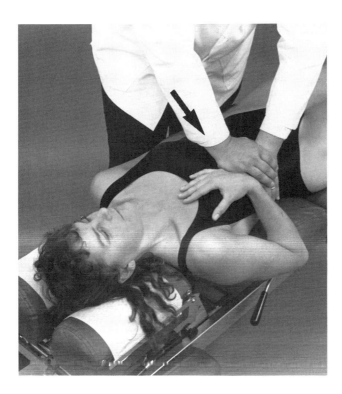

Figure 5.203 Covered thumb contact over the right anterior sixth rib to induce distraction in the right sixth costosternal articulation.

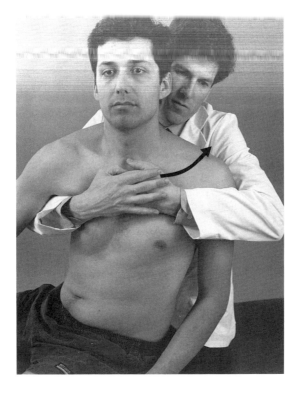

Figure 5.204 Hypothenar contact over the left third anterior rib to induce distraction in the third costosternal articulation.

SCP: Anterior rib just lateral to costosternal junction.

IH: Palm of superior hand reinforces dorsum of the contact hand.

VEC: Medial to lateral.

P: Slide laterally onto contact with the hypothenar of the contact hand and reinforce the contact with the palm of the indifferent hand. Develop distractive tension by tractioning laterally and rotating the patient toward the side of adjustive contact. At tension deliver a shallow impulse through both arms and the trunk. Avoid compression of the rib cage by inducing rotation and distraction during the adjustive thrust.

THE LUMBAR SPINE

The most important characteristic relative to the lumbar spine is that this area must bear tremendous loads because of the large, superimposed body weight, which interacts with forces generated by lifting and other activities involving powerful muscle actions. In addition to bearing formidable loads, the lumbar spine is largely responsible for trunk mobility thereby placing significant mechanical demands on this region.

Functional Anatomy

The body of a typical lumbar vertebra is a large, kidney-shaped structure designed to carry the heavy loads imposed by the upright posture. It is wider from side to side than from anterior to posterior. The anterior surface of the body is convex from side to side, while the posterior surface is concave

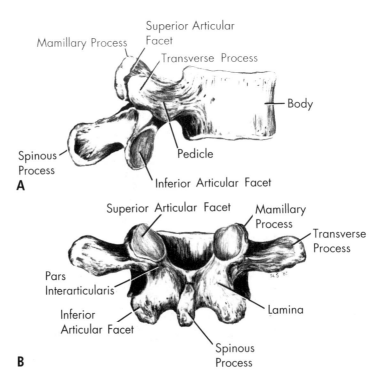

Figure 5.205 **(A)** Posterior and **(B)** side view of a lumbar segment. (From Dupuis and Kirkaldy-Willis,[77] with permission.)

from superior to inferior and from side to side. The superior and inferior surfaces are flat to slightly concave (Fig. 5-205).

The lumbar pedicles originate from the upper part of the body of the vertebra and extend horizontally and posteriorly. The pedicles are short and strong. The superior vertebral notch is shallow while the inferior vertebral notch is deep. The lumbar laminae are short, broad, and strong and run in a vertical plane (Fig. 5-205).

The thick and broad spinous processes are hatchet-shaped structures that point straight posteriorly. The transverse processes are long, slender, and flattened on their anterior and posterior surfaces. They originate from the lamina-pedicle junction and are considered to be quite frail. L3 has the longest of the lumbar transverse processes. The intervertebral foramen are large and triangular.

The articular processes are also large, thick, and strong. The superior articular processes are concave and face posterior and medial, while the inferior articular processes are convex and face anterior and lateral. The superior articular processes are wider apart and lay outside the inferior articular processes. The mammillary processes are located on the superior and posterior edge of the superior articular process. The lumbar facets lie primarily in the sagittal plane, but become more coronal at the lumbosacral junction (Fig. 5-206). This facet configuration limits rotational flexibility while allowing for greater mobility in flexion and extension (Fig. 5-207). The lumbar facets normally carry 10 percent of axial load and up to 33 percent in extended postures. The facets with their articular capsules provide up to 45 percent of the torsional strength of the lumbar spine.[28,29]

The lumbar intervertebral discs are well developed. The nucleus is localized somewhat posteriorly in the disc, and the disc height to body ratio is 1 : 3 (Fig. 5-208). This structure allows for more movement than the thoracic segments while maintaining a significant preload state, giving the disc greater resistance to axial compressive forces.

The lumbar spinal canal contains, supports and protects the distal portion of the lumbar enlargement of the spinal cord proximally (conus medularis)

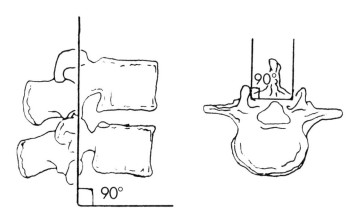

Figure 5.206 Lumbar facet planes. (From White and Panjabi,[1] with permission.)

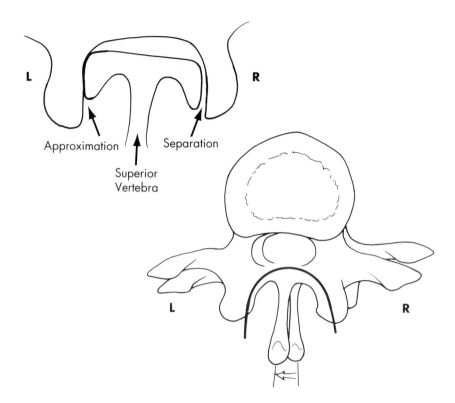

Figure 5.207 Right rotation of a lumbar segment showing effect of interlocking facets that cause the left facets to impact.

and the cauda equina with spinal nerves distally. This portion of the central nervous system is ensheathed in three meninges and tethered to the coccyx by the filum terminale. Because the cord itself ends at the level of L2, the nerve roots continue down the spinal canal as the cauda equina. The nerve roots exit the dura slightly above the foraminal opening, causing their course to be more oblique and their length to increase (Fig. 5-209). The dural sac and its contents are not freely mobile structures. A series of ligamentous

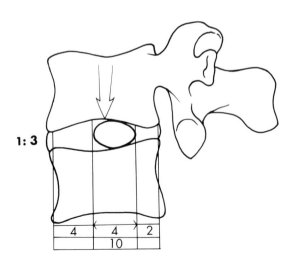

Figure 5.208 The location of the nucleus and disc height-to-body ratio in the lumbar spine.

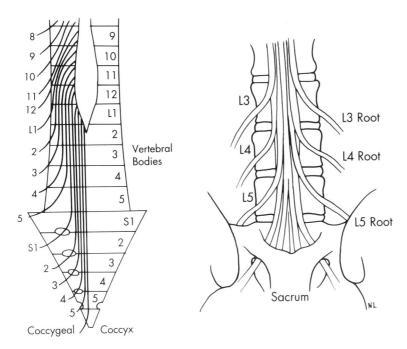

Figure 5.209 The course of the lumbar nerve roots.

attachments, called Hoffmann's ligaments, define a specific range of movement, thus stabilizing the dural sac within the foraminal canal (Fig. 5-210). Additionally, there will be changes in the spinal canal and cord during different movements and activities. When flexing from the neutral position the length of the spinal canal increases. This is because the instantaneous

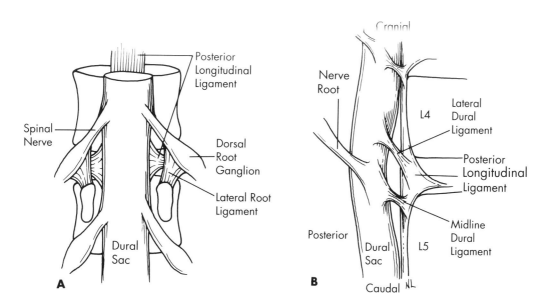

Figure 5.210 Hoffman's dural ligaments (A) posterior view and (B) lateral view with the posterior arch removed.

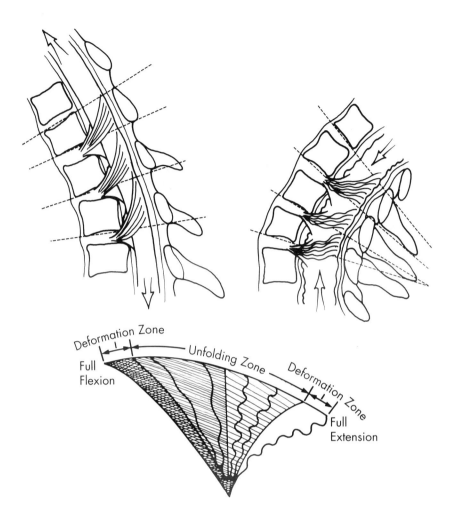

Figure 5.211 The effects of flexion (top left) and extension (top right) movements on the spinal canal and its contents (cord, meninges, and nerve roots).

axis of motion is located in the anterior aspect of the vertebral bodies. Similarly in extension, the canal length decreases. The spinal cord must follow the changes in the canal during these physiologic movements (Fig. 5-211). It accomplishes this through the mechanisms of folding and unfolding as well as elastic deformation. In the neutral position, the cord is folded somewhat like an accordion and has slight tension. During flexion, the cord will first unfold and then undergo elastic deformation. During extension the cord first folds upon itself, then undergoes elastic compression.

L5 is considered an atypical lumbar vertebra (Fig. 5-212). It has the largest circumference of all vertebrae and its body is thicker at its anterior aspect when compared with the posterior, though the overall thickness of the body is somewhat less than the bodies of the superior lumbar vertebrae. The transverse processes are short and thick. The spinous process is shorter and more rounded than the other lumbar vertebrae and the superior articulating

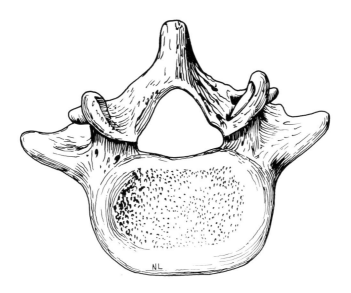

Figure 5.212 Structure of the L5 vertebra.

processes are directed more posteriorly and less medially. The inferior articulating processes are further apart and are oriented more in the coronal plane compared with the normal sagittal orientation of the remaining lumbar vertebrae.

Lumbar Curve

The secondary lordotic lumbar curve starts to develop when the child is about 9 to 12 months of age and beginning to sit up. As the child then later stands, the curve becomes established, usually by 18 months of age. The lumbar lordosis usually begins at the L1–2 level and gradually increases at each level caudally to the sacrum, with the apex of the curve centering around the L3–4 disc.[30] Moe et al. stated that the normal lumbar lordosis should be 40 to 60 degrees but failed to define the levels used for measurement.[31] The often ill-defined radiographic image of the superior aspect of the sacrum makes it difficult to use for measuring the lumbar lordosis. When using the inferior aspect of the L5 vertebral body and the superior aspect of the L1 vertebral body a normal range for the lumbar lordosis is 20 to 60 degrees[32,33] (Fig. 5-213).

In the upright bipedal posture, the lumbar curve, as well as the rest of the spine, is balanced on the sacrum. Therefore, changes in the sacral base angle can influence the depth of the anterior to posterior curves in the spine. The sacral base angle will increase with an anterior pelvic tilt, resulting in an increase in the lumbar lordosis, which places more weightbearing responsibility on the facets. The sacral base angle will decrease with a posterior pelvic tilt, resulting in a decrease in the lumbar lordosis, placing more weightbearing responsibility on the disc and reducing the spine's ability to absorb axial compression forces. Changes in the thoracic and cervical curve will occur, but, the extent and significance is difficult to predict.

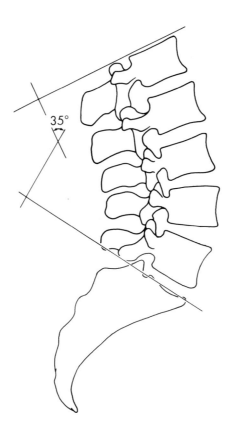

Figure 5.213 Measurement of the lumbar lordosis showing a 35° curve.

Range and Patterns of Motion (Table 5-9) (Fig. 5-24)

The lumbar spine is significantly more flexible in flexion and extension than any other lumbar movements. Approximately 75 percent of trunk flexion/extension occurs in the lumbar spine with approximately twice as much flexion occurring as extension. The first 60 degrees of torso flexion consists of lumbar spine sectional flexion as the pelvis is stabilized by the gluteal and hamstring muscles. After the lumbar flexion, the pelvis will begin to flex, producing an additional 30 degrees of motion. In contrast,

Table 5.9 Average Segmental Ranges of Motion for the Lumbar Spine

Vertebra	Combined Flexion and Extension	One Side Lateral Flexion	One Side Axial Rotation
L1–L2	12	6	2
L2–L3	14	6	2
L3–L4	15	8	2
L4–L5	16	6	2
L5–S1	17	3	1

(Adapted from White and Panjabi,[1] with permission.)

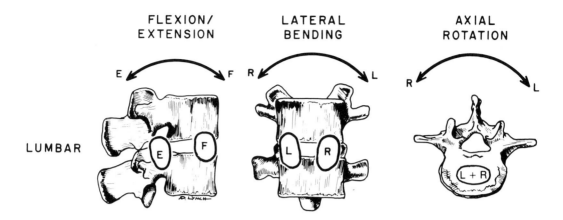

Figure 5.214 The approximate locations for the instantaneous axes of rotation for the six degrees of freedom in the lumbar segments. (From White and Panjabi,[1] with permission.)

lumbar lateral flexion exhibits only moderate mobility while axial rotation is quite limited. The majority of trunk rotation occurs in the thoracic spine.

Flexion/Extension

Combined segmental flexion/extension in the lumbar spine averages 15 degrees per segment, with motion increasing in a superior to inferior direction.[1,34] Lumbar flexion/extension combines sagittal plane rotation with an average 2–3 mm of sagittal plane translation in each direction.[1,35,36] White and Panjabi[1] have proposed that 1.5 mm be considered the upper limit for the radiographic investigation of clinical joint instability. Coupling of lateral flexion and rotation with flexion and extension have also been noted[24,36] but are considered by White and Panjabi[1] to be abnormal patterns suggestive of suboptimal muscle control.

The precise location of the instantaneous axis of rotation (IAR) for lumbar movements has not been established.[1] The IAR for flexion and extension are most commonly placed within the intervertebral disc of the subjacent vertebrae, with flexion located toward the anterior portion and extension toward the posterior (Fig. 5-214). During flexion the vertebra tilts and slides anteriorly as the inferior facets move superior and away from the lower vertebra. The disc is compressed anteriorly and stretched posteriorly. During extension the facets approximate one another, while the anterior longitudinal ligament, anterior portion of the joint capsule, and anterior portion of the disc are stretched (Fig. 5-215).

Lateral Flexion

Segmental lateral flexion averages approximately 6 degrees to each side. Movement is about the same for each segment, with the exception of the lumbosacral joint, which demonstrates about half the movement.[1,34] Lateral flexion in the lumbar spine is coupled with opposite side rotation (i.e., body rotation to the convexity and spinous deviation to the concavity). This leads to a pattern in which the spinous processes end up pointing in the same

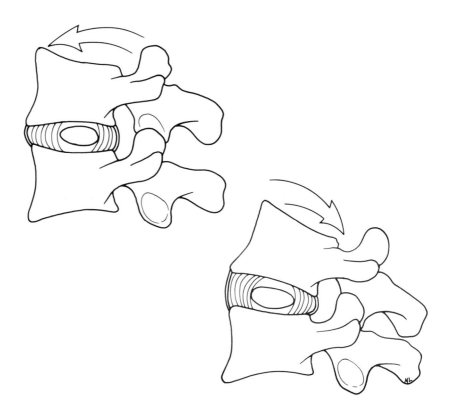

Figure 5.215 Flexion and extension movements of a lumbar segment.

direction as the lateral flexion (Fig. 5-216).[1,37] This pattern is opposite to that in the cervical and upper thoracic spine (Figs. 5-113, 114).

The instantaneous axis of rotation for lateral flexion is placed within the subadjacent disc space.[1] For left lateral flexion the axis is located on the right side, and with right lateral flexion on the left (Fig. 5-214). During lateral flexion the vertebra tilts and slides toward the concave side, producing a smooth continuous arc. The facets approximate on the concave side and separate on the convex side. The disc is compressed on the concave side and is stretched on the convex side. The ligamentum flavum, intertransverse ligament, and capsular ligaments are stretched on the convex side.

Grice and Cassidy[38,39] have studied the coupling movements for lateral flexion and have proposed classifying segmental lateral flexion into one of four commonly encountered patterns (Fig. 5-217). Additionally various pathomechanical theories have been proposed as possible explanations for each abnormal pattern. The first pattern, type I movement, exhibits the normal pattern of coupling in which lateral flexion is associated with axial rotation to the opposite side. This produces a pattern in which posterior body rotation occurs on the side opposite the lateral flexion and the spinous processes rotate toward the side of lateral flexion. Purportedly this pattern is represented when normal motor control is exerted through eccentric unilateral contraction of the quadratus lumborum muscle, though synergistic muscles act as a brake to prevent hypermobilities. Type I movement may still be abnormal if it is diminished or excessive (Fig. 5-217A).

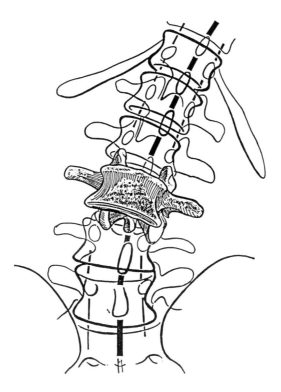

Figure 5.216 Coupling pattern of lateral flexion with contralateral rotation in the lumbar spine. (From Kapandji,[79] with permission.

Type II motion combines lateral flexion and axial rotation to the same side. This induces posterior body rotation on the side of lateral flexion and rotation of the spinous process to the side opposite the lateral flexion. A muscular imbalance of the sacrospinalis, especially the longissimus and spinalis portions, is proposed as the source of this abnormal pattern. The semi-slumped sitting posture may also produce this pattern of movement (Fig. 5-217B).

Type III movement is represented by aberrant segmental lateral flexion and normal coupled rotation. With type III movement the involved segment demonstrates no lateral flexion, with side bending or lateral flexion movement in the direction opposite the bending of the trunk. This pattern is theorized to result from faulty disc mechanics or overdominance of the quadratus lumborum or intertransversalis muscles (Fig. 5-217C).

The last pattern, Type IV, is represented by aberrant segmental rotation and lateral flexion. This pattern may also result from faulty disc mechanics or an imbalance in the psoas or multifidus muscles (Fig. 5-217D).

These patterns are primarily determined by evaluation of lateral bending functional X-ray studies. The use of lateral flexion and flexion–extension movement radiographs have been described (Fig. 3-23) and recommended for evaluation of segmental motion and instability.[38–56] While functional radiology should be considered an important potential tool in the evaluation of joint dysfunction, its limitations should also be realized. There is evidence to suggest that findings on lateral bending radiographs do not correlate well with back pain and other clinical findings.[48,57]

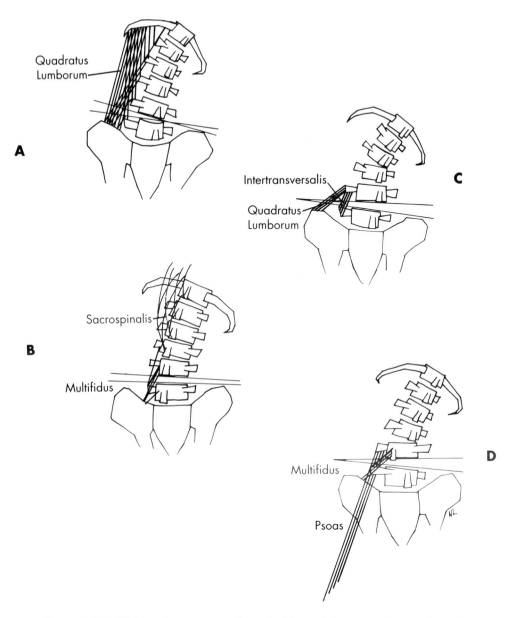

Figure 5.217 **(A)** Type I movement of coupled lateral flexion with contralateral rotation under the control of the quadratus lumborum muscle. **(B)** Type II movement of coupled lateral flexion with ipsilateral rotation under the control of the sacrospinalis and multifidus muscles. This pattern may be sectional, as shown here, or segmental. **(C)** Type III movement consisting of segmental aberrant lateral flexion owing to faulty disc mechanics and/or quadratus lumborum and intertransversalis muscles. **(D)** Type IV movement consisting of segmental aberrant lateral flexion and rotation owing to faulty disc mechanics and/or psoas and multifidus muscles.

Rotation

Axial rotation is quite limited in the lumbar spine. Segmental range of motion is uniform throughout the lumbar segments and averages only 2 degrees per motion segment[1,34] The sagittally oriented facet joints act as a significant barrier to rotational mobility. During rotation the facet joints glide apart on the side of rotation and approximate on the side opposite rotation (Fig. 5-207). The instantaneous axis for axial rotation is placed within the posterior nucleus and annulus[1] (Fig. 5-214).

Rotation of the lumbar spine is also consistently coupled with lateral flexion and slight sagittal plane rotation. The coupled lateral flexion varies between upper and lower lumbar segments. Rotation in the upper three segments (L1–L3) is coupled with opposite side lateral flexion. Rotation in the lower two segments (L4–S1) is coupled with same side lateral flexion.[24,58] The transitional change in coupling that occurs at the L4–L5 motion segment may be of clinical significance in predisposing this level to increased clinical instability and degenerative change.[1]

The pattern of coupled sagittal plane rotation depends on the starting position of the lumbar spine.[24] With the spine in a neutral starting position, the lumbar spine flexes at all levels when rotated. When the spine is rotated from a flexed posture it has a tendency to extend, and when rotated from an extended posture it has a tendency to flex. This pattern was also noted for lateral flexion leading to the generalization that "lateral bending or axial rotation has a tendency to straighten the spine (go toward neutral posture) from the flexed as well as the extended postures."[1]

Kinetics of the Lumbar Spine

The control of flexion movements is largely due to the eccentric contraction of the erector spinae (sacrospinalis) muscle (Fig. 5-218) though it is initiated by concentric contraction of the psoas and abdominals. The iliopsoas flexes the spine when the femur is fixed, and the abdominal muscles flex the spine when the pelvis is fixed. During the first 60 degrees of flexion the pelvis is locked by the gluteus maximus and hamstrings, but after 60 degrees the weight of the trunk overcomes the stabilizing force of the glutei and hamstrings and the pelvis rotates an additional 30 degrees at the hips. In full flexion all the muscles are relaxed except the iliocostalis thoracis and the trunk is supported by ligaments and passive muscle tension. The return to neutral is the reverse activity, with the pelvis moving first under the control of the hip extensors, followed by extension of the lumbar spine controlled by erector spinae muscles. Flexion is limited by the ligamentum flavum, posterior longitudinal ligament, posterior aspect of the capsular ligament, and interspinal ligament.

Extension is initiated by concentric contraction of the sacrospinalis. Again after the initial movement, gravity and eccentric activity of the abdominal muscles take over to be the major controlling force in extension. Extension is limited by the anterior longitudinal ligament, anterior annulus, and most significantly, by bony impact of the spinous processes and articular facets.

Lateral flexion is initiated by concentric contraction of the quadratus lumborum on the ipsilateral side and then immediately controlled by eccen-

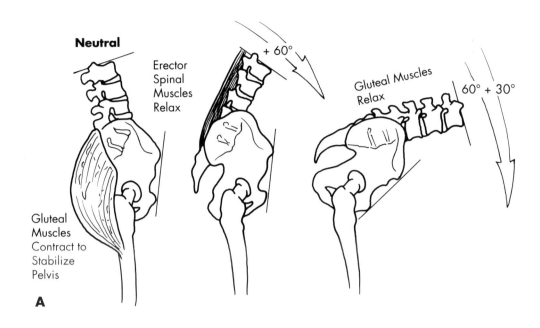

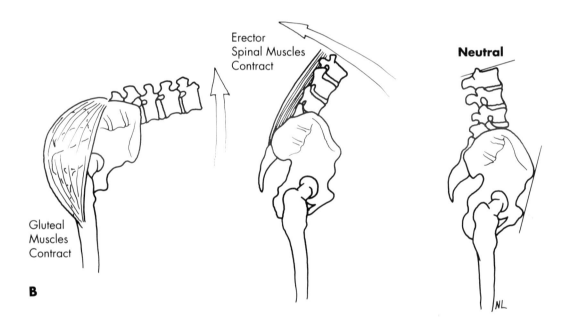

Figure 5.218 Flexion of the trunk. **(A)** The first 60 degrees of flexion involve eccentric contraction of the lumbar paraspinal muscles followed by an additional 30 degrees of hip flexion after relaxation of the gluteal muscles. **(B)** In extension the converse occurs.

tric activity of the contralateral quadratus lumborum. Lateral flexion movement is limited by impact of the articular facets on the side of bending, and the capsular ligaments, ligamentum flavum, intertransverse ligament, and deep lumbar fascia on the contralateral side. The theoretical explanations for lumbar coupled motion during lateral flexion include

It is not possible to bend a curved rod without some rotation

Lateral bending is controlled mainly by eccentric activity of the quadratus lumborum, which inserts posterior to the normal axis of motion. The normal axis is located in the posterior one-third of the disc. Therefore, normal muscular activity leads to rotation of the bodies posterior on the side of convexity and rotation of the spinous processes to the side of concavity.

Rotation is initiated by concentric activity of the abdominal obliques and assisted by concentric activity of the short segmental muscles (multifidus and rotatores) on the contralateral side. Rotational movements are controlled or limited by eccentric activity of the ipsilateral multifidus and rotatores (though mainly limited by facetal design) as well as the capsular, interspinous, and flaval ligaments. Balancing contraction of the contralateral muscles is important in maintaining the normal instantaneous axis of motion for axial rotation.

EVALUATION OF THE LUMBAR SPINE

Observation

The assessment of lumbar function should begin with an evaluation of lumbopelvic alignment and range of motion. The sacral base forms the foundation of the spine, and a functional or structural alteration in the pelvis or lower extremities may alter the alignment of the lumbar spine and segments above. Pelvic and hip alignment is evaluated by observing the alignment of the gluteal folds, posterior iliac spines (sacral dimples), and iliac crests. To palpate the alignment of the pelvis, place the thumbs on the posterior iliac spines and fingertips along the superior margin of the crests (Fig. 5-219). Compare each side for symmetry and their orientation to the greater trochanter for possible leg length inequality. Coronal plane alignment of the lumbar spine is evaluated by observing the orientation of the spinous process, status of the paraspinal muscles, and contours of the waist (Fig. 5-220). Scoliotic curvatures in the lumbar spine are frequently represented by muscle symmetry and increased paraspinal muscle mass on the convex side of scoliosis. Compensatory curvatures are common in the lumbar spine, and any noted deviations should be followed up with an assessment of leg length.

Sagittal plane orientation of the hips, pelvis, and lumbar spine is evaluated from the side. The lumbosacral angle, in large part, determines the angle of the lumbar curve and is often mirrored by the positioning of the pelvis. Anterior or posterior tilting of the pelvis usually results from alterations in the hip angle. Anterior pelvic tilt results from bilateral hip flexion, and posterior pelvic tilt results from bilateral hip extension (Fig. 5-221). Anterior

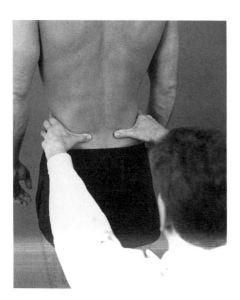

Figure 5.219 Observation of lumbopelvic alignment and posture with palpation of the posterior iliac spines and iliac crests.

pelvic tilt increases the lumbosacral angle and lumbar curve; posterior pelvic tilt reduces the lumbosacral angle and curve. The lumbar curve will also alter its angle relative to structural alteration in the thoracic curve. Congenitally straight thoracic curves often lead to straightening of the lumbar and cervical curves. Increased thoracic kyphosis may lead to accentuation of the lumbar and cervical curves.

Lumbopelvic movement should be observed for range and symmetry. Flexion, extension, and lateral flexion are usually assessed with the patient standing. Rotation is more effectively evaluated in the sitting position to fix the pelvis and prevent hip rotation. To assess flexion, the patient bends

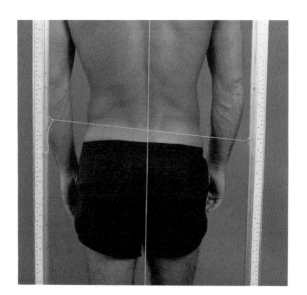

Figure 5.220 Posterior plumb line observation demonstrating pelvic unleveling, low on the right with a right convex curve in the lumbar spine.

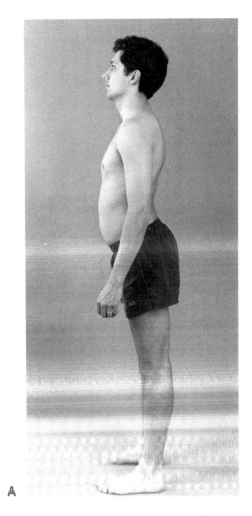
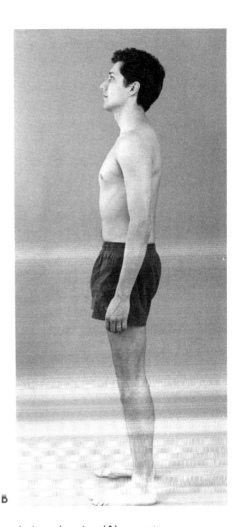

Figure 5.221 Observation of posture from a lateral view showing **(A)** an anterior pelvic tilt with lumbar hyperlordosis and **(B)** a posterior pelvic tilt with lumbar hypolordosis.

forward, and any limitations, painful arcs, or alterations in normal sequencing are observed. With normal range the patient should be able to come within several inches off the floor with the fingertips and the lumbar curve should reverse (Fig. 5-222). After the patient returns to neutral, the doctor should stabilize the patient's hips while extension is performed. Extension is significantly more limited than flexion, and mild midline lumbosacral discomfort is commonly associated with full extension. Lateral bending is evaluated by instructing patients to bend to one side while running their fingers down the lateral surface of the leg. It is important to insure that the patient does not axially rotate the trunk, bend the knee, or raise the foot off the floor while bending. The movement should be symmetric, and the doctor should record where the patient's fingertips pass relative to the

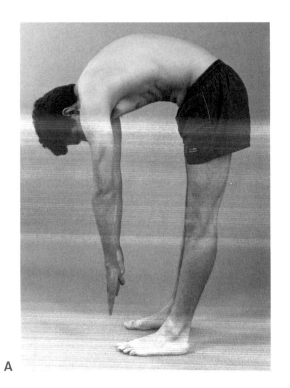

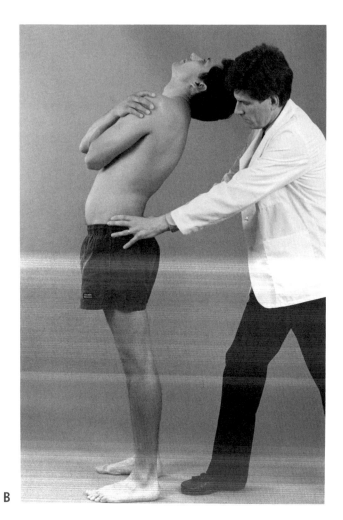

Figure 5.222 Observation of thoracolumbar ranges of motion: (**A**) flexion; (**B**) extension. (*Figure continues.*)

knees. A smooth C curve should be observed to the side of bending. Areas of regional restriction or increased movement may be noted by observing for a sudden break (bent stick configuration) in integrated movement.

To isolate movements of the lumbar spine from hip and thoracic movements, the doctor may employ inclinometric methods and measure movement between the thoracolumbar and lumbosacral regions. Table 5-10 lists the normal ranges for lumbar movement; the methods for measuring movement have been previously described (Fig. 3-10).

Static Palpation

To evaluate the bony and soft tissue structures of the lumbar spine, the patient is placed in the prone position and scanned for areas of potential tenderness, misalignment, or asymmetry. To scan the bony landmarks, use

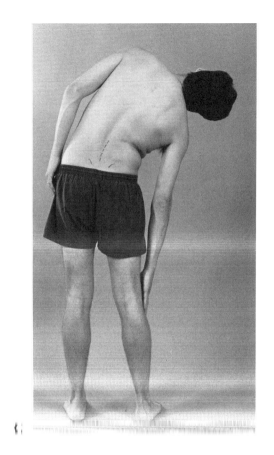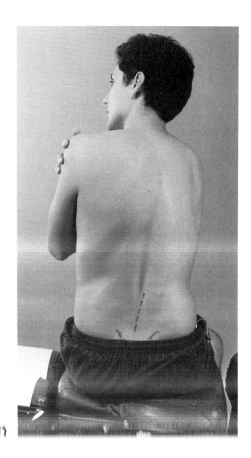

Figure 5.222 (*Continued*). (**C**) lateral flexion; (**D**) rotation.

the pads of the fingers or thumbs and palpate the spinous processes, interspinous spaces, and mammillary processes (Fig. 5-223). Palpation of the interspinous spaces is enhanced by placing a small roll under the abdomen
or elevating the lumbar and pelvic sections of an articulating table. The
mammillary processes are not distinctly palpable; rather the doctor feels
for a sense of firmness in the soft tissue as the contact passes over each
mammillary process. Rotational prominence of lumbar spinal segments is
perceived by a sense of fullness in the muscles over the top of the mammillary
processes and not by actual palpation of bony rotation.

Table 5.10 Global Ranges of Motion for the
            Lumbar Spine

Flexion	40°–60°
Extension	20°–35°
One Side Lateral Flexion	15°–25°
One Side Rotation	5°–18°

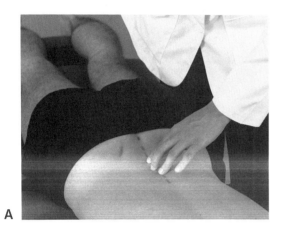
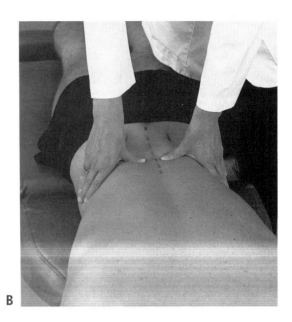

Figure 5.223 Palpation of lumbar (**A**) interspinous alignment and sensitivity and (**B**) paraspinal muscle tone, texture, and sensitivity.

Palpation of the lumbar paraspinal soft tissues is conducted by applying bilateral contacts with the palmar surfaces of the fingers or thumbs. Evaluation should incorporate an assessment of tone and texture of the erector spinae, quadratus lumborum, deep segmental muscles, and iliolumbar ligaments. The psoas muscle should also be palpated for tone and tenderness. The psoas is accessible for palpation in the supine position, and the belly becomes more evident by inducing hip flexion on the side of palpation.

Motion Palpation

Joint Play

The lumbar spine may be scanned in the sitting or prone position for sites of painful or restricted joint play. Sites of suspected abnormality should be further assessed with specific joint play tests. The same methods applied in the thoracic spine for assessing posterior to anterior glide and counter rotation may be applied to the lumbar spine (Fig. 5-224). Additional options include the evaluation of rotation with mammillary contacts, the assessment of lateral glide, and a side posture method for evaluating possible instability.

To assess rotational joint play with mammillary contacts, the doctor reaches around the patient with the cephalic hand and grasps the lower anterior rib cage while the caudal hand contacts the inferior mammillary process of the motion segment to be evaluated (Fig. 5-225). The hand contacting the rib cage induces gentle rotation of the trunk away from the table, and the doctor applies downward pressure through the contact hand. This method is designed to assess rotational gapping in the direction of trunk rotation, in the motion segment superior to the mammillary contact.

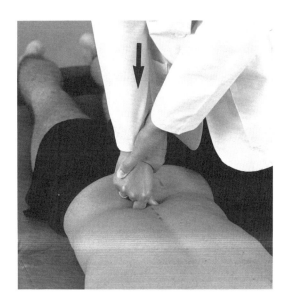

Figure 5.224 Lumbar joint play evaluation for posterior to anterior glide using a contact over the posterior aspect of the L4 spinous process.

Normal movement is represented by a sense of giving and forward movement on the side of contact.

Lateral glide of individual lumbar motion segments may be evaluated in the prone position by establishing a thumb contact against the lateral surface of adjacent spinous processes with the cephalic hand while the other hand grasps the patient's anterior medial thigh (Fig. 5-226). Movement is induced by applying medial pressure against the spinous process while the patient's leg is passively abducted. Normal movement is represented by segmental opening and closing at the spinous process away from the contact. This procedure can also be performed by moving the pelvic section of a flexion table from side to side.

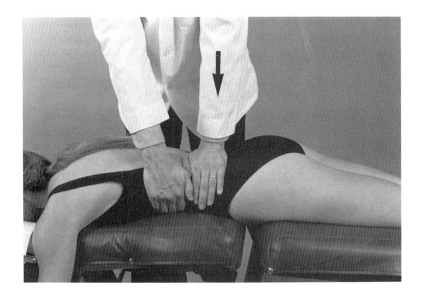

Figure 5.225 Lumbar joint play evaluation for unilateral posterior to anterior glide and gapping in the left L1–L2 articulation using a thenar contact over the posterior aspect of the left L2 mammillary process.

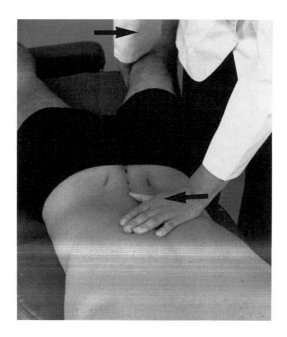

Figure 5.226 Lumbar joint play evaluation for lateral glide in the L3–L4 articulation using a thumb contact across the left L3–L4 interspinous space.

To evaluate segmental stability in side posture place the patient on either side with the upper thigh and knee flexed. Establish a fingertip contact over the spinous processes and interspinous spaces with the cephalic hand and straddle the patient's flexed knee (Fig. 5-227). Apply posterior shearing pressure through the patient's knee and gentle anterior pressure through the palpation hand. Feel for gliding between adjacent spinous processes. Excessive posterior glide (translation) of the inferior spinous process relative to the superior spinous process suggests possible clinical joint instability.

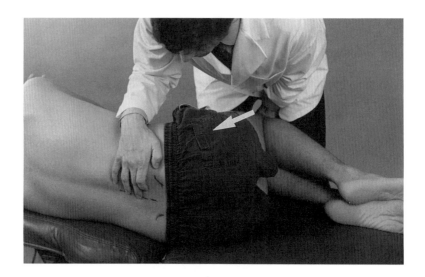

Figure 5.227 Side posture evaluation for lumbar instability with the doctor applying a force anterior to posterior along the line of the shaft of the patient's femur while palpating for increased translational movement between L3 and L4.

Lumbar Segmental Motion Palpation and End Play

Lumbar segmental motion may be evaluated in the sitting or side posture positions. Both postures are effective for assessing lumbar mobility, but side posture positions do not provide as much freedom for full trunk movement. This is especially true for the evaluation of lumbar lateral flexion and end play.

Sitting methods

For sitting evaluations place the patient on an adjusting bench or palpation stool with the arms crossed over the chest. The doctor may sit behind or stand beside the patient. Movement is controlled through contacts on the patient's shoulders.

Rotation. Lumbar segmental rotation is evaluated by establishing a thumb contact against the lateral surface of adjacent spinous processes. The contact is placed on the side of induced rotation so that the pad spans the interspinous space. The support hand reaches around the front of the patient and grasps the opposite forearm or is placed across the patient's shoulder and rotates the patient's trunk toward the side of contact (Fig. 5-228). During normal rotation the doctor should palpate the superior spinous process, rotating away from the spinous process below. Movement should occur in the direction of trunk rotation. If separation is not noted and adjacent spinous processes move together, segmental restriction should be suspected.

Lumbar segmental movement is quite limited in rotation (1 to 2 degrees), and the examiner may not be able to discriminate reductions of movement within these limits. Therefore the doctor should concentrate on whether

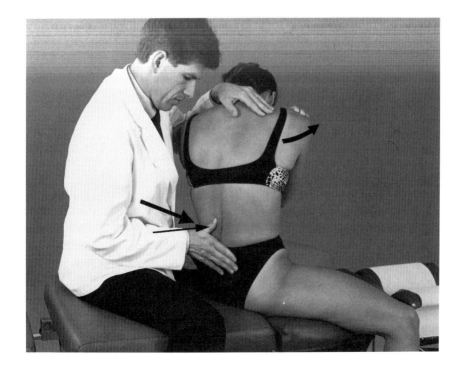

Figure 5.228 End feel evaluation for left rotation at the L2–L3 articulation using a thumb contact across the left L2–L3 interspace.

the segment moves from its neutral position (any shifting between adjacent spinous processes) and on the quality of end play movement.

Although the lumbar facets do provide a bony obstacle to rotation there is still some normal give to rotational end play. To assess end play the doctor applies additional overpressure at the end of passive motion. Contacts may be established against the superior spinous process on the side of induced rotation (Fig. 5-228) or over the mammillary process and posterior joint on the side opposite the induced rotation. Comparing the quality of end play between these two contacts may help in determining the side of joint restriction.

Lateral flexion. To assess lateral flexion, the palpation contact is also established against the lateral surface of adjacent spinous processes. The contact is placed on the side of desired lateral flexion and the patient is asked to bend toward the side of contact (Fig. 5-229). The doctor guides movement by applying downward pressure through the shoulder contact and medial pressure through the contact hand. The indifferent arm and contact arm must work together to maximize bending at the site of palpation. To induce lateral flexion in the lumbar spine the patient's upper trunk must be shifted sufficiently to the side of bending. During the performance of lateral flexion the doctor should feel the spine bend smoothly around the contact and the spinous process shift toward the opposite side (convex side).

End play evaluation is conducted by shifting the contact to the superior spinous process and applying additional overpressure at the end range of

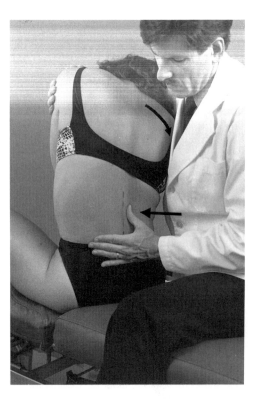

Figure 5.229 End feel evaluation for right lateral flexion at the L2–L3 articulation using a thumb contact across the right lateral aspect of the L2–L3 interspace.

motion. Lateral flexion end play is more elastic than rotation; a firm but giving response should be noted.

Flexion and extension. Lumbar flexion and extension is evaluated by establishing palpation contacts in the interspinous spaces with the doctor's fingertips or dorsal middle phalanx of the index finger (Fig. 5-230). Movement is induced by asking the patient to slouch and arch the lumbar spine. The indifferent arm and palpation hand help guide movement and insure that the apex of bending is accentuated at the level of palpation. During flexion the interspinous spaces should open, and during extension they should approximate.

Flexion end play is assessed by contacting the superior spinous process with the thumb and springing in an anterior and superior direction with the contact hand while applying downward pressure through the patient's shoulders (Fig. 5-231A). To induce extension, push anteriorly against the contact while inducing backward bending (Fig. 5-231B). Extension end play is inhibited by the impact of the spinous processes and has a more rigid quality than flexion.

Side posture methods
To conduct side posture mobility tests, patients are placed on their side with their down side arm crossed over the chest and resting on the opposite shoulder. The down side leg is extended along the length of the table and

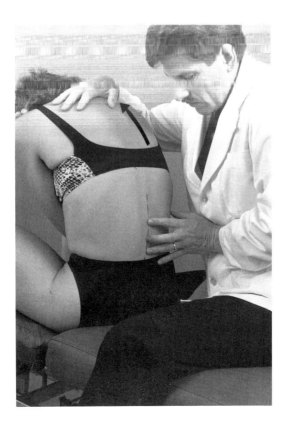

Figure 5.230 Movement evaluation of active and passive lumbar flexion with fingertip contacts in the L2–L3 and L3–L4 interspace.

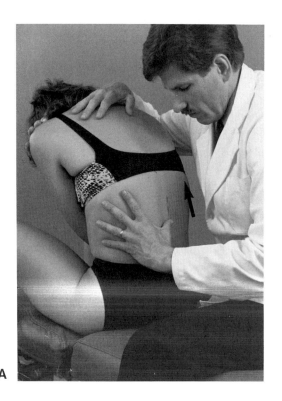 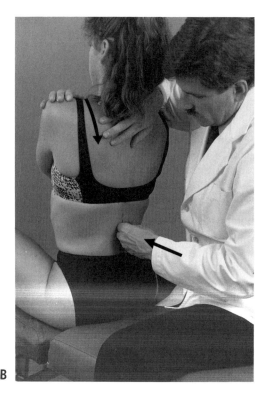

A

B

Figure 5.231 **(A)** End play evaluation for flexion at the L2–L3 articulation using a thumb contact over the inferior tip of the L2 spinous process. **(B)** Lumbar extension end play with a reinforced interphalangeal joint contact over the L2–L3 interspace.

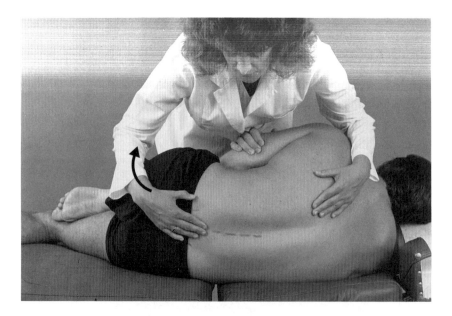

Figure 5.232 Side posture movement evaluation for **(A)** flexion. (*Figure continues.*)

the knee and hip of the opposite leg is flexed. The doctor controls movement through the patient's shoulders and by cradling the patient's flexed leg.

Flexion and extension. To evaluate flexion and extension, stand facing the patient and cradle the patient's flexed knee between your thighs. Palpate the interspinous space with the caudal hand and grasp the patient's shoulder with the cephalic hand and forearm. Induce flexion and extension by moving patient's knees superiorly and inferiorly and feel for opening and closing of the interspinous spaces (Fig. 5-232).

Lateral flexion. To assess lateral flexion use the caudal hand to establish a contact on the ischial tuberosity and gluteal soft tissues of the patient's up side hip. Place the fingertips or thumb of the doctor's cephalic hand on either side of adjacent spinous processes and interspinous space. To induce movement push headward against the patient's pelvis with the caudal hand while palpating for movement at the interspinal spaces (Fig. 5-233). On the concave side of bending the interspinous spaces should close and open on the convex side. If dysfunction is present the spinous processes do not move into the doctor's palpating fingers on the convex side (down side) or remain firm and do not glide away if palpating is done from the concave side (up side).

Rotation. Side posture lumbar rotation may be assessed by inducing movement through the patient's trunk or pelvis (Fig. 5-234). If the patient's trunk is used the indifferent contacts are established against the patient's up side shoulder. If the pelvis is used the indifferent contacts are established against the patient's thigh. To contact the torso, slide the forearm between the patient's arm and chest and contact the shoulder. When contacting the shoulder, have the patient grasp the opposite forearm with the up side hand or the shoulder will not provide enough resistance to induce rotation.

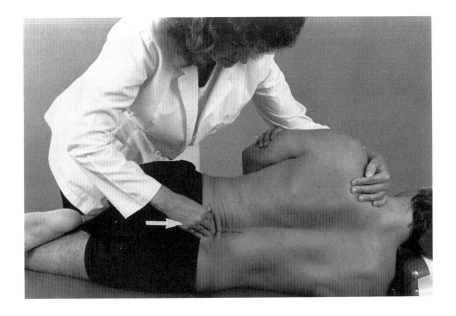

Figure 5.232 (*Continued*). (**B**) Extension of the L4–L5 motion segment using a fingertip contact over the L4–L5 interspace.

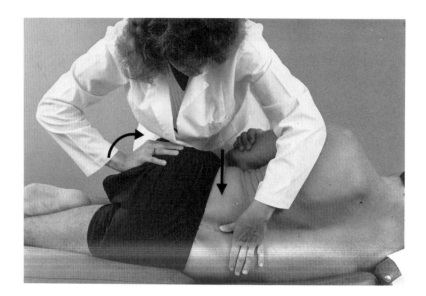

Figure 5.233 Side posture movement evaluation for lateral flexion of the L2–L3 motion segment using a thumb contact over the lateral aspect of the L2–L3 interspace.

To induce movement through the pelvis, contact the patient's up thigh with the dorsal surface of caudal ankle. For both methods locate the palpation contacts at the desired interspinous space with the middle finger or thumb of caudal hand.

To induce trunk movement apply posterior pressure against the patient's shoulder and forearm. To induce pelvic rotation, apply downward pressure against the patient's distal thigh. When movement is initiated through the trunk, the superior spinous process rotates away from the inferior spinous process in the direction of trunk rotation (toward the table). When movement is initiated with the pelvis, the inferior spinous process rotates away from the superior spinous process in the direction of pelvic rotation (away from the table).

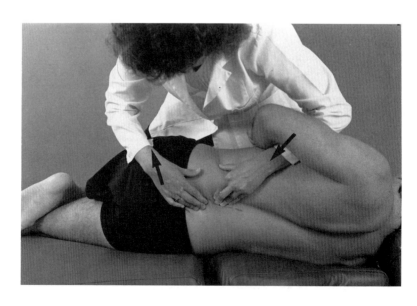

Figure 5.234 Side posture movement evaluation for left rotation of the L3–L4 motion segment using fingertip contacts over the left lateral surface of the L3 spinous process and right lateral surface of the L4 spinous process.

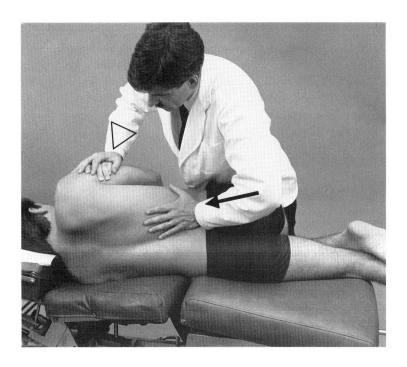

Figure 5.235 Side posture mammillary push adjustment.

ADJUSTMENTS OF THE LUMBAR SPINE

Side Posture Adjustments

Side posture lumbar adjustments are the most frequently applied adjustments for lumbar spinal dysfunction (Fig. 5-235). They offer freedom of movement to alter patient position and adaptability to methods that improve the doctor's leverage and mechanical advantage. Although they are difficult adjustments to perfect, one can reduce the frustration by understanding their mechanical principles and effects.

The specific level of joint tension is in large part determined by patient positioning. The level of segmental tension is regulated by the degree of induced lumbar flexion, lateral flexion, and the amount of counter rotation induced between the shoulders and pelvis (Fig. 5-236). The direction of adjustive thrust in relation to the direction of torso movement and pelvic movement is also critical to localizing the adjustive thrust. Adjustments that direct the adjustive thrust in the same direction as torso movement but opposite pelvic movement are defined as assisted adjustments. Adjustments that direct the adjustive thrust in a direction opposite the torso movement and in the same direction as pelvic movement are defined as resisted adjustments (Fig. 5-237). Assisted adjustments should develop maximal pre-adjustive tension in the motion segment inferior to the established contact, and resisted adjustments should develop maximal tension in the motion segment superior to the established contact.

The degree of torso movement is determined by the positioning of the patient's shoulders and the degree of pelvic movement is determined by the placement of the patient's pelvis. Various methods for positioning and

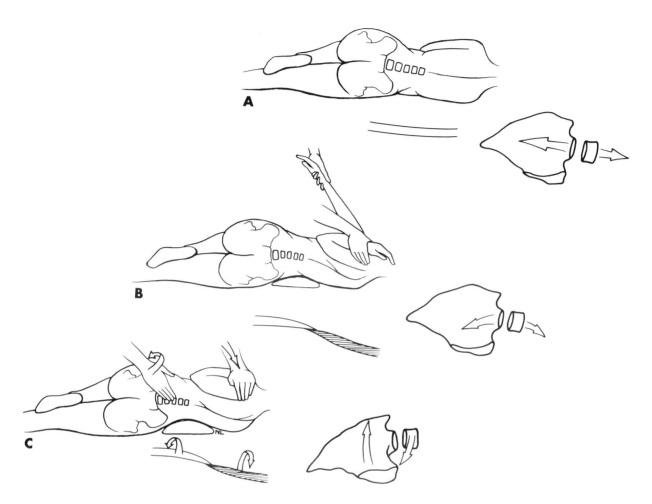

Figure 5.236 Side posture patient positioning. (**A**) Development of segmental flexion and distraction of the posterior joint by flexing the patient's upper knee and hip. (**B**) Development of lateral flexion by placing a pillow under the lumbar spine and pulling the patient's shoulder down and forward. (**C**) Counter rotation of the pelvis and shoulders to induce gapping distraction at the upper facet joint and centripetal distraction on the upper disc space.

contacting the patient's shoulders and pelvis are pictured in Figs. 5-238 to 5-240.

Proper utilization of body weight is also critical to the effective application of side posture adjusting. Side posture adjustments often demand the added force that is produced by incorporating the doctor's body weight in the development of pre-adjustive tension and adjustive thrusts.

Prone and Knee Chest Adjustments

Prone and knee chest adjustments are applied with specific short lever contacts (Fig. 5-241). They are especially suited to the treatment of extension restrictions or adjusting situations in which it is desirable to minimize rotation. Extension is easily induced in the prone or knee chest positions, and

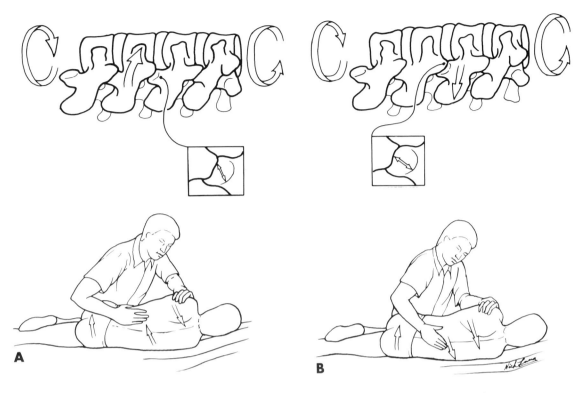

Figure 5.237 Side posture positioning for rotational dysfunction. (**A**) Resisted positioning with contact applied to the inferior vertebra to induce gapping in the joint superior to the contact. (**B**) Assisted positioning with contact applied to the superior vertebra to induce gapping in the joint inferior to the contact. Arrows on vertebrae indicate adjustive vectors and contact points.

the lumbar sagittal facet facings do not conflict with anteriorly directed adjustive vectors. The doctor also has the advantage of centering the body over the contact.

Since the knee chest positions are especially helpful in maximizing lumbar extension, the patient is vulnerable to hyperextension in this position. Therefore, the doctor must be skilled in the application of this procedure and deliver the adjustive thrust in a shallow and non-recoiling manner.

Sitting Lumbar Adjustments

Sitting lumbar adjustments (Fig. 5-242) conform to the same mechanical principles previously discussed for sitting thoracic adjustments. They employ assisted methods and develop maximal tension in the motion segment below the vertebra contacted. They are typically applied for lumbar rotation or combined rotation and lateral flexion dysfunction. The most frequent site of application occurs at the thoracolumbar region. Critical to their application is an understanding of the thoracolumbar transition to sagittal facet orientation and the impact this has on axial rotation and facet movements.

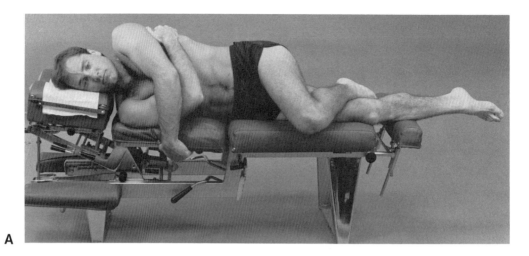

A

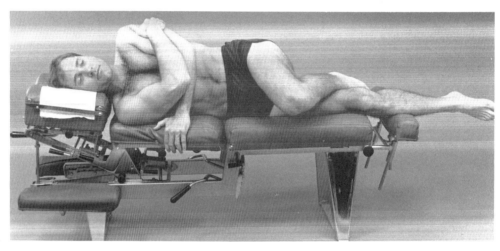

B

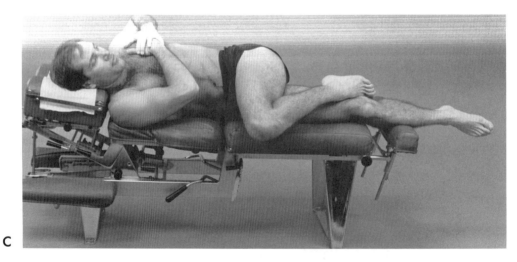

C

Figure 5.238 Optional patient arm positioning for side posture adjusting. (A) Forward positioning of the upper arm applied with flexible individuals to maintain neutral trunk positioning. (B) Midline positioning of the upper arm to accommodate neutral positions or positions incorporating trunk rotation. (C) Posterior positioning of the upper arm applied with large patients or specifically to induce posterior movement of the trunk.

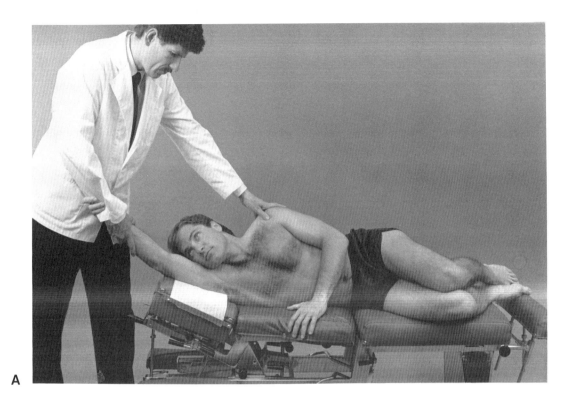

A

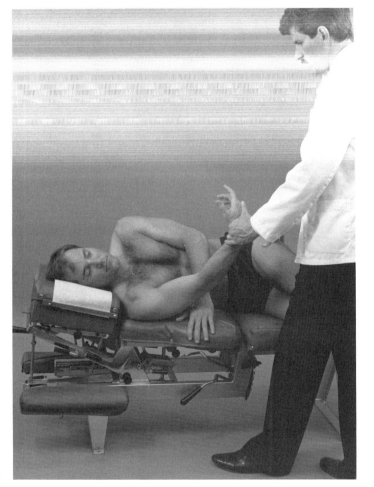

B

Figure 3.239 Movement of
the patient's lower arm to assist in the development of
lateral flexion. (**A**) Lateral
flexion away from the table
induced by pulling the arm
headward to place the pa-
tient on the lateral surface
of the shoulder (demon-
strated here for left lateral
flexion). (**B**) Lateral flexion
toward the table induced by
pulling the arm footward to
place the patient on the posterolateral surface of the
shoulder. Elevation of the
pelvic and lumbar sections
or a pillow placed under the
lumbar spine will assist in
the development of lateral
flexion toward the table.

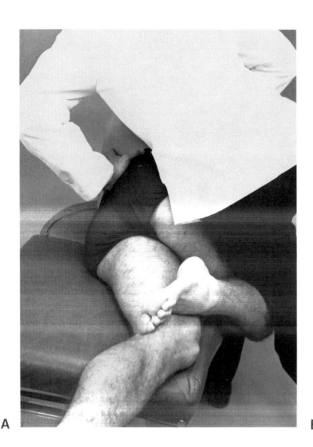 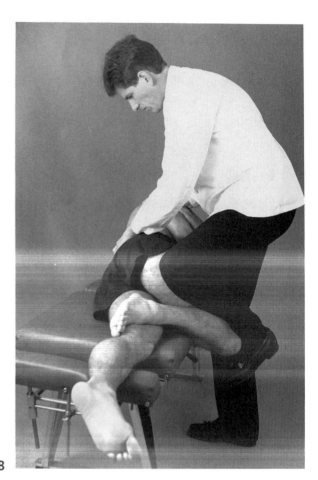

Figure 5.240 Optional leg contacts that may be employed in the application of side posture pelvic and lumbar adjustments. (**A**) Lateral thigh to thigh contact. (**B**) Shin to knee contact. (*Figure continues.*)

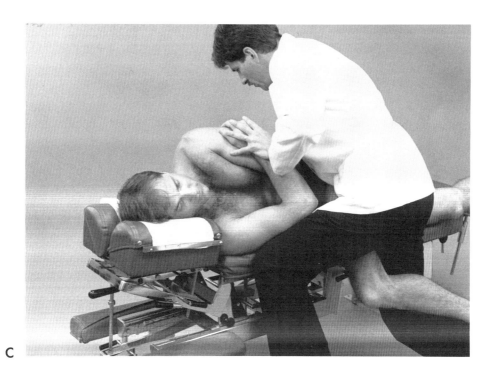

C

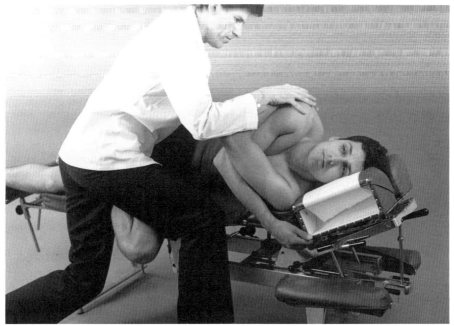

D

Figure 5.240 (*Continued*). **(C)** Straddling thigh contact. **(D)** Straddling flexed knee contact.

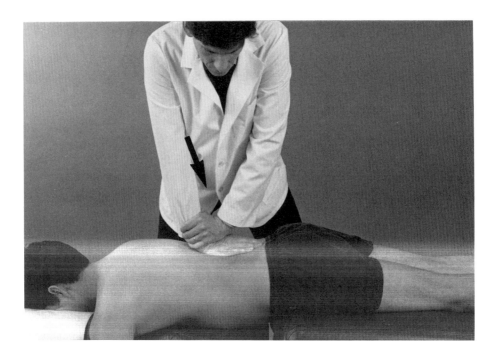

Figure 5.241 Prone unilateral hypothenar mammillary adjustment.

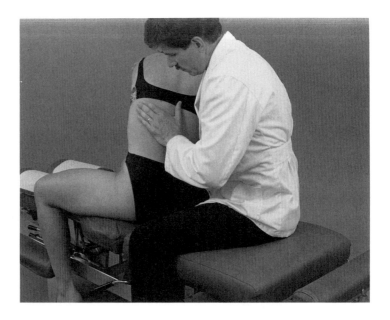

Figure 5.242 Sitting mammillary push adjustment.

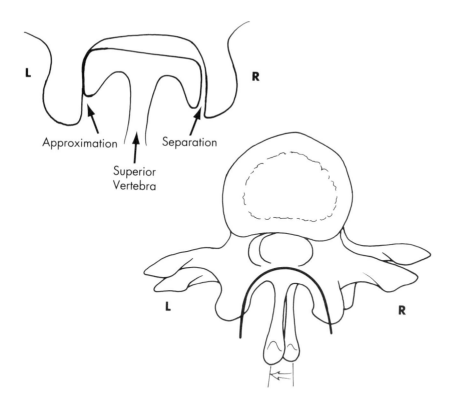

Figure 5.243 Illustration of right rotation demonstrating gapping of the right articulation and anterior glide and approximation of the left articulation.

ROTATIONAL ADJUSTMENTS

Rotational dysfunction of the lumbar spine theoretically may result from decreased mobility in the posterior joints on the side of rotational restriction or on the side opposite rotational restriction. Although the movements on each side are small, reduced play in either joint is potentially detrimental to joint function. Fixation in the joint on the side of rotational restriction may produce a loss of facetal separation. Fixation in the joint on the side opposite the rotational restriction may produce a loss of anterior glide of the inferior facet relative to the inferior facet (Fig. 5-243).

Whether the side of fixation can be clinically differentiated and to what degree each joint may be responsible for inducing rotational dysfunction is a matter of speculation. On the side opposite the direction of trunk rotation, the facets act as a major barrier to axial rotation. Bony impact of these structures are largely responsible for limiting lumbar rotation. As a result, functional changes in the periarticular soft tissues of these joints is unlikely to significantly affect the range of axial rotation. However, reduced play at the end of motion may still be a significant hindrance to normal joint function. In contrast, the joints on the side of trunk rotation are not limited by bony impact. Therefore, functional changes in these articulations may have a greater potential to limit joint movement.

To clinically differentiate the side of fixation, compare the end play quality of one side to the other. To accomplish this, push medially against the

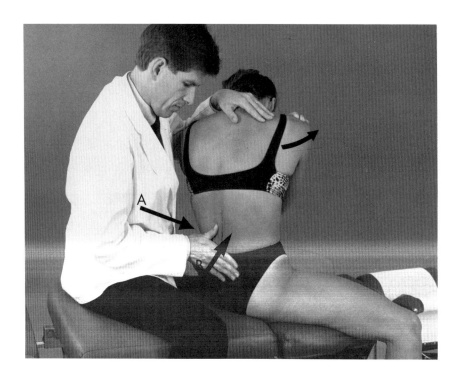

Figure 5.244 Palpation of left rotation end play at L2–L3; arrow *A* indicates contact on the left lateral surface of the L2 spinous process. Arrow *B* indicates site and vector for contact on the right mammillary process.

superior spinous process on the side of induced rotation and compare the quality of end play on that side to that induced by pushing anteriorly against the superior mammillary on the side opposite trunk rotation (Fig. 5-244).

Rotational dysfunction leading to a loss of gapping on the side of restricted rotation may be treated with side posture assisted or resisted methods. With both patient positions, the affected joint is placed away from the table and the patient is flexed, laterally flexed, and counter rotated at the level of dysfunction. With resisted methods the contact is established on the up side mammillary process or the down side of the spinous process of the inferior vertebra, and the thrust is delivered in the direction opposite the shoulder rotation. This method is applied to induce rotation and perpendicular gapping in the facet joint superior to the point of contact (Fig. 5-245). With assisted methods the contact is established on the spinous process of the superior vertebra and the thrust is delivered in the direction of shoulder rotation. This method is also applied to induce perpendicular facet gapping, but the point of distraction is directed to the articulation below the contact (Fig. 5-246). To incorporate forces applied in each of the previous two methods, apply a combination spinous push/pull adjustment (Fig. 5-247).

To induce rotation and perpendicular gapping in the sitting positions, simulate the position and contacts employed with side posture assisted spinous push adjustments. Contact the lateral surface of the superior spinous process on the side of rotational restriction (side of spinous rotation) and laterally flex the patient away from the contact as the torso is rotated in the direction of restriction (Fig. 5-248).

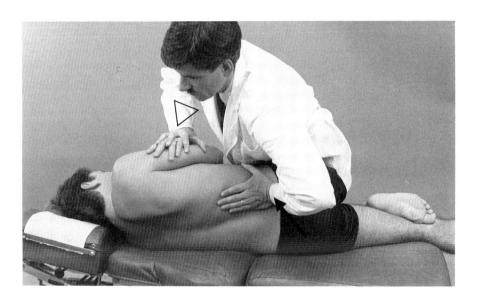

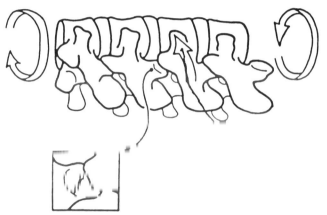

Figure 5.245 Resisted position with a hypothenar contact applied to the right L4 mammillary process to induce right rotation and gapping of the right L3–L4 articulation.

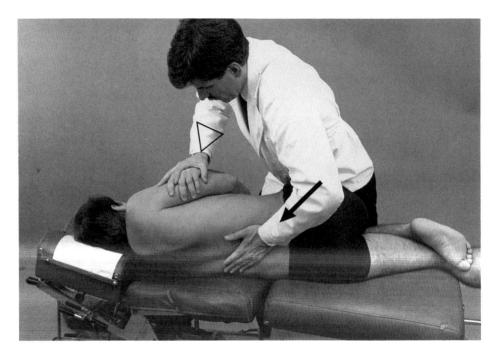

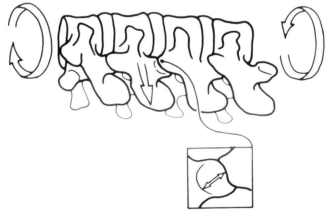

Figure 5.246 Assisted position with a hypothenar contact applied to the right L3 spinous process to induce right rotation and gapping of the right L3–L4 articulation.

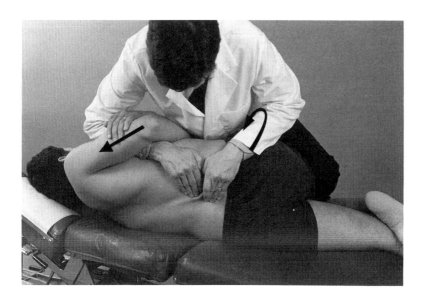

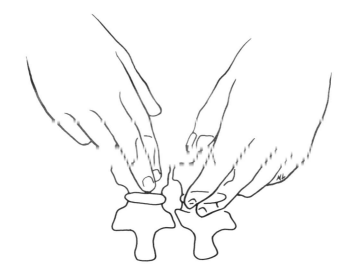

Figure 5.247 Digital contacts applied to the right lateral surface of the L3 spinous process and left lateral surface of the L4 spinous process to induce right rotation and gapping of the right L3–L4 articulation.

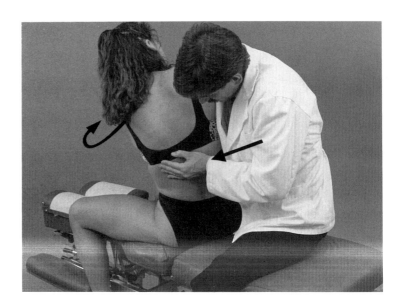

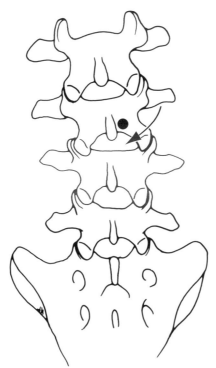

Figure 5.248 Assisted method with a hypothenar contact applied to the right lateral surface of the L3 spinous process to induce right rotation and gapping of the right L3–L4 articulation.

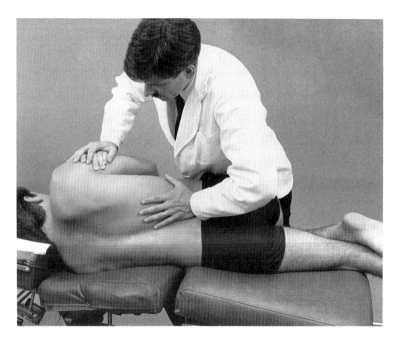

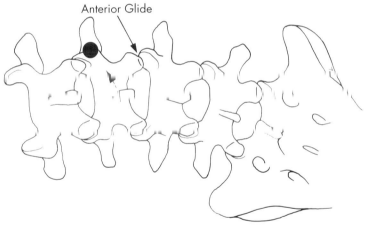

Anterior Glide

Figure 5.249 Neutral method with a hypothenar contact applied to the right L3 mammillary process (dot) to induce left rotation and anterior superior glide of the right L3–L4 articulation.

Rotational restrictions leading to a loss of anterior glide may be treated with neutral side posture mammillary push adjustments or assisted sitting mammillary push adjustments. The contacts are applied to the superior vertebra of the involved motions segment on the side of posterior body rotation (side opposite the rotational restriction). These methods are directed at distracting the motions segment inferior to the point of contact.

In the side posture method, take care to maintain the patient's relatively neutral position. Excessive posterior shoulder rotation opposes the direction of adjustive thrust and may place unwanted distractive tension at the joint above the desired level. Additionally the adjustive thrust should incorporate a superior inclination (Fig. 5-249). This serves to direct the thrust along

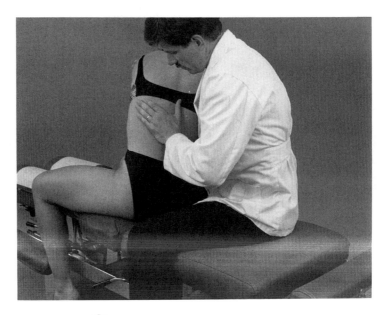

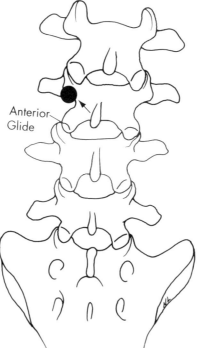

Anterior
Glide

Figure 5.250 Assisted method with a hypothenar contact applied to the left L3 mammillary (dot) to induce right rotation and/or right lateral flexion with anterior glide at the left L4–L5 articulation.

the plane of the lumbar sagittal facets and to traction the contacted segment away from the segment below.

When employing a sitting mammillary push adjustment, some lateral flexion must be induced away from the contact and incorporate a superior inclination to the adjustive thrust (Fig. 5-250). If the patient is laterally flexed toward the side of contact and the adjustive thrust is directed anteri-

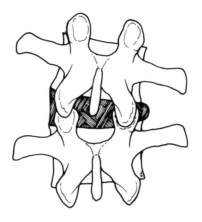

Figure 5.251 Illustration of right lateral flexion and inferior glide with approximation of the right articulation and superior glide with distraction of the left articulation.

orly without superior distraction, there is a risk of unnecessarily compressing the joint.

Lateral Flexion Adjustments

Lateral flexion dysfunction in the lumbar spine may result from a loss of disc closure and inferior glide of the facet on the side of lateral flexion dysfunction (open wedge) and/or contralateral superior glide on the side opposite the lateral flexion restriction (closed wedge) (Fig. 5-251).

Lateral flexion dysfunction is commonly treated with side posture adjustments but may also be treated in sitting positions. In side posture positions the adjustive contacts are established on the spinous process or the mammillary processes. Seated patient positions are used with spinous process contacts with pillows and/or positioning of the lumbar and pelvic sections to induce the lateral flexion postures. The patient is placed on the side opposite the lateral flexion restriction (side of closed wedge) and the patient is laterally flexed away from the table (laterally flexed toward the doctor) (Fig. 5-252). After tension is developed the doctor thrusts posterior to anterior and lateral to medial to induce segmental lateral flexion and inferior glide and closure of the up side facets and disc and separation of the down side facets.

When employing mammillary contacts, the side of patient placement depends on whether the maximum effect is to be facet distraction or disc closure. When superior glide is desired, the patient is placed with the closed wedge side up (side of lateral flexion restriction). The patient is laterally flexed toward the table to distract the up side joint. A roll may be placed under the patient to assist in the development of distraction. The contacts are established on either the upper or lower vertebra. With a contact on the superior vertebra, the thrust is delivered anteriorly and superiorly in the direction of trunk bending to distract the joint below the contact (Fig. 5-253). With an inferior vertebra contact, the thrust is directed anteriorly and inferiorly to distract the joint above the contact. Upper vertebra contacts are more commonly applied and easier on the doctor's wrist.

When mammillary contacts are applied to accentuate disc closure, the patient is placed with the open wedge side up (side of lateral flexion restric-

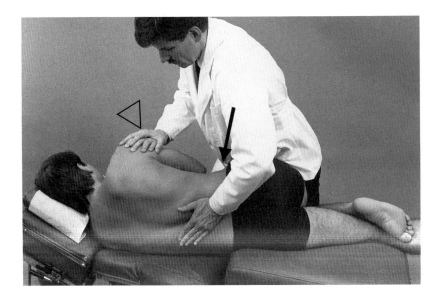

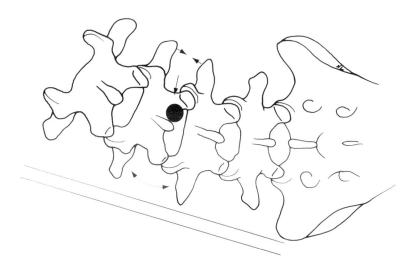

Figure 5.252 Assisted method with a hypothenar contact applied to the right lateral surface of the L3 spinous process (dot) to induce right lateral flexion with approximation of the right L3–L4 articulation and distraction of the left L3–L4 articulation.

tion). The patient is laterally flexed away from the table, and the doctor thrusts posterior to anterior, lateral to medial, and superior to inferior to induce inferior glide of the facets and disc closure (Fig. 5-254).

Flexion and Extension

Flexion dysfunction is commonly treated in the side posture position with contacts established over the spinous processes. The spine is flexed at the level of dysfunction and contacts are applied to the superior or inferior vertebra of the involved motion segment to induce separation of the interspinous space and posterior joints. With assisted methods the contact is established on the superior vertebra and the thrust is delivered anteriorly and superiorly. With resisted methods the contact is applied to the inferior vertebra and the thrust is delivered anteriorly and inferiorly. Resisted meth-

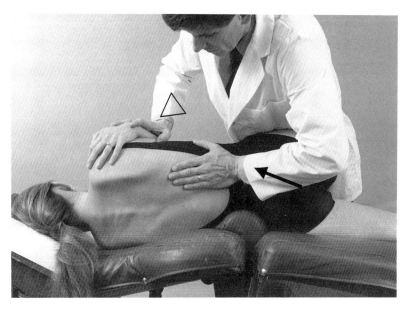

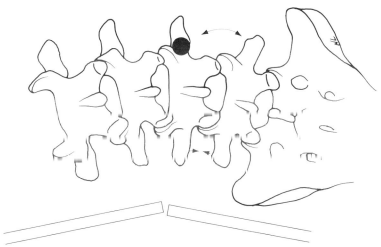

Figure 5.253 Assisted method with a hypothenar contact applied to the right L4 mammillary process (dot) to induce left lateral flexion distraction at the right L4–L5 articulation.

ods are not commonly applied except at the lumbosacral junction, where the contacts are established on the sacral apex (Fig. 5-255).

Extension dysfunction may also be treated in side posture position with spinous contacts. In this case the involved motion segment is allowed to extend and the doctor establishes contacts over the superior or inferior spinous process and directs the adjustive thrust to induce approximation of the posterior joints and disc and distraction of the anterior elements (Fig. 5-256).

As mentioned previously, prone or knee chest adjustments may be especially efficient in the delivery of lumbar extension adjustments. They are applied with unilateral or bilateral contacts, depending on whether you wish to extend one side or both sides simultaneously. The contacts may be established over the spinous processes but are more commonly applied over the mammillary processes.

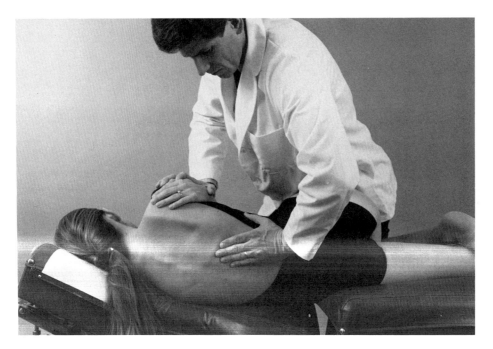

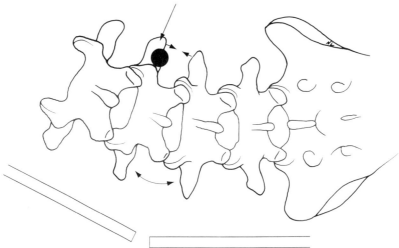

Figure 5.254 Assisted method with a hypothenar contact applied to the right L3 mammillary (dot) to induce right lateral flexion with approximation of the right L3–L4 articulation and distraction of the left L3–L4 articulation.

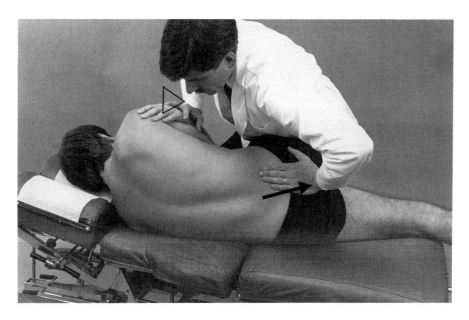

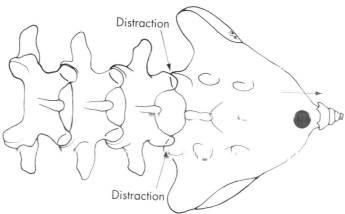

Figure 5.255 Resisted method with a hypothenar contact applied to the sacral apex (dot) to induce flexion and distraction of the L5–S1 articulation.

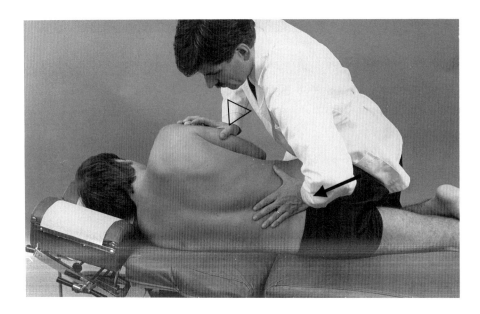

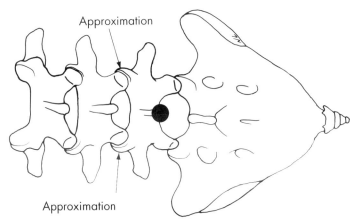

Figure 5.256 Resisted method with a hypothenar contact applied to the L5 spinous process (dot) to induce extension and approximation of the L4–L5 articulation.

Side Posture Lumbar Adjustments

Mammillary push (Fig. 5-257)

IND: Restricted rotation and/or lateral flexion, L1–L5. Rotation and/or lateral flexion malpositions, L1–L5.

PP: The patient lies in side posture with the head supported on the elevated cervical section or pillow. The patient's down side arm is crossed over the chest with the hand resting on the opposite shoulder

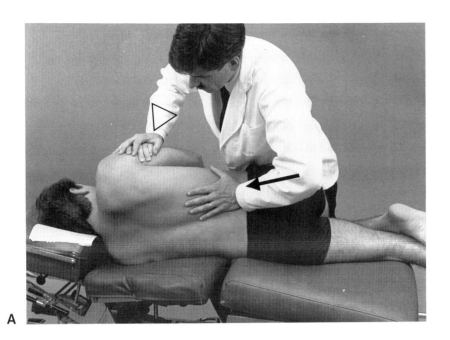

A

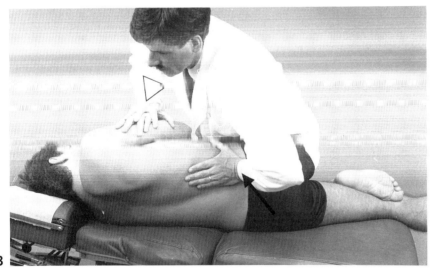

B

Figure 5-267 (A) Neutral method with a hypothenar contact applied to the right L4 mammillary process to induce right rotation and anterior glide of the right L4–L5 articulation. **(B)** Resisted method with a hypothenar contact applied to the right L4 mammillary process to induce right rotation and gapping of the right L3–L4 articulation. (*Figure continues.*)

or lateral rib cage. The patient's down side leg is extended along the length of the table and the upper leg and thigh are flexed. The patient's foot is placed over the popliteal space of the down side leg. Optional arm and leg positions are covered in Figures 5-238 to 240.

DP: Stand in a fencer stance angled approximately 45 degrees to the patient. Support the patient's pelvis by contacting the patient's thigh with the inferior thigh (Fig. 5-240A) or by straddling the patient's upper leg between the thighs (Figs. 5-240C and D).

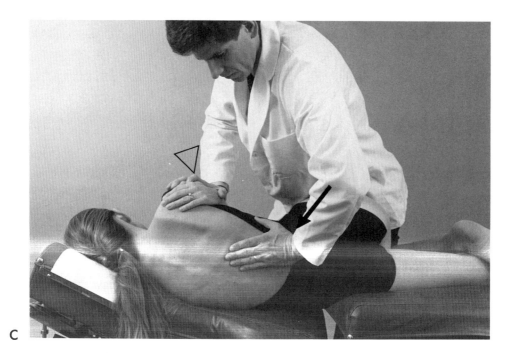

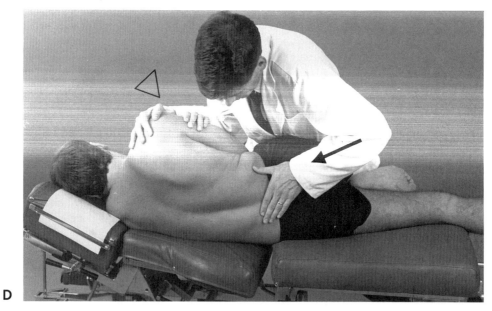

Figure 5.257 (*Continued*). (**C**) Assisted method with a hypothenar contact applied to the right L4 mammillary process to induce right lateral flexion with approximation of the right L4–L5 articulation and distraction of the left L4–L5 articulation. (**D**) Resisted method with a hypothenar contact applied to the right sacral base to induce right lateral flexion with approximation of the right L5–S1 articulation and distraction of the left L5–S1 articulation. (*Figure continues.*)

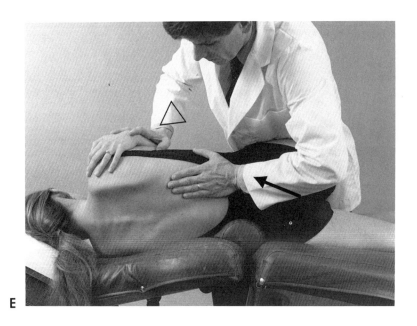

E

Figure 5.257 (*Continued*). (**E**) Assisted method with a hypothenar contact applied to the right L3 mammillary process to induce left lateral flexion with distraction of the right L3–L4 articulation.

CP: Hypothenar (pisiform) of the caudal hand with the fingers running parallel to the spine.

SCP: Mammillary process.

IH: The indifferent hand contacts the patient's up shoulder and overlapping hand.

VEC: The adjustive vectors are described below.

P: Ask the patient to lie on the appropriate side and to straighten the down leg. Position the patient's shoulders and flex the upper thigh to distract the interspinous space of the dysfunctional motion segment. Establish the vertebral and thigh contacts develop and pre-adjustive tension. At tension generate an impulse thrust by dropping your body weight and thrusting through the shoulder.

Rotation restrictions

Neutral position. To induce rotation from a neutral position place the patient on the side opposite the posterior body rotation (side of rotational restriction) and minimize rotation between the patient's shoulders and pelvis. Establish the segmental contact by sliding laterally onto the superior vertebra on the side of posterior body rotation. For example, if the L4 body is rotated posterior on the right (left rotation restriction), the contact should be established on the right L4 mammillary (Fig. 5-257A). At tension deliver an impulse thrust anteriorly and superiorly parallel to lumbar facetal planes.

Resisted position. To effect rotation with a resisted method, place the patient on the side opposite the rotational restriction (side of posterior body rotation) and contact the mammillary of the inferior vertebra on the side of rotational restriction. For example, when treating an L3–L4 right rotation restriction (L3 left posterior body rotation), place the patient on the left side and contact the right L4 mammillary (Fig. 5-257B).

To develop pre-adjustive tension rotate the patient's posteriorly, laterally flex the trunk toward the adjusting bench, and counter rotate the patient's pelvis anteriorly. This should induce gapping distraction in the motion segment ipsilateral and superior to the point of contact.

Shoulder rotation and lateral flexion are induced by pulling the patient's down arm anteriorly and inferiorly (Fig. 5-238B). Lateral flexion of the patient may be assisted by elevating the thoracolumbar section of an articulating adjustive bench or by placing a roll under the patient's lumbar spine.

Forward rotation of the patient's pelvis is aided by downward traction along the patient's flexed thigh and hip by the doctor's anterolateral thigh (Fig. 5-240A) or lower abdomen (Fig. 5-240C and D).

The degree of shoulder rotation depends on the area treated. It is greater in the upper lumbars as compared to the lower lumbars. Excessive counter rotation through the shoulders may be unnecessarily uncomfortable to the patient and may be traumatic to the intercostal muscles.

At tension deliver an impulse thrust through the body and contact arm. The adjustive vector follows the movement of the pelvis and should not be directed straight anteriorly. Thrusts directed anteriorly have a tendency to induce segmental extension instead of rotation and gapping distraction. The contact must remain light, and the vector must reinforce the pelvic rotation by incorporating a strong medial to lateral component (Fig. 5-257B).

Resisted adjustive methods may also be used to treat rotational restriction coupled with opposite side lateral flexion restrictions (PRI, PLI; LPS, RPS).

Lateral flexion restrictions. Mammillary push adjustments for lateral flexion dysfunction are commonly treated with assisted patient positions. The patient is laterally flexed in the direction of restriction with the contact established on the superior or inferior vertebra. The side of contact is determined by the side of desired mechanical effect. To maximize forces of approximation, contact the side of lateral flexion restriction (open wedge side) (Figs. 5-257C and D). To maximize forces of distraction, contact the side opposite the lateral flexion restriction (closed wedge side) (Fig. 5-257E).

When contacting the open wedge side, place the patient on the side opposite the lateral flexion restriction (closed wedge) and laterally flex the patient away from the table. Lateral flexion is induced by elevating the patient's shoulders and pulling headward on the down arm (Fig. 5-239A). The thoracolumbar section of an articulating adjusting bench may be lowered and released to aid in the production of lateral bending (Fig. 5-257C and D). Establish the contact on the superior vertebra or on the inferior vertebra. At tension deliver an impulse thrust anteriorly, medially, and inferiorly with a superior vertebral contact (Fig. 5-257C) and anteriorly, medially and superiorly with an inferior vertebra contact (Fig. 5-257D). This superior vertebral contact method is commonly applied in Gonstead technique to treat rotational restrictions coupled with opposite side lateral flexion restrictions (PRI, PLI; LPS, RPS).

When contacting the closed wedge side, place the patient on the side of lateral flexion restriction (open wedge) and laterally flex the patient toward the table. The thoracolumbar section of the adjustive bench may be elevated or a roll may be placed under the patient's lumbar spine to assist in the development of lateral flexion (Fig. 5-257E). Deliver the adjustive thrust superiorly and anteriorly.

Spinous push (Fig. 5-258)

IND: Restricted flexion, extension, rotation, and lateral flexion L1–S1. Rotation, flexion, extension, and lateral flexion malpositions, L1–S1.

 PP: The patient lies in the basic side posture position.

 DP: Stand in a fencer stance angled approximately 45 degrees to the patient. Support the patient's pelvis by contacting the patient's thigh with the inferior thigh.

 CP: Hypothenar of inferior hand with fingers angled across the spine.

SCP: Lateral margin of the superior spinous process.

 IH: The indifferent hand contacts the patient's up side shoulder and overlapping hand.

VEC: Lateral to medial and posterior to anterior.

  P: Ask the patient to lie on the appropriate side and to straighten the down side leg. Position the patient's shoulders and flex the upper thigh to distract the interspinous space of the dysfunctional motion segment. Establish the vertebral and thigh contacts and develop pre-adjustive tension. Generate the spinous push adjustive thrust by dropping your body weight while thrusting through the shoulder. This adjustment is typically delivered with a non-pause thrust.

Spinous push adjustments utilize assisted patient positions for rotation and lateral flexion restrictions and assisted or resisted positions for flexion or extension restrictions.

Rotation restrictions. To effect rotation place the patient on the side opposite the rotation restriction (side opposite spinous rotation). Rotate the shoulders posteriorly in the direction of restriction and laterally flex the trunk toward the adjusting bench. Induce the shoulder rotation and lateral flexion by pulling the patient's down arm anteriorly and inferiorly (Fig. 5-258A).

Establish the segmental contact and remove superficial tissue slack by sliding medially onto the lateral surface of the superior spinous process (side of spinous rotation). The contact must remain light and well padded or it becomes painful.

Develop pre-adjustive tension by rotating the patient's shoulders and contacted vertebra posteriorly while the patient's pelvis and segments below are rotated anteriorly. The forward rotation of the patient's pelvis is aided by downward traction along the patient's flexed thigh and hip by your anterolateral thigh.

At tension deliver an impulse thrust through the body and shoulder aided by a simultaneous high velocity downward torquing impulse with the wrist.

Lateral flexion restrictions. When treating pure lateral flexion dysfunction, place the patient on the side opposite the lateral flexion restriction (side of open wedge) and laterally flex the patient away from the table. Induce lateral flexion by pulling cephalically on the patient's down side shoulder while lowering and releasing the thoracolumbar section of an articulated

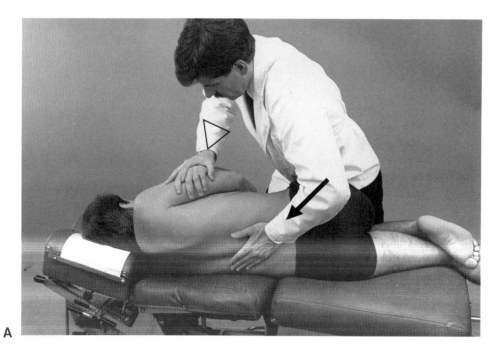

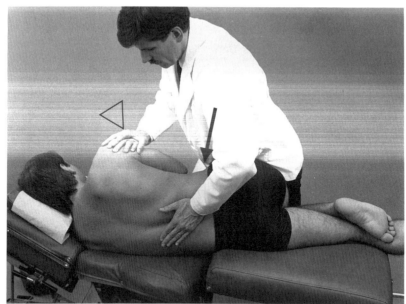

Figure 5.258 **(A)** Assisted method with a hypothenar contact applied to the right lateral surface of the L3 spinous process to induce right rotation and gapping of the right L3–L4 articulation. **(B)** Assisted method with a hypothenar contact applied to the right lateral surface of the L3 spinous process to induce right lateral flexion with approximation of the right L3–L4 articulation and distraction of the left L3–L4 articulation. (*Figure continues.*)

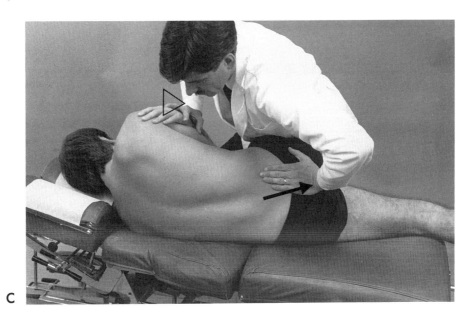

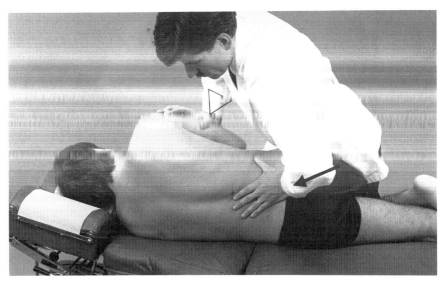

Figure 5.258 (*Continued*). (**C**) Resisted method with a hypothenar contact applied to the sacral apex to induce flexion and distraction of the L5–S1 articulation. (**D**) Resisted method with a hypothenar contact applied to the spinous process of L5 to induce extension and approximation of the L4–L5 articulation.

adjusting bench (Fig. 5-258B). Establish the adjustive contact and remove superficial tissue slack by sliding medially onto the lateral surface of the superior spinous process (side of spinous rotation). Develop pre-adjustive tension by transferring additional weight through your trunk into the spinous contact. At tension deliver a body drop and pectoral thrust aided by a simultaneous high velocity downward torquing impulse with the wrist.

Flexion restrictions. To treat flexion dysfunction, place the patient on either side and flex the upper hip to induce segmental flexion. Establish the segmental contact with the proximal midline palmar surface on your caudal hand.

When employing an assisted method, slide superiorly to contact the inferior tip of the superior spinous process and thrust superiorly and anteriorly.

When employing a resisted method, slide inferiorly to contact the inferior vertebra and thrust anteriorly and inferiorly. The resisted approach is commonly applied only when treating lumbosacral flexion restriction with a sacral contact (Fig. 5-258C).

Extension restrictions. To treat extension dysfunction use the same contacts as described for flexion dysfunction but allow the lumbar spine to move into extension.

With an assisted approach, contact the superior vertebra and thrust anteriorly and inferiorly. With a resisted approach, contact the inferior vertebra and thrust anteriorly and superiorly. To induce extension at the lumbosacral junction with an inferior vertebral contact, contact the sacral base at the level of S1 and thrust anteriorly and slightly superiorly (Fig. 5-258D).

Spinous pull (Fig. 5-259)

IND: Restricted rotation or combined restrictions in rotation and opposite side lateral flexion, L1–L5. Rotation or combined rotation and ipsilateral flexion malpositions, L1–L5.

PP: The patient lies in the basic side posture position with the foot of the patient's flexed leg hooked behind the popliteal space of the down leg.

DP: Stand facing the patient with your inferior thigh contacting the patient's thigh (Fig. 5-259B) or with the distal surface of your leg contacting the patient's flexed knee (long lever contact) (Fig. 5-259A, Fig. 5-240B).

CP: Fingertips (digital contacts) of first three fingers of your inferior hand with the forearm resting along the patient's posterolateral buttock and hip.

SCP: Lateral surface of the spinous process.

IH: Your indifferent hand contacts the patient's up side shoulder and overlapping hand.

VEC: Lateral to medial pulling movement to induce axial rotation.

P: Ask the patient to lie on the appropriate side and to straighten the down side leg. Flex the patient's upper thigh to distract the interspinous space of the dysfunctional motion segment. Then establish contacts on the spinous process and the patient's flexed leg. The spinous contacts are established by hooking the down side of the

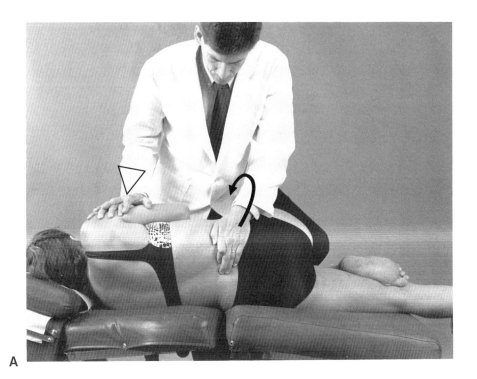

A

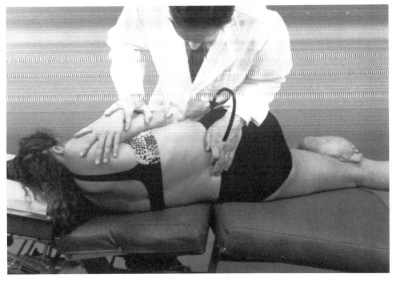

B

Figure 5.259 A digital contact applied to the left lateral surface of the L4 spinous process to induce (**A**) left rotation and gapping of the left L4–L5 articulation using a neutral method and (**B**) right rotation and gapping of the right L3–L4 articulation using a resisted method.

spinous process with the second, third, and fourth fingers while the forearm rests against the patient's posterolateral buttock and hip. Contacts on the leg are established with the distal surface of your tibia against the patient's knee or with your inferior thigh.

At tension a pulling impulse is generated by extending your contact shoulder while simultaneously inducing anterior pelvic rotation.

With a long lever contact, induce anterior pelvic rotation by quickly extending your contact knee (Fig. 5-259A). With a thigh to thigh contact, produce anterior pelvic rotation when you drop your body weight by flexing your hips and knees (Fig. 5-259B).

Rotation restriction. This adjustment may be delivered from a neutral or resisted patient posture. Resisted methods may be more effective in developing rotational tension.

Neutral. When applying the neutral patient position, place the patient on the side of rotational restriction and establish a contact on the down side of the superior spinous process (side of spinous rotation) (Fig. 5-259A).

Develop pre-adjustive tension by anteriorly rotating the patient's pelvis with your leg and forearm, while applying cephalic traction to the patient's shoulder.

Resisted. With a resisted method, place the patient on the side opposite the restriction (side opposite spinous rotation) and establish the segmental contact on the down side of the inferior spinous process. For example, when treating a right rotation restriction (left posterior body rotation) at the L3–L4 motion segment, place the patient on the left side and contact the left side of the L4 spinous process (Fig. 5-259B).

Develop pre-adjustive tension by rotating the patient's shoulders posteriorly in the direction of segmental restriction as you rotate the patient's pelvis anteriorly with your leg and forearm. Induce posterior shoulder rotation and lateral flexion of the patient's trunk toward the table by pulling the patient's down arm anteriorly and inferiorly.

Resisted spinous pull adjustments may also be applied for combined rotational and opposite side lateral flexion restrictions (PRS, PLS; LPI, RPI). The contacts and positioning are the same, but lateral flexion toward the adjusting bench is maximized. This may be accomplished by raising the thoracolumbar section of an articulating adjusting bench or by placing a roll under the patient's lumbar spine.

Spinous push-pull (Fig. 5-260)

IND: Restricted rotation or combined restrictions in rotation and opposite side lateral flexion, L1–L5. Rotation or combined rotation and ipsilateral lateral flexion malpositions, L1–L5.

PP: The patient lies in the basic side posture position with the foot of the patient's flexed leg hooked behind the popliteal space of the down leg.

DP: Stand facing the patient with your inferior thigh contacting the patient's thigh (Fig. 5-260A) or with the distal surface of your leg contacting the patient's flexed knee (long lever contact) (Fig. 5-260B).

CP: The fingertips (digital) of cephalic hand reach under the patient's up arm to contact the lateral surface of the superior spinous process. The fingertips of caudal hand hook the inferior spinous process while the forearm contacts the patient's posterolateral buttock and thigh.

SCP: Adjacent spinous processes.

VEC: The superior hand thrusts (pushes) lateral to medial and inferior to

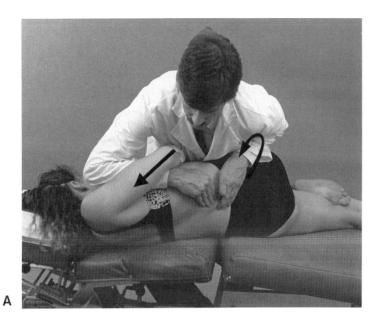

A

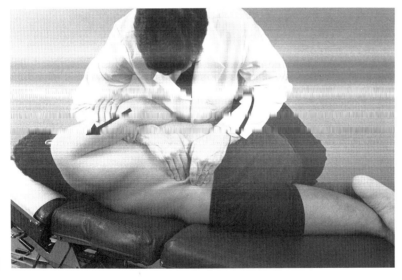

B

Figure 5.200 Digital contacts applied to the right lateral surface of the L2 spinous process and left lateral surface of the L3 spinous process to induce right rotation and gapping of the right L2–L3 articulation using (**A**) a thigh to thigh contact and (**B**) a shin to knee contact.

superior. The inferior hand thrusts (pulls) lateral to medial in the opposing direction.

P: Place the patient in side posture. Flex the patient's upper thigh to distract the interspinous space of the dysfunctional motion segment. Rotate the patient's shoulders posteriorly in the direction of segmental restriction and flex the trunk laterally toward the adjusting bench.

The doctor establishes appropriate contacts on adjacent spinous process and develops local joint tension by counter rotating the pelvis, shoulders, and segmental contacts. As the shoulders are rotated posteriorly the patient's pelvis and contacted vertebra are counter rotated

Figure 5.261 Digital contact applied to the left lateral surface of the L2 spinous process to induce left rotation and gapping of the left L2–L3 articulation and distraction of the right L2–L3 articulation.

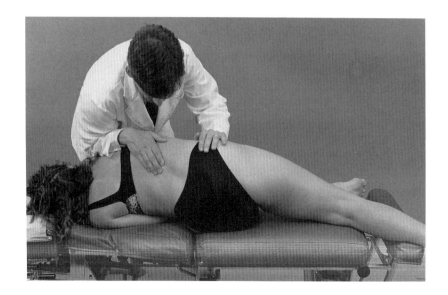

anteriorly. This should induce distraction in the motion segment between the established contacts. Posterior shoulder rotation is greater when treating upper lumbar dysfunction as compared with lower lumbar dysfunction.

At tension deliver a high velocity counter torquing thrust through both contact hands reinforced by a body drop thrust and shoulder thrust through your cephalic shoulder. Take care not to apply undue pressure to the patient's lateral rib cage with the superior forearm contact.

Reverse lumbar roll (Fig. 5-261)

IND: Restricted rotation, L1–L5. May be employed as slow stretch for the sacrospinalis muscle group.

  PP: The patient lies in a modified side posture position on the anterior surface of the down side shoulder. The patient's down side leg is flexed while the upper leg is extended back off the edge of the table.

  DP: Stand in front of the patient facing medial and inferior in modified fencer stance.

  CP: The fingertips of cephalic hand hook the spinous process with reinforcement and traction through your forearm along the patient's rib cage.

SCP: Spinous process with reinforcement along the rib cage.

  IH: Caudal hand contacts the anterior ilium, tractioning the pelvis posterior and inferior.

VEC: Lateral to medial and inferior to superior.

  P: Place the patient in a modified side posture position, lying on the anterior surface of the shoulder. Establish segmental joint tension by rotating the pelvis posteriorly as the trunk and contacted segment is counter rotated anteriorly. At tension deliver a thrust very similar to the spinous push pull. Pull the forearm contact toward you reinforcing it by a short body drop. The stabilization hand gently counter thrusts posteriorly against the pelvis to prevent anterior rotation. Take care to avoid compression of the patient's rib cage. This is an assisted adjustive approach and should bring maximal tension to the motion segment below the established contact.

Prone Lumbar Adjustments

Bilateral thenar mammillary (Fig. 5-262)

IND: Restricted extension or flexion, L1–L5. Extension or flexion malpositions, L1–L5.

  PP: The patient lies prone.

  DP: Stand in a fencer stance facing cephalad on either side of the patient.

  CP: Bilateral thenar contacts parallel to the spine with fingers fanned and running medial to lateral.

SCP: Mammillary processes.

VEC: Posterior to anterior.

   P: The patient lies prone. Establish bilateral thenar contacts and develop joint tension by transferring additional body weight into the contacts. At tension deliver a combined impulse thrust through the arms, trunk, and body. The thrust may be applied with a lumbar drop section. The thrust must be shallow to avoid hyperextension of the back.

Extension restrictions. When treating extension dysfunction, release and lower the thoracic section to assist in the development of segmental exten-

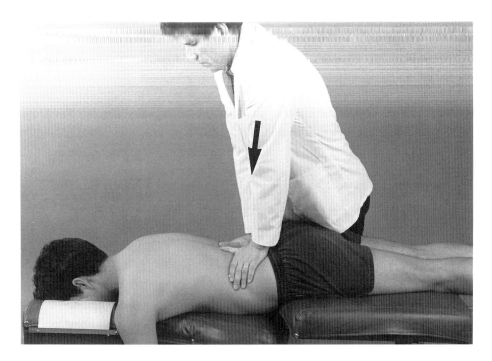

Figure 5.262 Bilateral hypothenar contacts applied to the mammillary processes of L3 to induce extension at the L3–L4 articulation.

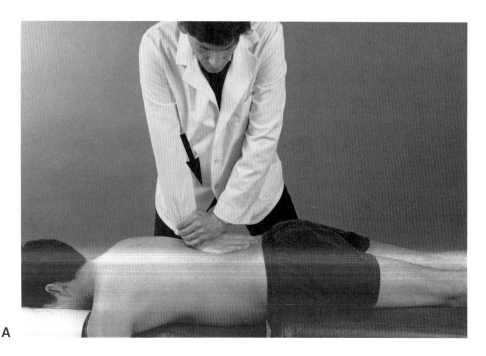

Figure 5.263 (**A**) Hypothenar contact applied to the right L1 mammillary process to induce extension, extension and left rotation, and anterior glide at the L1–L2 articulation. (*Figure continues.*)

sion. Establish the contacts on the superior or inferior vertebra of the involved motions segment. When contacting the superior vertebra, the adjustive thrust is delivered anteriorly and slightly inferiorly. When contacting the inferior vertebra, the thrust is delivered anteriorly and slightly superiorly.

Flexion restrictions. When treating flexion dysfunction a lumbar roll is placed under the patient's abdomen or the adjusting tables thoracolumbar section is elevated. The adjustive contacts are established on the superior vertebra and the adjustive thrust is delivered anteriorly and superiorly.

Unilateral hypothenar mammillary (Fig. 5-263)

IND: Restricted lateral flexion and/or rotation coupled with restricted extension, L1–L5. Rotation and/or lateral flexion malpositions coupled with flexion malpositions, L1–L5.

PP: The patient lies prone.

DP: Stand in a fencer stance or square stance on side of adjustive contact.

CP: Hypothenar (pisiform) with arched hand and fingers running parallel to the spine.

SCP: Mammillary process.

IH: Your indifferent hand reinforces the contact or reaches around to grasp the anterior ilium or rib cage on the side of adjustive contact.

VEC: Posterior to anterior and superior to inferior or inferior to superior, depending on the restriction treated.

P: The patient lies prone with the thoracic section released and lowered to assist in the development of segmental extension. Remove super-

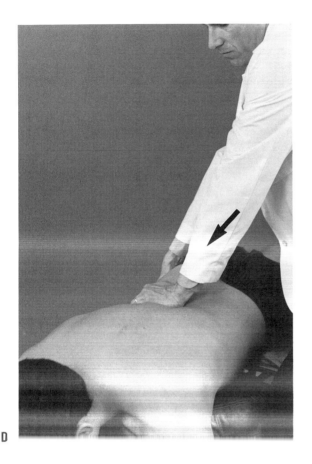

D

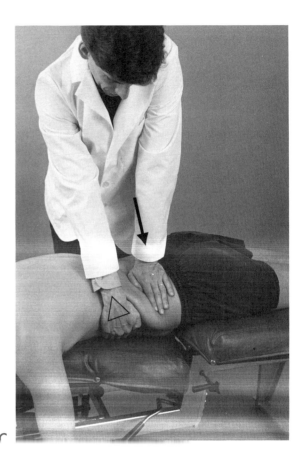

C

Figure 5-263 (Continued). **(B)** Hypothenar contact applied to the right L1 mammillary process to induce left rotation and anterior glide at the right L1–L2 articulation, indifferent hand on ASIS. **(C)** Thenar contact applied to the left L2 mammillary process to induce left rotation and gapping at the left L1–L2 articulation, indifferent hand on rib cage.

ficial tissue slack and establish adjustive contact. Develop pre-adjustive tension by transferring additional body weight into the contact. Deliver an impulse thrust through the arms, trunk, and body. The thrust may be applied with a lumbar drop section.

When treating combined extension and/or rotation or lateral flexion dysfunction, you may establish a contact on the superior or inferior vertebra of the dysfunctional motion segment. The superior vertebra contact is the method traditionally applied.

With superior vertebral contacts, the contact is established on the side opposite the rotation restriction (the side of posterior body rotation). The contact may be reinforced with the indifferent hand or the indifferent hand may contact the ipsilateral anterior ilium. When applying a reinforcing contact, stand on the side of adjustive contact (Fig. 5-263A). If the indifferent hand contacts the ilium or rib cage, stand on the side opposite the adjustive contact (Fig. 5-263B,C).

When utilizing an ilial contact, develop pre-adjustive tension by lifting and tractioning inferiorly against the ilium as the weight of your trunk is transferred anteriorly and superiorly against the contact. The counter distractive tension through the ilium should be limited and the patient's pelvis should not be rotated off the table more than 1 to 2 in. Deliver the thrust with an impulse and body drop thrust through the contact hand.

When employing a resisted method and an inferior vertebral rather than a superior vertebral contact, stand on the side opposite the rotational restriction. The caudal hand establishes the segmental contact and the cephalic hand reaches around to gently counter rotate the rib cage (Fig. 5-263C). At tension deliver a shallow thrust through the mammillary contact while the contact on the rib cage remains stationary. This adjustment is designed to induce distraction in the articulation superior to the segmental contact.

Hypothenar spinous (Fig. 5-264)

IND: Restricted extension coupled with rotation and/or lateral flexion restrictions, L1–L5. Flexion malpositions coupled with rotation and/or lateral flexion malpositions, L1–L5.

PP: The patient lies prone.

DP: Stand in a modified fencer stance or square stance on the side of adjustive contact.

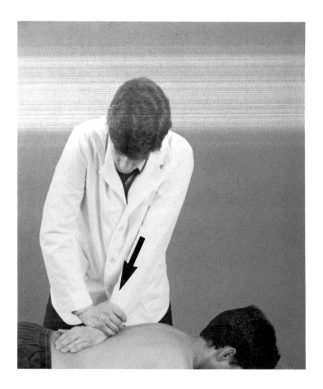

Figure 5.264 Hypothenar contact applied to the left L2 spinous process to induce extension, left lateral flexion, and left rotation of the L2–L3 articulation.

CP: Mid hypothenar.

SCP: Lateral proximal surface of the spinous process of the superior vertebra.

IH: Supports contact hand on the dorsal surface with fingers wrapped around the wrist.

VEC: Posterior to anterior, lateral to medial, and superior to inferior.

P: The patient lies prone with the thoracolumbar section released and lowered to assist in the development of segmental extension. Establish a fleshy hypothenar contact against the spinous process on the side of rotation restriction (side of spinous rotation). The contact is developed by sliding medially onto the spinous while inducing a slight clockwise or counter clockwise torquing movement depending on the restriction treated.

Develop pre-adjustive tension by transferring additional body weight into the contacts. At tension deliver an impulse thrust through the arms, trunk, and body. The thrust must be shallow to avoid hyperextension of the back. The thrust may be applied with a lumbar drop section.

This adjustment is commonly applied in the treatment of coupled restrictions in rotation and same side lateral flexion (PRS, PLS; LPI, RPI).

Knee Chest Lumbar Adjustments

Hypothenar spinous (Fig. 5-265)

IND: Restricted extension, lateral flexion, and/or rotation, L1–L5, Flexion, rotation, and/or lateral flexion malpositions, T4–T12.

PP: Position the patient in the knee chest position with the chest support placed so the patient's pelvis is slightly lower than the thoracic spine. The patient's femurs should be angled between 95 degrees and 110 degrees.

DP: Stand at the side of the table in a square stance typically on the side of the contact. You may also stand in a fencer stance facing caudally.

CP: Mid hypothenar.

SCP: Lateral surface of the spinous process.

IH: Supports contact hand on the dorsal surface with fingers wrapped around the wrist.

VEC: Posterior to anterior, lateral to medial, and superior to inferior.

P: The indifferent hand first raises the patient's abdomen to make the spinous processes more prominent and available for establishing the contacts (Fig. 5-265A). The patient is then instructed to allow the abdomen to drop and, at tension, an impulse thrust is delivered (Fig. 5-265B). The patient is vulnerable to hyperextension in this adjustment and the thrust must be shallow and non-recoiling.

Hypothenar transverse (Fig. 5-266)

IND: Restricted extension, rotation, and/or lateral flexion, T4–T12. Rotation and/or lateral flexion malpositions, T4–T12.

PP: Position the patient in the knee chest position with the chest support

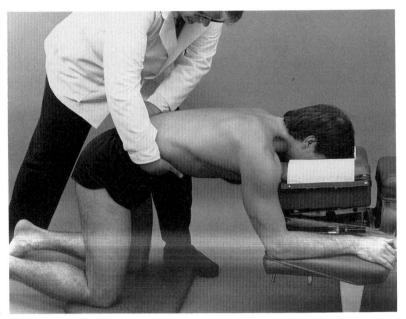

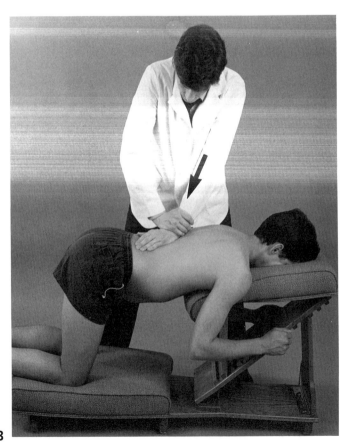

Figure 5.265 Knee chest adjustment. (A) Development of the adjustive contact and utilization of an adjusting bench in circumstances where a knee chest table is not available. (B) Hypothenar contact applied to the left L1 spinous process to induce extension, left lateral flexion, and left rotation of the L1–L2 articulation.

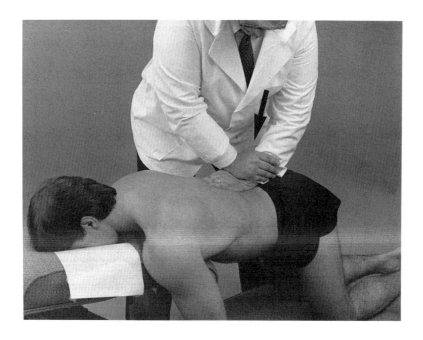

Figure 5.266 Hypothenar contact applied to the right L4 mammillary process to induce extension, extension and left rotation, and anterior glide at the L4–L5 articulation.

placed so the patient's pelvis is slightly lower than the thoracic spine. The patient's femurs should be angled between 95 and 110 degrees.

DP: Stand at the side of the table in a square stance, typically on the side of the contact. You may also stand in a fencer stance facing caudally.

CP: Hypothenar (pisiform).

SCP: Mammillary process.

IH: Supports contact hand on the dorsal surface with fingers wrapped around the wrist. The indifferent hand may be placed on the opposite side to stabilize or impart an assisting impulse.

VEC: Posterior to anterior for extension restriction or flexion malposition; lateral to medial, superior to inferior and posterior to anterior for rotation and/or lateral flexion restrictions or malpositions.

P: The indifferent hand first raises the patient's abdomen. Establish a contact on the mammillary process. Then instruct the patient to allow the abdomen to drop and, at tension, deliver an impulse thrust. The patient is vulnerable to hyperextension in this adjustment and the thrust must be shallow and non-recoiling. If the indifferent hand delivers an assisting thrust, it is directed posterior to anterior and superior to inferior or inferior to superior, depending on the coupled lateral flexion restriction.

Sitting Lumbar Adjustments

Sitting lumbar (Fig. 5-267)

IND: Restricted rotation and/or lateral flexion T12–L5; may be coupled with restricted extension or flexion. Rotation and/or lateral flexion malpositions T12–L5; may be coupled with flexion or extension malpositions.

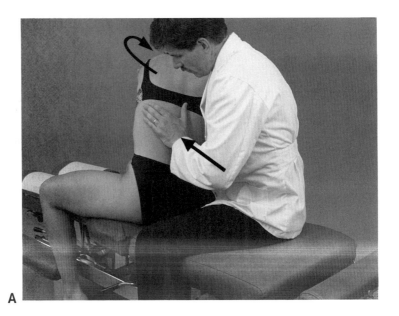

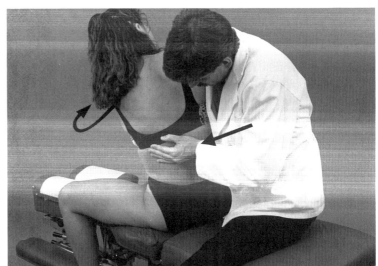

Figure 5.267 Hypothenar contact applied to the left mammillary process of L2 to induce (**A**) right rotation and/or right lateral flexion with superior glide and distraction of the left L2–L3 articulation, and (**B**) right rotation and gapping of the right L2–L3 articulation.

PP: The patient sits with legs straddling the adjusting bench with knees locked against each side. The arms are folded across the chest with hands grasping the opposing shoulders.

DP: The doctor may sit behind the patient, straddle the bench or stand at the caudal end of the bench. In the standing position the doctor may support his elbow against his anterior ilium.

CP: Hypothenar (pisiform) of contact hand.

SCP: Mammillary or spinous process of superior vertebra.

IH: The indifferent hand reaches around the patient to clasp the patient's opposite arm.

VEC: Contact hand thrusts laterally and posterior to anterior as the indifferent hand pulls anterior to posterior.

P: The patient is asked to sit with crossed arms. Pre-adjustive tension is typically developed by flexing, laterally flexing and rotating the patient in the direction of joint restriction (assisted method). Once tension is established an impulse thrust is delivered through the contact hand assisted by a pulling and twisting thrust generated through the doctor's indifferent arm and trunk. The direction of induced lateral flexion and the point of adjustive contact is dependent on the restriction being treated.

Although this adjustment may be applied in all lumbar regions it is probably most effectively applied in the upper lumbars and lower thoracics.

Rotation restrictions. When treating rotational dysfunction the doctor may establish contacts on the spinous process or mammillary process.

When using a mammillary contact, establish the contact on the superior vertebra on the side opposite the rotation restriction (side of posterior body rotation). Develop pre-adjustive tension by flexing, rotating, and laterally flexing the patient away from the side of contact (Fig. 5-267A). At tension, deliver an adjustive thrust anteriorly, laterally, and superiorly. This method is applied to induce maximal distraction in facet joint ipsilateral and inferior to the point of contact. It is also applied to treat restrictions in rotation and same side lateral flexion (e.g., right or left rotation restriction coupled with the corresponding right or left lateral flexion restriction).

To employ a spinous process contact, slide medially and establish a fleshy mid-hypothenar contact on the lateral surface of the spinous process on the side of induced rotation (side of spinous rotation). Develop pre-adjustive tension by flexing, rotating, and laterally flexing the patient away from the side of contact (Fig. 5-267B).

At tension deliver an adjustive thrust medially to induce rotation. This contact should induce maximal distraction in the facet joint ipsilateral and inferior to the side of spinous contact, therefore inducing distraction in the facet joints on the side opposite the transverse process contact. This method is also commonly applied when treating combined restrictions in rotation and opposite side lateral flexion (e.g., right or left rotation restriction coupled with the opposing right or left lateral flexion restriction).

Lateral flexion restrictions. Lateral flexion dysfunction is treated by contacting the mammillary process of the superior vertebra on the side opposite the lateral flexion restriction (closed disc wedge side) (Fig. 5-267A). Develop pre-adjustive tension by flexing, laterally flexing, and rotating the patient away from the side of contact. At tension deliver an adjustive thrust superiorly, laterally, and anteriorly.

THE PELVIC JOINTS

Probably the least understood and most controversial function of any area in the musculoskeletal system is that of the bones and joints that compose the pelvic mechanism. The two sacroiliac joints posteriorly, together with the pubic symphysis anteriorly, form a three-joint complex with much the same function as the typical vertebral functional unit. There is now no doubt that the sacroiliac joints are mobile diarthrodial joints that are important to the statics and dynamics of posture and gait. They must provide support for the trunk while functioning to guide movement and help absorb the compressive force associated with locomotion and weight bearing.

Grieve[59] believes that this articulation, together with the cranio-vertebral region and other transitional areas, is of prime importance in understanding the conservative treatment of vertebral joint problems. Moreover, dysfunction of the sacroiliac joint is often ignored by other health care practitioners as an insignificant feature of musculoskeletal problems. The sacroiliac dysfunctional syndrome is, however, a legitimate clinical entity that is separate from painful low back conditions associated with lumbar facet syndrome, sciatica, or disc conditions.[59-63]

Functional Anatomy of the Sacroiliac Joints

The pelvic complex comprises the two innominate bones with the sacrum between. The ilium, ischium, and pubic bone fuse at the acetabulum to form each innominate (Fig. 5-268). The sacrum is a fusion of the five sacral segments and is roughly triangular in shape, giving it the appearance of a wedge inserted between the two innominate bones (Fig. 5-269). The sacral

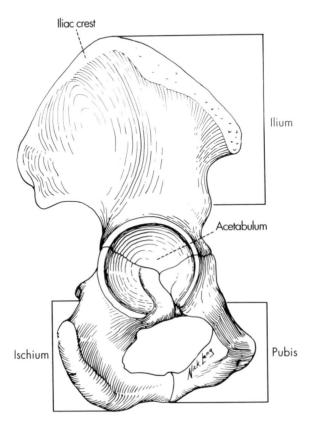

Figure 5.268 Lateral view of the right innominate showing the ilium, ischium, and pubic contributions to the acetabulum.

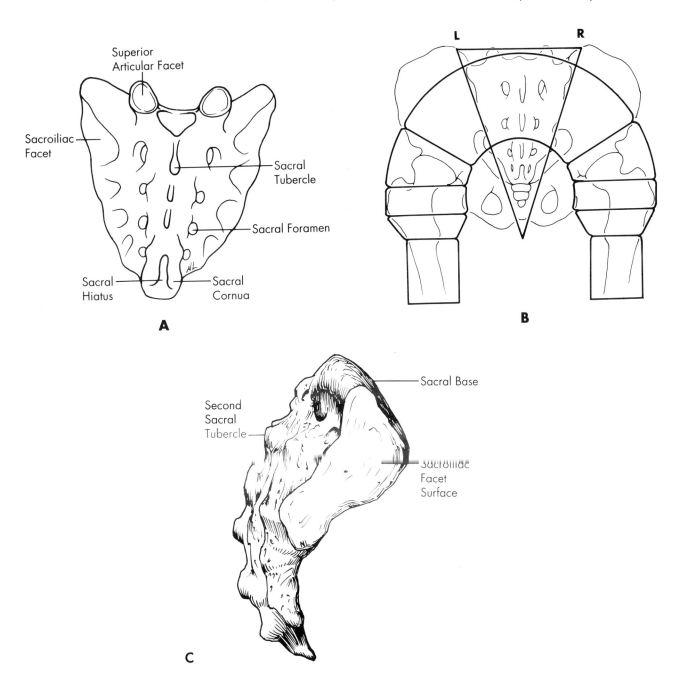

Figure 5.269 The sacrum (**A**) viewed from the posterior is triangular and serves as a (**B**) keystone in the arch between the two columns formed by the lower extremities. (**C**) Lateral view of the sacrum.

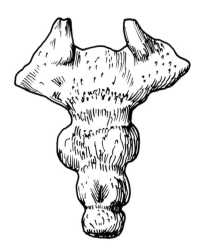

Figure 5.270 The coccyx.

base has two superior articulating facets: the sacral promontory, which projects upwards to articulate with the fifth lumbar vertebra, and the apex, which points downwards to articulate with the coccyx.

The vertebral foramen leads into the sacral canal. The two sacral alae have a margin on their lateral aspect. The tubercles on the posterolateral aspect correlate with transverse processes. The sacral tubercles, located in the midline, correlate with the spinous processes of the unfused vertebra. The apex of the sacrum is oval and articulates with the coccyx by means of a disc. By around age 30, this disappears and the two structures are essentially fused together. The sacral crests contain articular tubercles, which correlate with the articular processes of the unfused vertebra. The fifth sacral vertebra contains the cornua by which the sacrum articulates with the coccyx, which comprises four fused vertebrae (Fig. 5-270).

The shape and configuration of the posterior joints are important to their function, as well as for the manipulative procedures designed to influence dysfunction. The sacroiliac articulation is a true synovial joint, having a joint cavity containing synovial fluid and enclosed by a joint capsule. The articular surface is described as auricular (ear-shaped), a letter C, or a letter L lying on its side (Fig. 5-271). The articular surfaces have different contours, which develop into interlocking elevations and depressions. This bony configuration produces what has been termed a keystone effect of the sacrum, effectively distributing axial compressive forces through the pelvic mechanism (Fig. 5-269B). Forces from the lower extremities divide, heading upward toward the spine and anteriorly toward the pubic symphysis, while downward forces of gravity on the spine split to both sides (Fig. 5-272).

The morphologic configuration of the sacroiliac joints are not static and are extremely variable from individual to individual.[64,65] At birth the joints are undeveloped, smooth, and flat. Only after the individual becomes ambulatory do the joints begin to take on their adult characteristics. In the teenage years the joint surfaces begin to roughen and develop their characteristic grooves and ridges. In the third to fourth decades this process is well established, and by the fifth and sixth decades the joint surfaces may be

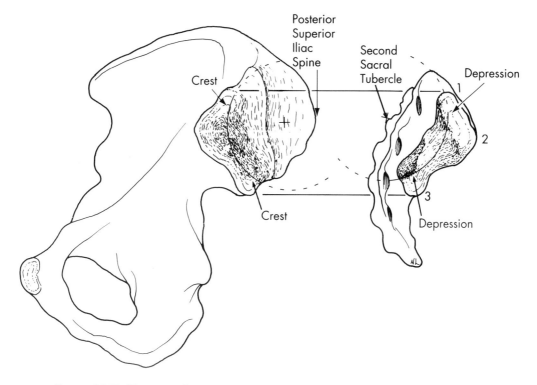

Figure 5.271 The auricular shaped surfaces of the posterior joints of the sacroiliac articulation.

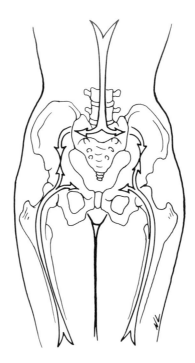

Figure 5.272 Forces from
gravity above meet with
forces from the lower ex-
tremities at the sacroiliac
and hip articulations.

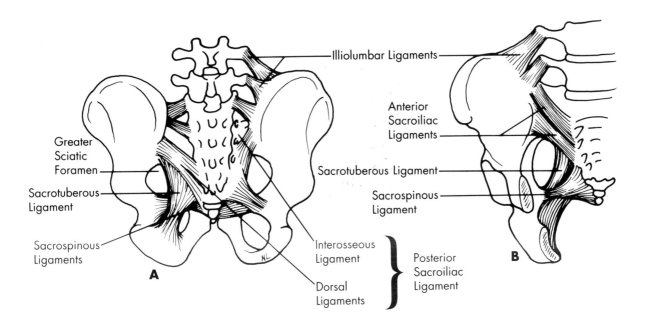

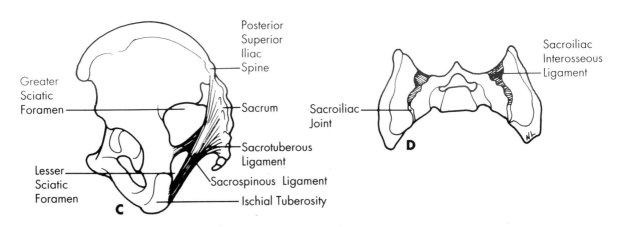

Figure 5.273 The ligaments of the posterior sacroiliac articulations: (**A**) posterior view; (**B**) anterior view; (**C**) lateral view; (**D**) transverse section.

very eroded. In later years a high percentage of male patients will have developed interarticular adhesions across the sacroiliac joints and will have lost sacroiliac joint motion.[64,65]

A number of strong ligaments aid in stabilizing the pelvic mechanism (Fig. 5-273). The posterior sacroiliac ligaments run from the sacrum to the iliac tuberosity and posterior superior iliac spine (PSIS). They are continuous

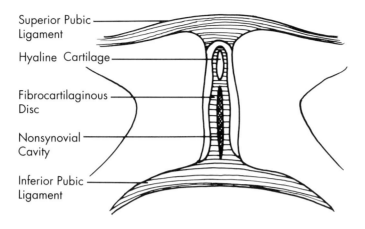

Figure 5.274 The pubic symphysis, anterior joint of the sacroiliac three-joint complex.

laterally with the sacrotuberous ligament and medially with the thoracolumbar fascia. The sacrotuberous ligament extends from the lower portion of the sacrum obliquely downward to the ischial tuberosity. It is continuous caudally with the tendon of the long head of the biceps femoris. The anterior sacroiliac ligament consists of numerous bands attaching from the lateral edge of the sacrum to the auricular surface of the ilium. The sacrospinous ligament is triangular and extends from the lower lateral edge of the sacrum and the upper edge of the coccyx to the ischial spine. The sacrotuberous and sacrospinal ligaments limit posterior movement of the sacral apex; the posterior sacroiliac ligament limits anterior movement of the sacral base.

Anteriorly, the pubic bones are joined by the symphysis pubis, a cartilaginous joint containing a fibrocartilaginous interpubic disc (Fig. 5-274). The superior pubic ligament connects the pubic bones superiorly; the inferior pubic ligament connects the lower borders of the symphysis pubis, forming the upper boundary of the pubic arch. Anteriorly, there is evidence of connective tissue layers passing from one bone to another. They are interlaced with fibers of the external oblique aponeuroses and the medial tendons of the rectus abdominous muscles. Posteriorly, there is also some fibrous tissue that is continuous with the periosteum of both pubic bones. The inguinal ligament, the lower reflected aponeurotic margin of the external oblique muscle, extends from the anterior superior iliac spine to the pubic tubercle.

While some of the strongest muscles of the body surround the sacroiliac joint, none are intrinsic to it or act upon it directly.[59] This is not to say, however, that the surrounding muscle mass may not influence the mechanical behavior of the joint or respond to the stresses applied to it.

Sacroiliac Motions

Though it has become accepted that the sacroiliac is a truly moveable joint, there is still much controversy as to exactly how it moves, how much it moves, and where axes of motion might be located. A number of different hypotheses and models of pelvic mechanics have been proposed, but the one developed by Illi[66] still maintains the most credence and influence.[63,67–73] This model presents the sacroiliac joint as most active during locomotion,

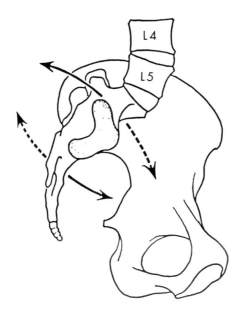

Figure 5.275 The sagittal plane movement of flexion and extension of the sacroiliac articulation.

with movement occurring primarily in the oblique sagittal plane (Fig. 5-275). Translational movements, superior to inferior and anterior to posterior, may also occur but are considered abnormal. During locomotion the sacroiliac joints flex and extend in unison with the corresponding hip joint. In the process of ambulating, each sacroiliac joint goes through two full cycles of alternating flexion and extension. Movements of flexion or extension in one joint are mirrored by the opposite movement at the other joint. Illi's model of sacroiliac motion proposes that compensatory movements at the sacrum and lumbosacral junction occur to help absorb the pelvic torsion induced by these opposing movements of flexion and extension. He suggests that as one innominate flexes (the PSIS moves posterior and inferior) the ipsilateral sacral base moves anterior and inferior, and as the other innominate extends (moves anterior and superior) the sacral base on that side moves posterior and superior (Fig. 5-276). If the described actions of the sacrum are envisioned as one continuous motion, then a picture of an oblique and horizontal figure-eight, rocking movement of the sacrum becomes apparent (Fig. 5-277). He further postulates that alternating movements of flexion act through the iliolumbar ligament to dampen motion at L5 and hence the whole spine.[71] As the ilium moves posterior, L5 is pulled posterior and inferior through tension in the iliolumbar ligament, and the rest of the lumbar spine undergoes coupled motion in slight rotation and lateral flexion (Type I movement).

There has been an unfortunate tendency in the chiropractic profession to refer to the complimentary ipsilateral anterior inferior and posterior superior sacral movements as extension and flexion. This has led to the confusing situation in which the same restriction in sacroiliac movement may be referred to interchangeably as flexion and extension restrictions. For example, during sacroiliac flexion, if the PSIS is the point of reference

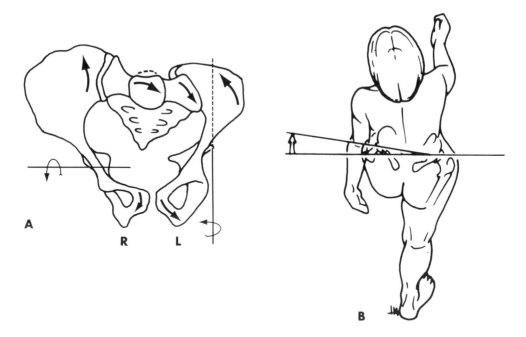

Figure 5.276 Movements of the pelvic joints during gait. (A) Anterior view: as the left innominate moves posterior, a pivoting motion occurs at the pubic symphysis, the left sacral base moves anterior and inferior, and in the (B) posterior view, the pelvis rotates anteriorly about the lumbosacral articulation. The opposite movements occur on the other side.

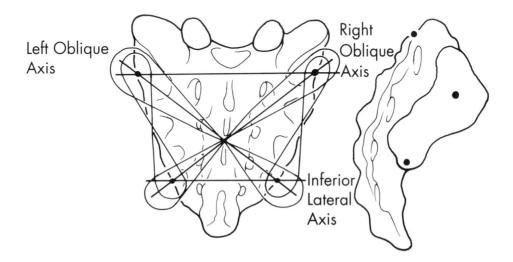

Figure 5.277 The proposed axes of motion in the sacroiliac articulation allow a "gyroscopic" figure-eight movement.

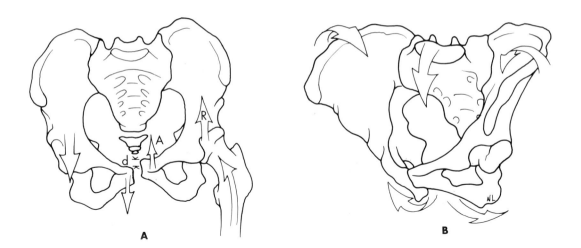

Figure 5.278 While the usual movement of the pubic symphysis is rotation about a transverse axis, the mechanisms exist for (A) shear and (B) separation or compression of the pubes; Fig. B also demonstrates mutation of the sacral base and extension of the lumbosacral articulation.

and perceived to be limited in its posterior and inferior movement, the restriction is described as a sacroiliac flexion restriction. However, if the sacral base is the point of reference and a loss of complimentary ipsilateral anterior inferior movement of the sacral base is perceived, then the same sacroiliac restriction is labeled as an extension restriction.

The obvious confusion with this approach is that both of these movements occur during sacroiliac flexion and it is not possible for a joint to both flex and extend at the same time. The basis of this misunderstanding probably relates to the fact that the sacrum articulates with both the sacroiliac joint and the lumbosacral joint. Lumbosacral extension does involve anterior inferior movement of the sacral base, but the same movement relative to the ilium occurs during sacroiliac flexion, not extension. Pure sagittal plane movements of the sacral base anterior inferior (nutation) and posterior inferior (counter nutation) do occur, but only during trunk flexion and extension and when changing from the upright, seated, and recumbent positions. These movements are appropriately labeled as flexion and extension, but they are defined relative to the lumbosacral articulation, not the sacroiliac joints (Fig. 5-278B).

To avoid confusion, we suggest applying the descriptions of flexion and extension to joint movement, not movement of the sacrum in space. If anterior glide of the sacral base is restricted at the lumbosacral articulation, then it should be referred to as a lumbosacral extension restriction, but if the movement restriction is perceived to be across the sacroiliac joint, it should be referred to as a sacroiliac flexion restriction.

Observing the sacroiliac joints from the posterior and using the PSIS and posterior sacral base as reference points, sacroiliac flexion and extension movements may be described as follows.

1. Flexion of the sacroiliac incorporates posterior inferior movement of the PSIS and ipsilateral anterior inferior movement of the sacral base.
2. Extension of the sacroiliac incorporates anterior superior movement of the PSIS and ipsilateral posterior superior movement of the sacral base (Fig. 5-276).

It is also important to understand and appreciate that with flexion and extension movements at the posterior sacroiliac joints, motion of the pubic symphysis in rotation about a transverse axis must occur. Though this twisting type of motion is considered the only normal motion at the pubic symphysis, small amounts of translational movements forward, backward, up, and down may occur. Large translational movements of the pubic symphysis in a superior to inferior and anterior to posterior direction may also occur but are considered abnormal and present only with an unstable pelvic complex (Fig. 5-278).

Abnormal movement and malpositions of the pubic symphysis have been described.[74] A vertical shear where the pubic bone on one side is higher than the other occurs and can be palpated as well as seen on x-ray.[75] Separation of the pubic symphysis, though less often encountered and occurring mainly in pregnancy, can also be palpated and visualized on x-ray. Rarely, an anterior displacement occurs and is identified with palpation. Palpable pain may occur in dysfunctional patterns of the pubic symphysis.

EVALUATION OF THE PELVIC COMPLEX

The examination of the pelvic complex should incorporate an assessment of alignment, tone, texture, and tenderness of the pelvic ring and its related soft tissues. Also, the sacroiliac joints should be examined for mobility.

Observation

The alignment of the pelvic ring and sacroiliac joints should be assessed in standing, sitting, and prone positions. Standing postural evaluation has been previously described within the section on evaluation of the lumbar spine (Figs. 5-219 through 221). Sitting and prone evaluation of pelvic alignment incorporates an evaluation of the same pelvic landmarks and provides the doctor the opportunity to compare alignment in weightbearing and non-weightbearing positions. For example, a low iliac crest standing and sitting may identify a discrepancy in bony symmetry of the innominates versus a discrepancy in leg length. A low iliac crest in the standing position that appears high in the prone position may indicate the presence of sacroiliac dysfunction and a functional short leg versus an anatomic short leg.

Static Palpation

The palpatory assessment of pelvic bony and soft tissue structures is primarily conducted in the prone position. To evaluate the bony landmarks, establish bilateral contacts with the thumbs or fingertips and compare the contour and alignment of the iliac crests, posterior iliac spines (PSIS), sacral base, and sacral apex (Fig. 5-279). The palpatory depth of the sacral base just

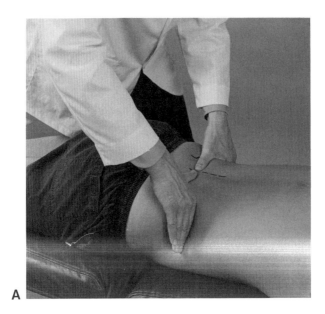

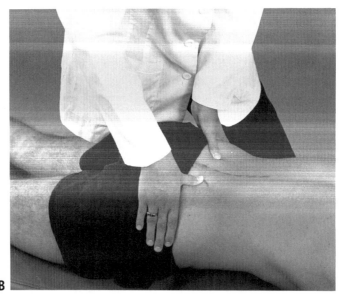

Figure 5.279 Prone palpation of the bony landmarks of the pelvis: **(A)** palpation of the alignment of the iliac crests; **(B)** palpation of the alignment of the PSISs. (*Figure continues.*)

medial to the PSIS and the distance between the second sacral tubercle and the PSIS should be evaluated on each side and compared (Fig. 5-279).

Incorporated into the evaluation of the bony structures of the pelvis is an evaluation of comparative leg length. Anatomic discrepancies in length may predispose the patient to pelvic dysfunction, and functional leg length inequality is considered a potential significant sign of sacroiliac subluxation/dysfunction. Leg length is traditionally evaluated in the prone position by observing the comparative length of the heels or medial malleoli. If discrepancies are noted, the legs should be elevated to 90 degrees to screen

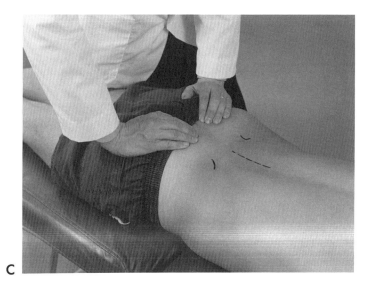

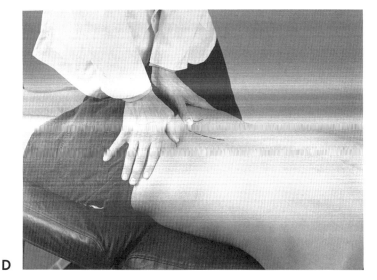

Figure 5.279 (*Continued*). (**C**) Palpation of the alignment of the sacral apex; and (**D**) palpation of the sacral sulcus, noting the depth and alignment of the sacral base.

for a shortened tibia (Fig. 5-280). The elevated feet must be maintained in neutral upright position. Internal or external rotation of the hip induces a false indication of tibial shortening. In cases of suspected sacroiliac dysfunction and associated functional leg length inequality, the doctor should also evaluate and compare leg length in the supine and sitting positions. Functional leg length inequality that is secondary to sacroiliac subluxation/dysfunction may reverse from the supine to sitting position, whereas anatomic leg length inequality or functional inequality secondary to dysfunction at other sites likely will not (Fig. 5-281).

Flexion (PI) or extension (AS) malpositions of one innominate as compared with the other are possible indications of pelvic dysfunction. These positions of distortion may be identified with the aid of palpation and

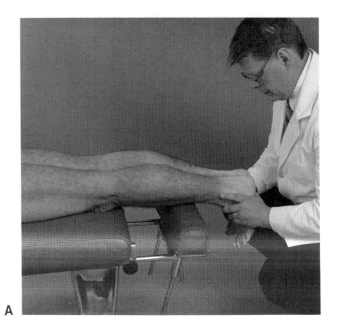

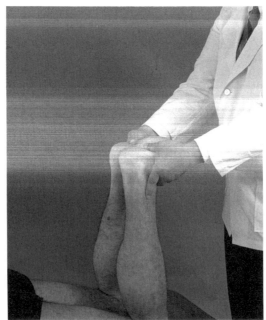

Figure 5.280 Prone evaluation of leg length: (A) knees extended and (B) knees flexed.

Table 5.11 Clinical Findings Associated With a Pelvic Distortion

Posterior Innominate Flexion Malposition	Anterior Innominate Extension Malposition
PSIS prominent, medial, and inferior	PSIS anterior, lateral, and superior
Gluteal fold low	Glutal fold high
ASIS elevated	ASIS lowered
Sacral base anterior and inferior	Sacral base posterior and superior
Sacral apex deviated contralaterally	Sacral apex deviated ipsilaterally
L5 rotated posteriorly ipsilaterally	
Ipsilateral convexity of lumbar lateral curve	
Functional leg length deficiency	

observation. Table 5-11 lists the clinical findings that have been empirically reported by the chiropractic profession to reflect each distortion. However, remember that identification of altered alignment is not confirmation of dysfunction. The evaluation of alignment, like all physical procedures, is prone to examiner error, and congenital asymmetries of the pelvis are not uncommon.

The soft tissues of the lumbosacral, sacroiliac, and gluteal regions are also palpated with the palmar surfaces of the fingers or thumbs. In the patient complaining of low back pain, it is important to carefully distinguish between several common sites of dysfunction. Pain arising in the sacroiliac joint, iliolumbar ligaments, posterior lumbosacral joints, or adjacent gluteal soft tissues may all be responsible for the subjective complaint of generalized lumbosacral or sacroiliac pain. The sacroiliac ligaments are palpated just medially to the PSIS, and the iliolumbar ligaments between the L5 transverse process and iliac crest. Pain arising from the myofascial origins of the gluteal and piriformis muscles are identified by exploring their attachments along the PSIS and sacral ala (Fig. 5-282).

Joint Play

Sitting Joint Play

To assess sitting joint play of the sacroiliac joint, place the patient in the sitting position with the arms relaxed on the lap. Sit behind the patient, shifted slightly to the contralateral side. Establish the palpation contact with the thumb along the medial aspect of the PSIS with the supporting forearm placed across the patient's shoulders (Fig. 5-283). Guide the patient in lateral flexion away from the side of contact until tension at the SI joint is felt. At tension apply additional downward pressure through the indifferent arm coupled with lateral pressure from the contact thumb. Slight give should be perceived during evaluation, and abnormal resistance or pain may be associated with sacroiliac dysfunction.

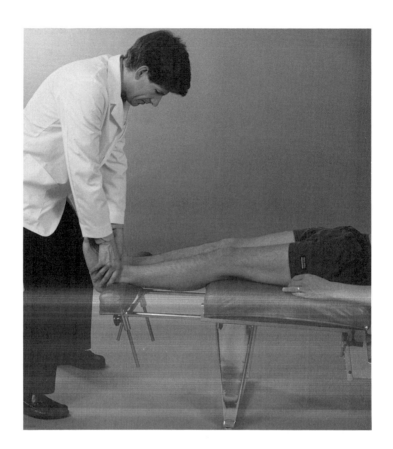

Figure 5.281 Supine evaluation of leg length: (**A**) lying
supine. (*Figure continues.*)

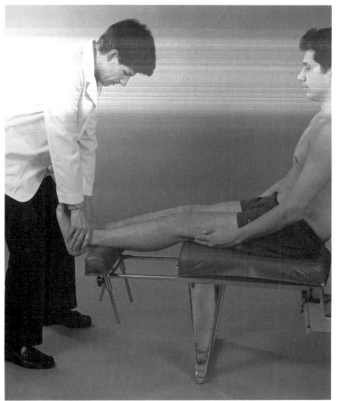

Figure 5.281 (*Contin-
ued*). (**B**) sitting. (*Figure continues.*)

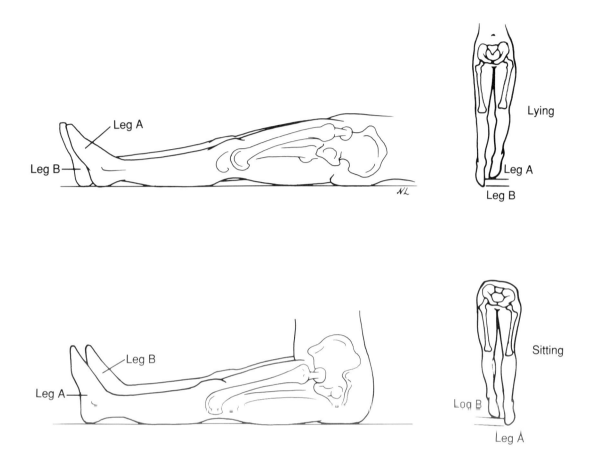

Figure 5.281 (*Continued*). (**C**) Changes in leg length observed from the lying to the sitting position may indicate a sacroiliac dysfunction. On the side of the relative posterior innominate (leg A), the acetabulum is displaced anteriorly, creating a leg deficiency when lying supine, which lengthens upon sitting. (Modified from Gatterman,[76] with permission.)

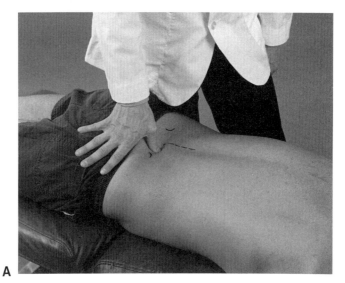

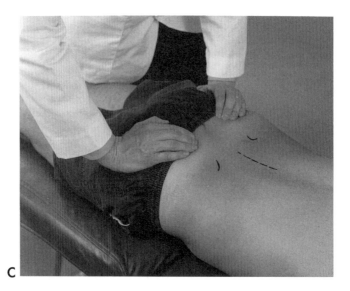

Figure 5.282 Palpation of the lumbosacral and gluteal soft tissues. (**A**) Palpation for tenderness of the right iliolumbar ligament. (**B**) Palpation of the origins of the gluteal muscles. (**C**) Palpation of the origins of the piriformis muscles.

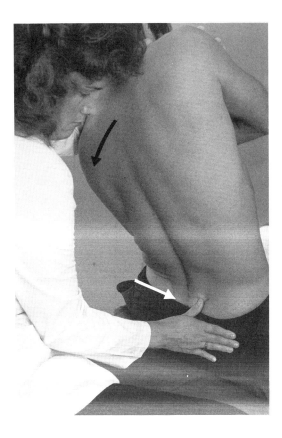

Figure 5.283 Thumb contact applied to the right PSIS to evaluate joint play of the right sacroiliac articulation.

Side Posture Joint Play

The sacroiliac joint can be stressed for flexion and extension movements in the side posture position. Contact the ASIS with the cephalic hand and the ischial tuberosity with the caudal hand to induce flexion (posterior inferior movement) of the sacroiliac joint. By contacting the PSIS and the inferior aspect of the anterior portion of the innominate, the sacroiliac joint can be stressed to induce extension (anterior superior movement) (Fig. 5-284).

Prone Joint Play

Sacroiliac flexion

To evaluate flexion joint play reach across with the caudal hand and cup the patient's anterior ilium. Then palpate the sacroiliac joint with the cephalic hand by locating the fingertips just medial to the PSIS over the dorsal aspect of the ipsilateral sacral ala (sulcus of the SI joint) (Fig. 5-285). To execute the procedure, pull posterior with the anterior ilial contact and palpate for posterior glide of the ilium.

The same movement may be assessed by applying counter pressure on each side of the joint. To perform this variation, establish a contact on the sacral base with the thenar or hypothenar of the cephalic hand and a contact on the lower ischium with the palmar surface of the caudal hand (Fig.

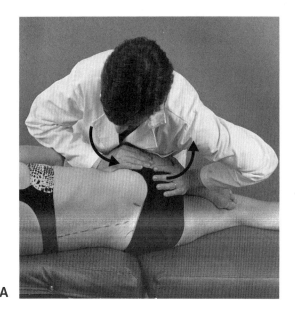
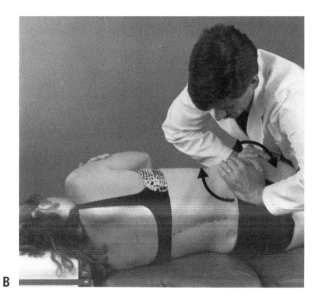

Figure 5.284 Side posture position to stress the right sacroiliac articulation (**A**) anterior to posterior (flexion), and (**B**) posterior to anterior (extension).

5-286). After establishing the contacts, lean body weight into the patient and apply anterior superior pressure through the sacral contact and anterior inferior pressure through the ischial contact. Although movement is subtle, separation should be perceived between the contacts. Pain and/or increased or decreased joint play indicates sacroiliac dysfunction.

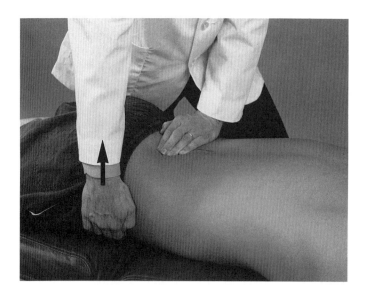

Figure 5.285 Anterior to posterior pressure applied to the right ilium and digital contacts applied to the right sacroiliac joint assess for the presence of flexion joint play.

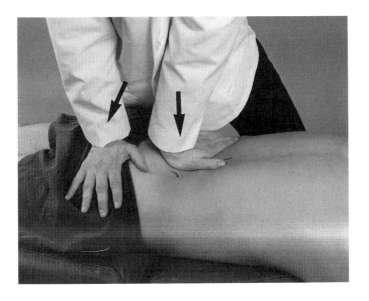

Figure 5.286 Counter pressure is applied to the right sacroiliac joint with a thenar contact over the right sacral base and a calcaneal contact over the right lower ilium to assess flexion joint play.

Sacroiliac extension

To assess extension, contact the sacral apex with the caudal hand and the sulcus of the SI joint with the cephalic hand (Fig. 5-287). As the caudal hand pushes the apex of the sacrum anteriorly, the palpating hand feels for posterior movement of the sacral base in relation to the ilium. To modify this procedure for the application of counter pressure, establish a contact on the sacral apex with the hypothenar of the caudal hand and a contact on the ipsilateral PSIS with the hypothenar of the cephalic hand (Fig. 5-288). Apply anterior and superior pressure against the ilium and anterior and inferior movement against the sacral apex. Normal movement is reflected

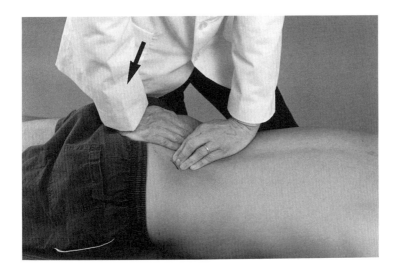

Figure 5.287 Posterior to anterior pressure is applied to sacral apex while a digital contact over the right sacroiliac joint is used to assess extension joint play.

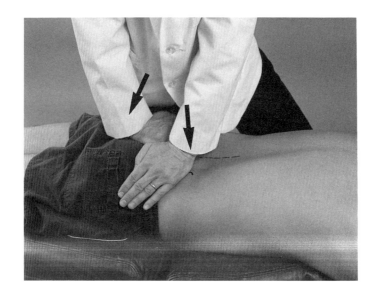

Figure 5.288 Counter pressure applied through a hypothenar contact over the right PSIS and a hypothenar contact over the sacral apex to assess extension joint play in the right sacroiliac joint.

by a sense of give and separation into extension. Pain and/or increased or decreased play indicates sacroiliac dysfunction.

Inferior sacral glide

The patient is placed in the prone position, and the doctor reaches across the patient with the heel of the caudal hand to contact the patient's lower ischium. The ulnar side of the cephalic hand contacts the superior dorsal surface of the sacrum, also on the contralateral side (Fig. 5-289). To execute the procedure, apply caudal pressure against the sacrum as counter stabilizing pressure is maintained against the ischium. Pain or discomfort during the test may indicate sacroiliac dysfunction.

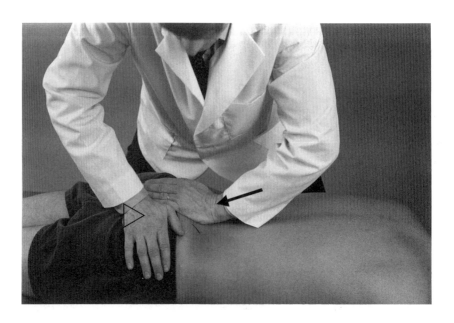

Figure 5.289 Hypothenar contact applied to the right sacral base exerts pressure inferiorly against counter pressure applied by a calcaneal contact over the right ischium to assess inferior sacral glide.

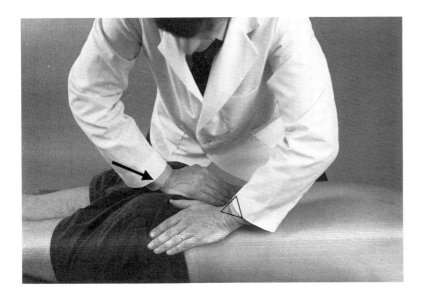

Figure 5.290 Hypothenar contact applied to the right inferior margin of the sacrum exerts pressure superiorly against counter pressure applied by a calcaneal contact over the right iliac crest to assess superior sacral glide.

Superior sacral glide

The patient is placed in the prone position. The doctor reaches across the patient with the ulnar side of the caudal hand to contact the inferolateral margin of the sacrum. The cephalic hand stabilizes the iliac crest with a broad contact (Fig. 5-290). Cephalic pressure is applied against the sacral contact as counter pressure is maintained against the ilium. Pain or discomfort during the test may also indicate sacroiliac dysfunction.

Pelvic Motion Palpation

Screening Mobility Tests

Piedau's sign

With the patient standing or sitting on a flat surface, contact the sacral apex with the thumbs and each PSIS with the fingertips (Fig. 5-291). Make an initial comparison of height and ask the patient to bend forward. If the

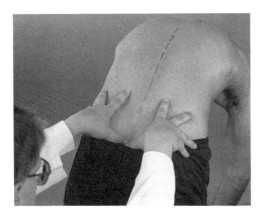

Figure 5.291 Digital contacts over the PSISs and thumb contacts over the sacral apex. With forward flexion these contacts should separate, indicating that the sacral base can move posteriorly. The converse is true with extension.

PSISs were uneven at the start and the lower PSIS glides higher than the contralateral PSIS, then the test is considered positive. Dysfunction is suspected on the side that went from the initially lower position to the more superior position. It is assumed that the involved side is hypomobile and rises higher with forward flexion because the sacroiliac joint is not free to glide along its articular surface. Additionally, if the PSISs were even at the start, on flexion a separation of the PSISs from the sacral apex should be perceived, indicating the sacral base has moved posterior. The converse occurs with extension.

Sacral push

The patient is asked to sit with arms relaxed on the thighs. The doctor sits behind the patient and establishes bilateral thumb contacts across the patient's SI joints and sacral ala (Fig. 5-292). The patient is then asked to extend back and rotate around the doctor's thumbs. With proper SI and lumbosacral joint motion the doctor's thumbs should move symmetrically forward with the patient's sacral base. Restricted anterior gliding of the sacral base may indicate sacroiliac dysfunction.

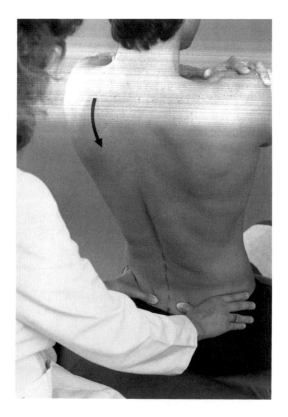

Figure 5.292 Thumb contacts push posterior to anterior over the sacral base on both sides to assess anterior glide of the sacrum.

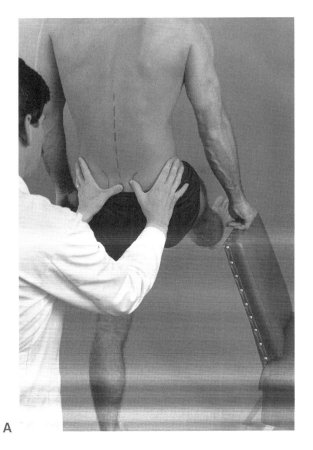 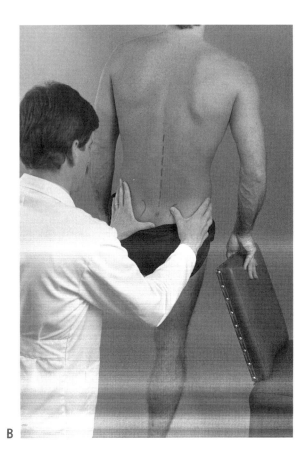

A   B

Figure 5.293 Standing sacroiliac joint evaluation for right upper joint movement. After thumb contacts are established over the right PSIS and sacral tubercle, the patient flexes the **(A)** ipsilateral hip to assess SI joint flexion (approximation of finger and thumb) and **(B)** the contralateral hip to assess SI joint extension (separation of finger and thumb).

Standing SI Tests

Upper SI mobility

The patient is asked to stand holding a support for balance. The doctor stands or sits behind the patient and establishes thumb contacts on the patient's PSIS and second (or first) sacral tubercle (Fig. 5-293). The patient is then instructed to raise the ipsilateral leg to approximately 90 degrees. This induces flexion of the hip and sacroiliac joint. With normal movement the doctor's thumbs approximate as the PSIS moves posterior and inferior toward the relatively stationary second sacral tubercle (Fig. 5-293A). Sacroiliac flexion restrictions should be suspected when the thumbs do not approximate and the pelvis rotates obliquely around the opposite hip.

After flexion has been evaluated, the patient is instructed to raise the contralateral leg to a level above 90 degrees. This induces posterior nodding

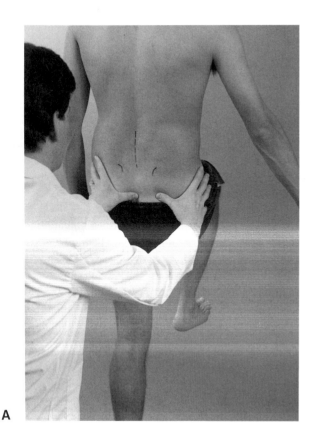
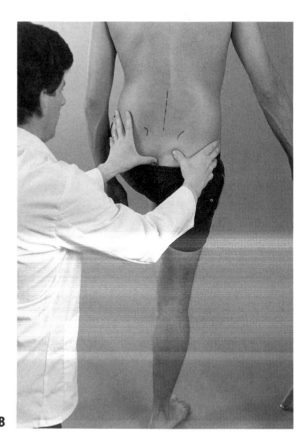

A

B

Figure 5.294 Standing sacroiliac joint evaluation for right lower joint move-ment. After thumb contacts are established over the right sacral apex and the soft tissue lateral to the sacral apex in line with the PSIS the patient flexes the (**A**) ipsilateral hip to assess SI joint flexion (separation of thumbs) and (**B**) the contralateral hip to assess SI joint extension (separation of thumbs).

of the sacral base and sacroiliac extension on the side of palpation. With normal movement, the doctor's thumbs move apart as the PSIS moves anterior and superior away from the second sacral tubercle (Fig. 5-293B).

Lower SI Mobility

To assess mobility of the lower sacroiliac joint the palpation contacts are moved down to the sacral apex and adjacent ischium (Fig. 5-294). The patient is again instructed to raise the ipsilateral leg to approximately 90 degrees. Flexion in the lower joint is assessed and the doctor's thumbs should separate as the ischium moves anterior and superior relatively to the sacral apex (Fig. 5-294A). Extension of the lower sacroiliac joint is evaluated by elevating the opposite leg to a level above 90 degrees. Normal extension of the lower joint is also reflected by separation of the sacral and ischial contacts (Fig. 5-294B).

Pubic Symphysis Dysfunction

The symphysis is not a synovial joint and as such does not demonstrate significant movement. However, some degree of shifting and shearing movement at the symphysis is probably present with locomotion and occurs by virtue of its fibrocartilaginous structure. As a result dysfunction at this joint may contribute to pelvic dysfunction. The question then remains, if the symphysis is capable of contributing to sacroiliac dysfunction how does one determine if the symphysis should be manipulated? Although methods for assessing glide are presented, it is doubtful that mobility at the symphysis is palpable and pain on stress testing may be more indicative of dysfunction. The decision is based on the clinical impression of the doctor, which is formulated from all the physical findings. It is appropriate that manipulation of the symphysis pubes occur on a trial-and-error basis, after contraindications have been ruled out, in cases that are not responding as expected.

Evaluation of the Pubic Symphysis

The patient lies in the supine position while the doctor palpates the anterior aspect of each pubic bone with the index fingers of both hands, noting changes in anterior to posterior and superior to inferior alignment from one side to the other (Fig. 5-295). Then stress the symphysis anterior to posterior, superior to inferior, and inferior to superior, noting the direction that causes the most pain as well as any movement abnormality. Finally, ask the patient to actively tilt the pelvis sideways or alternately elongate and shorten the legs as you palpate for subtle shifting between the two pubic bones.

Evaluation of the Coccyx

With the patient prone, palpate over the sacrococcygeal joint space for abnormal alignment and tenderness. Apply posterior to anterior stress to the sacrococcygeal joint with double thumbs to induce a gliding joint play movement. Misalignment with tenderness or loss of posterior to anterior joint play movement, or both, is characteristic of dysfunction.

ADJUSTMENTS OF THE PELVIS

Movement at the sacroiliac joint occurs primarily in the semi-sagittal plane along the angle of the joint's articular surface.[69,70,72,75] These movements occur primarily during locomotion and when changing from supine to sitting or sitting to standing positions. They involve movements of the ilium and sacrum in reciprocally opposing directions[66] and have been referred to previously as movements of flexion and extension.[71,72] To treat sacroiliac flexion or extension dysfunction, adjustive contacts may be applied on the ilium or the sacrum. Flexion dysfunction is treated by contacting the ilium and inducing posterior and inferior movement of the ilial articular surface relative to the ipsilateral sacral articular surface, or by contacting the sacrum and inducing anterior inferior movement of the sacral articular surface relative to the ipsilateral ilial articular surface. Extension dysfunction is induced by contacting the ilium and inducing anterior superior movement

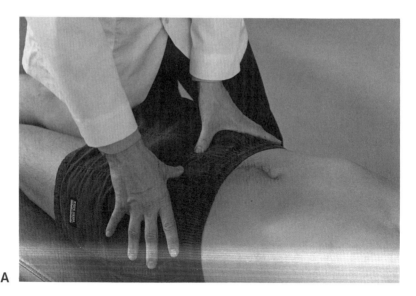

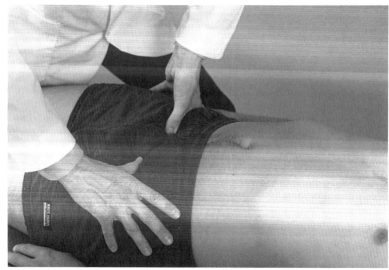

Figure 5.295 Palpation of the pubic symphysis for pain and displacement. (**A**) An anterior to posterior pressure is applied to assess anterior displacement and posterior glide. (**B**) Superior to inferior and inferior to superior pressure is applied to assess for superior or inferior displacement and glide.

of the ilial articular surface relative to the ipsilateral sacral articular surface, or by contacting the sacrum and inducing posterior superior movement of the sacral articular surface relative to the ilial articular surface. These adjustments may be applied in a variety of patient positions and may incorporate methods that establish adjustive contacts on both sides of the articular surfaces.

Side Posture Pelvic Adjustments

Side posture sacroiliac adjustments are the most common manipulative methods employed for treating sacroiliac joint dysfunction. Like lumbar side posture adjustments, they offer flexibility in patient position and added leverage. They do, however, potentially produce unwanted rotational tension in the lumbar spine. This can be minimized by limiting counter rotation of the patient's shoulders and by emphasizing traction and tension on the sacroiliac joint through the contact hand.

Prone Pelvic Adjustments

Prone pelvic adjustments can be efficient alternatives to side posture pelvic adjustments. They do not produce the pre-adjustive joint distraction of side posture adjustments but may be more appropriate for situations in which side posture position would unduly stress the lumbar spine.

Symphysis Adjustments

The adjustive procedures that are applied to the pubic symphysis use an initial patient contraction of specific muscles against resistance supplied by the doctor. The muscle contraction first pulls on the symphysis in the desired direction and when, or if, tolerated by the patient, an impulse thrust is applied. This is not a synovial joint and cavitation is not possible. Therefore a joint release will not occur. Sometimes, a noise will be heard or felt that probably is a soft tissue release or a tendinous snap.

Coccyx Adjustments

Coccygeal pain may occur after a fall or postpartum and can be very persistent. The benefits of coccygeal adjustment will either be realized very quickly or it will likely not be effective at all. The external contact uses a tissue pull procedure and is probably less effective but more comfortable for the patient. The internal contact has the doctor placing a finger intrarectally to establish a contact on the anterior aspect of the coccyx. Use of latex gloves is necessary to provide a sanitary barrier. Appropriate patient gowning and draping as well as a thorough explanation of the procedure is important to maintain professional boundaries.

Side Posture Pelvic Adjustments

Hypothenar ilium (PI ilium) (Fig. 5-296)

IND: Restricted sacroiliac extension. Flexion malposition of the ilium (PI).

  PP: The patient lies in the basic side posture position.

  DP: Stand in a fencer stance angled approximately 45 degrees to the patient. Support the patient's pelvis by contacting the patient's thigh with your inferior thigh or by straddling the patient's bent upper leg between your thighs.

  CP: Hypothenar (pisiform) of caudal hand.

SCP: Medial margin of the PSIS.

  IH: The indifferent hand contacts the patient's up side shoulder and overlapping hand.

VEC: Posterior to anterior, medial to lateral, and inferior to superior.

    P: Place the patient in side posture with the involved side up. Flex the upper thigh to between 60 degrees and 80 degrees. Establish the ilial and thigh contacts and develop pre-adjustive tension by distracting and extending the involved sacroiliac joint.

       Produce joint distraction by lowering your body weight through

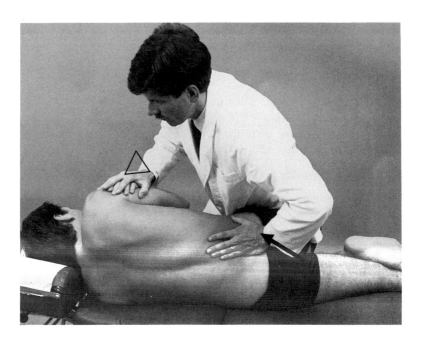

Figure 5.296 Hypothenar contact established over the right PSIS to induce extension of the upper right sacroiliac joint (PI ilium).

the thigh contact. Produce joint extension by leaning anteriorly and cephalically through the torso and contact. The indifferent hand stabilizes the patient's shoulder and applies gentle traction cephalically and posteriorly; take care to avoid excessive posterior rotation of the patient's upper torso.

At tension generate an impulse thrust by dropping the body weight and thrusting through the shoulder.

Hypothenar sacral base (PS sacrum) (Fig. 5-297)

IND: Restricted sacroiliac flexion. Unilateral posterior superior malposition of the sacrum.

PP: The patient lies in the basic side posture position.

DP: Stand in a fencer stance angled approximately 45 degrees to the patient. Support the patient's pelvis by contacting the patient's thigh with your inferior thigh or by straddling the patient's bent upper leg between your thighs.

CP: Hypothenar (pisiform) of the caudal hand.

SCP: Superior sacral base just medial to the PSIS on the side of sacroiliac dysfunction.

IH: The indifferent hand contacts the patient's up side shoulder and overlapping hand.

VEC: Posterior to anterior and slightly inferior to superior.

P: Place the patient in side posture with the dysfunctional sacroiliac against or away from the table. Flex the upper thigh to between 60 degrees and 80 degrees. Establish the ilial and thigh contacts and develop pre-adjustive tension by distracting and flexing the involved sacroiliac joint. The indifferent hand stabilizes the patient's shoulder

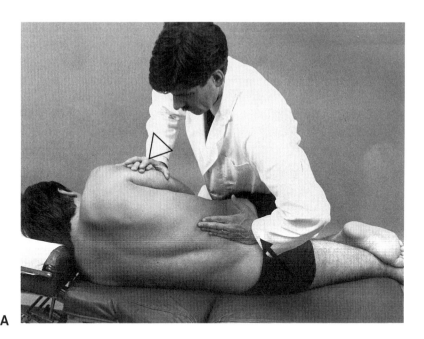

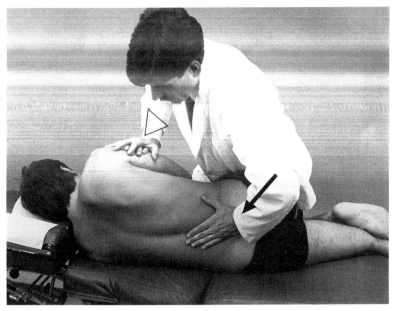

Figure 5.297 Hypothenar contact established over the **(A)** right and **(B)** left side of the sacral base to induce posterior to anterior movement of the sacral base on the side of contact.

and applies gentle traction cephalically and posteriorly; take care to avoid excessive posterior rotation of the patient's upper torso.

Dysfunctional side up. The patient lies on the side opposite the dysfunctional sacroiliac joint. Induce sacroiliac flexion by pushing the sacral base forward. Produce sacroiliac joint distraction by lowering your body weight through the thigh contact (Fig. 5-297A). At tension generate an impulse thrust by dropping your body weight and thrusting anteriorly through your shoulder.

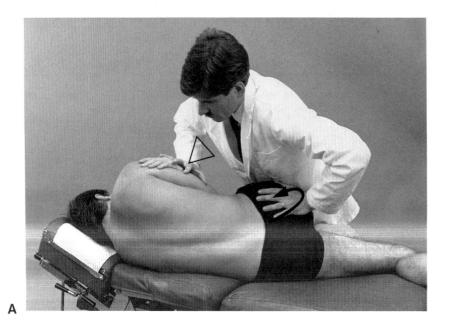

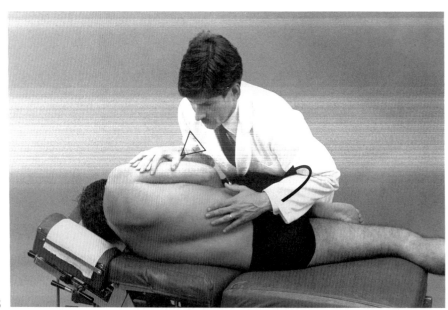

Figure 5.298 To induce flexion (AS ilium) of the right sacroiliac joint. **(A)** A hypothenar contact or **(B)** a forearm contact is established over the posterior aspect of the ischial tuberosity. (*Figure continues.*)

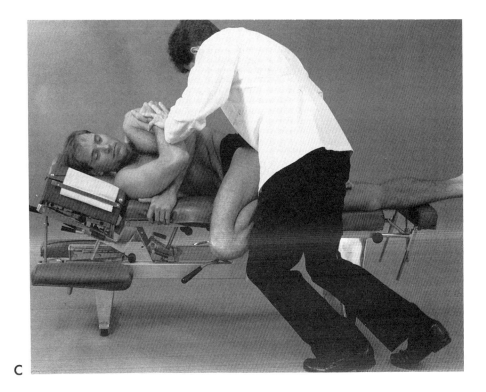

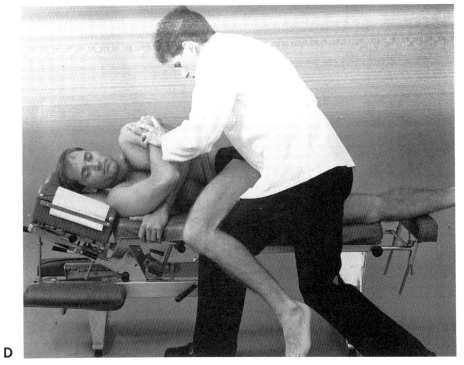

Figure 5.298 (*Continued*). The doctor's leg contacts are modified in this adjustment to a (**C**) double thigh to shin or (**D**) split leg, knee to popliteal fossa to prestress the sacroiliac into flexion.

Dysfunctional side down. The patient lies on the side of sacroiliac joint dysfunction. Establish the adjustive contact on the sacral base on the down side and rotate the patient slightly further toward you. At tension generate an anteriorly directed impulse thrust through your trunk and shoulder along the plane of the sacroiliac articulation (Fig. 5-297B). (A thenar contact may be substituted for the hypothenar contact.)

Hypothenar ischium (AS ilium) (Fig. 5-298)

IND: Restricted sacroiliac flexion. Extension malposition of the ilium (AS).
 PP: The patient lies in the basic side posture position.
 DP: Stand in a low fencer stance straddling the patient's flexed upper knee. Support the patient's flexed leg against the proximal anterior thigh of your caudal leg. Your lower abdomen may rest against the patient's posterior lateral buttock and hip.
 CP: Soft broad hypothenar contact of the caudad hand with the fingers spread and pointing cephalad (Fig. 5-298A).
SCP: Medial inferior ischium.
 IH: The cephalad hand stabilizes the patient's upper shoulder, maintaining spinal flexion.
VEC: Posterior to anterior.
  P: Place the patient in side posture with the involved side up. Slightly flex the patient's trunk and flex the upper thigh above 90 degrees. Establish a broad soft contact along the superior medial margin of the ischium.

   Pre-adjustive tension is produced by inducing sacroiliac distraction and flexion. Sacroiliac distraction is induced by dropping the patient's flexed thigh toward the floor and by lowering the doctor's body weight against the patient's flexed hip. Sacroiliac flexion is induced by pulling inferiorly with the contact hand as the doctor pushes cephalically against the patient's flexed leg with his caudal leg.

   At tension an impulse thrust is delivered anteriorly through the trunk, lower extremities and shoulder. A slight variation of this procedure may be employed by using a forearm contact instead of a hypothenar contact (Fig. 5.298B). Optional doctor stances and leg contacts may also be used in this adjustment (Fig. 5.298C,D).

Hypothenar sacral apex (AI sacrum) (Fig. 5-299)

IND: Restricted sacroiliac extension. Unilateral anterior inferior malposition of the sacrum.
 PP: The patient lies in the basic side posture position.
 DP: Stand in a low fencer stance straddling the patient's flexed upper knee. Support the patient's flexed leg against the proximal anterior thigh of your caudal leg. Your lower abdomen may rest against the patient's posterior lateral buttock and hip.
 CP: Hypothenar of the caudal hand with fingers pointing cephalad (Fig. 5-299A).
SCP: Apex of the sacrum.
 IH: Superior hand stabilizes the patient's upper shoulder maintaining spinal flexion.

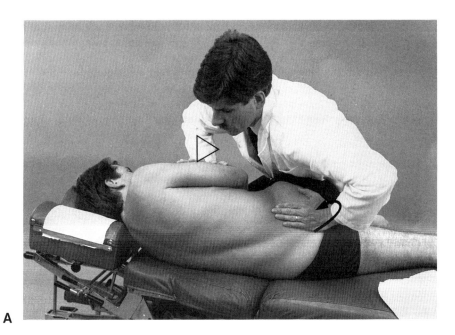

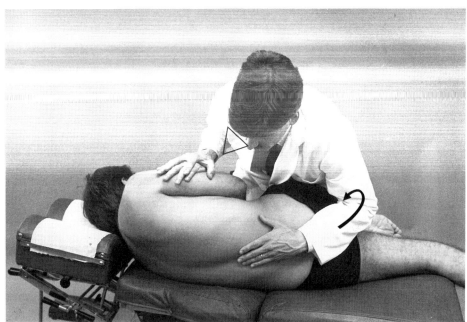

Figure 5.299 (A) A hypothenar contact or (B) a forearm contact is established over the sacral apex to induce sacral extension.

VEC: Posterior to anterior.

P: Place the patient in side posture with the involved side down. Slightly flex the patient's trunk and flex the upper thigh above 90 degrees. Establish a broad soft contact along the up side of the sacral apex.

Develop pre-adjustive tension by inducing lumbosacral flexion and anterior pelvic rotation. This produces posterior nodding and rotation of the sacral base on the down side and extension of the down side sacroiliac joint. Induce anterior pelvic rotation by dropping the patient's flexed thigh toward the floor and by lowering your body weight against the patient's flexed hip. Induce posterior nodding of the sacral base by pulling inferiorly with the contact hand against the sacral apex as you push cephalically against the patient's flexed leg with your caudal leg.

At tension deliver an impulse thrust anteriorly through the trunk, lower extremities, and shoulder. A slight variation of this procedure may be employed by using a forearm contact instead of a hypothenar contact (Fig. 5-299B).

Prone Pelvic Adjustments

Hypothenar ilium sacral apex (PI ilium or AI sacrum) (Fig. 5-300)

IND: Restricted sacroiliac extension. PI malposition of the ilium and/or unilateral AI malposition of the sacrum.

PP: The patient lies prone.

DP: Stand in a modified fencer stance on the side opposite the dysfunction.

CP: Hypothenar contacts of both hands.

SCP: Medial superior margin of the PSIS and sacral apex (Fig. 5-300A).

VEC: Posterior to anterior, inferior to superior, and medial to lateral with the PSIS contact. Posterior to anterior, superior to inferior, and medial to lateral with the sacral apex contact.

P: Position the patient in the prone position. Reach across the patient with the caudal hand and establish a hypothenar contact on the contralateral PSIS. With the cephalic hand reach inferiorly to establish a contact on the sacral apex.

Develop pre-adjustive tension by leaning anteriorly and superiorly with the iliac contact and anteriorly and inferiorly with the sacral contact. A pelvic block may be positioned under the greater trochanter to assist in the development of sacroiliac extension.

At tension deliver a high velocity thrust combined through the arms, trunk, and body.

When using this adjustment with a drop table, place the patient's anterior superior iliac spines in the break between the adjusting table's pelvic and lumbar sections. The adjustive thrust should not be delivered until appropriate drop piece tension has been established.

If desired a PI ilium or sacroiliac extension restriction may be treated with a unilateral contact on the PSIS. With this method you may stand on either side of the patient (Fig. 5-300B).

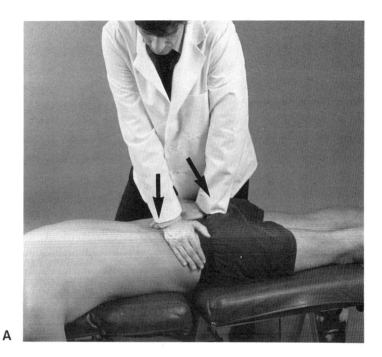

A

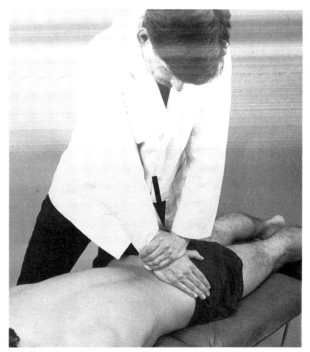

B

Figure 5.300 Adjustment for restricted extension in the left sacroiliac joint using
(**A**) bilateral contacts over the left PSIS and sacral apex, and (**B**) a unilateral
contact over the PSIS.

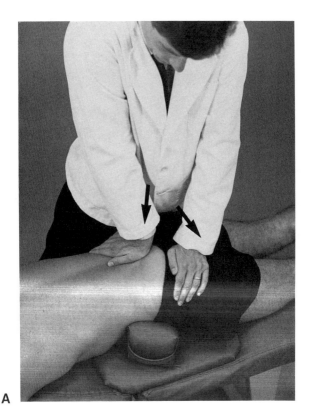

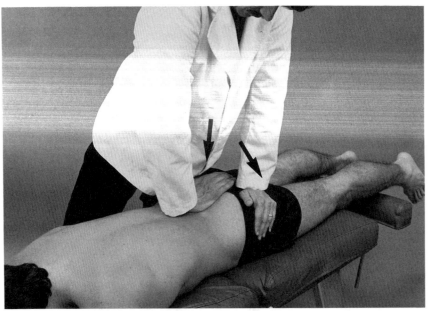

Figure 5.301 Adjustment for restricted flexion of the left sacroiliac joint using contacts over the left ischial tuberosity and sacral base **(A)** with blocks, **(B)** without blocks. (*Figure continues.*)

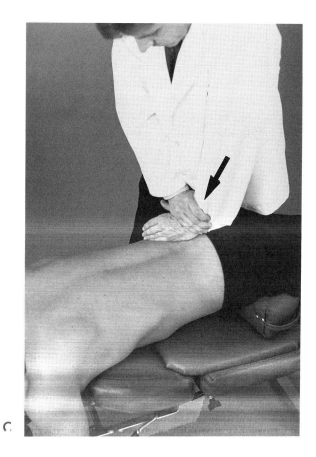

Figure 5.301 (*Continued*). (**C**) Using a unilateral sacral base contact.

Hypothenar ischium sacral base (AS ilium or PS sacrum) (Fig. 5-301)

IND: Restricted sacroiliac flexion. AS malposition of the ilium and/or unilateral PS malposition of the sacrum.

PP: The patient lies prone.

DP: Stand in a modified fencer stance on the side opposite the dysfunction.

CP: Proximal palmar surface of the caudal hand for ischial contact and thenar or hypothenar eminence of cephalic hand for sacral base contact (Figs. 5-301A and B).

SCP: Inferior ischium and proximal sacral base.

VEC: Posterior to anterior and superior to inferior with ischial contact. Posterior to anterior and inferior to superior with sacral contact.

P: Position the patient in the prone position. Reach across the patient with the caudal hand and establish a palmar contact on the inferior ischium. With the thenar or hypothenar of the cephalic hand contact the superior margin of sacral base just medial to the PSIS on the same side.

Develop pre-adjustive tension by leaning anteriorly and inferiorly with the ischial contact and anteriorly and superiorly with the sacral contact. A pelvic block may be positioned under the ASIS to assist in the development of sacroiliac flexion (Fig. 5-301A).

At tension deliver a high velocity combined thrust through the arms, trunk, and body.

When using this adjustment with a drop table, place the patient's anterior superior iliac spines at the superior end of the table's pelvic section. The adjustive thrust should not be delivered until appropriate drop piece tension has been established.

If desired a PS sacral subluxation or sacroiliac flexion restriction may be treated with a unilateral contact on the involved PS sacral base. With this method you may stand on either side of the patient (Fig. 5-301C).

Genu ilium (PI ilium) (Fig. 5-302)

IND: Restricted sacroiliac extension. PI malposition of the ilium.
 PP: The patient lies prone.
 DP: Stand in a fencer stance on the side opposite the dysfunction.
 CP: Hypothenar of cephalic hand.
SCP: Medial superior margin of the PSIS.
 IH: The caudal hand grasps the patient's distal thigh on the same side as the adjustive contact.
VEC: Posterior to anterior, inferior to superior, and medial to lateral.
  P: Position the patient in the prone position. Reach across the patient with the cephalic hand and establish a hypothenar contact on the contralateral PSIS. With the caudal hand reach across the patient and grip the patient's contralateral thigh just proximal to the knee.

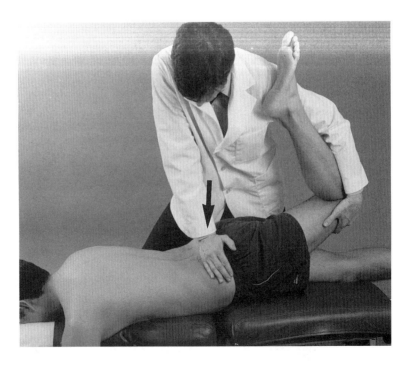

Figure 5.302 Contact over the left PSIS while extending the hip to induce extension of the left sacroiliac joint.

Develop joint tension by leaning into the contact and gently extending the patient's thigh. Accompanying hip extension is minimal and should not induce significant rotation of the pelvis off the table.

At tension deliver an impulse thrust through the ilial contact, reinforced by a shallow lift with the thigh contact. The thrust through the hip must be shallow. It is possible to overextend the hip, damaging the capsule and its adjacent soft tissues. This adjustment is contraindicated in patients with hip pathology or meralgia paresthetica.

When using this adjustment with a drop table, place the patient's anterior superior iliac spines in the break between the adjusting table's pelvic and lumbar sections. The adjustive thrust should not be delivered until appropriate drop piece tension has been established.

Pelvic Blocking

Pelvic blocking—prone (Fig. 5-303)

IND: AS or PI malposition of the ilium.
  PP: The patient lies prone with a firm surface (padded board) under the pelvic area.
  DP: The doctor has a passive role; place padded wedges (pelvic blocks) under both sides of the pelvis.
  CP: Padded wedge (pelvic block).
SCP: ASIS and anterior to the ischial tuberosity.
   P: Position the patient in the prone position on a padded board. Place a padded wedge under the ASIS on the side of the anterior innominate and another under the anterior aspect of the ischial tuberosity on the side of the posterior innominate to develop sacroiliac flexion.

No thrust is given; gravity provides the force applied over time

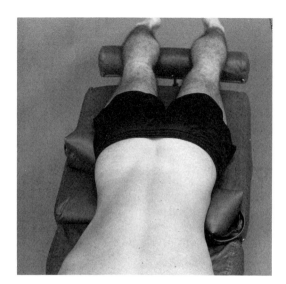

Figure 5.303 Prone pelvic blocking for a left AS and right PI distortion pattern using gravity over time to induce movement at the sacroiliac joints. There is no thrust.

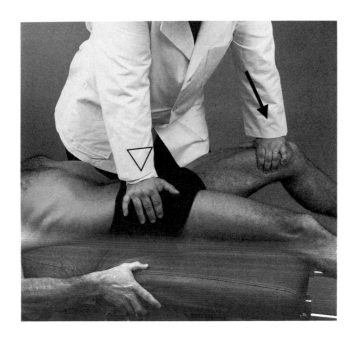

Figure 5.304 Left superior pubes adjustment.

(up to 8 minutes). This procedure does not fit the definition of an adjustment because of lack of high velocity thrust.

Supine Symphysis Adjustments

Hypothenar thigh (superior pubes) (Fig. 5-304)

IND: Restricted inferior glide of the pubes. Superior malposition of the pubes.

PP: The patient lies supine with the side of involvement at the edge of the table. The corresponding leg hangs off the table. The PSIS is just on the table.

DP: Stand on the involved side facing footward, assuming a fencer's stance.

CP: A palmar contact of the caudal hand.

SCP: Distal femur of the involved side leg.

IH: The cephalad hand establishes a palmar contact over the uninvolved side ASIS.

VEC: Superior to inferior.

P: While stabilizing the pelvis with the indifferent hand, the contact hand applies an anterior to posterior stress on the patient's thigh. Ask the patient to attempt to raise the thigh against the resistance and after 4 to 5 seconds deliver a slight and shallow impulse thrust downward to the distal thigh. After the adjustment is applied, the patient should relax, maintaining the adjustive position for approximately 1 to 2 minutes.

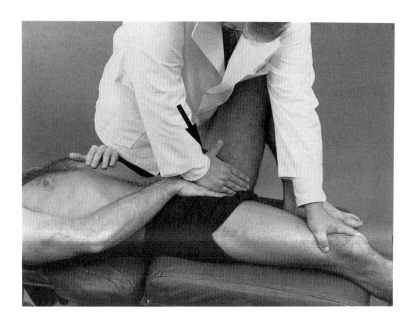

Figure 5.305 Right anterior pubes adjustment; also an alternative for a right superior pubes.

Hypothenar pubes (anterior pubes) (Fig. 5-305)

IND: Restricted posterior glide of the pubes. Anterior malposition of the pubes (alternate procedure for superior pubes).

PP: The patient lies supine with uninvolved knee and hip flexed and the foot flat on the table.

DP: Stand on the uninvolved side facing obliquely footward.

CP: A hypothenar, knife-edge contact of the cephalad hand.

SCP: Anterior aspect of the involved pubic ramus (superior aspect for a superior pubes).

IH: The caudal hand either reinforces the contact hand with fingers wrapped around the wrist or establishes a palmar contact over the knee of the uninvolved leg and applies additional flexion stress.

VEC: Anterior to posterior (superior to inferior).

P: At tension, deliver a quick and shallow impulse thrust anterior to posterior or superior to inferior to the involved pubes. This technique is best done with the use of a pelvic drop section.

Hypothenar ilium—ischium (inferior pubes) (Fig. 5-306)

IND: Restricted superior glide of the pubes. Inferior malposition of the pubes.

PP: The patient lies supine with the involved side knee and hip fully flexed.

DP: Stand on the side of the table opposite the side of involvement, leaning over the patient with your upper body contacting the anterior aspect of the patient's tibia.

CP: The caudal hand grasps the patient's lower ischium while the cepha-

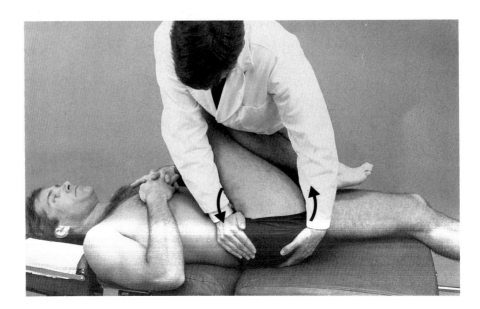

Figure 5.306 Right inferior pubes adjustment.

lad hand reaches over the patient and contacts the ASIS on the side of involvement.

VEC: Posterior to anterior and inferior to superior with the caudal hand and anterior to posterior with the cephalic hand.

 P: Develop pre-adjustive tension by applying body weight to the patient's flexed leg. At tension, deliver a pulling impulse thrust with the caudal hand while the cephalic hand thrusts posteriorly. Your body weight should be maintained over the flexed leg for a few seconds after the adjustment is applied.

Pubic distraction (Fig. 5-307)

IND: Painful restriction with pubic separation movement. Approximation (compression) of the pubes. Tenderness over the pubic tubercles, adductor muscles, and adductor tubercles.

 PP: The patient lies supine flexing both knees and hips to rest the feet flat on the table and close to one another.

 DP: Stand at or kneeling on the foot end of the table facing the patient.

 CP: Palmar contacts of both hands.

SCP: Medial aspects of both knees.

VEC: Medial to lateral.

 P: Separate the patient's knees, crossing and placing both forearms between the knees, contacting the medial aspects of the patient's knees. Ask the patient to squeeze the knees together for approximately 5 seconds or until sufficient adductor muscle fatigue occurs. Then deliver a shallow impulse thrust to both knees.

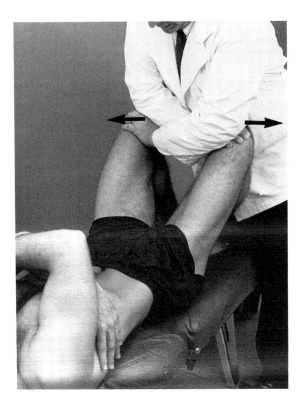

Figure 5.307 Pubic distraction.

Coccyx Adjustments

External coccyx (Fig. 5-308)

IND: Restricted coccyx movement, malposition of the coccyx, coccygodynia.

PP: The patient lies in the prone position with the thoracic and pelvic pieces raised or a Dutchman's roll placed under the ASIS; the buttocks should be appropriately draped.

DP: Stand at the side of the table, assuming a fencer's stance facing cephalad.

CP: The thumb contact of the cephalad hand.

SCP: The base of the coccyx (skin to skin).

IH: The pisiform-hypothenar contact of the caudad hand is established over the thumbnail of the contact hand, with the fingers lying loosely over the dorsum of the contact hand.

VEC: Inferior to superior.

P: Draw tissue slack out in a cephalad direction with both hands. At tension, deliver an impulse thrust cephalad and slightly posterior to anterior over the coccygeal base, producing a mixed tissue pull and osseous adjustive technique.

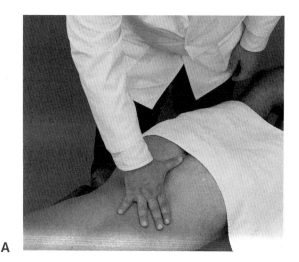 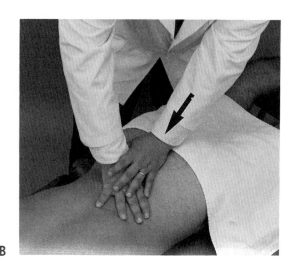

Figure 5.308 External coccyx adjustment: (**A**) tissue pull, thumb contact taken, and (**B**) reinforced contact with thrust headward.

Internal coccyx (Fig. 5-309)

IND: Restricted coccyx movement, malposition of the coccyx, coccygodynia.

PP: The patient lies in the prone position with the thoracic and pelvic pieces raised or a Dutchman's roll placed under the ASIS.

DP: Stand at the side of the table, assuming a fencer's stance facing cephalad.

CP: A digital contact with a gloved and lubricated middle finger of the caudad hand.

SCP: The anterior surface of coccyx, intra-rectally.

IH: A palmar-calcaneal contact of the cephalad hand over the upper half of the sacrum.

VEC: Superior to inferior.

P: The intra-rectal contact applies tension to the coccyx inferiorly and slightly posteriorly. Deliver an impulse thrust through the indifferent hand on the sacrum as a body drop inferior to superior and posterior to anterior effectively creates a long axis distraction at the sacrococcygeal articulation.

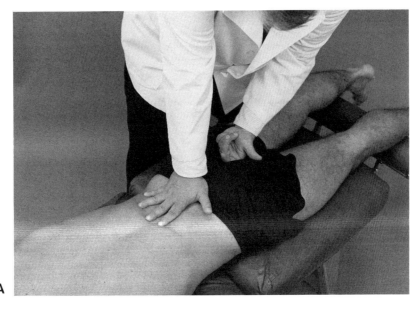

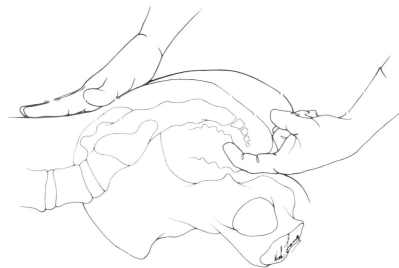

Figure 5.309 **(A)** Simulation of an internal coccyx adjustment; **(B)** illustration of contacts.

REFERENCES

1. White AA, Panjabi MM: Clinical Biomechanics of the Spine. 2nd Ed. JB Lippincott, Philadelphia, 1990

2. Harrison DD: Ideal normal upright static spine. In: CBP Technique, an overview. Presented at the Sixth Annual Conference on Research and Education, Consensus Conference. Self-published, 1990

3. Panjabi M, Dvorak J, Duranceau J et al: Three-dimensional movements of the upper cervical spine. Spine 13:726, 1988

4. Harrison DL, Harrison DD: Chiropractic: Spinal Mechanics and Human Biophysics. p. 30. Harrison Chiropractic Seminars, Inc., Sunnyvale, CA, 1980

5. Jackson R: The Cervical Syndrome. Charles C Thomas, Springfield, Illinois, 1977

6. Pal GP, Sherk HH: The vertical stability of the cervical spine. Spine 13:447, 1988

7. Pierce VW: Results. Chirp Publications, Dravosburg, PA, 1979

8. Jochumsen OH: The curve of the cervical spine. JACA 7:549, 1970

9. Suh CH: Computer model of the spine. In Haldeman S (ed): Modern Developments in the Principles and Practice of Chiropractic. Appleton-Century-Crofts, East Norwalk, CT, 1980

10. Lysell E: Motion in the cervical spine. Acta Orthop Scand Suppl 123:00, 1969

11. Rasch PJ, Burke RK: Kinesiology and Applied Anatomy. 5th Ed. Lea & Febiger, Philadelphia, 1974

12. Krag MH, Seroussi RE, Wilder DG et al: Internal displacement: distribution from in vitro loading of human thoracic and lumbar spinal motion segments: experimental results and theoretical predictions. Spine 12:1001, 1987

13. White AA, Johnson RM, Panjabi MM et al: Biomechanical analysis of clinical stability in the cervical spine. Clin Orthop 109:85, 1975

14. MacRae JE: Roentgenometrics in Chiropractic. Canadian Memorial Chiropractic College, Toronto, 1974

15. Bernhardt M, Bridwell KH: Segmental analysis of the sagittal plane alignment of the normal thoracic and lumbar spines and the thoracolumbar junction. Spine 14:717, 1989

16. Bradford S: Juvenile kyphosis. p. 347. In Bradford DS, Lonstein JE, Moe JH, Ogilvie JW, Winter RB (eds): Moe's Textbook of Scoliosis and Other Spinal Deformities. WB Saunders, Philadelphia, 1987

17. Pratt NE: Clinical Musculoskeletal Anatomy. JB Lippincott, Philadelphia, 1991

18. Kendall HO, Kendall FP, Boyton DA: p. 153. In: Posture and Pain. Robert E. Krieger, Huntington, New York, 1952

19. Jahn WT, Griffiths JH, Hacker RA: Conservative management of Scheuermann's juvenile kyphosis. J Manipulative Physiol Ther 1:228, 1978

20. Gatterman MI, Panzer DM: Disorders of the thoracic spine. p. 201. In: Gatterman MI: Chiropractic Management of Spine Related Disorders. William & Wilkins, Baltimore, 1990

21. Panjabi MM, Krag MH, Dimnet JC et al: Thoracic spine centers of rotation in the sagittal plane. J Orthop Res 1:387,1984

22. Panjabi MM, Brand RA, White AA: Three dimensional flexibility and stiffness properties of the human thoracic spine. J Biomech 9:185, 1976

23. Miles M, Sullivan WE: Lateral bending at the lumbar and lumbosacral joints. Anat Rec 139:387, 1961

24. Panjabi MM, Yamamoto I, Oxland T et al: How does posture affect the coupling? Spine 14:1002, 1989

25. Hollinsted WH, Cornelius R: Textbook of Anatomy. 4th Ed. Harper & Row, Philadelphia, 1985

26. Davis PR: The thoracolumbar mortise joint. J Anat 89:370, 1955

27. Maigne R: Low back pain from thoracolumbar origin. Arch Phys Med Rehabil 61:389, 1980

28. King AI, Prassad P, Ewing CL: Mechanism of spinal injury due to caudocephalad acceleration. Orthop Clin North Am 6:19, 1975

29. Adams MA, Hutton WC: The effects of posture on the role of the apophyseal joints in resisting intervertebral compression forces. J Bone Joint Surg 62(B)358, 1980

30. Bernhardt M, Bridwell KH: Segmental analysis of the sagittal plane alignment of the normal thoracic and lumbar spines and the thoracolumbar junction. Spine 14:717, 1989

31. Moe JH, Winter RB, Bradford DS, Lonstein JE: Kyphosis-lordosis: general principles. p. 325. In: Scoliosis and other spinal deformities. WB Saunders, Philadelphia, 1978

32. DeSmet AA: Radiographic evaluation. p. 23. In DeSmet AA (ed): Radiology of Spinal Curvature. CV Mosby, St. Louis, 1985

33. Propst-Proctor SL, Bleck EE: Radiographic determination of lordosis and kyphosis in normal and scoliotic children. J Pediatr Orthop 3:344, 1983

34. Pearcy M, Portek I, Shepard J: Three dimensional x-ray analysis of normal movement in the lumbar spine. Spine 9:294, 1984

35. Pearcy MJ: Stereo radiography of normal lumbar spine motion. Acta Orthop Scand 56:212 (suppl), 1985

36. Posner I, White AA, Edwards WT et al: A biomechanical analysis of the clinical stability of the lumbar and lumbosacral spine. Spine 7:374, 1982

37. Miles M, Sullivan WE: Lateral bending at the lumbar and lumbosacral joints. Anat Rec 139:387, 1961

38. Grice A: Radiographic, biomechanical and clinical factors in lumbar lateral flexion: part 1. J Manipulative Physiol Ther 2:26, 1979

39. Cassidy JD: Roentgenological examination of the functional mechanics of the lumbar spine in lateral flexion. JCCA 20:13, 1976

40. Bronfort G, Jochumsen OH: The functional radiographic examination of patients with low-back pain: a study of different forms of variations. J Manipulative Physiol Ther 7:89, 1984

41. Dimnet J, Fischer LP, Gonon G, Carret JP: Radiographic studies of lateral flexion in the lumbar spine. J Biomech 11:143, 1978

42. Dupuis PR, Yong-Hing K, Cassidy JD, Kirkaldy-Willis WH: Radiologic diagnosis of degenerative lumbar spinal instability. Spine 10:262, 1985

43. Dvorak J, Panjabi MM, Chang DG et al: Functional radiographic diagnosis of the lumbar spine. Spine 16:562, 1991

44. Dvorak J, Panjabi MM, Novotny JE et al: Clinical validation of functional flexion-extension roentgenograms of the lumbar spine. Spine 16:943, 1991

45. Frymoyer JW, Frymoyer WW, Wilder DG, Pope MH: The mechanical and kinematic analysis of the lumbar spine in normal living human subjects in vivo. J Biomech 12:165, 1979

46. Hanley EN, Matteri RE, Frymoyer JW: Accurate roentgenographic determination of lumbar flexion-extension. Clin Orthop Rel Res 115:145, 1976

47. Korpi J, Poussa M, Heliovaara M: Radiographic mobility of the lumbar spine and its relation to clinical back motion. Scand J Rehabil Med 20:71, 1988

48. Phillips RB, Howe JW, Bustin G et al: Stress x-rays and the low back pain patient. J Manipulative Physiol Ther 13:127, 1990

49. Sandoz RW: Technique and interpretation of functional radiography of the lumbar spine. Ann Swiss Chiro Assoc 3:66, 1965

50. Shaffer WO, Spratt KF, Weinstein J et al: The consistency and accuracy of roentgenograms for measuring sagittal translation in the lumbar vertebral motion segment: an experimental model. Spine 15:741, 1990

51. Soini J, Antti-Poika I, Tallroth K et al: Disc degeneration and angular movement of the lumbar spine: comparative study using plain and flexion-extension radiography and discography. J Spinal Disorders 4:183, 1991

52. Stokes IAF, Wilder DG, Frymoyer JW, Pope MH: Assessment of patients with low-back pain by biplanar radiographic measurement of intervertebral motion. Spine 6:233, 1981

53. Tanz SS: Motion of the lumbar spine. Am J Roentgenol 69:399, 1953

54. Van Akkerveeken PF, O'Brien JP, Park WM: Experimentally induced hypermobility in the lumbar spine. Spine 4:236, 1979

55. Vernon H: Static and dynamic roentgenography in the diagnosis of degenerative disc disease: a review and comparison assessment. J Manipulative Physiol Ther 5:163, 1982

56. Weitz EM: The lateral bending sign. Spine 6:388, 1981

57. Haas M, Nyiendo J, Peterson C et al: Lumbar motion trends and correlation with low back pain. Part 1. A roentgenological evaluation of coupled lumbar motion in lateral bending. J Manip Physiol Ther 15:145, 1992

58. Pearcy MJ, Tibrewal SB: Axial rotation and lateral bending in the normal lumbar spine measured by three-dimensional radiography. Spine 9:582, 1984

59. Grieve GP: Common Vertebral Joint Problems. 2nd Ed. Churchill Livingstone, Edinburgh, 1988

60. Cox HH: Sacroiliac subluxations as a cause of backache. Surg Gynecol Obstet 45:637, 1927

61. Jessen AR: The sacroiliac subluxation. ACA J Chiro 7(S):65, 1973

62. Cyriax E: Minor subluxations of the sacroiliac joints. Br J Phys Med 9:191, 1934

63. Dontigney RL: A review. Physical Therapy 65:35, 1985

64. Solonen KA: The sacroiliac joint in the light of anatomical, roentgenological and clinical studies. Acta Orthop Scand Suppl 26:9, 1957

65. Bowen V, Cassidy JD: Macroscopic and microscopic anatomy of the sacroiliac joint from embryonic life until the eighth decade. Spine 6:620, 1986

66. Illi F: The Vertebral Column: Lifeline of the Body. National College of Chiropractic, Chicago, 1951

67. Otter R: Review study of differing opinions expressed in the literature about the anatomy of the sacroiliac joint. Eur J Chiro 33:221, 1985

68. McGregor M, Cassidy JD: Post-surgical sacroiliac joint syndrome. J Manipulative Physiol Ther 6:1, 1983

69. Grieve GP: The sacroiliac joint. Physiotherapy 62:384, 1976

70. Frigerio NA, Stowe RR, Howe JW: Movement of the sacroiliac joint. Clin Orthop 100:370, 1974

71. Grice AS, Fligg DB: Biomechanics of the pelvis. Denver Conference monograph. ACA Council of Technic, Des Moines, 1980

72. Grice AS: Mechanics of walking, development and clinical significance. JCCA 16:15, 1972

73. Schafer RC, Faye LJ: Motion palpation and chiropractic technic—principles of dynamic chiropractic. Motion Palpation Institute, Huntington Beach, CA, 1989

74. Greenman P: Principles of Manual Medicine. Williams & Wilkins, Baltimore, 1989

75. Sturesson B, Selvik G, Uden A: Movements of the sacroiliac joints: a roentgen stereophotogrammetric analysis. Spine 14:162, 1989

76. Gatterman MI: Chiropractic Management of Spine Related Disorders. Williams & Wilkins, Baltimore, 1990

77. Dupuis PR, Kirkaldy-Willis WH: The spine: integrated function and patho-physiology. p. 673. In Cruess RL, Rennie WRJ (eds): Adult Orthopaedics. Churchill Livingstone, New York, 1984

78. Basmajian JV: Manipulation, Traction and Massage. 3rd Ed. Williams & Wilkins, Baltimore, 1985

79. Kapandji IA: The Trunk and the Vertebral Column. Vol. 3, p. 135. In: The Physiology of the Joints. 2nd Ed. Churchill Livingstone, Edinburgh, 1974

SUGGESTED READINGS

The following citations represent sources for many of the evaluative and technique procedures discussed in this chapter. While some procedures have been modified or may appear as a variation, most are described in one or more of these texts. They are presented in alphabetical order.

Basmajian JV (ed): Manipulation, Traction and Massage. 3rd Ed. Williams & Wilkins, Baltimore, 1985

Beatty HG: Anatomical Adjustive Technique. 2nd Ed. Self-published. Denver, 1937

Donnatelli R, Wooden MJ (eds): Orthopedic Physical Therapy. Churchill Livingstone, New York, 1989

Eder M, Tilscher H: Chiropractic Therapy, Diagnosis and Treatment. Aspen Publishers, Rockville, MD, 1990

Gatterman MI: Chiropractic Management of Spine Related Disorders. Williams & Wilkins, Baltimore, 1990, p. 201

Gillet H, Leikens M: Belgian Chiropractic Research Notes. 10th Ed. Self-published, Brussels, 1973

Greco MA: Chiropractic Technique Illustrated. Jari Publishing, New York, 1953

Greenman PE: Principles of Manual Medicine. Williams & Wilkins, Baltimore, 1989

Grieve GP: Common Vertebral Joint Problems. 2nd Ed. Churchill Livingstone, Edinburgh, 1988

Grove AB: Chiropractic Technique: a Procedure of Adjusting. Self-published, Strauss Printing and Publishing, Madison, WI, 1979

Herbst RW: Gonsted Chiropractic Science and Art. Sci-Chi Publications, Mt. Horeb, WI, 1968

Hertling D, Kessler RM: Management of Common Musculoskeletal Disorders: Physical Therapy Principles and Methods, 2nd Ed. JB Lippincott, Philadelphia, 1990

Hoag J (ed): Osteopathic Medicine. Blakiston, New York, 1969

Hoppenfeld S: Physical Examination of the Spine and Extremities. Appleton-Century-Crofts, East Norwalk, CT, 1976

Janse JJ, Houser RH, Wells BF: Chiropractic Principles and Technic. National College of Chiropractic, Chicago, 1947

Kenna C, Murtagh J: Back Pain and Spinal Manipulation: A Practical Guide. Butterworths, London, 1989

Kirk CR, Lawrence DJ, Valvo NL: States Manual of Spinal, Pelvic and Extra-Vertebral Technic. 2nd Ed. National College of Chiropractic, Lombard, Illinois; Waverly Press, Baltimore, 1985

Nwuga VC: Manipulation of the Spine. Williams & Wilkins, Baltimore, 1976

Schafer RC, Faye LJ: Motion Palpation and Chiropractic Technic—Principles of Dynamic Chiropractic. Motion Palpation Institute, Huntington, CA, 1989

Stoddard A: Manual of Osteopathic Technique. Hutchinson, London, 1959

Wadsworth CT: Manual Examination and Treatment of the Spine and Extremities. Williams & Wilkins, Baltimore, 1988

6
Extraspinal Techniques

Thomas F. Bergmann

Although the musculoskeletal system accounts for over half the body's mass, it remains the most clinically overlooked system in the body. The extremity joints are lever–hinge complexes that translate forces into motion, but in so doing, can also amplify forces negatively to the neuromusculoskeletal system. The mechanical principles that determine what functions the body can do are the same regardless of the activity, whether athletic, recreational, occupational, or an everyday task.

Understanding biomechanics (the application of mechanical laws to living structures) is paramount when confronted with a clinical dysfunctional process affecting the musculoskeletal system and, specifically, a peripheral joint. The joint, its ligamentous structures, and capsule form the hinge for the bony lever to move about when a force from the muscles is provided. Proper joint function depends on the integrity of the soft tissues and the alignment of the bony joint surfaces.

By incorporating biomechanical principles in clinical practice, the chiropractor will better understand the nature and extent of the manipulative lesion as well as how the patient's neuromusculoskeletal system is influenced locally and globally. Moreover, mechanisms for the dysfunctional changes will become apparent, as will the extent and effect of the patient's adaptational process.

THE TEMPOROMANDIBULAR JOINT

The weight of the head must be balanced and stabilized atop the spine. A biomechanical relationship exists between the forces developed in stabilization of the cervical spinal segments, tension in the deep cervical fascia, movements of the temporomandibular joints (TMJs), activity of the hyoid bone muscles, as well as the structures of the shoulder girdle (Fig. 6-1). More importantly, postural stresses, muscle tone, malocclusion of the teeth, and joint dysfunction have clinical relationships with neck pain, headache, orofacial pain, and abnormalities of chewing and swallowing. An association is formed between two of the body's most complicated joint systems—the

523

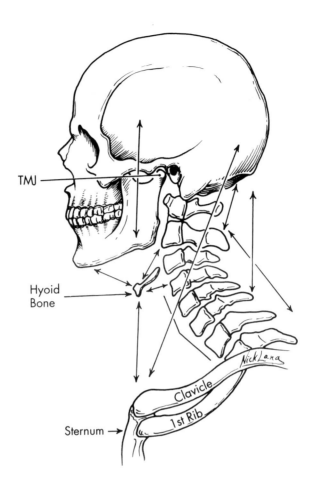

Figure 6.1 Biomechanical relationship necessary to stabilize the head and cervical spine segments. Arrows indicate direction of muscle pull. (Adapted from Grieve G: Common Vertebral Joint Problems. 2nd Ed. Churchill Livingstone, Edinburgh, 1988, p. 26.)

TMJ and the atlanto-occipital joint. Both of these joint systems should be evaluated in patients complaining of head and neck pain.

The craniomandibular complex is composed of the TMJ, the teeth, muscles of mastication, and hyoid bone. The TMJ is one of the most active joints in the body, moving more than 2,000 times per day in its functions of mastication, swallowing, respiration, and speech.

The head is tethered to the body by the muscles that move the TMJ and the atlanto-occipital joint. Head posture depends on the tone of these muscles, thus developing an intimate association between movements of the head and mandible. Because of this relationship, a change in either cervical spine posture, head posture, or mandibular rest position can create a change in the others.

Functional Anatomy

Osseous Structures

The mandible, the largest and the strongest bone of the face, articulates with the temporal bones while accommodating the lower teeth (Fig. 6-2). The body of the mandible runs horizontally and has two rami posteriorly.

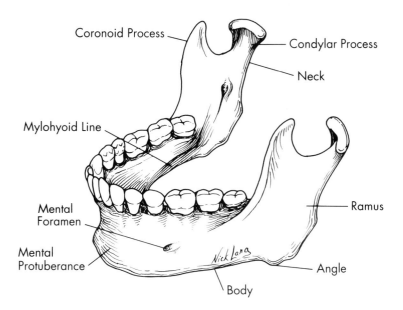

Coronoid Process

Condylar Process

Neck

Mylohyoid Line

Mental Foramen

Mental Protuberance

Ramus

Angle

Body

Nick Lang

Figure 6.2 The mandible. (Modified from Hertling and Kessler,[1] with permission.)

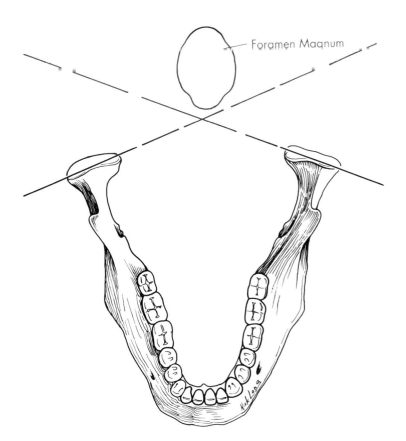

Foramen Magnum

Nick Lang

Figure 6.3 Line drawn through the axes of the mandibular condyles will intersect just anterior to the foramen magnum. (Modified from Hertling and Kessler,[1] with permission.)

The rami are perpendicular to the body and form a palpable angle inferiorly. Each ramus has two processes: the coronoid process, serving as a point of attachment for muscles, and the condylar process, for articulation with the temporal bone via the intra-articular disc. Lines drawn through the axis of each condyle will intersect just anterior to the foramen magnum, the significance of which is in visualizing a line of correction for manipulative procedures (Fig. 6-3). The temporal bone has a concave mandibular fossa with the convex articular eminence just anterior to it.

Functionally, the mandibular fossa serves as a receptacle for the condyles when the joint is in a closed packed position (teeth approximated). During opening, closing, protrusion, and retrusion, the convex surface of the condyle must move over the convex surface of the articular eminence (Fig. 6-4). The existence of the intra-articular disc compensates functionally for the incongruity of the two opposing convex surfaces.[1] The disc also separates the joint into an upper and lower portion, or compartment, each with synovial linings. The outer edges of the disc are connected to the joint capsule.

Ligamentous Structures

Four ligaments serve as secondary stabilizers for the joint. They are the articular capsule, temporomandibular ligament, stylomandibular ligament, and sphenomandibular ligament (Fig. 6-5). The primary function of the joint capsule is to enclose the joint, but because the disc is tethered to it, it also causes the disc to move forward when the condyle moves forward. The temporomandibular ligament is the main suspensory ligament of the mandible during opening movements of the jaw. It also prevents excessive forward, backward, and lateral movements. The stylomandibular ligament prevents excessive anterior movement of the mandible and as such serves as a stop for the mandible in extreme opening. The sphenomandibular ligament functions as a suspensory ligament for the mandible during wide opening of the joint.

A mandibular-malleolar ligament connecting the neck and anterior process of the malleus to the medioposterior aspect of the joint capsule has been reported.[2,3] The clinical significance of this structure lies in making an anatomic connection between the TMJ and the middle ear.

Musculature

The prime movers of the mandible in elevation are the temporalis, masseter, and medial pterygoid muscles (Table 6-1, Fig. 6-6). The posterior fibers of the temporalis also retract the mandible while maintaining the condyles posteriorly. The superficial fibers of the masseter protrude the jaw, while the deep fibers act as a retractor. The deep fibers also attach to the lateral aspect of the joint capsule. The medial pterygoid can protrude the mandible as well as deviate the jaw laterally (Fig. 6-7).

The major depressors of the mandible are the lateral pterygoid, suprahyoid, and infrahyoid muscles. The lateral pterygoid also attaches to the mandibular condyle and the intra-articular disc, thereby serving as a significant stabilizer of the joint. It is the primary muscle used in opening the mouth but can also assist in lateral movements and protrusion. Of clinical importance is its frequency of involvement in cases of TMJ dysfunction.

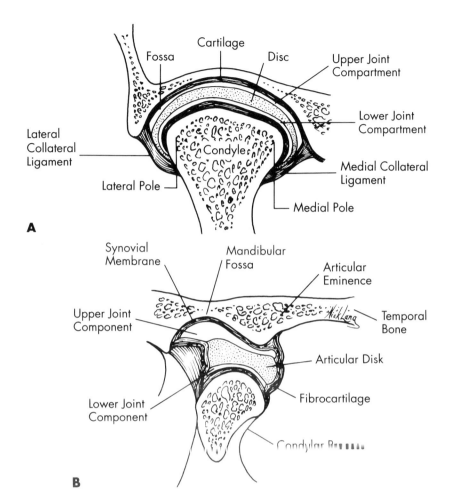

Figure 6.4 **(A)** A coronal (frontal) section through the temporomandibular joint in the closed position. **(B)** A sagittal section through the temporomandibular joint in the open position.

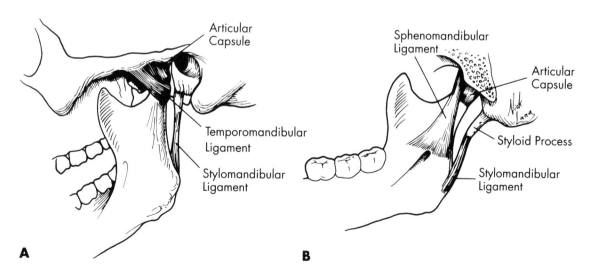

Figure 6.5 **(A)** Lateral and **(B)** medial views of the left temporomandibular joint showing the ligamentous structures.

Table 6.1 Actions of the Muscles of the Temporomandibular Joint

Action	Muscles
Mandibular elevation (closing)	Temporalis, masseter, medial pterygoid
Mandibular depression (opening)	Lateral pterygoid, suprahyoid, infrahyoid
Protrusion (anterior glide)	Superficial fibers of the masseter, medial pterygoid, lateral pterygoid
Retrusion (posterior glide)	Temporalis, deep fibers of the masseter
Lateral glide	Medial pterygoid, lateral pterygoid
Hyoid elevation	Stylohyoid, mylohyoid
Hyoid depression	Infrahyoid

The suprahyoid muscle group is composed of the digastric, stylohyoid, geniohyoid, and the mylohyoid muscles (Fig. 6-8). The digastric muscle pulls the mandible down and posteriorly. The stylohyoid muscle initiates and assists jaw opening but also draws the hyoid bone upward and backward when the mandible is fixed. The geniohyoid muscle pulls the mandible down and back. The mylohyoid muscle elevates the floor of the mouth and assists in depressing the mandible when the hyoid is fixed or in elevating the hyoid when the mandible is fixed.

The prime function of the infrahyoid muscle group—composed of the sternohyoid, thyrohyoid, and omohyoid muscles—is to stabilize or depress the hyoid bone. This action then allows the suprahyoid muscles to act on the mandible.

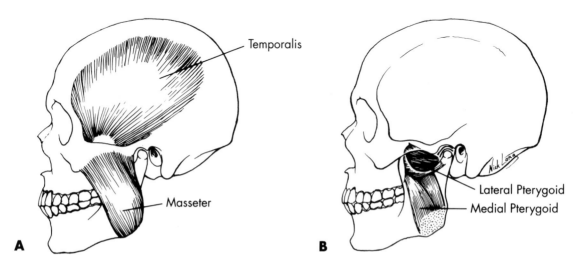

Figure 6.6 Intrinsic musculature of the mandible. **(A)** The left temporalis and masseter, externally. **(B)** The left medial and lateral pterygoid, with proximal mandible removed.

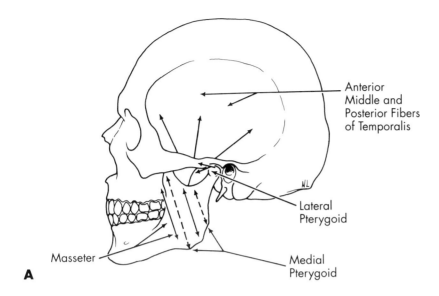

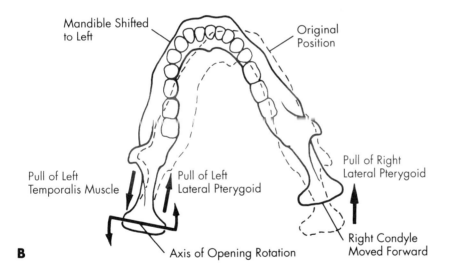

Figure 6.7 The directions of muscular pull in the temporo-mandibular joint. (**A**) Opening, closing, and anterior glide. (**B**) Left lateral deviation.

Biomechanics

Posture and Alignment

In the normal, relaxed, and inactive state of the TMJ, referred to as the *mandibular postural rest position,* the teeth should not touch. Instead, there should be an intra-occlusal space, termed *the freeway space,* of approximately 3 to 5 mm. This position is the result of the equilibrium between the muscle tone of the mandibular elevators and the force of gravity. Moreover, it is influenced by the state of the anterior and posterior neck muscles, head posture, and inherent elasticity of the mandibular muscles. This resting

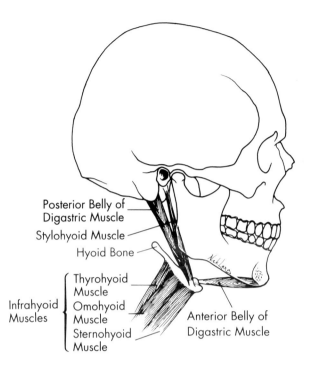

Figure 6.8 The suprahyoid and infrahyoid muscle groups of the mandible.

posture is decreased in people who brux, or clench, their teeth and is increased in mouth breathers. Disturbances in the resting position may impact on the remodeling or reparative processes, leading to an unhealthy TMJ system.

The position of the mandible when the teeth are fully occluded is termed the *intercuspal position* and is directly influenced by the state of the dentition. In this position, the condylar location is influenced by the dentition, which may differ from that imposed by muscle action. Furthermore, the intercuspal position may influence the mandibular resting posture by disturbing the balance of the musculature, which in turn can affect the head posture and cervical spine function. Therefore, the state of the dentition should not be ignored in patients presenting with chronic neck pain.

The TMJ undergoes the coupled motions of rotation and translation. Rotational movement of the condyle occurs about a transverse axis beween the condyle and the intra-articular disc. This movement causes the first 12 to 15 mm of mandibular opening and closing. Translational movement of the condyle consists of a downward and forward gliding movement of the disc–condyle complex and depends on the synchronous movement of disc and condyle (Fig. 6-9). Rotational movements occur mainly in the inferior (subdiscal) joint space, while translational movements occur mainly in the superior (supradiscal) joint space.

Mandibular movement is a dynamic combination of opening, closing, anterior glide (protrusion), posterior glide (retrusion), and lateral glide. Mandibular opening involves the contraction of the lateral pterygoids and

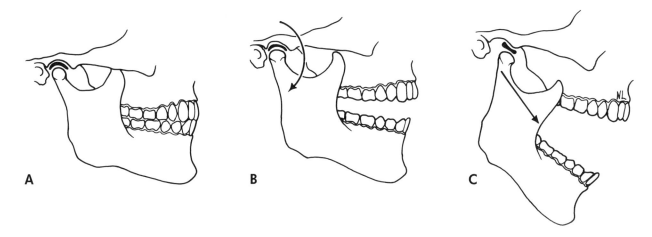

Figure 6.9 Mandibular movement is a complex relationship of rotational and translational movements. (**A**) Closed position. (**B**) Initial opening is rotational. (**C**) Full opening requires translation forward.

digastrics, with assistance from the suprahyoid and infrahyoid muscles. Indirectly, the posterior cervical muscles must contract to prevent neck flexion and permit the mandible to drop away from the cranium. The first few degrees of opening are rotational movements about a transverse axis. Then the condyle and disc complex must translate forward over the articular eminence, allowing condylar rotation to continue. The closing sequence is the reverse. The condyle and disc complex translate posteriorly with condylar rotation, which brings the joint to its resting position or intercuspal position. The masseter, medial pterygoid, and temporalis muscles are responsible for this action. Table 6-2 lists the osteokinematic and arthrokinematic movements of the TMJ.

Lateral glide of the mandible involves a pivoting rotation of the condyle on the side to which the mandible is moving and a translation of the other condyle. For lateral glide to the right, the left lateral pterygoid and the anterior bellies of both the digastrics contract, causing the left condyle to move downward, forward, and medially. Meanwhile, contraction of the right

Table 6.2 Arthrokinematic and Osteokinematic Movements of the Temporomandibular Joint

Osteokinematic Movements		Arthrokinematic Movements
Mandibular elevation and depression	40–60 mm of incisor separation	A combination of spin and glide occurring in the upper and lower joint compartments
Mandibular retraction and protrusion	5–10 mm of incisor separation	Glide movement occurring in the upper joint compartment
Mandibular lateral deviation	5–10 mm of incisor separation	Glide, spin, and angulation occur mostly in the upper compartment but also in the lower joint space

Table 6.3 Close-Packed and Loose-Packed (Rest) Positions for the Temporomandibular Joint

Close-Packed Position	Loose-Packed Position
The maximal intercuspal position, in which all teeth make full contact with one another—clenched	The "freeway space" position of slight mandibular opening, which occurs because of equilibrium between jaw-opening and jaw-closing muscles

temporalis and the right lateral pterygoid rotate the right condyle in the fossa and displace the mandible to the right. Table 6-3 identifies the close-packed and loose-packed positions for the TMJ.

Evaluation

Problems affecting the TMJ can be broadly classified into developmental abnormalities, intracapsular diseases, and dysfunctional conditions (Table 6-4). Developmental abnormalities include hypoplasia, hyperplasia, impingements of the coronoid process, chondromas, and ossification of ligaments such as the stylohyoid ligament (Eagle's syndrome). The intracapsular diseases include degenerative arthritis, osteochondritis, rheumatoid arthritis, psoriatic arthritis, synovial chondromatosis, infections, steroid necrosis, gout, and metastatic tumors.[4] Developmental abnormalities and intracapsular diseases must be ruled out using appropriate evaluative procedures including diagnostic imaging and clinical laboratory studies. The focus here is on the dysfunctional conditions affecting the TMJ, which are categorized as extracapsular (myofascial pain syndromes and muscular imbalance); capsular (sprain or strain, hypomobility and hypermobility, and synovial folds); and intracapsular (disc displacement and disc adhesions).

Inspect the face and jaw, looking for bony or soft tissue asymmetry, alignment of the teeth, and evidence of swelling (Fig. 6-10). Observe the jaw during opening and closing to identify excursional deviations and the presence of clicking[5–7] (Fig. 6-11). Ask the patient whether the movements are painful. Normal opening should accommodate three of the patient's

Table 6.4 Classification of Problems Affecting the Temporomandibular Joint

Developmental Abnormalities	Intracapsular Diseases	Dysfunctional
Hypoplasia	Degenerative arthritis	Extracapsular
Hyperplasia	Osteochondritis	Myofascial pain syndrome
Impingement of the coronoid process	Inflammatory arthritis (Rheumatoid, psoriatic, gout)	Muscular imbalance (strain, spasm)
Chondromas	Synovial chondromatosis	Capsular
Ossification of ligaments (i.e., Eagle's syndrome)	Infections	Sprain
	Metastatic tumors	Hypomobility
		Hypermobility
		Synovial folds
		Intracapsular
		Disc displacement
		Disc adhesions

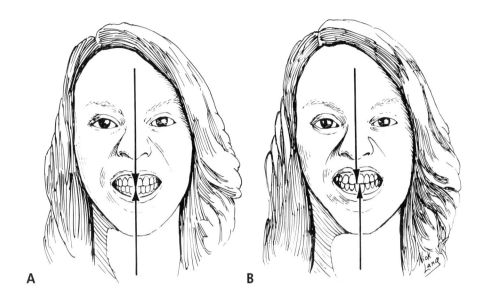

Figure 6.10 Intercuspal alignment. **(A)** Normal. **(B)** Left lateral deviation.

fingers inserted between the incisors. If not, hypomobility or closed lock that is due to disc displacement is suspected. If opening beyond three fingers occurs, hypermobility is likely (Fig. 6-12).

Palpate the joint by placing the fifth digit into the patient's external auditory meatus with the palmar surface forward (Fig. 6-13). Before placing the finger into the ear, push on the tragus to determine if the external ear canal is painful. The position of the condyles and intra-articular clicking can be felt from within the external canal. The lateral aspect of the joint and capsule can be palpated externally for position, pain, and movement disorders (Fig. 6-14). Palpate the muscles to determine changes in tone, texture,

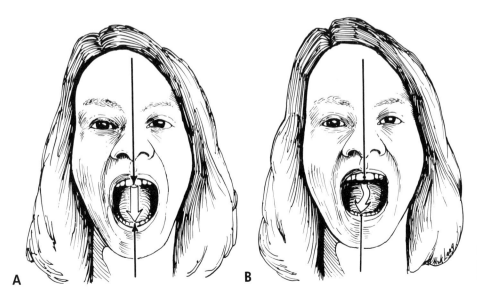

Figure 6.11 Mandibular gait pattern. **(A)** Normal. **(B)** Deviation.

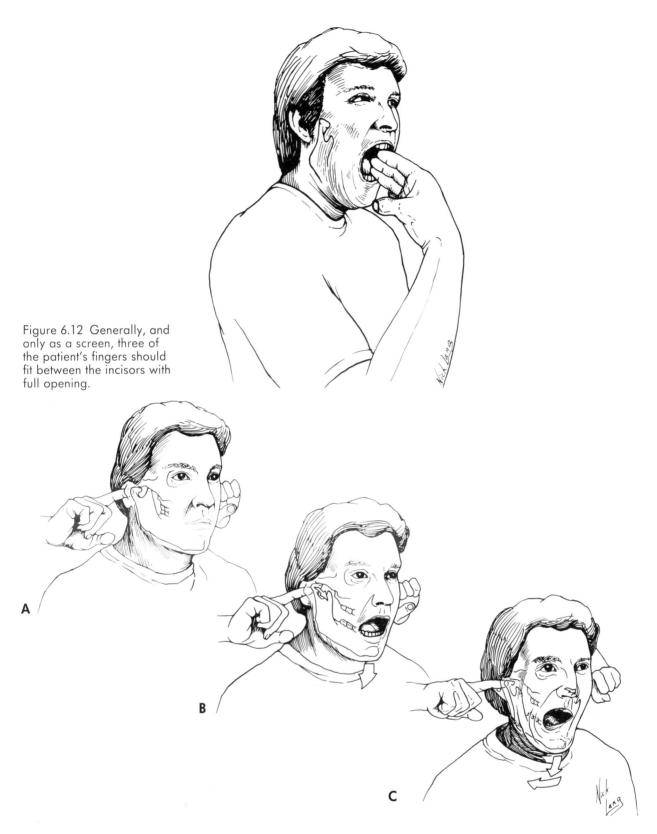

Figure 6.12 Generally, and only as a screen, three of the patient's fingers should fit between the incisors with full opening.

Figure 6.13 Palpation of temporomandibular joint. **(A)** Finger is placed in external auditory meatus. **(B)** Movement of condyle is palpated on opening and closing. **(C)** Asymmetric joint movement.

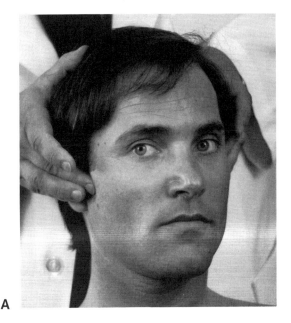

A

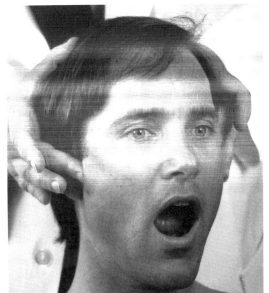

B

Figure 6.14 External palpation of temporomandibular joint space. **(A)** Jaw closed. **(B)** Jaw open.

and tenderness. The lateral pterygoid can be palpated intraorally by following the buccal mucosa to the medial aspect of the TMJ and just proximal to the tonsils (Figs. 6-15 and 6-16). Note the position and movement of the hyoid bone as well as the state of the associated soft tissues.

Perform accessory motions of the TMJ by placing the gloved thumbs intraorally over the lower teeth and wrapping the fingers around the mandible externally (Fig. 6-17). Apply passive stress in long axis distraction, lateral

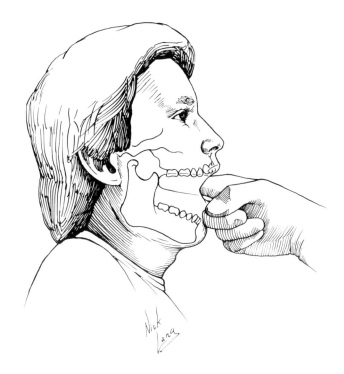

Figure 6.15 Palpation of pterygoid muscles with intraoral contact.

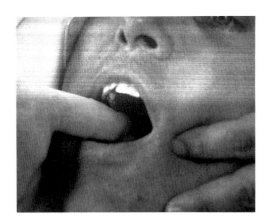

Figure 6.16 Intraoral palpation of the pterygoid muscles.

Table 6.5 Accessory Joint Movements of the Temporomandibular Joint

Long axis distraction
Lateral glide
Anterior glide
Posterior glide

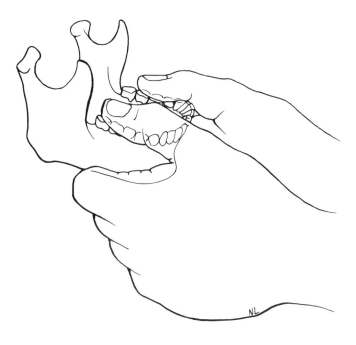

Figure 6.17 Double-thumb, intraoral contact on mandible.

glide, and anterior to posterior glide (Table 6-5). Normally, a springing end feel is perceived (Fig. 6-18).

A general survey of the oral cavity should be done to rule out dental or oral lesions. Ask the patient to close the teeth together quickly and sharply.

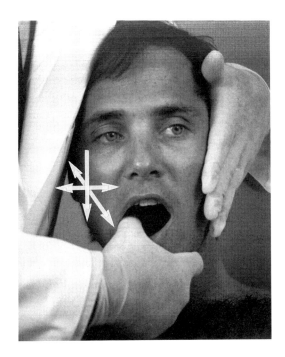

Figure 6.18 Accessory joint movement evaluation for the temporomandibular joint.

Normally, this is not painful, and a broad clicking of the dental surface should be heard. If local pain is produced or only a faint, single striking sound is heard, a dental source is indicated (acute malocclusion, tooth abscess, periodontal disease), and a referral to a dentist is advised.

Adjustive Procedures

The manipulative techniques used to treat TMJ disorders aim to restore normal joint mechanics, which will then allow full, and it is hoped, pain-free functioning of the mandible. Two basic types of adjustive procedures are used for the different forms of TMJ dysfunction: distraction and translation techniques.

Abbreviations used in illustrating technique

IND, indications PP, patient's position DP, doctor's position SCP, segmental contact point (on patient) CP, contact point (on doctor) IH, indifferent hand VEC, vector P, procedure	→ Arrows on photographs indicate direction of force. ▲ Triangles on photographs indicate stabilization.

Distraction Techniques

Distraction procedures create a slow and controlled joint gapping or separation of the joint surfaces. Typically, they require an intraoral contact, making the use of rubber gloves necessary.

Long axis distraction[1,5,6] *(Fig. 6-19)*

IND: Reduce an acutely dislocated disc, treat loss of accessory joint movements, stimulate mechanoreceptors, and influence disc nutrition.

 PP: The patient is supine, mouth slightly open; a head belt or assistant may be used to stabilize the patient's head.

 DP: With gloved hands, stand at the side of the table facing the patient on the side of the joint dysfunction.

SPC: Lower teeth on uninvolved side.

 CP: Use your cephalad hand with thumb contact on the lower teeth of the affected side; wrap your fingers around the mandible externally, with the index fingers along the body of the mandible.

 IH: Use your caudal hand, if jaw excursion allows, to reinforce the CP with a thumb contact on top of the CP. If this is not possible, place the thumb on the lower teeth of the other side.

VEC: Long axis distraction.

  P: Ask the patient to swallow, then apply distraction to the joint surfaces caudally. For an acute anterior dislocation of the disc (Fig. 6-20), tip

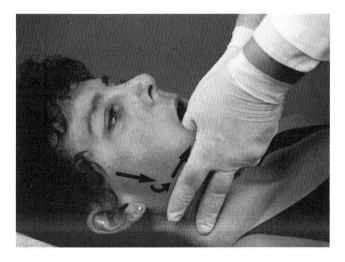

Figure 6.19 Long axis distraction manipulation of the temporomandibular joint.

the condyle anteriorly to position it under the disc and add a posterior to anterior force. For an acute posterior dislocation of the disc, tip the condyle posterior to position it under the disc and add an anterior to posterior force.

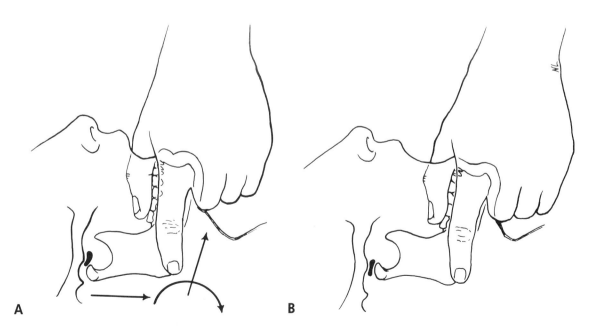

Figure 6.20 Distraction technique for an anterior dislocated disc for the temporomandibular joint. (**A**) starting position. (**B**) Distraction of the condyle with tilt and anterior translation under the disc.

For loss of specific accessory joint movements and for stimulation of mechanoreceptors, this procedure can be done with the addition of lateral glide movements or dorsal–ventral glide movements, or both.

When a synovial fold becomes entrapped, pain will be produced when the disc moves medially or the condyle moves laterally. To reduce the entrapped fold of synovial tissue, the distraction technique must be combined with contraction of the patient's ipsilateral masseter muscle.

Plica entrapment reduction technique[5] (Fig. 6-21)

IND: Plica entrapment (synovial fold).
  PP: The patient is seated, head stabilized, with the mandible deviated away from the involved side.
  DP: Stand at the side of the patient.
SCP: Lower teeth on involved side.
  CP: Establish the thumb contact over the lower teeth, with fingers grasping the mandible.
VEC: Long axis distraction.
   P: Apply a long axis distraction force while maintaining the mandible in lateral deviation away from the problem. Then ask the patient to move the mandible (contracting the deep fibers of the masseter) toward the affected side against the applied resistance.

Translational Techniques

Translational adjustive techniques use a line of correction parallel to the plane of the joint surfaces. Additionally, a compressive loading force may be applied. The primary affect of this procedure is to move the disc posteriorly,

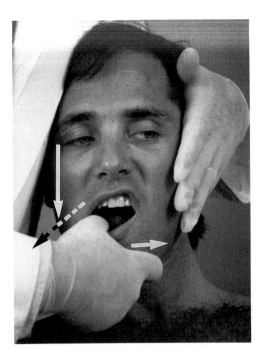

Figure 6.21 Manipulation for plica entrapment of the left temporomandibular joint.

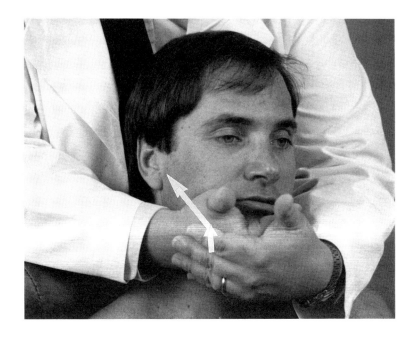

Figure 6.22 Anterior to posterior translational manipulation for the right temporomandibular joint.

which is specifically indicated for releasing minor disc adhesions (intracapsular adhesions). Translational techniques use extraoral contacts, and gloves are not necessary.

Anterior to posterior translation[5,7] (Fig. 6-22)

IND: Release intracapsular discal adhesions, restore accessory joint movements, stimulate mechanoreceptors, and stimulate stretch receptors of the lateral pterygoid muscle.

PP: The patient sits.

DP: Stand behind the patient with a rolled towel or pillow placed between you and the patient to support the cervical spine.

SCP: Ramus of the mandible.

CP: Your ipsilateral hand takes a knife edge, palmar contact over the ramus of the mandible while the fingers cradle the chin.

IH: Your contralateral hand reinforces over the CP.

VEC: Anterior to posterior, along the line of the articular eminence (Fig. 6-23).

P: First apply a compressive loading force (inferior to superior), then deliver the thrust as an impulse anterior to posterior and along the line of the articular eminence. To distract the patient's attention and to prevent jamming of the teeth, have the patient open his mouth and slowly close it; make the adjustment when he is closing.

Lateral to medial translation[1,5] (Fig. 6-24)

IND: Restore accessory joint movements, stimulate mechanoreceptors, and stimulate stretch receptors of the lateral pterygoid muscle.

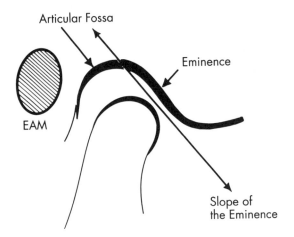

Figure 6.23 The slope of the articular eminence must first be established because this will determine or influence the direction of a translational thrust. External palpation of the eminence is used to determine the slope. (Modified from Curl,[5] with permission.)

PP: The patient is supine with the head turned slightly, affected side up.
DP: Stand at the side of the table toward the side of contact.
SCP: Neck of the mandible.
CP: Establish a double thumb contact over the neck of the mandible.
VEC: Lateral to medial.
P: Deliver an impulse thrust in a lateral to medial direction.

Lateral to medial translation—seated (Fig. 6-25)

IND: Restore accessory joint movements, stimulate mechanoreceptors, and stimulate stretch receptors of the lateral pterygoid muscle.

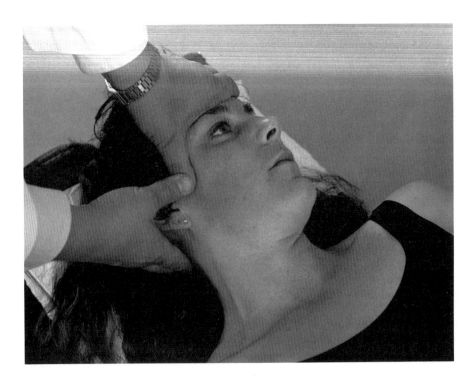

Figure 6.24 Supine lateral to medial translation manipulation of the right temporomandibular joint.

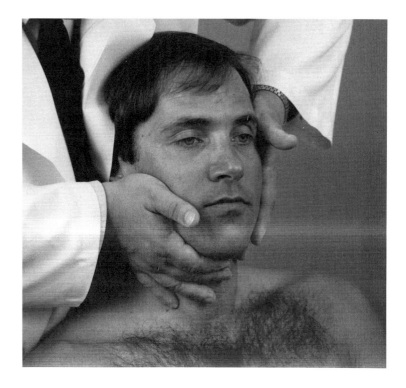

Figure 6.25 Seated lateral to medial translation manipulation of the temporomandibular joint.

PP: The patient sits.
DP: Stand behind the patient and slightly to the side of involvement.
SCP: Proximal mandible.
CP: With your ipsilateral hand, establish a thenar contact over the proximal aspect of the mandible just distal to the joint space.
IH: Use the contralateral hand to apply a broad palmar contact on the uninvolved side of the face and head.
P: With the patient's jaw relaxed (teeth not clenched), deliver an impulse thrust in a lateral to medial direction.

One of the greatest difficulties encountered when adjusting the TMJ is the patient's inability to adequately relax the jaw muscles. Furthermore, it is detrimental to the joint to overstretch the upper joint compartment; therefore, care must be taken when using intraoral contacts.

THE SHOULDER

The primary role of the shoulder is to place the hand in a functional position. To achieve this function, a great deal of joint mobility is necessary, which requires complex anatomy and biomechanics. The shoulder is not one joint but a relationship of anatomic and physiologic joints forming a four-joint complex. The glenohumeral joint is a true anatomic joint and forms the shoulder proper. The sternoclavicular and acromioclavicular joints are also true anatomic joints formed between the manubrium of the sternum, the

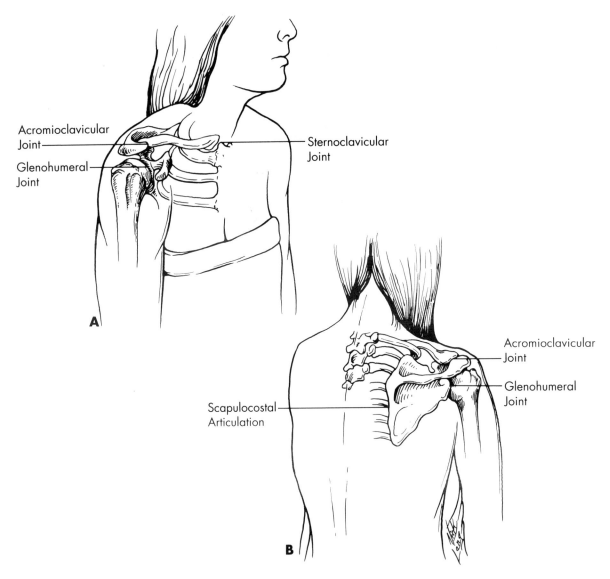

Figure 6.26 The four joints that make up the shoulder complex. The osseous structures of the shoulder, **(A)** anterior view, and **(B)** posterior view.

clavicle, and the acromium process of the scapula, respectively. The scapulocostal joint lacks a joint capsule and is therefore considered a physiologic joint that is necessary to allow the smooth gliding of the scapula over the ribs (Fig. 6-26).

Functional Anatomy

Osseous Structures

The convex articular surface of the proximal humerus is directed slightly posterior, medial, and superior and is met by the articular surface of the glenoid fossa of the scapula (Fig. 6-27). A 45-degree angle is formed between

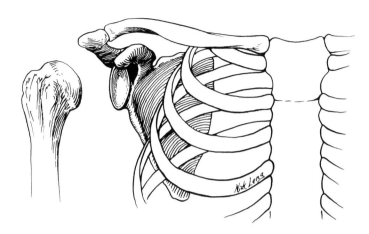

Figure 6.27 The proximal humerus articulates with the shallow glenoid fossa of the scapula.

the articular surface and the shaft of the humerus. The glenoid fossa is not a deep impression into the bone of the scapula, and by itself is incongruous with the humeral head. The glenoid labrum is a fibrocartilaginous rim that encircles the fossa and provides a greater surface area of contact for the humerus, which helps to provide some stability (Fig. 6-28).

The clavicle, which is S-shaped, provides for more movement during elevation of the arm. The distal third of the clavicle is concave anteriorly, which directs the distal articular surface anterior and somewhat superior. The proximal end of the clavicle articulates with the upper and lateral edge

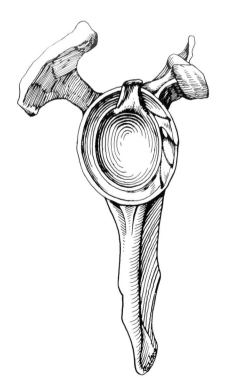

Figure 6.28 The glenoid fossa of the right scapula.

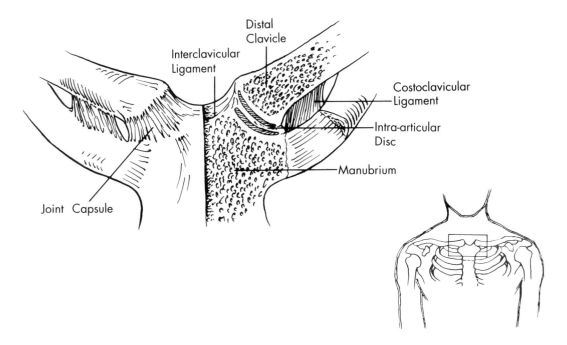

Figure 6.29 A coronal section through the sternoclavicular joints.

of the manubrium and the superior surface of the first rib costocartilage (Fig. 6-29). An intra-articular disc is present between the clavicle and manubrium joint surfaces and is important in preventing medial dislocations of the clavicle.

The scapula lies at a 30-degree angle away from the coronal plane and forms a 60-degree angle with the clavicle (Fig. 6-30). It has the coracoid process for muscular attachment projecting anteriorly and lying just medial to the glenoid fossa. The spine of the scapula arises from the medial border at about the T3 level and courses laterally and superiorly, ending as the acromion process.

Ligamentous Structures

Many ligaments are associated with the shoulder, connecting one bone to another and providing a secondary source of joint stability (Fig. 6-31). With the varied movements the shoulder can perform, these ligaments will either become slack or taut. Remember that a ligament is painlessly palpated unless it is injured or stretched.

The glenohumeral joint capsule is thin, lax, and redundant, with folds anteriorly when the arm is at rest. The glenohumeral ligaments provide some reinforcement to the joint capsule anteriorly while helping to check external rotation and possibly abduction. The coracohumeral ligament runs from the coracoid process to the greater tubercle, reinforces the superior aspect of the capsule, and checks external rotation and possible extension.

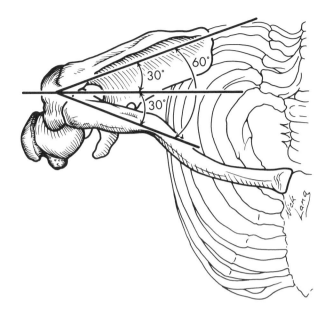

Figure 6.30 Apical view of the shoulder complex showing the relationship between the scapula and clavicle.

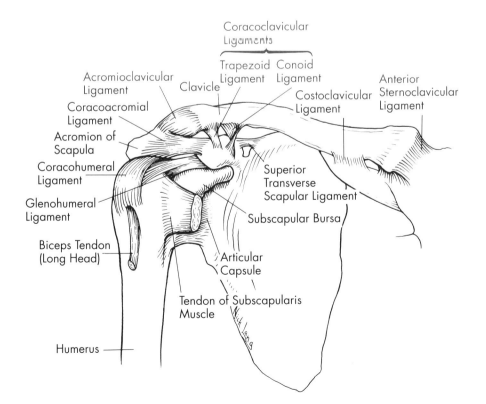

Figure 6.31 The ligaments of the shoulder complex.

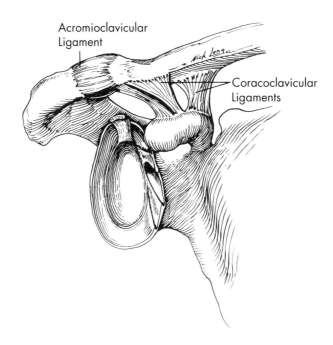

Figure 6.32 Ligaments of the acromioclavicular joint.

The transverse humeral ligament attaches across the greater and lesser tubercles and serves to contain the tendon of the long head of the biceps muscle.

The acromioclavicular ligament strengthens the superior aspect of the joint capsule. It is intrinsically weak, however, and gives way when a force is applied to the acromion process or glenohumeral joint from above (Fig. 6-32). The major stabilizing ligaments of the acromioclavicular joint are the coracoclavicular ligaments, which include the conoid and trapezoid ligaments. The conoid ligament twists on itself as it connects between the coracoid process and clavicle. It prevents excessive superior movement of the clavicle on the acromion as well as retraction of the scapula by not allowing the scapuloclavicular angle to widen. Furthermore, the conoid ligament tightens on humeral abduction, causing axial rotation of the clavicle that is necessary for full elevation of the arm. The trapezoid ligament also connects between the coracoid process and the clavicle but lies distal to the coronoid ligament. Its role is to check lateral movement of the clavicle, thereby preventing overriding of the clavicle on the acromion process. The trapezoid ligament also prevents excessive scapular protraction by not allowing the scapuloclavicular angle to narrow.

The sternoclavicular joint capsule is reinforced anteriorly and posteriorly by the anterior and posterior sternoclavicular ligaments, respectively (Fig. 6-32). The interclavicular ligaments reinforce the capsule superiorly. Lying just lateral to the joint, the costoclavicular ligament attaches between the clavicle and first rib and serves to check elevation of the clavicle. Its posterior fibers prevent medial movement while the anterior fibers prevent lateral movement of the clavicle.

Musculature

Owing to the high degree of mobility and the numerous muscles necessary to provide stability to the joint, eight or nine bursas are found about the shoulder joint to reduce friction between the moving parts. Irritation to the bursas leading to an inflammatory response is a common clinical occurrence. Of specific clinical significance are the subscapular bursas and the subacromial or subdeltoid bursas (see Fig. 6-31). The subscapular bursa lies beneath the subscapularis muscle and overlies as well as communicates with the anterior joint capsule. Distension of this bursa occurs with articular effusion. The subacromial or subdeltoid bursa extends over the supraspinatus tendon and under the acromion process and deltoid muscle (Fig. 6-33). It is susceptible to impingement beneath the acromial arch, and inflammation often follows supraspinatus tendinitis.

A review of the location and function of the numerous muscles that stabilize and supply the force for performing the varied movements of the shoulder is necessary to understand the dysfunctional conditions that affect the shoulder joint complex (Table 6-6). While muscle tendons tend to lend stability to the joint, they do not prevent downward dislocation. The rotator cuff is composed of the supraspinatus, infraspinatus, teres minor, and subscapularis muscles. It is most notably the horizontal running fibers that prevent dislocation as they check the lateral excursion of the glenoid cavity, which in turn allows downward movement of the humerus. The factors preventing downward dislocation include the slope of the glenoid fossa, which forces the humerus laterally as it is pulled down; tightening of the upper part of the capsule and of the coracohumeral ligament; and the activity of the supaspinatus muscle working with the posterior fibers of the deltoid.

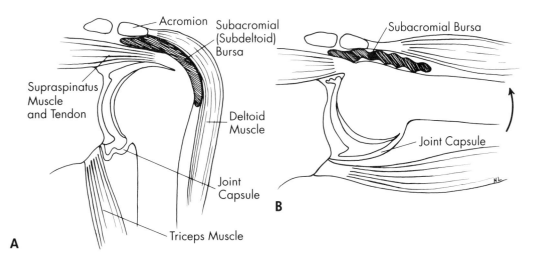

Figure 6.33 Subacromial bursa. (**A**) With humerus pendulous. (**B**) With humerus abducted. (Modified from Hertling and Kessler,[1] with permission.)

Table 6.6 Actions of the Muscles of the Shoulder Joint Complex

Action	Muscles
Flexion	Anterior deltoid, coracobracialis, pectoralis major—clavicular
Extension	Latissimus dorsi, teres major, posterior deltoid
Abduction	Middle deltoid, supraspinatus, serratus anterior (scapular stability)
Adduction	Pectoralis major, latissimus dorsi
External rotation	Infraspinatus, teres minor, posterior deltoid
Internal rotation	Subscapularis, pectoralis major, latissimus dorsi, teres major, anterior deltoid
Scapula stabilization	Trapezius, serratus anterior, rhomboids
Scapula retraction (medial glide)	Rhomboid major and minor
Scapula elevation	Trapezius, levator scapulae

The tendon of the long head of the biceps is unique in its relation to the joint in that it originates from within the joint capsule. It arises from the upper margin of the glenoid fossa as a continuation of the glenoid labrum. It penetrates the capsule and passes through the intertubercular groove, which has been converted to a tunnel by the transverse humeral ligament. The passage through the capsule, over the humeral head, and between the two tubercles is facilitated by a tubular sheath of synovial membrane.

Shoulder abduction can be artificially divided into two phases of movement, each involving different muscles to a more or less degree. Shoulder movement is fluid, however, and the various muscular actions and motions run into one another. The first phase of movement, from 0 to 90 degrees of abduction, involves a coupling of the deltoid and supraspinatus muscles that draws the humerus up. To go further, the scapula and shoulder girdle must also move. In phase 2, the serratus anterior along with the upper and lower trapezius tip the scapula so that the inferior angle moves lateral and the acromion process is elevated. This allows movement between 90 and 180 degrees.

Forward flexion of the shoulder begins with the contraction of the anterior fibers of the deltoid, coracobrachialis, and clavicular division of the pectoralis major muscles. Up to 60 degrees of flexion can occur before the scapula and shoulder girdle must move. Again, the serratus anterior and the upper and middle trapezius contract, tipping the scapula, raising the acromion process, and causing axial rotation at the acromioclavicular and sternoclavicular joints.

Internal (medial) rotation is accomplished by contraction of subscapularis, teres major, pectoralis major, latissimus dorsi, and the anterior deltoid muscles. For extreme ranges of internal rotation, the scapula will abduct from the pull of the serratus anterior and the pectoralis minor muscles.

The external (lateral) rotator muscles, in comparison to the internal rotators, are quite weak but are still very important to normal function of the upper limb. Clinically, they are easily strained. The infraspinatus, teres minor, and to a lesser degree, posterior deltoid muscles are responsible for external rotation of the humerus, with the rhomboids and trapezius muscles adducting the scapula for extreme movement.

Shoulder extension is accomplished by contraction of the latissimus dorsi, teres major, and posterior deltoid muscles, with some adduction of the scapula from contraction of the middle trapezius and rhomboid muscles.

Adduction of the humerus is accomplished by contraction of the latissimus dorsi, teres major, and pectoralis major muscles, with the rhomboids adducting the scapula.

Biomechanics

Scapulohumeral Rhythm

For the arm to be abducted from the side to overhead, motion of the scapula must be simultaneous and synchronous. During the first 30 degrees of abduction, the scapula seeks a stable position on the rib cage through contraction of the trapezius, serratus anterior, and rhomboid muscles (Fig. 6-34). Beyond 30 degrees, 2 degrees of glenohumeral movement occurs for every 1 degree of scapulocostal movement. Thus, each 15 degrees of arm abduction results from 10 degrees of glenohumeral joint movement and 5 degrees of scapulocostal joint movement. Rotation of the scapula during abduction also enhances mechanical stability by bringing the glenoid fossa directly under the humeral head.

Acromioclavicular Joint

Arm abduction also requires axial rotation of the clavicle. For every 10 degrees of arm abduction, the clavicle must elevate 4 degrees. After 90 degrees of arm abduction (60 degrees of humeral abduction and 30 degrees of scapular rotation), the clavicle rotates to accommodate the scapula through its full 60 degrees of motion. This is achieved through the S-shape of the clavicle.[9] The acromioclavicular joint usually has a meniscus that functionally divides the joint. Rotational movements occur through the conoid ligament and between the acromion and the meniscus. Hinging movements occur between the meniscus and the clavicle.[10]

Glenohumeral Joint

The rotator cuff muscles pull the humerus inferiorly (depression) while the glenohumeral joint capsule creates external rotation during abduction to permit the greater tuberosity to pass under the acromion and coracoacromial ligament (Fig. 6-35). Carefully evaluate patients complaining of loss of full abduction with or without pain to determine whether the humerus is displaced superiorly and/or has lost inferior glide movements because of capsular ligament fibroadhesions or improper functioning of the rotator cuff muscles.

During shoulder movements away from the body (flexion, abduction, and extension), the superior aspect of the glenohumeral joint capsule becomes lax, so that it can no longer maintain joint integrity against external forces. The rotator cuff muscles carry the responsibility for keeping the humerus

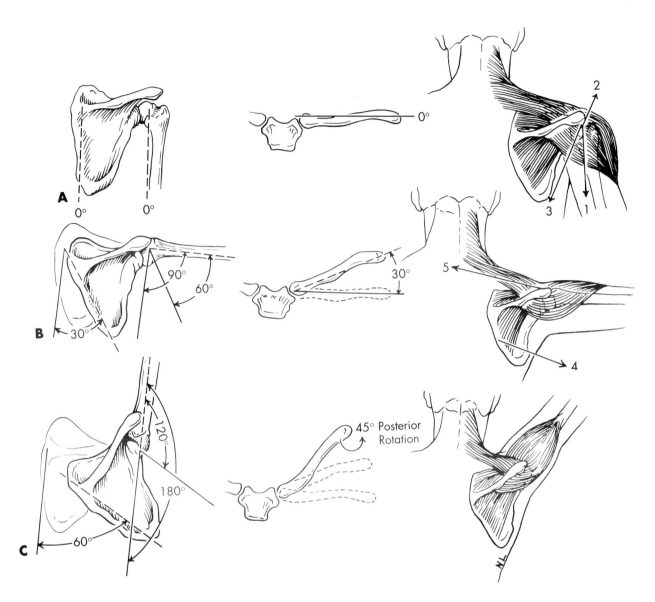

Figure 6.34 Scapulohumeral rhythm. **(A)** shoulder at 0-degree abduction, with scapula, humerus, and clavicle in neutral positions. The weight of the extremity (1) is balanced by a force couple comprising an upward pull from the deltoid muscle (2) and a downward pull from rotator cuff muscles plus the pressure and friction of the humeral head (3). **(B)** Shoulder at 90-degree abduction, with 30-degree scapular rotation and 60-degree humeral abduction; clavicle elevates 30 degrees; serratus anterior muscle (4) and upper trapezius muscle (5) force couple balance and rotate scapula. **(C)** Shoulder at 180-degree abduction, with 60-degree scapular rotation and 120-degree humeral abduction; clavicle rotates 45 degrees to reach an additional 30-degree elevation. (Modified from Wadsworth,[8] with permission.)

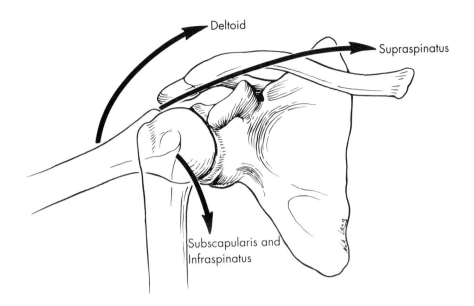

Figure 6.35 The actions of the rotator cuff muscles in shoulder abduction.

oriented to the glenoid fossa. Table 6-7 identifies the normal ranges of motion for the shoulder joint complex, while Table 6-8 describes the close-packed and loose-packed positions of the shoulder joints.

The minimally constrained, ball-and-socket glenohumeral joint allows for a significant amount of movement but is also suceptible to injury and instability. Rotational movements are the most frequent surface motion, though combinations of gliding and rolling also occur.[10] For other movements, the humeral ball must displace with respect to the glenoid fossa.

Sternoclavicular Joint

Considerable gliding movements occur at the sternoclavicular joint, with the costoclavicular ligament serving as fulcrum during shoulder motion.

Table 6.7 Arthrokinematic and Osteokinematic Movements of the
           Shoulder Joints

Osteokinematic Movements (Degrees)		Arthrokinematic Movements
Glenohumeral flexion	120	Rotation and glide
Glenohumeral extension	55	Rotation and glide
Glenohumeral abduction	120	Roll and glide
Glenohumeral adduction	45	Roll and glide
Glenohumeral internal rotation	90	Rotation
Glenohumeral external rotation	90	Rotation
Clavicle internal and external rotation	10	Rotation
Clavicle elevation and depression	5	Roll and glide
Clavicle abduction and adduction	10	Roll and glide
Scapula internal and external rotation	25	Rotation and glide

Table 6.8 Close-Packed and Loose-Packed (Rest) Positions for the Shoulder Joints

Articulation	Close-Packed Position	Loose-Packed Position
Glenohumeral	Full abduction with external rotation	55 Degrees of abduction with 30 degrees of horizontal adduction
Acromioclavicular	90 Degrees of abduction	Physiologic rest position
Sternoclavicular	Full arm elevation	Physiologic rest position

Similar to the acromioclavicular joint, in the sternoclavicular joint the meniscus divides the joint into two functional units. Anterior to posterior gliding occurs between the sternum and the meniscus, while superior to inferior gliding occurs beween the clavicle and the meniscus.[10] Rotation of the clavicle about its long axis is also possible. A reciprocal motion occurs between the sternoclavicular joint and acromioclavicular joint during glide motions but not during rotational motions.

Evaluation

The acromioclavicular joint is relatively weak and inflexible for the constant burden and repeated stresses it bears. A force applied to the acromion process or the glenohumeral joint from above causes the scapula to rotate around an axis located at the coracoid process. The acromioclavicular ligament, being intrinsically weak, gives way and the joint disrupts. A second mechanism of injury comes with a downward force of greater intensity, which lowers the clavicle on the first rib, with the rib becoming a fulcrum. Both the acromioclavicular and coracoclavicular ligaments tear, causing a complete acromioclavicular separation. This usually happens with a fall on the point of the shoulder or a fall on the hand of an outstretched arm. The sternoclavicular and costoclavicular ligaments also may be sprained during shoulder trauma.

Rotator cuff muscle strains are caused by falls on an outstretched arm, impingement against the coracoacromial arch, and minor or repetitive stresses to a compromised tendon. Most injuries are to the supraspinatus tendon.

Because of the relatively poor blood supply near the insertion of the supraspinatus, nutrition to this area may not meet the demands of the tendon tissue. An inflammatory response arises in the tendon, creating a tendinitis that probably is due to the release of enzymes and resultant dead tissue acting as a foreign body. The body may react by laying down scar tissue or even calcific deposits. This is then referred to as calcific tendinitis.

Bursitis as a primary condition resulting from local trauma is fairly rare. As a secondary progression from tendinitis, however, it is very common. Acute bulging of the tendon compresses the bursa against the coracoacromial arch, resulting in inflammation and swelling of the bursa. This will produce severe limitation of motion as well as severe pain. The subacromial or subdeltoid bursae are most frequently involved.

Capsulitis (adhesive capsulitis, frozen shoulder) is a further progression of tendinitis-bursitis clinical phemomenon with resultant adherence of the bursal walls, causing the supraspinatus and deltoid muscles to become "stuck together." Continued immobility leads to capsular tightening and eventual capsular fibrosis. Degenerative joint disease, rheumatoid arthritis, immobilization, and reflex sympathetic dystrophy also cause capsular tightening that may lead to capsulitis.

The shoulder and arm are common sites for referred pain from the cervical spine, myocardium, gall bladder, liver, diaphragm, and braest. Usually, the history will suggest the origin of pain. Moreover, many of the muscles responsible for shoulder movement and proper function receive innervation from the C5 or C6 nerve root, again signifying the importance of evaluating the cervical spine.

To begin the evaluation of the shoulder, observe the shoulder posture for the presence of asymmetry of shoulder heights, position of scapulae, and position of the humerus. Inspect the soft tissues for signs of atrophy and swelling.

Identify osseous symmetry and pain production through static palpation of the sternoclavicular joint, clavicle, coracoid process, acromioclavicular joint, acromion process, greater tuberosity, bicipital groove, lesser tuberosity, spine of the scapula, and the borders and angles of the scapula. Tone, texture, and tenderness changes should be identified through soft tissue palpation of the bursa, pectoralis major, biceps, deltoid, trapezius, rhomboids, levator, latissimus dorsi, serratus anterior, rotator cuff muscles, and teres major.

Evaluate accessory joint motions for each of the four-component articulations when joint dysfunction is suspected (Table 6-9).

Table 6.9 Accessory Joint Movements of the
          Shoulder Joint Complex

Joint	Movement
Glenohumeral	Long axis distraction
	Anterior to posterior glide
	Posterior to anterior glide
	Internal rotation
	External rotation
	Medial to lateral glide
	Inferior glide in flexion
	Inferior glide in abduction
Sternoclavicular	Inferior to superior glide
	Superior to inferior glide
	Anterior to posterior glide
	Posterior to anterior glide
Acromioclavicular	Inferior to superior glide
	Superior to inferior glide
	Anterior to posterior glide
	Posterior to anterior glide
Scapulocostal	Lateral to medial glide
	Medial to lateral glide
	Clockwise rotation
	Counterclockwise rotation

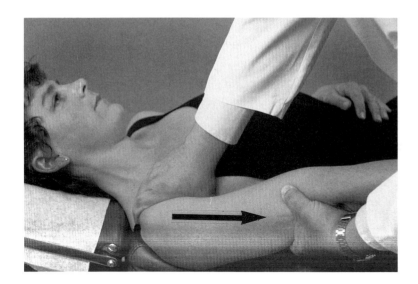

Figure 6.36 Assessment of long axis distraction of the glenohumeral joint.

Assess long axis distraction of the glenohumeral joint with the patient in the supine position and the involved arm at side of body. Stand at the side of the table and use the inside hand to stabilize the scapula in the patient's axilla. Use the other hand to grasp the humerus and stress it caudally, feeling for a springing motion (Fig. 6-36).

Evaluate anterior to posterior glide with the patient supine and the involved arm slightly abducted. Standing between the patient's arm and table, grasp the outer aspect of the distal humerus with your inside hand and grasp the anterior aspect of proximal humerus with your outside hand.

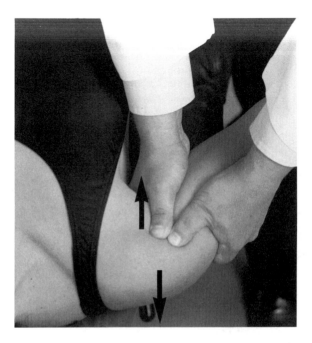

Figure 6.37 Assessment of anterior to posterior and posterior to anterior glide of the glenohumeral joint.

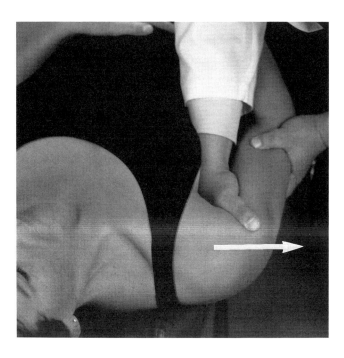

Figure 6.38 Assessment of medial to lateral glide of the glenohumeral joint.

Stress the proximal humerus, anterior to posterior. Conduct posterior to anterior glide with the hands reversed, stressing the proximal humerus posterior to anterior (Fig. 6-37).

Medial to lateral glide can be done with the patient in the supine position. Grasp the medial aspect of the proximal humerus with one hand while stabilizing the distal humerus at the elbow with the other hand. Using the elbow as a fulcrum, stress the proximal humerus medial to lateral (Fig. 6-38).

Assess internal and external rotation with the patient in the supine position with the involved arm slightly abducted. Stand at the side of the table and use both hands to grasp the proximal humerus. Stress the humerus internally and externally (Fig. 6-39).

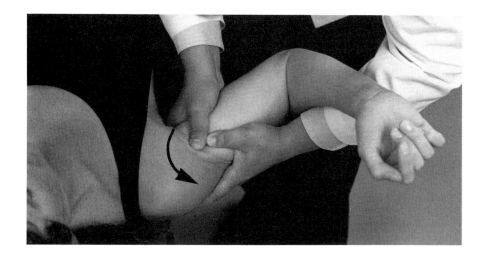

Figure 6.39 Assessment of external rotation of the glenohumeral joint.

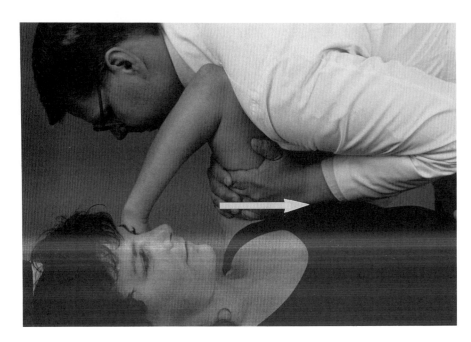

Figure 6.40 Assessment of inferior glide in flexion of the glenohumeral joint.

Evaluate inferior glide in flexion with the patient in the supine position and the involved arm flexed to 90 degrees. Stand at the side of table, interlace the fingers of both hands around the proximal humerus, and rest the patient's elbow against your shoulder. Using the patient's elbow against your shoulder as a fulcrum, stress the patient's shoulder inferiorly (Fig. 6-40).

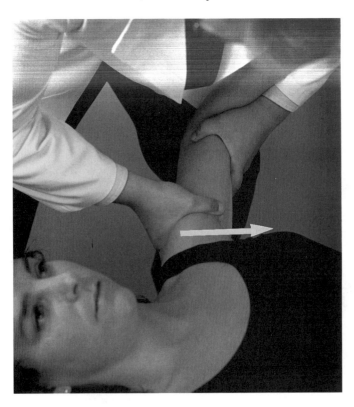

Figure 6.41 Assessment of inferior glide in abduction of the glenohumeral joint.

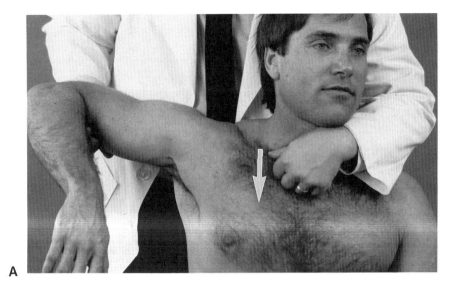

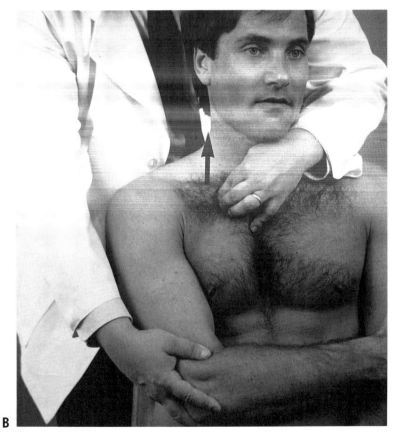

Figure 6.42 Assessment of the sternoclavicular joint. (**A**) Superior to inferior glide. (**B**) Inferior to superior glide. (*Figure continues.*)

Perform inferior glide in abduction with the patient in the supine position with the involved arm abducted to 90 degrees. Stand at the head of the table, and place the cephalad hand on the superior aspect of the proximal humerus while grasping the inferior aspect of the elbow with the other hand. Then stress the proximal humerus inferiorly (Fig. 6-41).

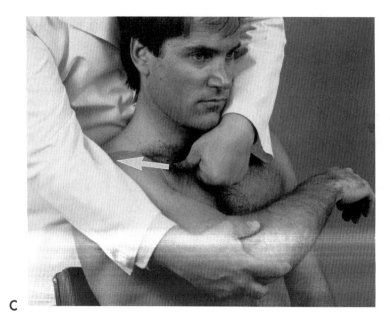

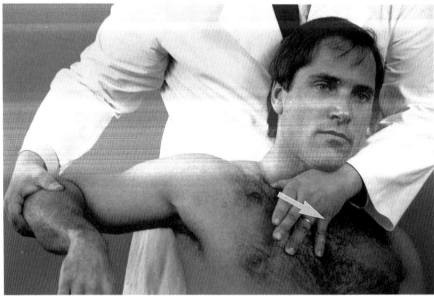

Figure 6.42 (*Continued*). (**C**) Anterior to posterior glide. (**D**) Posterior to anterior glide.

The sternoclavicular joint has accessory movements in inferior glide, superior glide, posterior glide, and anterior glide. For evaluation of each of these movements, stand behind the seated patient. Reach in front of the patient's neck and use a thumb contact on the proximal clavicle to stress it inferiorly, superiorly, posteriorly, and anteriorly (Fig. 6-42).

Evaluate the acromioclavicular joint for accessory movements standing at the patient's side with the patient seated. Grasp the distal clavicle with one hand and stabilize the scapula and shoulder with the other hand. Then stress the distal clavicle anteriorly, posteriorly, inferiorly, and superiorly (Fig. 6-43).

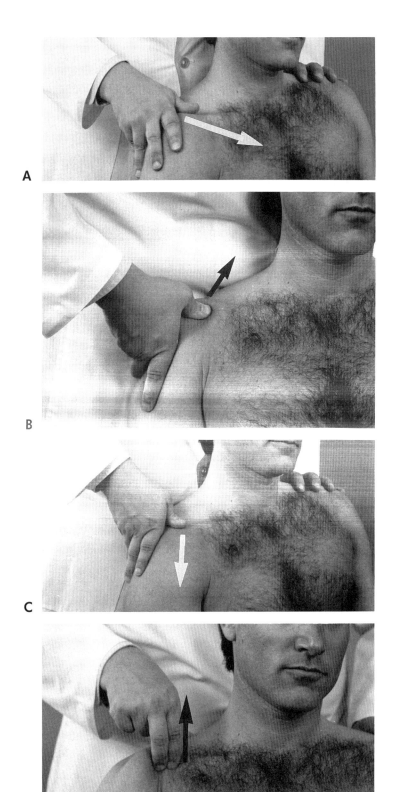

Figure 6.43 Assessment of the acromioclavicular joint. (**A**) Posterior to anterior glide. (**B**) Anterior to posterior glide. (**C**) Superior to inferior glide. (**D**) Inferior to superior glide.

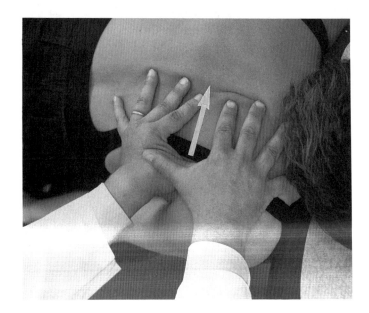

Figure 6.44 Assessment of the scapulocostal articulation for lateral to medial glide.

The scapulocostal joint, although not an anatomic joint, also undergoes a stress evaluation. The findings are somewhat different in that a springing end feel or joint-play movement is not expected. The stress evaluation is used to determine the integrity of the subscapular soft tissues and the supporting musculature. Decreased movement is still the positive finding. The movements assessed are medial glide, lateral glide, and rotation in both directions. Perform the evaluation standing at the side of the table with the patient lying in the prone position. For medial glide, bring the patient's arm to rest along the side of the body and use both hands to contact the lateral aspect (axillary border) of the scapula. Stress the scapula medially (Fig. 6-44). For rotational glide moving the inferior angle medially, place the

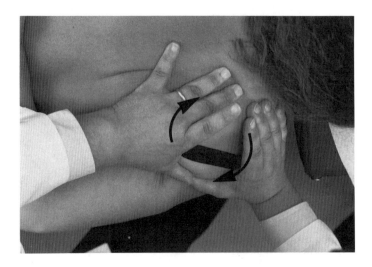

Figure 6.45 Assessment of the scapulocostal articulation for rotation-glide, inferior angle, medial.

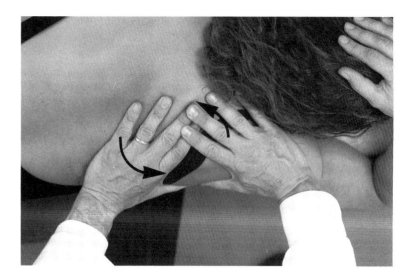

Figure 6.46 Assessment of the scapulocostal articulation for rotation-glide, inferior angle, lateral.

patient's arm in the small of the back, and use both hands to grasp the scapula such that the caudal hand thumb hooks the lateral aspect of the inferior angle. With both hands, twist the scapula so that the inferior angle is stressed medially (Fig. 6-45). For rotational glide moving the inferior angle laterally, place the patient's hand behind the head, and use both hands to grasp the scapula such that the cephalad hand thumb hooks the medial aspect of the inferior angle. With both hands, twist the scapula so that the inferior angle is stressed laterally (Fig. 6-46). For medial to lateral glide, the patient's arm hangs off the table; stand on the opposite side of the table, and use both hands to contact the medial aspect (vertebral border) of the scapula. With both hands, stress the scapula laterally (Fig. 6-47).

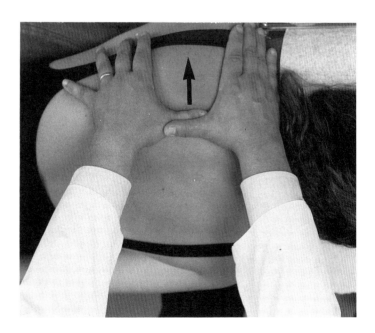

Figure 6.47 Assessment of the scapulocostal articulation for medial to lateral glide.

Adjustive Techniques

Glenohumeral Joint

Long axis distraction (Fig. 6-48)

IND: Palpable point tenderness at the superior aspect of the humerus and/
or the supraspinatus tendon, loss of long axis accessory movement,
superior misalignment of humerus.

PP: The patient is supine with the involved arm alongside the body.

DP: Stand on the involved side, bring the patient's arm into slight abduction, then straddle the arm such that your slightly bent knees can
grasp the patient's distal humerus just proximal to the epicondyles.

SCP: The patient's axilla.

CP: With your inside hand, establish a thumb-web contact in the patient's
axilla while applying downward pressure with your fingers on the
shoulder girdle to stabilize it against the table.

IH: With your outside hand, use a digital contact over the lateral aspect
of the joint to monitor for movement.

VEC: Long axis distraction.

P: While maintaining the shoulder girdle against the table and applying
slight superior pressure with the CP, make a quick "bunny hop"
movement by extending both knees and drawing the humerus into
long axis distraction.

Anterior to posterior distraction of the humerus—sitting (Fig. 6-49)

IND: Point tenderness over the anterior aspect of the joint, loss of anterior
to posterior accessory movement, anterior misalignment of the humerus, history of previous anterior dislocation of the glenohumeral
joint.

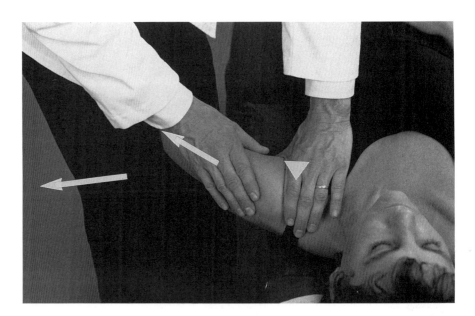

Figure 6.48 Adjustment for long axis distraction of the glenohumeral joint.

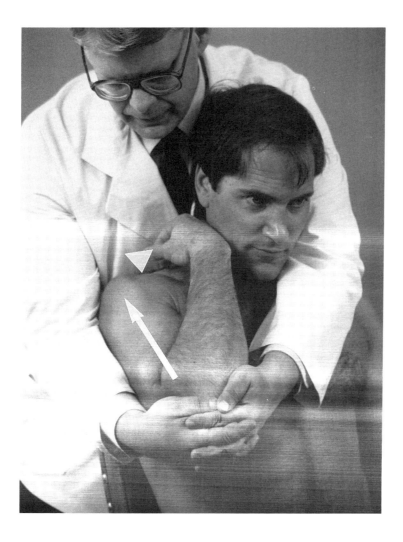

Figure 6.49 Adjustment for anterior to posterior glide of the glenohumeral joint in the sitting position.

PP: The patient sits with the arm in forward flexion, elbow bent, and hand resting on the opposite shoulder if internal rotation is also desired or on the same shoulder if external rotation is also desired.

DP: Stand behind the patient, slightly to the side of involvement, and stabilizing the patient's shoulder girdle against the torso.

SCP: The olecranon process.

CP: With your ipsilateral hand, use a palmar contact to cup the patient's elbow.

IH: With your other hand, reinforce the CP.

VEC: Anterior to posterior.

P: Using both hands, remove the articular slack and give a very quick and shallow thrust primarily in the axis of the humerus.

Anterior to posterior humerus—supine (Fig. 6-50)

IND: Point tenderness over the anterior aspect of the joint, loss of anterior to posterior accessory movement, anterior misalignment of the hum-

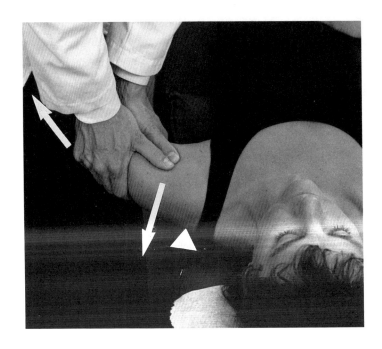

Figure 6.50 Adjustment for anterior to posterior glide of the glenohumeral joint in the supine position.

erus, history of previous anterior dislocation of the glenohumeral joint.

PP: The patient lies in the supine position with the involved arm in slight abduction and the glenohumeral joint positioned off the edge of the table.

DP: Stand at the side of the table, and straddle the affected arm such that the patient's epicondyles are held between your knees.

SCP: Proximal humerus.

CP: With both hands, grasp the proximal humerus with thumbs together in the midline.

VEC: Anterior to posterior.

P: With your knees, provide slight distraction while applying an impulse thrust anterior to posterior with both hands.

Posterior to anterior humerus (Fig. 6-51)

IND: Palpable tenderness of the posterior aspect of the glenohumeral joint, rotator cuff tendons, and/or inferior and lateral glenohumeral ligaments; loss of posterior to anterior accessory movements; posterior misalignment of the humerus.

PP: The patient lies in the prone position with the involved arm in slight abduction and the glenohumeral joint positioned off the edge of the table.

DP: Stand at the side of the table, and straddle the patient's affected arm with the epicondyles held between your knees.

SCP: Proximal humerus.

CP: With both of your hands, grasp the proximal humerus with thumbs together in the midline.

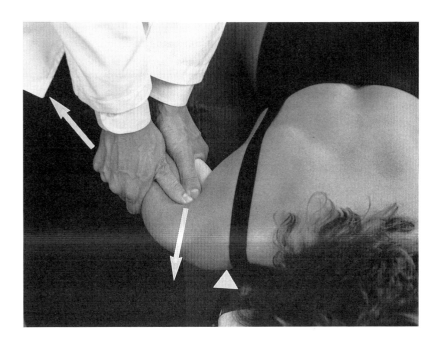

Figure 6.51 Adjustment for posterior to anterior glide of the glenohumeral joint.

VEC: Posterior to anterior.
   P: With your knees, provide slight distraction while applying an impulse thrust posterior to anterior with both hands.

Inferior glide in flexion–standing (Fig. 6-52)
IND: Palpable tenderness at the superior aspect of the humerus and/or supraspinatus tendon; loss of accessory movements in inferior glide

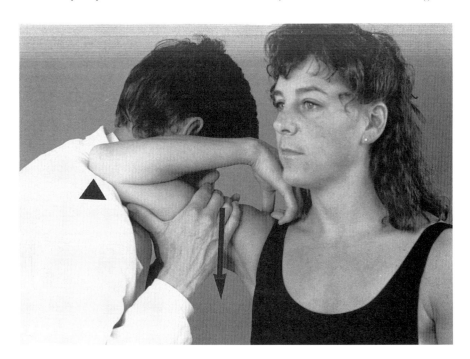

Figure 6.52 Adjustment for inferior glide in flexion of the glenohumeral joint in the standing position.

in flexion; glenohumeral capsular adhesions; a history of trauma that drove the humerus superior.

PP: The patient stands with feet spread at least shoulder distance apart (or farther if the patient is taller than the doctor); the involved arm is flexed to 90 degrees, and the elbow is flexed so that the hand will rest on the patient's shoulder.

DP: Stand in front of the patient and off to the affected side; your legs should be spread appropriately for balance as well as to align to the patient's height.

SCP: Proximal humerus.

CP: First place the patient's elbow on your shoulder, then using both hands, grasp the proximal humerus with your fingers interlaced on the superior aspect of the joint capsule while your thumbs wrap into the axilla.

VEC: Superior to inferior.

P: First draw away from the patient, creating a joint separation, and then apply a downward pressure to remove articular slack; give a thrust in the superior to inferior direction.

Inferior glide in flexion—supine (Fig. 6-53)

IND: Palpable tenderness at the superior aspect of the humerus and/or supraspinatus tendon; loss of accessory movements in inferior glide in flexion; glenohumeral capsular adhesions; a history of trauma that drove the humerus superior.

PP: The patient is supine with the involved arm raised to 90 degrees flexion and the elbow bent such that the hand can rest on the shoulder.

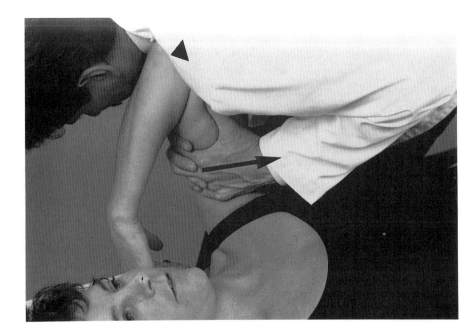

Figure 6.53 Adjustment for inferior glide in flexion of the glenohumeral joint in the supine position.

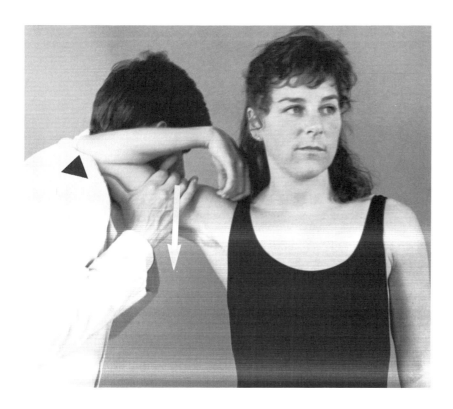

Figure 6.54 Adjustment for inferior glide in abduction of the glenohumeral joint in the standing position.

DP: Stand on the involved side in a lunge position facing headward, allowing the patient's elbow to rest against your shoulder.
SCP: Proximal humerus.
CP: Grasp the proximal humerus with both hands using interlaced fingers over the superior aspect of the glenohumeral joint.
VEC: Superior to inferior.
P: Using the patient's elbow on your shoulder as a pivot point, apply superior to inferior joint distraction with both hands, finishing with an impulse thrust superior to inferior.

Inferior glide in abduction—standing (Fig. 6-54)

IND: Intracapsular adhesions, decreased shoulder range of motion and specifically abduction, pain over the supraspinatus tendon and supraspinatus tendonitis, pain over the subdeltoid or subacromial bursa and bursitis.
PP: The patient stands with legs at least shoulder distance apart, with the involved arm abducted to 90 degrees and the elbow flexed such that the hand will rest on the patient's shoulder.
DP: Stand with legs apart so that the patient's elbow can rest on your shoulder.
SCP: Proximal humerus.
CP: Grasp the proximal humerus with interlaced fingers on the superior aspect and thumbs in the axilla.

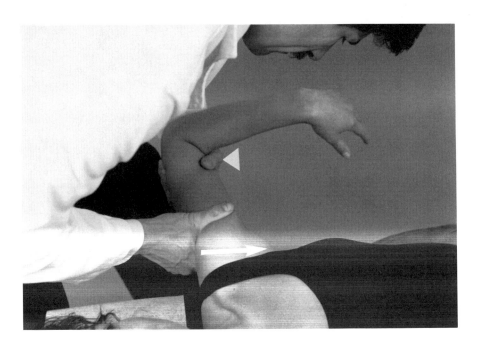

Figure 6.55 Adjustment for inferior glide in abduction of the glenohumeral joint in the supine position.

VEC: Superior to inferior.
  P: Back away from the patient to distract the joint while applying a downward pressure with the hands to remove articular slack. Give an impulse thrust in the superior to inferior direction.

Inferior glide in abduction—supine (Fig. 6-55)

IND: Intracapsular adhesions, decreased shoulder range of motion and specifically abduction, pain over the supraspinatus tendon and supraspinatus tendonitis, pain over the subdeltoid or subacromial bursa, and bursitis.
 PP: The patient is supine with the involved arm abducted to 90 degrees.
 DP: Stand on the involved side at the head of the table, facing footward.
SCP: Superior aspect of the proximal humerus.
 CP: Establish a web contact over the superior aspect of the proximal humerus with the cephalad hand.
 IH: With your caudal hand, grasp the distal aspect of the patient's humerus.
VEC: Superior to inferior.
  P: Your indifferent hand serves as a pivot point, stabilizing the disal humerus and elbow, while your cephalad hand removes articular slack, finishing with an impulse-type thrust in a superior to inferior direction.

Internal rotation (Fig. 6-56)

IND: Restricted internal rotation accessory joint movement, intercapsular adhesions, mobilization of the shoulder.
 PP: The patient is supine with the affected arm abducted slightly away from the patient's body and the edge of the table in internal rotation.

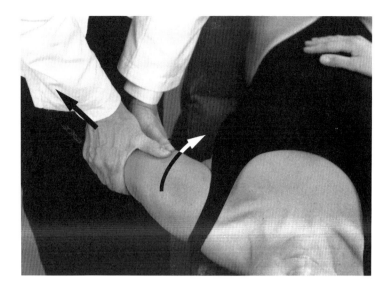

Figure 6.56 Adjustment for internal rotation of the glenohumeral joint. External rotation is done with the same procedure but different thrust.

DP: Stand on the involved side, facing headward and straddling the patient's affected arm such that your knees can squeeze the distal humerus just above the epicondyles.

SCP: Proximal humerus.

CP: Grasp the patient's proximal humerus with interlaced fingers of both hands.

VEC: Rotational—internal rotation.

P: Your hand contacts first turn the humerus into internal rotation removing articular slack; simultaneously, straighten both knees, applying a long axis distraction to the glenohumeral joint.

External rotation (Fig. 6-56, 6-39)

IND: Restricted external rotation accessory joint movement, intercapsular adhesions, and mobilization of the shoulder.

PP: The patient is supine with the affected arm abducted slightly away from his body and the edge of the table, holding the arm in external rotation.

DP: Stand on the involved side, facing headward and straddling the patient's affected arm such that your knees can squeeze the distal humerus just above the epicondyles.

SCP: Proximal humerus.

CP: With your hand, grasp the patient's proximal humerus with interlaced fingers.

VEC: Rotational—external rotation.

P: Use both hands to turn the humerus into external rotation; simultaneously, straighten both knees, to create a long axis distraction to the glenohumeral joint.

External rotation in abduction (Fig. 6-57)

IND: Decreased external rotation accessory joint movement, intercapsular adhesions, and mobilization of the glenohumeral joint.

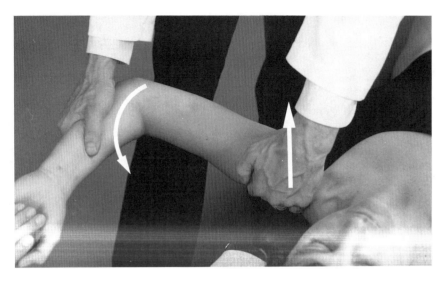

Figure 6.57 Adjustment for external rotation in abduction of the glenohumeral joint.

PP: The patient is supine with the affected arm abducted to 90 degrees and the elbow flexed to 90 degrees.

DP: Stand in a lunge position on the side of involvement, facing the patient.

SCP: Spine of the scapula.

CP: With your inside hand, apply a digital contact over the spine of the scapula.

IH: With your outside hand, grasp the patient's proximal forearm.

VEC: Rotational—external rotational.

P: With your indifferent hand, externally rotate the patient's humerus by pushing down on the patient's forearm to remove articular slack. At the point of full external rotation, pull up sharply on the spine of the scapula with your contact hand.

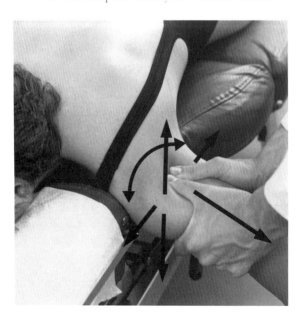

Figure 6.58 Glenohumeral mobilization in the prone position.

Glenohumeral mobilization—prone (Fig. 6-58)

IND: Intercapsular adhesions and mobilization of the shoulder.

 PP: The patient lies prone with the affected arm hanging down and off the side of the table.

 DP: Kneel at the side of the table facing the patient.

SCP: Proximal humerus.

 CP: With both hands, grasp the patient's proximal humerus with your thumbs together on the posterior aspect of the humerus while your fingers wrap around and into the axilla on the underside of the humerus.

VEC: Circumduction.

  P: Using both hands, first distract the glenohumeral joint in the long axis of the humerus followed by movements of the humerus toward and away from you, headward and footward, and in a figure-8 motion.

Glenohumeral mobilization—supine (Fig. 6-59)

IND: Intercapsular adhesions in the glenohumeral joint, mobilization of the shoulder.

 PP: The patient is supine with the affected arm outstretched.

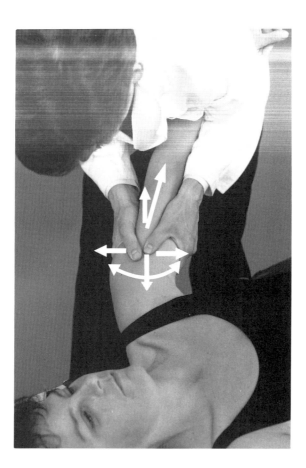

Figure 6.59 Glenohumeral mobilization in the supine position.

DP: Stand in a lunge position on the affected side, facing the head of the table.
SCP: Humerus.
CP: With your inside hand, grasp the patient's arm to hold the patient's forearm against your thoracic cage.
IH: With your outside hand, make a palmar contact on the posterior aspect of the shoulder and scapula to provide support and lift during the mobilization.
VEC: Circumduction and distraction.
P: Use body weight to assist in producing a mild distraction and circumduction movement of the shoulder in all directions.

Glenohumeral mobilization—pendular abduction (Fig. 6-60)

IND: Intercapsular adhesions in the glenohumeral joint, mobilization of the shoulder, and adhesive capsulitis.
PP: The patient is supine with the affected arm slightly abducted and the forearm flexed to 90 degrees pointing upward.
DP: Stand at the side of the table on the involved side, facing the patient.
SCP: The hand.
CP: With both hands, grasp the patient's hand.
VEC: Superior to inferior, passive rocking.
P: Instruct the patient to relax the arm as much as possible. Raise the

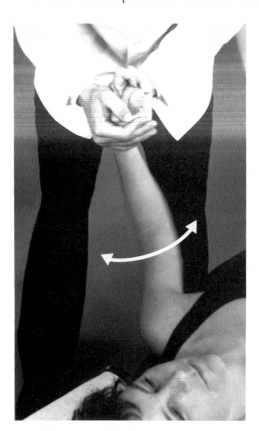

Figure 6.60 Glenohumeral mobilization using pendular abduction.

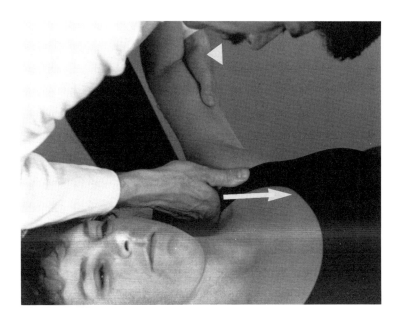

Figure 6.61 Adjustment for superior to inferior glide of the acromioclavicular joint in the supine position.

arm away from the table so that it can swing freely. Induce a pendular motion in the glenohumeral joint by rocking the forearm headward and footward, increasing the arc of abduction motion, as tolerated.

Acromioclavicular Joint

Superior to inferior glide—supine (Fig. 6-61)

IND: Point tenderness over the superior aspect of the acromioclavicular joint, restricted superior to inferior accessory movement of the distal clavicle, and acromioclavicular joint separation.

PP: The patient is supine with the affected arm abducted to 90 degrees.

DP: Stand at the head of the table, facing footward off to the side of the affected arm.

SCP: Superior aspect of the distal clavicle.

CP: Establish an index contact with the inside hand over the superior aspect of the distal clavicle.

IH: With your outside hand, grasp the humerus at midshaft.

VEC: Superior to inferior.

P: As your indifferent hand draws the humerus into long axis distraction and abduction, apply a superior to inferior impulse thrust with your contact hand.

Superior to inferior glide—sitting (Fig. 6-62)

IND: Point tenderness over the superior aspect of the acromioclavicular joint, restricted superior to inferior accessory movement of the distal clavicle, and acromioclavicular joint separation.

PP: The patient sits with the affected arm abducted.

DP: Stand behind the patient and off to the side of the affected arm.

SCP: Superior aspect of the distal clavicle.

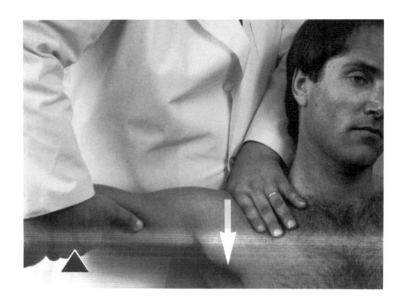

Figure 6.62 Adjustment for superior to inferior glide of the acromioclavicular joint in the seated position.

CP: With your inside hand, apply a web contact over the superior aspect of the distal clavicle.

IH: With your outside hand, grasp the patient's distal forearm.

VEC: Superior to inferior.

P: While your indifferent hand uses the patient's forearm as a lever to distract and abduct the shoulder joint, deliver a superior to inferior impulse thrust with your contact hand.

Inferior to superior glide (Fig. 6-63)

IND: Point tenderness at the inferior aspect of the acromioclavicular joint and decrease in inferior to superior accessory joint movement of the distal clavicle.

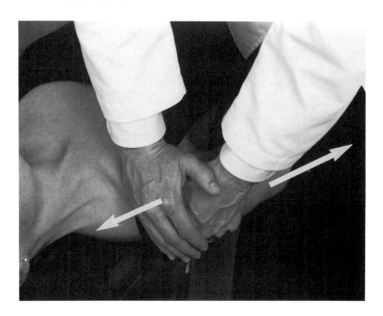

Figure 6.63 Adjustment for inferior to superior glide of the acromioclavicular joint.

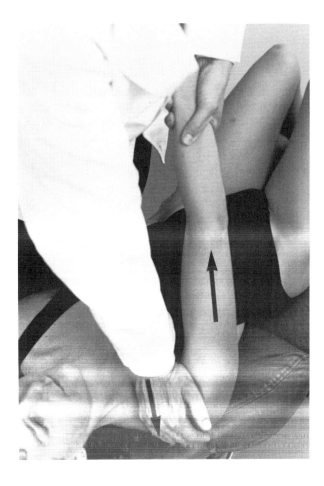

Figure 6.64 Adjustment for anterior to posterior glide of the acromioclavicular joint.

PP: The patient is supine with the affected arm straight and slightly abducted.

DP: Stand at the side of the table, straddling the patient's affected arm such that your knees can grasp the distal humerus above the patient's epicondyles.

SCP: Inferior aspect of the distal clavicle.

CP: With your inside hand, apply a thumb contact on the inferior aspect of the proximal clavicle.

IH: With your outside hand, place a pisiform contact over the thumbnail of the contact hand.

VEC: Inferior to superior.

P: As you straighten your knees to create a long axis distraction of the shoulder joint, use both hands to deliver an impulse thrust inferior to superior to the distal clavicle.

Anterior to posterior glide (Fig. 6-64)

IND: Point tenderness at the anterior aspect of the acromioclavicular joint, palpable anterior displacement of the distal clavicle, and restricted anterior to posterior accessory joint movement of the proximal clavicle.

PP: The patient is supine with the affected arm straight and forward flexed to about 60 degrees.

DP: Stand at the side of the table opposite the involved side.

SCP: Anterior aspect of the distal clavicle.

CP: With your cephalad hand, establish a pisiform hypothenar contact over the anterior aspect of the distal clavicle.

IH: With your indifferent hand, grasp the outer aspect of the distal forearm.

VEC: Anterior to posterior.

P: As you distract the shoulder anterior and inferior with your indifferent hand, apply an impulse thrust anterior to posterior to the distal clavicle, with your contact hand.

Posterior to anterior glide (Fig. 6-65)

IND: Restricted posterior to anterior accessory joint movement of the distal clavicle and mobilization of the acromioclavicular joint.

PP: The patient is supine with the affected arm straight, flexed to approximately 60 degrees, and slightly abducted.

DP: Stand at the side of the table on the affected side, facing headward between the patient's affected arm and the table.

SCP: Posterior and superior aspect of the distal clavicle.

CP: With your inside hand, place the digital contact of the index and middle fingers over the posterosuperior aspect of the distal clavicle.

IH: With your outer hand, grasp the patient's distal forearm.

VEC: Posterior to anterior.

P: With your indifferent hand, distract the shoulder anteriorly and, while maintaining distraction, flex the arm, raising it past 90 degrees. As the articular slack is taken out, use your contact hand to deliver

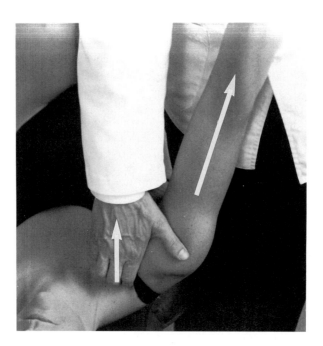

Figure 6.65 Adjustment for posterior to anterior glide of the acromioclavicular joint.

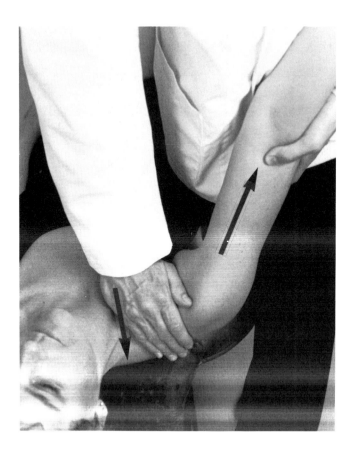

Figure 6.66 Adjustment for anterior to posterior glide of the sternoclavicular joint.

a very quick and shallow impulse thrust posterior to anterior to the distal clavicle (lifting the distal clavicle).

Sternoclavicular Joint

Anterior to posterior glide (Fig. 6-66)

IND: Point tenderness at the anterior aspect of the sternoclavicular joint, restricted anterior to posterior accessory movement of the proximal clavicle, and sternoclavicular joint separation.

PP: The patient is supine with the involved arm flexed forward to approximately 60 degrees.

DP: Stand on the side of the table on the side of involvement, facing headward.

SCP: Anterior aspect of the proximal clavicle.

CP: Use your inside hand to apply a pisiform–hypothenar contact over the anterior aspect of the proximal clavicle.

IH: With your outside hand, grasp the outer aspect of the distal humerus at the epicondyles.

VEC: Anterior to posterior.

P: With your indifferent hand, distract the shoulder anteriorly, raising the shoulder and scapula off the adjusting table. As the articular

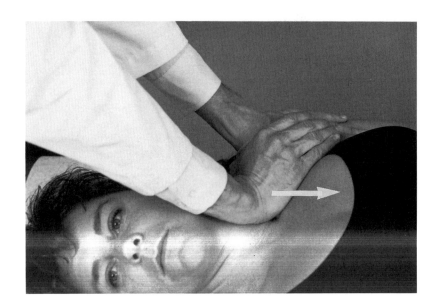

Figure 6.67 Adjustment for superior to inferior glide of the sternoclavicular joint.

slack is removed, deliver an impulse thrust anterior to posterior over the proximal clavicle with the contact hand.

Superior to inferior glide (Fig. 6-67)

IND: Point tenderness at the superior aspect of the sternoclavicular articulation, a loss of superior to inferior accessory motion of the proximal clavicle, and a palpable superior displacement of the proximal clavicle.

PP: The patient is supine with the involved arm abducted to 90 degrees, and the hand placed under the head.

DP: Stand at the head of the table, facing footward.

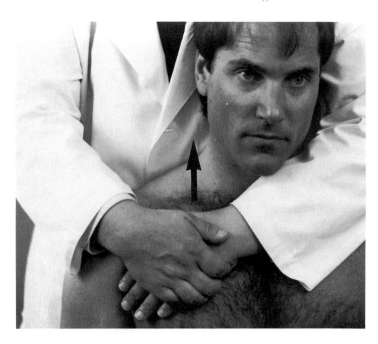

Figure 6.68 Adjustment for inferior to superior glide of the sternoclavicular joint in the seated position.

SCP: Superior aspect of the proximal clavicle.

CP: With your ipsilateral hand, place a thumb contact on the superior aspect of the proximal clavicle.

IH: With your contralateral hand, place a pisiform–hypothenar contact over the thumb contact.

VEC: Superior to inferior.

P: Deliver an impulse thrust with both hands in a superior to inferior direction on the proximal clavicle.

Inferior to superior glide—sitting (Fig. 6-68)

IND: Pain in the sternoclavicular joint and loss of inferior to superior accessory joint movement of the proximal clavicle.

PP: The patient sits with arms relaxed.

DP: Stand behind the patient.

SCP: Inferior aspect of the proximal clavicle.

CP: With your contralateral hand, establish a thenar contact on the inferior aspect of the proximal clavicle.

IH: With your ipsilateral hand, take a calcaneal contact over the thenar contact for reinforcement.

VEC: Inferior to superior.

P: Stabilize the patient's torso against the back of the chair and/or your body. Deliver an impulse thrust with both hands in an inferior to superior direction.

Inferior to superior glide—supine (Fig. 6-69)

IND: Pain in the sternoclavicular joint, loss of inferior to superior accessory joint movement of the proximal clavicle.

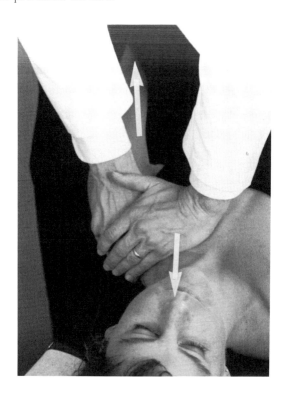

Figure 6.69 Adjustment for inferior to superior glide of the sternoclavicular joint in the supine position.

PP: The patient is supine with the affected arm slightly abducted.

DP: Stand on the affected side, straddling the patient's arm and grasping the forearm between your knees.

SCP: Inferior aspect of the proximal clavicle.

CP: With your outside hand, place a thumb contact on the inferior aspect of the proximal clavicle.

IH: With your inside hand, place a pisiform–hypothenar contact over the thumb contact for reinforcement.

VEC: Inferior to superior.

P: Use the leg contact on the patient's arm to distract the shoulder girdle footward. When articular slack has been removed, apply an impulse thrust through both hands in an inferior–superior direction on the proximal clavicle.

Posterior to anterior glide (Fig. 6-70)

IND: Pain in the sternoclavicular joint, loss of posterior to anterior accessory joint movement of the proximal clavicle, and a palpable posterior displacement of the proximal end of the clavicle.

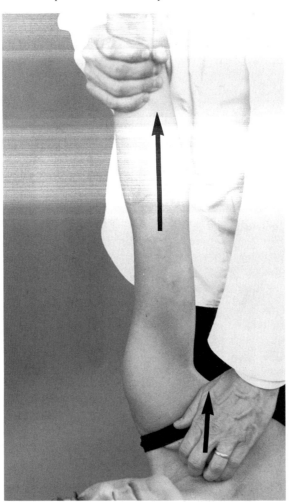

Figure 6.70 Adjustment for posterior to anterior glide of the sternoclavicular joint.

PP: The patient is supine.

DP: Stand at the side of the table on the affected side, facing headward.

SCP: Posterior and superior aspect of the proximal clavicle.

CP: With your inside hand, apply the digital contact of the index and middle fingers over the posterosuperior aspect of the proximal clavicle.

IH: Grasp the patient's distal forearm with your outer hand.

VEC: Posterior to anterior.

P: With your indifferent hand, distract the shoulder anteriorly and, while maintaining distraction, flex the arm, raising it past 90 degrees. As the articular slack is taken out, use your contact hand to deliver a very quick and shallow impulse thrust posterior to anterior to the proximal clavicle (lifting the proximal clavicle).

Sternoclavicular joint distraction—sitting (Fig. 6-71)

IND: Pain in the sternoclavicular joint, generalized decrease in movement of the sternoclavicular joint, and displacement of the intra-articular meniscus.

PP: The patient sits with the affected arm abducted to approximately 90 degrees.

DP: Stand behind the patient and slightly to the side of involvement.

SCP: Proximal clavicle.

CH: With your ipsilateral hand, reach under the patient's affected arm to support the patient's arm on your forearm. Make digital contact with the index and middle fingers on the proximal end of the clavicle.

IH: With your contralateral hand, make a thenar contact over the manubrium of the sternum with the forearm lying across the contralateral clavicle.

VEC: Distraction.

P: With your indifferent hand, stabilize the manubrium and opposite shoulder girdle against the back of the chair and/or your body, while your contact hand draws the affected clavicle medial to lateral and

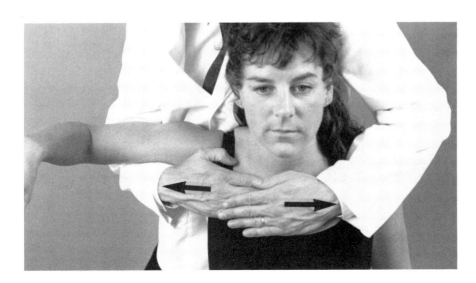

Figure 6.71 Distraction of the sternoclavicular joint in the seated position.

your arm draws the patient's affected shoulder slightly anterior to posterior. When articular slack is removed, give a quick and shallow impulse thrust, separating the proximal clavicle from the manubrium.

Sternoclavicular joint distraction—supine (Fig. 6-72)

IND: Pain in the sternoclavicular joint, generalized decrease in movement of the sternoclavicular joint, and displacement of the intra-articular meniscus.

PP: The patient is supine with a rolled towel or small cylindrical pillow placed under the upper thoracic spine. The affected arm is abducted to approximately 90 degrees.

DP: Stand on the affected side in a lunge position, facing headward.

SCP: Distal clavicle.

CP: With your outside hand, place a thenar contact over the distal clavicle and grasp the deltoid area.

IH: With your inside hand, place a thenar contact over the manubrium of the sternum with the thumb pointing headward and the fingers pointing laterally across the contralateral clavicle.

VEC: Distraction.

P: With your indifferent hand, stabilize the patient's manubrium and opposite shoulder against the table, applying a downward pressure. The pillow or rolled towel serves as a fulcrum as you apply a shallow impulse thrust to the distal clavicle and shoulder to distract the proximal clavicle from the manubrium.

Scapulocostal Articulation

Lateral to medial glide (Fig. 6-73)

IND: Dysfunctional scapulohumeral rhythm, subscapular adhesions, and subscapular dull aching pain.

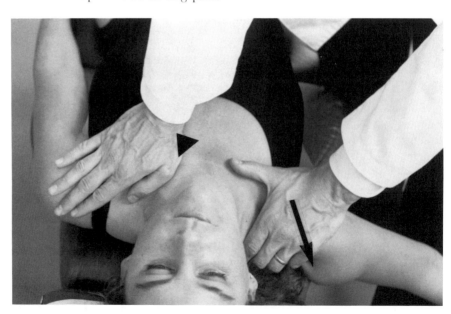

Figure 6.72 Distraction of the right sternoclavicular joint in the supine position.

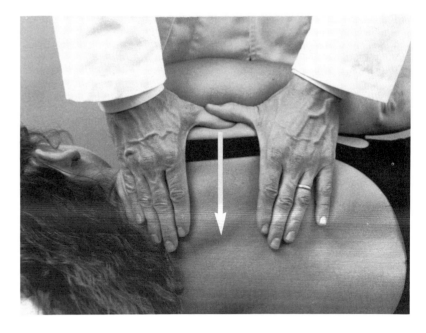

Figure 6.73 Manipulation for lateral to medial glide of the scapulocostal articulation.

PP: The patient is in a side-lying position with the affected side up and arm resting on the side.

DP: Stand at the side of the table facing the patient.

SCP: Lateral border of the scapula.

CP: With both hands, establish a thumb, thenar, and calcaneal contact over the axillary (lateral) border of the scapular with the fingers pointing toward the spine.

VEC: Lateral to medial.

P: Draw the scapula from lateral to medial, and when the end of passive movement is reached, give an impulse thrust from lateral to medial.

Medial to lateral glide (Fig. 6-74)

IND: Dysfunctional scapulohumeral rhythm, subscapular adhesions, and subscapular dull aching pain.

PP: The patient is in a side-lying position with the affected arm hanging forward in front of the table.

DP: Stand at the side of the table to the front of the patient in a lunge position, facing headward.

SCP: Medial border of the scapula.

CP: Use your caudal hand to apply a knife-edge contact over the vertebral (medial) border of the affected scapula, with fingers over the spine and body of the scapula.

IH: With your cephalad hand, establish a calcaneal contact over the vertebral border of the other scapula and fingers over the body of the scapula.

VEC: Medial to lateral.

P: Use both hands in opposing directions to draw passive movement from medial to lateral, and administer an impulse thrust primarily through the contact hand from medial to lateral.

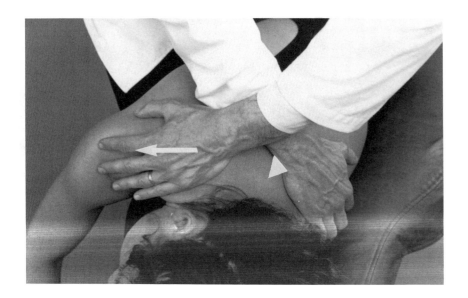

Figure 6.74 Manipulation for medial to lateral glide of the right scapulocostal articulation.

Rotation—inferior angle, lateral to medial (Fig. 6-75)

IND: Dysfunctional scapulohumeral rhythm, subscapular adhesions, and subscapular dull aching pain.

PP: The patient is in a side-lying position with the affected side up and affected arm placed behind the back with the fist in the small of the back.

DP: Stand at the side of the table facing the patient.

SCP: Lateral aspect of the inferior angle of the scapula.

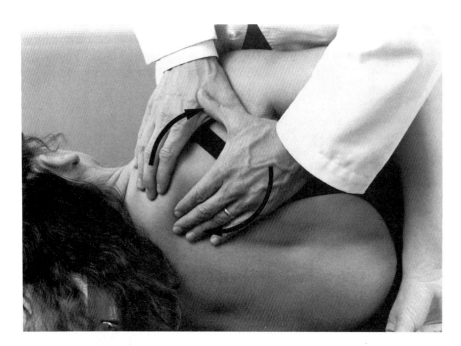

Figure 6.75 Manipulation for rotation of the scapulocostal articulation moving the inferior angle in a lateral to medial direction.

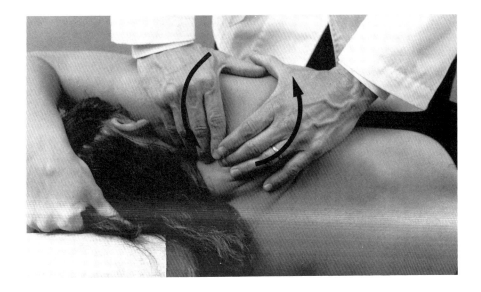

Figure 6.76 Manipulation for rotation of the scapulo-costal articulation moving the inferior angle in a medial to lateral direction.

CP: With your caudal hand, apply a thenar contact on the lateral aspect of the inferior angle of the scapula, with the fingers lying across the scapula pointing toward the spine.

IH: With your cephalad hand, place a thenar contact on the superior aspect of the spine of the scapula, with the fingers pointing toward the inferior angle.

VEC: Rotational.

P: Use both hands to induce a rotational twisting action using an impulse-type thrust to drive the inferior angle of the scapula lateral to medial.

Rotation—inferior angle medial to lateral (Fig. 6-76)

IND: Dysfunctional scapulohumeral rhythm, subscapular adhesions, and subscapular dull aching pain.

PP: The patient is in a side-lying position with the affected side up and affected arm abducted with the hand behind his head.

DP: Stand at the side of the table facing the patient.

SCP: Medial aspect of the inferior angle of the scapula.

CH: With your caudal hand, establish a pisiform–hypothenar contact on the medial aspect of the inferior angle of the scapula, with the fingers pointing toward the axilla.

IH: With your cephalad hand, grasp the spine of the scapula.

VEC: Rotational.

P: Use both hands to create a rotational, twisting action using an impulse-type thrust to drive the inferior angle medial to lateral.

THE ELBOW

Though outwardly, the elbow appears to be a simple singular joint, it is actually an intricate mechanism that depends on the integrated action of three bones, forming three distinct articulations. This peripheral three-joint complex must work together to enable the movements of flexion and extension, as well as pronation and supination of the forearm and hand. Performance of the unique manual skills of the upper extremity depends largely on the proper functioning of the bones, ligaments, and muscles around the elbow joint.

Functional Anatomy

Osseous Structures

The cylindric shaft of the humerus becomes flattened and spreads out distally to form the medial and lateral epicondyles. The distal end of the humerus contains two articular surfaces; the trochlea, which resembles an hourglass on its side, and the capitulum, which is spherical (Fig. 6-77). The radial fossa and coronoid fossa on the anterior surface and the olecranon fossa on the posterior surface serve to allow an increased range of flexion and extension by delaying impact of the respective bony prominences on the humeral shaft.[9] The proximal end of the ulna contains the coronoid process and olecranon process with the trochlear notch lying between. This surface of the ulna articulates with the trochlea of the humerus. The trochlear articular surface is asymmetric, which directs the ulna, and hence the forearm, into an abducted position on full extension. The forearm will form

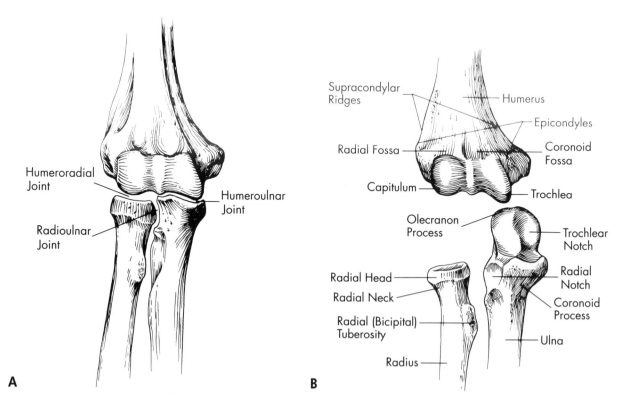

A   **B**

Figure 6.77 Anterior view of the right elbow. **(A)** The three joints. **(B)** The osseous structures.

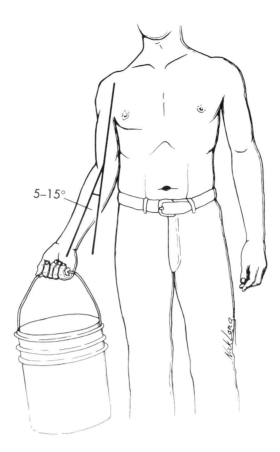

5–15°

Figure 6.78 The carrying angle, a valgus angle ranging from 5 to 15 degrees.

an angle with the arm ranging from 5 to 15 degrees, which is commonly referred to as *the carrying angle* (Fig. 6-78).

The superior surfce of the radial head is concave to accept the spherical capitulum. The radial or bicipital tuberosity protrudes anteromedially just distal to the head of the radius.

Ligamentous Structures

Beside the joint capsule that encloses the three-joint complex (humeroulnar joint, radiohumeral joint and radioulnar joint), three primary ligaments stabilize the elbow. The annular ligament encircles the head of the radius and maintains its contact with the ulna. It is lined with articular cartilage so that the radial head has an articular surface with the ulna, humerus, and annular ligament (Fig. 6-79). The medial and lateral collateral ligaments reinforce the joint capsule of the elbow. They restrict medial and lateral angulation and glide of the ulna on the humerus. Each collateral ligament spreads from its respective epicondyle attachment to reinforce the angular ligament anteriorly while providing medial and lateral stability through attachments to the radius and ulna, respectively.

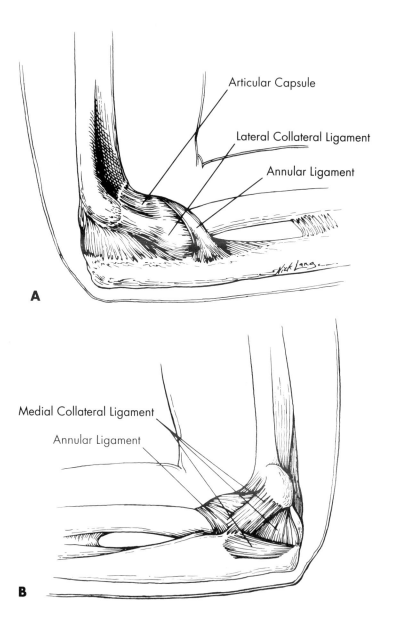

Figure 6.79 The ligaments of the elbow. (A) Lateral view. (B) Medial view.

Musculature

Several significant muscle groups cross the elbow joint and, therefore, serve as predominant stabilizers of the elbow (Table 6-10). The wrist flexors cross the elbow to attach at the medial epicondyle, and the wrist extensors cross the elbow to attach to the lateral epicondyle. Tendons from both of these muscles blend into the fibers of their respective collateral ligaments. Although these muscles cross the elbow joint, their primary function is wrist movement. Elbow flexion is accomplished by the brachialis, brachioradialus, and biceps brachii muscles. Extension of the elbow occurs through the action on only one muscle, the triceps brachii, though the anconeus is thought to

Table 6.10 Actions of the Muscles of the Elbow

Action	Muscles
Flexion	Brachialis
Flexion in supination	Biceps
Rapid flexion or flexion with loads	Brachioradialis
Extension	Triceps, anconeus
Supination	Supinator, biceps
Pronation	Pronator quadratus
Rapid promation or pronation with loads	Pronator teres
Medial stability and some extension	Wrist flexors
Lateral stability and some flexion	Wrist extensors

provide some extension. Supination of the forearm is produced by the contraction of the supinator and, to a lesser degree, the biceps. The pronator quadratus and pronator teres muscles provide the contractive force for the pronation of the forearm.

The olecranon bursa lies between the skin and the olecranon process to reduce friction between the large bony process and the skin (Fig. 6-80). A bicipitoradial bursa lies between the tendon of the biceps muscle and the radius.

Biomechanics

The elbow joint is a modified hinge, classified as a compound paracondylar joint in that one bone, the humerus, articulates with two others that lie side by side, by way of two distinct facets.[11] Flexion and extension movements occur between the trochlea of the humerus and the trochlear notch of the ulna. Within a single joint cavity lie the hinged (ginglymus) humeroulnar articulation, the gliding (plane) humeroradial articulation, and the pivotal

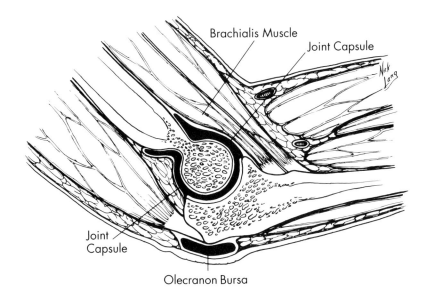

Figure 6.80 Sagittal section through the elbow showing the olecranon bursa.

Brachialis Muscle

Joint Capsule

Joint Capsule

Olecranon Bursa

Table 6.11 Arthrokinematic and Osteokinematic Movements of the Elbow Joints

Osteokinematic Movements (Degrees)		Arthrokinematic Movements
Flexion	135–165	Roll and glide
Extension	0–5	Roll and glide
Supination	90	Rotation and glide
Pronation	90	Rotation and glide

(trochoid) superior radioulnar articulation.[8] Table 6-11 shows the normal ranges of motion for the elbow joint.

Flexion and extension movements occur around an axis that passes through the centers of arcs described by the trochler sulcus and the capitulum, permitting 145 degrees active and 160 degrees passive movement from full extension to flexion (Fig. 6-81). Extension with supination is the closed packed position for the humeroulnar joint, whereas the closed packed position for the humeroradial joint is at 90 degrees of flexion with 5 degrees of supination. For the elbow to move from extension to flexion, the radius and ulna must undergo roll and glide movements in relation to the capitullum and the trochlea, respectively. Active flexion is limited by compression of the soft tissues in the anterior aspect of the forearm and arm, with passive flexion being limited by the tension of the posterior joint capsule and tension in the triceps. Extension is limited by contact of the olecranon process in the olecranon fossa.

The anatomic and mechanical arrangement of the superior radioulnar joint accounts for the uniqueness of this joint but also adds difficulty to its treatment. Eighty percent of the articular surface is composed of a fibro-osseous ring that is part of the annular ligament as opposed to true articular cartilage.

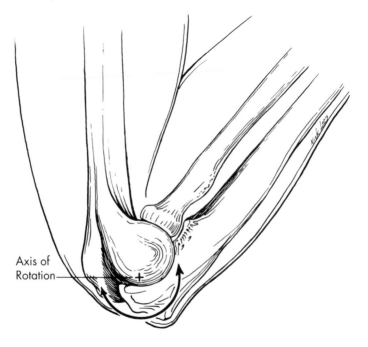

Axis of Rotation

Figure 6.81 Flexion of the elbow.

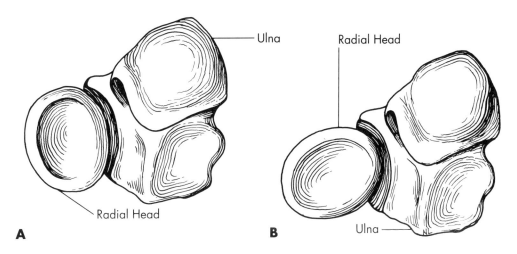

Figure 6.82 Transverse section through the proximal radioulnar articulation. **(A)** Pronation. **(B)** Supination.

The mechanical axis for forearm pronation and supination movements is a line passing from the center of the radial head to near the styloid process of the ulna distally. Normally, between 175 and 180 degrees of movement occur from pronation to supination. This motion is primarily the function of the humeroradial joint and the proximal radioulnar joint (Fig. 6-82).

As mentioned, when the arm is extended in its anatomic position, the longitudinal axis of the arm and forearm forms a lateral (valgus) angle at the elbow known as *the carrying angle.* The normal carrying angle measures approximately 5 degrees in men and between 10 and 15 degrees in women. An increased angulation can be caused by epiphyseal damage secondary to lateral epicondylar fracture and may cause a delayed nerve palsy, which presents as an ulnar nerve distribution in the hand. A decrease in the carrying angle, called *a gunstock deformity,* is often the result of trauma such as a supracondylar fracture in childhood.

Arthrokinematics of the elbow are dictated by the spiral shape of the articular surface of the trochlea. Flexion and extension movements are impure swing movements that couple adduction with flexion and abduction with extension. The close-packed and loose-packed positions for the elbow joints are identified in Table 6-12.

Table 6.12 Close-Packed and Loose-Packed (Rest) Positions for the Elbow Joints

Articulation	Close-Packed Position	Loose-Packed Position
Humeroulnar	Full extension in supination	70 Degrees of flexion with 10 degrees of supination
Humeroradial	90 Degrees of flexion with 5 degrees of supination	Full extension and supination
Proximal radioulnar	5 Degrees of supination	35 Degrees of supination with 70 degrees of flexion

Evaluation

The elbow is exposed to numerous traumatic events that can lead to joint injury and dysfunction. A common cause of elbow problems is a result of muscle activity across the joint. Lateral epicondylitis results from such activity of the wrist extensors. The extensor mass, and especially the deeply located extensor carpi radialus, rubs and rolls over the lateral epicondyle and radial head during forced contraction of the muscle. The forced contractions of the muscle group produce tugs on the origin, resulting in microtears in the tendon and a pulling away of the periosteum. This, coupled with the irritation of soft tissue rubbing over bony prominences, results in a painful elbow condition. Typically, a pain pattern extending down the forearm, following the extensor muscle group, and point tenderness over the lateral epicondyle both occur. The pain will be intensified by resisted extension of the wrist and fingers as well as by shaking hands. The pain may progress to the point that the patient has difficulty picking up a coffee cup or turning a door knob. The action of the back hand stroke in tennis has been a frequent cause, hence the name *tennis elbow*.

Medial epicondylitis occurs as a result of forced muscle activity of the wrist flexors. The clinical picture is much the same as for lateral epicondylitis, but the pain is medial and follows the wrist flexors. It has been referred to as *golfer's elbow*, being associated with forced flexion during a golf swing.

Subluxation of the radial head can occur in a young person who is forcibly pulled up from the floor by grabbing the wrist. This action creates a traction on the annular ligament on one side by the pull of the arm and on the other side by the pull of the body. This condition, *pulled elbow*, or *nursemaid's elbow*, results in a limitation of supination with tenderness over the radial head. The patient's arm will usually hang limp at the side, the hand in pronation, and the patient refuses to move it.

Trauma to the posterior aspect of the elbow, either by a fall on the flexed elbow or by recurrent irritation, can lead to inflammation of the olecranon bursa. Swelling will be visible and palpable and will result in pain on palpation and movement. Olecranon bursitis is frequently seen in individuals, such as students, who lean on their elbows on a hard surface for long periods of time. The ligamentous stability of the elbow can be breached, causing an elbow sprain in hyperextension, hyperabduction, and hyperadduction.

The ulnar nerve is vulnerable to trauma as it passes through the ulnar groove at the medial aspect of the elbow. It can be contused by a direct blow, stretched by a valgus force to the elbow, trapped in scar tissue following trauma to the elbow, and irritated by bone spurs. Any or all of these processes can create a peripheral entrapment of the ulnar nerve known as *cubital tunnel syndrome*. Elbow pain may or may not be associated with this problem. The cardinal symptoms of ulnar nerve injury are tingling and burning of the little finger and ulnar half of the ring finger. Motor function of the opponens digiti minimi and interosseous muscles also may be impaired.

The effective treatment and management of patients with elbow problems obviously depends on first establishing the nature and extent of the lesion, being aware of which anatomic structures have been potentially injured. The elbow is largely derived from C6 and C7 and may, therefore, be a site

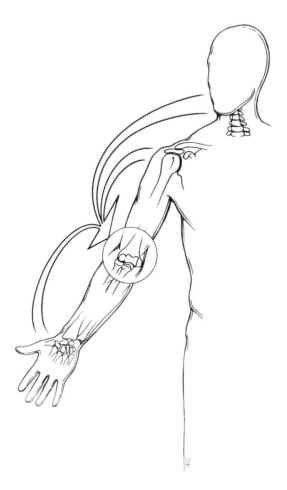

Figure 6.83 The elbow may be the site of referred pain as well as the source of referral.

of referred pain, as well as a source for referral of pain to other structures from these segments (Fig. 6-83).

To begin the evaluation of the elbow, observe the elbow for evidence of swelling, symmetry of contours, posture, and attitude. Also note functional use of the arm during gait, changing positions, and other activities. Evaluate the carrying angle by having the patient straighten his supinated elbows (anatomic position), and measure the angle from the junction of the longitudinal axis of the upper arm and forearm.

Identify osseous symmetry and pain production through static palpation of the radial head, medial epicondyle, lateral epicondyle, olecranon process, and fossa. Structural integrity of the elbow joint can be evaluated through the relationship of the olecranon process to the humeral epicondyles. With the elbow extended and viewed from posterior, the three landmarks should lie in a horizontal line. Then flex the elbow to 90 degrees; the three landmarks should form an isosceles triangle with the apex pointing down (Figs. 6-84 and 6-85). Any appreciable deviation from this alignment may indicate some anatomic problem and requires further investigation.[12]

Identify tone, texture, and tenderness changes through soft tissue palpa-

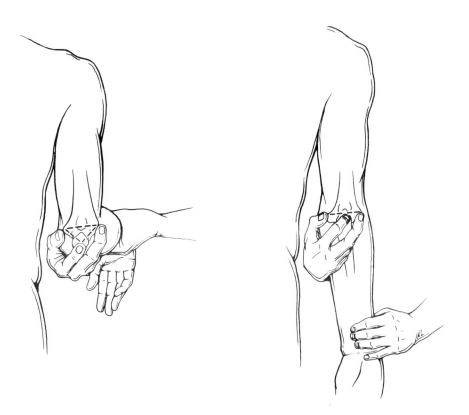

Figure 6.84 Palpational relationship between the epicondyles and olecranon process in a normal elbow.

tion of the olecranon bursa, the collateral ligaments, annular ligament, ulnar nerve, wrist flexor muscle group, wrist extensor muscle group, triceps, brachial radialus, and biceps.

Evaluate accessory joint motions for the elbow articulations (Table 6-13) to determine the presence of joint dysfunction.

Figure 6.85 Palptional relationship between the epicondyles and olecranon process. (A) Flexion. (B) Extension.

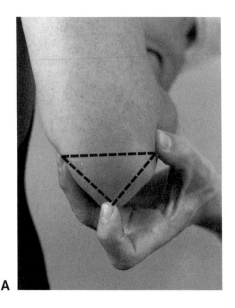

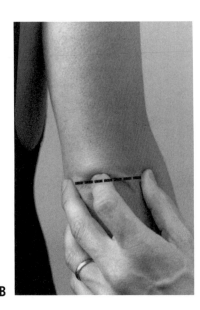

A   B

Table 6.13 Accessory Joint Movements of the Elbow Joint

Long axis distraction
Medial to lateral glide
Lateral to medial glide
Posterior to anterior glide in extension
Anterior to posterior glide—radioulnar joint
Posterior to anterior glide—radioulnar joint
Posterior to anterior glide—radioulnar joint in pronation

Assess long axis distraction, primarily of the humeroulnar joint, with the patient sitting or supine with his elbow bent slightly. Stand to the side of involvement, facing the patient, and use your inside hand to stabilize the humerus while your outside hand grasps the distal forearm. Then stress the forearm along its long axis, feeling for a springing end feel (Fig. 6-86).

Evaluate medial to lateral glide of the humeroradial and humeroulnar joints with the patient seated, the affected arm extended at the elbow and flexed at the shoulder. Stand facing the patient on the medial side of the affected arm. Stabilize the patient's arm against your body by your outer arm while your inside hand takes a calcaneal contact over the medial aspect of the elbow joint. With the forearm stabilized, stress the elbow, medial to lateral, assessing for the presence of a springing joint play movement (Fig. 6-87).

Assess lateral to medial glide of the humeroradial and humeroulnar joint with the patient in a seated position, the affected arm extended at the elbow and flexed at the shoulder. Stand facing the patient on the lateral aspect of the affected arm. Stabilize the patient's forearm using the inside arm to hold the patient's arm against your body. Your outside arm takes a calcaneal contact over the lateral aspect of the elbow joint. With the patient's forearm stabilized against your body, stress the elbow, lateral to medial, determining the presence of a springing joint play movement (Fig. 6-88).

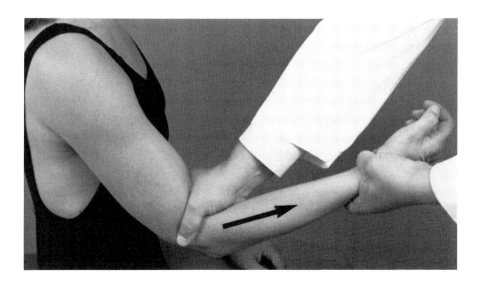

Figure 6.86 Assessment of long axis distraction of the humeroulnar joint.

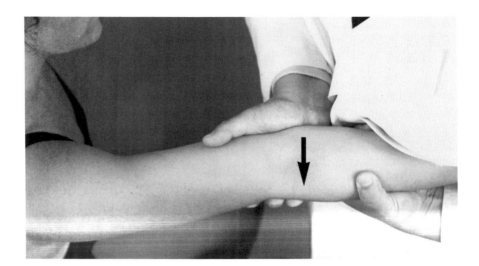

Figure 6.87 Assessment of medial to lateral glide of the humeroulnar joint.

Evaluate posterior to anterior glide of the humeroulnar joint in extension with the patient sitting with the affected arm extended at the elbow and flexed at the shoulder. Stand facing the patient on the lateral side of the affected arm. Form a ring with your thumb and index finger of your outside hand and place it over the posterior aspect of the olecranon process. Rest your other hand on the anterior aspect of the distal forearm. With very little downward pressure on the distal forearm, apply a gentle posterior to

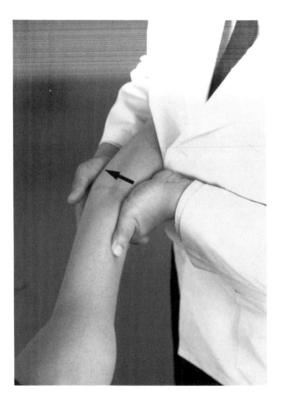

Figure 6.88 Assessment of lateral to medial glide of the humeroulnar joint.

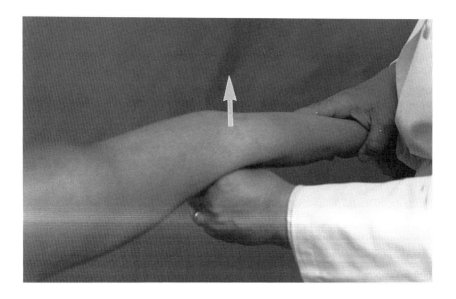

Figure 6.89 Assessment of posterior to anterior glide of the humeroulnar joint.

anterior stress to the olecranon process, looking for a springing joint play movement (Fig. 6-89).

Assess anterior to posterior and posterior to anterior glide of the radioulnar joint with the patient in the seated position, the affected arm extended at the elbow and flexed at the shoulder. Stand facing the patient on the lateral aspect of the affected arm. With your inside arm, stabilize the patient's forearm against your body and grasp the distal humerus and proximal ulna. With your outside hand, hold the radial head between the thumb and index finger. While stabilizing the ulna and humerus, stress the radial head, anterior to posterior and posterior to anterior, determining the presence of a springing joint play movement (Fig. 6-90).

Evaluate posterior to anterior glide of the radioulnar joint in pronation with the patient in the seated position, the affected arm extended at the

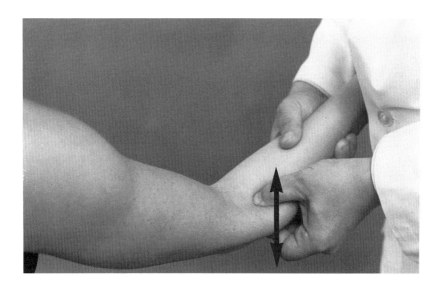

Figure 6.90 Assessment of anterior to posterior and posterior to anterior glide of the radioulnar joint.

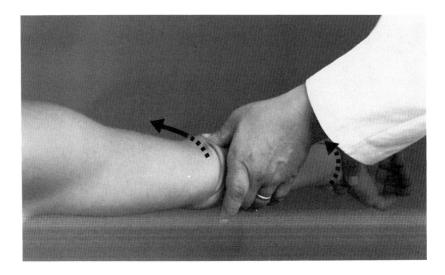

Figure 6.91 Assessment for posterior to anterior glide in pronation of the radial head.

elbow and flexed at the shoulder. Stand facing the lateral aspect of the affected arm. With your outside hand, grasp the distal forearm with digital contacts of the index, middle, and ring finger on the posterior aspect of the radius. With your inside hand, place a thumb contact on the posterior aspect of the radial head. Use your outside hand to pronate the forearm. At the contact over the radial head, you should first perceive a rotational movement of the radial head, and at the end point of movement, apply a posterior to anterior stress to the radial head to determine the presence of a springing end-feel movement (Fig. 6-91).

Adjustive Techniques

Long axis distraction—sitting (Fig. 6-92)

IND: Vague pain around the elbow, compressive injury to the elbow such as caused by a fall on an outstretched arm, and loss of joint separation in the long axis.

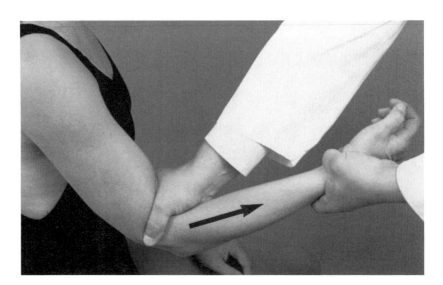

Figure 6.92 Adjustment for long axis distraction of the humeroradial joint in the seated position.

PP: The patient sits with the affected arm in slight elbow flexion.

DP: Stand facing the patient.

SCP: Proximal forearm.

CP: Grasp the patient's proximal forearm with your inside hand.

IH: Apply a web contact over the distal humerus with your outside hand.

VEC: Long axis of the forearm.

P: With your distal hand, stabilize the humerus while your contact hand delivers an impulse-type thrust in the long axis of the forearm. This procedure can also be used to mobilize the elbow by applying sustained traction followed by pronation and supination movements.

Long axis distraction—supine (Fig. 6-93)

IND: Vague pain around the elbow, compressive injury to the elbow such as caused by a fall on an outstretched arm, and loss of joint separation in the long axis.

PP: The patient is supine with the affected arm slightly abducted.

DP: Stand on the affected side, facing headward, and straddle the patient's forearm, such that your knees can grasp the patient's distal forearm.

SCP: Distal humerus.

CP: Use both hands to grasp the patient's distal humerus.

VEC: Long axis of forearm.

P: Use both hands to stabilize the humerus and then straighten both knees to create long axis distraction at the elbow.

Medial to lateral glide—sitting (Fig. 6-94)

IND: Medial elbow joint capsule or collateral ligament pain, lateral epicondylar pain, ulnar nerve paresthesia, olecranon process displaced toward the medial epicondyle, and loss of medial to lateral accessory joint movement.

PP: The patient sits with the affected arm flexed at the shoulder.

DP: Stand facing the patient and on the medial aspect of the patient's affected arm.

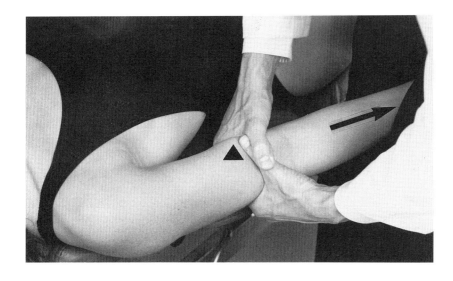

Figure 6.93 Adjustment for long axis distraction of the humeroradial joint in the supine position.

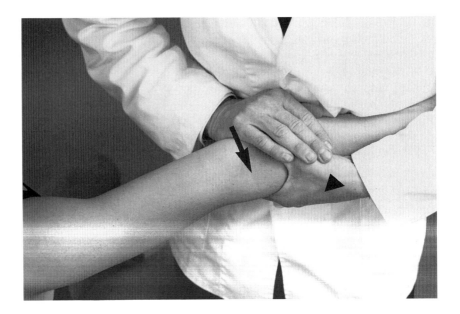

Figure 6.94 Adjustment for medial to lateral glide of the elbow in the seated position.

SCP: Medial aspect of the proximal ulna.

CP: With your inside hand, establish a calcaneal contact over the medial aspect of the proximal ulna, just distal to the medial aspect of the elbow joint space. The fingers will rest in the anticubital fossa and over the proximal anterior forearm.

IH: With your outside hand, contact the lateral aspect of the forearm so that your arm can stabilize the patient's forearm against your body.

VEC: Medial to lateral.

P: As your indifferent hand stabilizes the forearm, drawing it into slight distraction and elbow extension, induce an impulse thrust medial to lateral with your contact hand.

Medial to lateral glide—supine (Fig. 6-95)

IND: Medial elbow joint capsule or collateral ligament pain, lateral epicondylar pain, ulnar nerve paresthesia, olecranon process displaced toward the medial epicondyle, and loss of medial to lateral accessory joint movement.

PP: The patient is supine with the affected arm abducted slightly.

DP: Stand at the side of the table facing headward and straddling the patient's affected arm such that your knees can grasp the patient's distal forearm.

SCP: Lateral aspect of the proximal ulna.

CP: Use your inside hand to apply a web contact over the lateral aspect of the proximal ulna just distal to the medial elbow joint space. Wrap your fingers around the posterior aspect of the elbow with the thumb in the anticubital fossa.

IH: With your outside hand, grasp the lateral aspect of the forearm, distal to the other contact.

VEC: Medial to lateral.

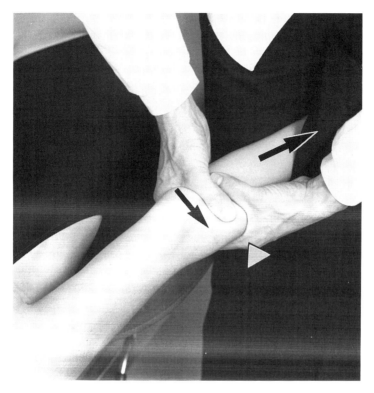

Figure 6.95 Adjustment for medial to lateral glide of the elbow in the supine position.

P: Straighten your knees to create distraction at the elbow joint, simultaneously applying a medial to lateral thrust with your contact hand as you supply an opposite vector with your indifferent hand.

Lateral to medial glide—sitting (Fig. 6-96)

IND: Lateral elbow joint capsule or collateral ligament pain, medial epicondylar pain, olecranon process displaced toward the lateral epicondyle, and loss of lateral to medial accessory joint motion.

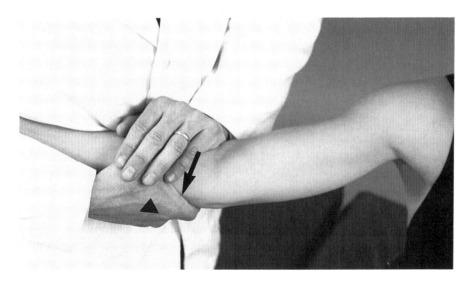

Figure 6.96 Adjustment for lateral to medial glide of the elbow in the seated position.

PP: The patient sits with the affected arm flexed at the shoulder.

DP: Stand facing the patient on the lateral side of the patient's affected arm.

SCP: Lateral aspect of the elbow joint and proximal radius.

CP: With your outer hand, establish a calcaneal contact over the radial head and lateral aspect of the elbow joint.

IH: With your inner hand, grasp the patient's proximal forearm so that the patient's forearm is held against your body.

VEC: Lateral to medial.

P: With your indifferent hand and body, stabilize the forearm and apply a slight distractive force while delivering an impulse thrust in a lateral to medial direction with your contact hand.

Lateral to medial glide—supine (Fig. 6-97)

IND: Lateral elbow joint capsule or collateral ligament pain, medial epicondylar pain, olecranon process displaced toward the lateral epicondyle, and loss of lateral to medial accessory joint motion.

PP: The patient is supine with the affected arm abducted slightly at the shoulder.

DP: Stand facing headward, straddling the patient's affected arm such that your knees can squeeze the distal forearm.

SCP: Lateral aspect of the elbow joint and proximal radius.

CP: Using your outside hand, apply a web contact over the lateral aspect of the proximal radius just distal to the lateral elbow joint space. Wrap your fingers around the posterior aspect of the elbow with the thumb in the anticubital fossa.

IH: With your inside hand, grasp the medial aspect of the forearm, distal to the other contact.

VEC: Lateral to medial.

P: Straighten your knees to create distraction at the elbow joint, simulta-

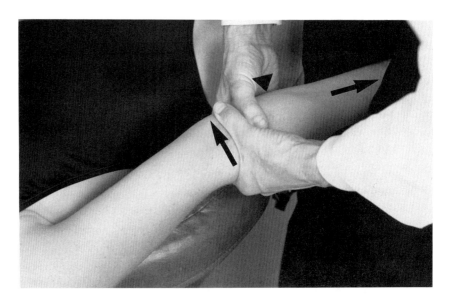

Figure 6.97 Adjustment for lateral to medial glide of the elbow in the supine position.

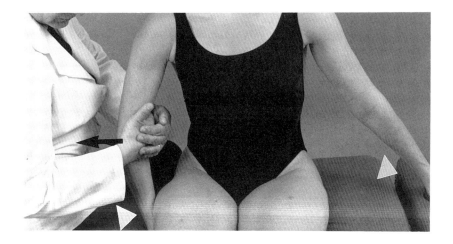

Figure 6.98 Adjustment for anterior to posterior glide of the radial head.

neously applying a lateral to medial thrust with your contact hand as you supply an opposite vector with your indifferent hand.

Anterior to posterior glide—radial head (Fig. 6-98)

IND: Lateral elbow pain, pain on pronation and supination, and decreased anterior to posterior glide of the radial head.

 PP: The patient sits on a chair or on the edge of an adjusting table, sitting on the palmar aspect of the hand on the affected side.

 DP: Either straddle the table facing the patient on the affected side, or squat next to the patient seated on a chair.

SCP: Anterior aspect of the radial head.

 CP: Using your forward hand, establish a pisiform–hypothenar contact on the anterior aspect of the radial head.

 IH: Reinforce your contact hand with your posterior hand.

VEC: Anterior to posterior.

  P: The patient's body weight on the patient's hand stabilizes the upper extremity, while the doctor delivers an impulse thrust with both hands, anterior to posterior, to the radial head.

Posterior to anterior glide of the radial head in pronation (Fig. 6-99)

IND: Pain at the radial head, lateral elbow joint pain, lateral epicondylar pain, and loss of posterior to anterior accessory joint movement of the radial head in pronation.

 PP: The patient sits with the affected arm flexed at the elbow and pronated.

 DP: Stand on the affected side of the patient.

SCP: Posterior aspect of the radial head.

 CP: Use your proximal hand to apply a thumb contact on the posterior aspect of the radial head with your fingers lying across the posterior aspect of the elbow.

 IH: Grasp the patient's distal forearm with a digital contact of all fingers on the posterior aspect of the radius.

VEC: Posterior to anterior.

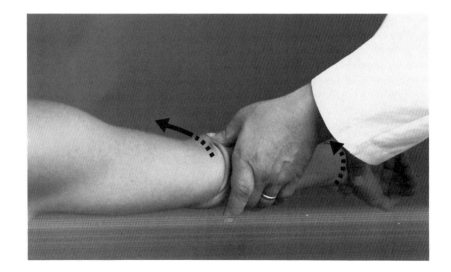

Figure 6.99 Adjustment for posterior to anterior glide in pronation of the radial head.

P: Use your indifferent hand to move the elbow from a flexed and supinated position to an extended and pronated position. Repeat this procedure several times so that the patient will relax the elbow. When the patient's elbow is fully extended and fully pronated, deliver a very shallow but quick impulse thrust, in a posterior to anterior direction against the radial head, with your contact hand.

Anterior to posterior glide—ulna (Fig. 6-100)

IND: Elbow pain, painful flexion and extension, hyperextension trauma to the elbow, and decreased anterior to posterior movement of the ulnohumeral joint.

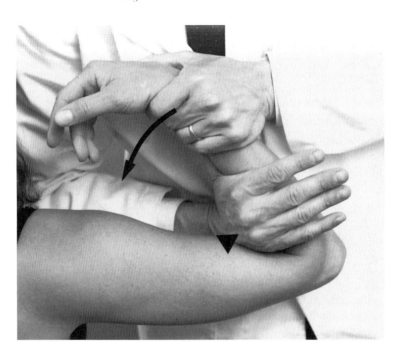

Figure 6.100 Adjustment for anterior to posterior glide of the ulna.

PP: The patient sits with the affected arm flexed at the shoulder and flexed at the elbow.

DP: Stand facing the patient.

SCP: Proximal ulna.

CP: With your inside hand, establish a knife-edge contact over the proximal ulna in the anticubital fossa.

IH: Grasp the proximal forearm with your outer hand.

VEC: Anterior to posterior.

P: Using your indifferent hand, flex the patient's elbow over your contact hand until articular slack is removed. Accomplish the thrust with your indifferent hand moving the forearm toward the patient's shoulder while your contact hand delivers an anterior to posterior thrust over the proximal ulna.

Posterior to anterior glide—radial head (Fig. 6-101)

IND: Pain at the radial head, lateral elbow joint pain, lateral epicondylar pain, and loss of posterior to anterior accessory joint movement of the radial head.

PP: The patient sits on a chair or on the edge of an adjusting table, sitting on the palmar aspect of the hand on the affected side.

DP: Either straddle the table facing the patient on the affected side, or squat next to the patient seated on a chair.

SCP: Posterior aspect of the radial head.

CP: With your forward hand, establish a pisiform–hypothenar contact on the posterior aspect of the radial head.

IH: Grasp the proximal ulna with your posterior hand.

VEC: Posterior to anterior.

P: The patient's body weight on the patient's hand stabilizes the upper extremity. While your indifferent hand stabilizes the ulna, deliver

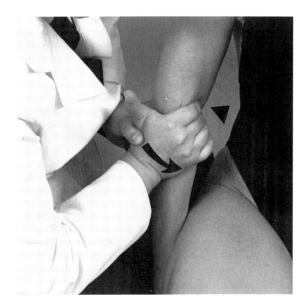

Figure 6.101 Adjustment for posterior to anterior glide of the radial head.

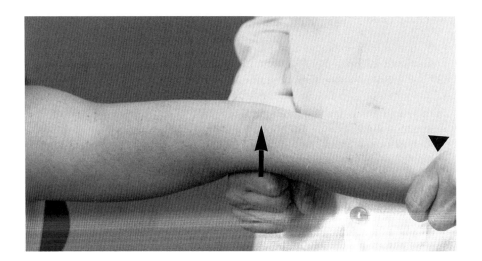

Figure 6.102 Adjustment for posterior to anterior glide of the ulna in extension.

an impulse thrust, posterior to anterior to the radial head, with the contact hand.

Posterior to anterior glide—ulna, full extension (Fig. 6-102)

IND: Elbow pain, loss of full extension, and loss of posterior to anterior glide of the humeroulnar joint.

PP: The patient sits with the affected arm extended at the elbow and flexed at the shoulder.

DP: Stand facing the patient on the lateral side of the affected arm.

SCP: The olecranon process.

CP: Form a ring with thumb and index finger of your outside hand, and place it over the posterior aspect of the olecranon process.

IH: Rest your other hand on the anterior aspect of the distal forearm.

VEC: Posterior to anterior.

P: With very little downward pressure on the distal forearm, apply a gentle posterior to anterior stress to the olecranon process, finishing with a very shallow impulse thrust.

WRIST AND HAND

An intricate interaction of numerous structures in the wrist and hand is necessary to produce the remarkable dexterity and precision that characterize this joint complex.[8] The entire upper limb is apparently subservient to the hand in its use as a means of expression, a tactile organ, and a weapon. The study of the hand is inseparable from that of the wrist and the forearm, which function as a single physiologic unit, with the wrist being the key joint.[1] By far the most important musculoskeletal function of the hand is its ability to grasp objects. Because the hand is the main manipulative organ of the body, performing many different types of functions, it should not be overlooked in the evaluation for dysfunction.

Functional Anatomy

Osseous Structures

Interestingly, although the ulna plays a highly significant role in the function of the elbow, it is secondary in the wrist; whereas the radius, having a secondary role in the elbow, has a dominant part in the wrist. The radius flares to become much larger at the distal end, terminating with a lateral extension, the radial styloid process. The distal end of the ulna also ends in a styloid process, but it is much smaller in comparison to the radial styloid. The distal aspects of the radius and ulna form an articulation with the proximal row of carpal bones, directly, in the radius, and indirectly, via an intracapsular disc in the ulna. The eight carpal bones that make up the wrist are arranged in two rows and greatly enhance the hand's mobility. The proximal row, from medial to lateral, consists of the scaphoid, lunate, triquetrum, and pisiform. The pisiform overlies the triquetrum, which forms an articulation with the proximal ulna via the interarticular disc. The scaphoid and lunate articulate directly with the radius. The distal row of carpals, from lateral to medial, consists of the trapezium, trapezoid, capitate, and hamate. The proximal and distal rows of carpal bones collectively form an intercarpal joint, though some movement also occurs between the individual carpal bones (Fig. 6-103).

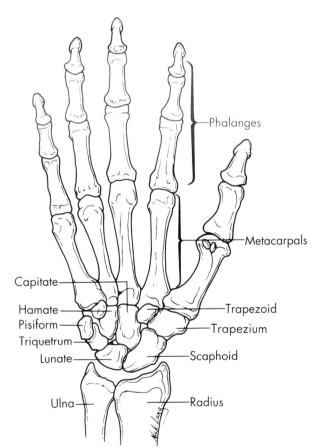

Figure 6.103 Palmar view of the osseous structures of the wrist and hand.

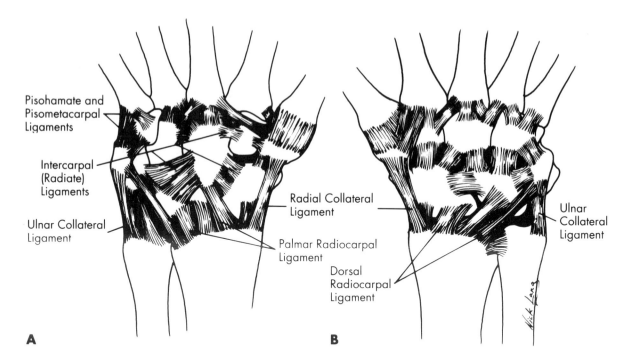

Figure 6.104 The ligaments of the wrist. **(A)** Palmar view. **(B)** Dorsal view. (Modified from Hertling and Kessler,[1] with permission.)

The base of each of the five metacarpals articulates with the distal row of carpals. Five proximal phalanges articulate with each of the metacarpals, followed by a middle and distal phalanx for each of the fingers and a distal phalanx for the thumb.

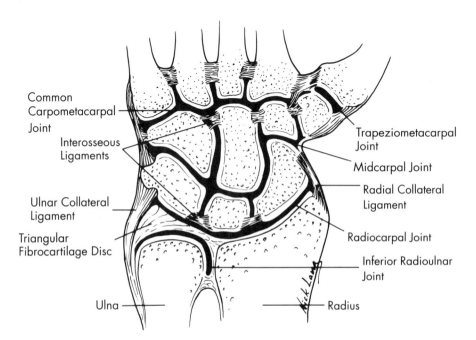

Figure 6.105 Coronal section through right wrist showing intercarpal joints and ligaments.

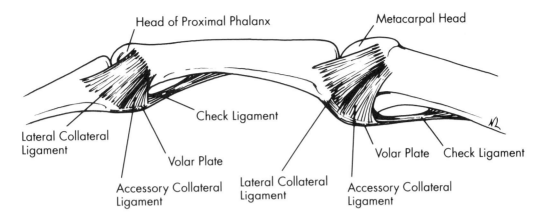

Figure 6.106 Lateral view of the ligaments of the finger.

Ligamentous Structures

The numerous ligaments of the wrist, many of which are unnamed, are not all separate entities. They form a criss-cross pattern of connections between the radius and ulna to the carpals, between the carpals, from the carpals to the metacarpals, and between the metacarpals (Fig. 6-104). The volar radiocarpal and radioulnar carpal ligaments strengthen the joint capsule and wrist anteriorly, while the dorsal radiocarpal ligament provides support posteriorly (Fig. 6-105). Radial collateral and ulnar collateral ligaments stabilize the wrist laterally and medially, respectively. Collateral ligaments also support the metacarpophalangeal and the interphalangeal joints (Fig. 6-106).

Table 6.14 Actions of the Muscles of the Wrist and Hand

Actions	Muscles
Wrist flexion	Flexor carpi radialis, abductor pollicis longus, palmaris longus, flexor pollicis longus, flexor carpi ulnaris, flexor digitorum superficialis and profundus
Wrist extension	Extensor carpi radialis, extensor digitorum, extensor carpi ulnaris, extensor pollicis longus
Wrist adduction (ulnar deviation)	Extensor carpi ulnaris, flexor carpi ulnaris
Wrist abduction (radial deviation)	Extensor carpi radialis, abductor pollicis longus, extensor pollicis longus and brevis
Finger flexion	Flexor digitorum superficialis and profundus
Finger extension	Extensor digitorum, extensor digiti minimi, extensor indicis
Finger abduction	Interosseous muscles

Musculature

Extrinsic and intrinsic muscles function for the wrist and hand (Table 6-14). The wrist flexors and extensors are located in the forearm, attached to the epicondyles of the humerus. As the muscles head distally, their tendons are enclosed in sheaths that offer a smooth environment for sliding. Intrinsic muscles include the interosseous and lumbricales muscles as well as those responsible for the movements of the thumb and little finger. Six passageways transport the extensor tendons through fibro-osseous tunnels. Fibrous bands running from the retinaculum to the carpal bones form the tunnels (Fig. 6-107). The flexor retinaculum spans between the scaphoid, trapezium, hamate, and pisiform. It forms a tunnel out of the carpal arch to allow passage of the median nerve and the flexor tendons (Fig. 6-108).

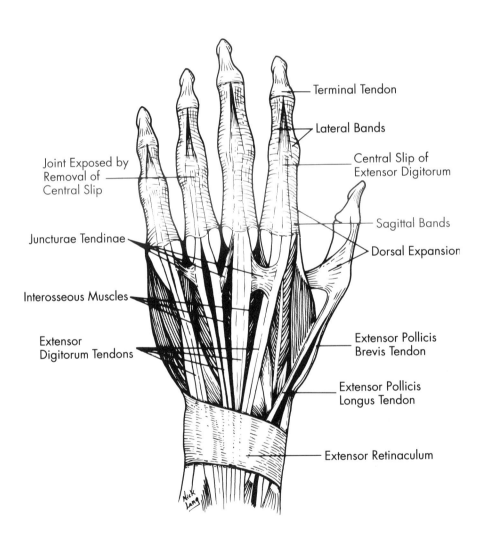

Figure 6.107 Dorsal view of left hand showing location of extensor tendons and dorsal interosseous muscles.

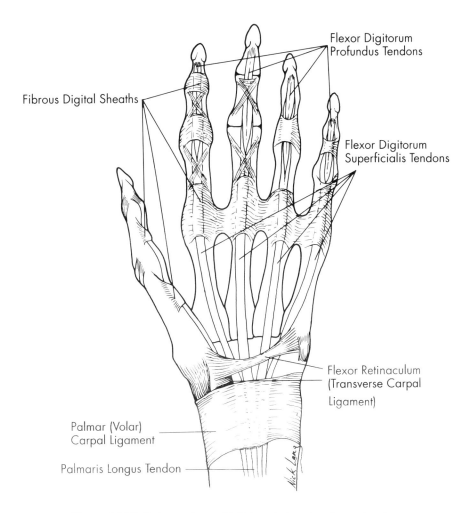

Flexor Digitorum
Profundus Tendons

Fibrous Digital Sheaths

Flexor Digitorum
Superficialis Tendons

Flexor Retinaculum
(Transverse Carpal
Ligament)

Palmar (Volar)
Carpal Ligament

Palmaris Longus Tendon

Figure 6.108 Palmar view of left hand showing flexor tendons.

Biomechanics

The complex movements of the wrist are accomplished by the distal radioulnar joint, the radiocarpal joint, and the midcarpal joint. The radiocarpal and midcarpal joint produce the motion at the wrist joint. Wrist flexion and extension as well as radial and ulnar deviation are thought to occur around an axis of movement that passes through the capitate (Fig. 6-109). However, the multiplicity of wrist articulations and the complexity of joint motion make it difficult to calculate the precise instantaneous axis of motion.[10] The close-packed position for the wrist is full extension (Table 6-15). The wrist can undergo approximately 160 degrees of flexion and extension, with extension being slightly greater. Sixty degrees of radial and ulnar deviation are possible, and ulnar deviation is almost twice as great as radial deviation (Fig. 6-110). Radial deviation is limited by contact of the scaphoid against

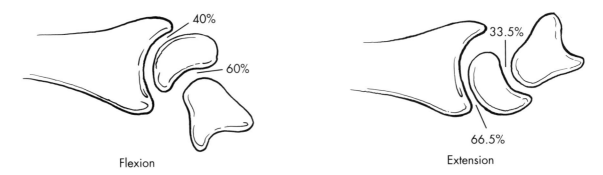

Flexion

Extension

Figure 6.109 Most wrist flexion occurs at the intercarpal joint, while most wrist extension occurs in the radiocarpal joint.

the radial styloid process. Ranges of motion for the wrist and hand are listed in Table 6-16.

With dorsiflexion of the wrist, a supinatory rotation of the carpal bones also occurs, which is due mostly to the scaphoid moving more with respect to the radius while the lunate and triquetrum relate to the ulna. Furthermore, when moving from flexion to dorsiflexion, the distal row of carpals becomes close-packed with respect to the scaphoid first. This results in the scaphoid moving with the distal row into dorsiflexion, necessitating movement between the scaphoid and lunate as full dorsiflexion is approached. With extension of the wrist, the proximal row of carpals rolls and glides anteriorly with respect to the radius and ulna, while the distal row of carpals moves similarly with respect to the proximal row of carpals. The converse is true of wrist flexion; the proximal row moves posteriorly relative to the radius and ulna, as the proximal row moves posteriorly relative to the proximal row of carpals.

Radial and ulnar deviation involve rotary movements between the proximal row of carpals and the radius, as well as between the proximal row and

Figure 6.110 Dorsal view of the right wrist. (A) With ulnar deviation, some extension of proximal carpals occurs. (B) With radial deviation, some flexion of the proximal carpal occurs. TP, trapezium; TZ, trapezoid; C, capitate; H, hamate; TQ, triquetrum; S, scaphoid; L, lunate.

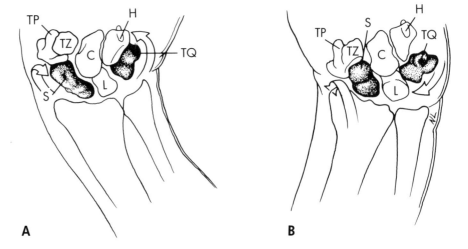

Table 6.15 Close-Packed and Loose-Packed (Rest) Positions for the Wrist and Hand Joints

	Close-Packed Position	Loose-Packed Position
Wrist	Full dorsiflexion	Palmer flexion with slight ulnar deviation
Hand	Full extension	Flexion with slight ulnar deviation

distal row of carpals. Moreover, during radial deviation, the proximal row combines pronation, flexion, and ulnar glide movements with respect to the radius as the distal row combines supination, extension, and ulnar glide movements with respect to the proximal row. Ulnar deviation has the opposite movements.[1,9]

The hand must be able to change its shape to grasp objects. Three physiologic, functional arches running in different directions provide the means for the wrist and hand to conform to a position for grasping (Fig. 6-111). Transversely, an arch through the carpal region corresponds to the concavity of the wrist, and distally the metacarpal arch is formed by the metacarpal heads. Longitudinal arches are formed along each finger by the corresponding metacarpal bone and phalanges. Obliquely, arches are formed by the thumb during opposition with the other fingers. These arches allow coordinating synergistic digital flexion and opposition of the thumb and little finger.

The wrist provides a stable base for the hand, and its position controls the length of the extrinsic muscles to the digits. The muscles stabilize the wrist as well as provide for the fine movements of the hand to place it in its functioning position. The positioning of the wrist has a significant influence

Table 6.16 Arthrokinematic and Osteokinematic Movements of the Wrist and Hand Joints

Osteokinematic Movements (Degrees)		Arthrokinematic Movements
Wrist flexion	80	Roll and glide
Wrist extension	70	Roll and glide
Ulnar deviation	30	Roll and glide
Radial deviation	20	Roll and glide
MCP flexion	90	Roll and glide
MCP extension	30–45	Roll and glide
PIP flexion	100	Roll and glide
PIP extension	0	Roll and glide
DIP flexion	90	Roll and glide
DIP extension	10	Roll and glide
Finger abduction	20	Roll and glide

DIP, distal interphalangeal joint; MCP, metacarpophalangeal joint; PIP, proximal interphalangeal joint.

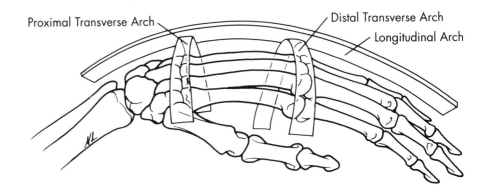

Figure 6.111 The three physiologic arches of the wrist and hand. (Modified from Nordin and Frankel,[10] with permission.)

on the strength of the fingers. For most effective action of the extrinsic muscles of the fingers, the wrist usually must move in a direction opposite the movement of the fingers.

The naturally assumed position of the hand to grasp an object, or the position from which optimal function is most likely to occur, is termed *the functional position* (Fig. 6-112). The functional position occurs when the wrist is extended 20 degrees and ulna deviated 10 degrees, the fingers are flexed at all of their joints, and the thumb is in midrange position with the metacarpophalangeal joint moderately flexed and the interphalangeal joints slightly flexed. Prehensile functions of the hand are unique and fundamental characteristics (Fig. 6-113).

Evaluation

The wrist and hand are prone to injuries from trauma, commonly, a fall on the outstretched hand. The radial side of the wrist and hand tends to take the majority of the force from such a trauma. Displacement, instability, and rotary subluxation of the scaphoid often occur, creating pain on dorsiflexion of the wrist and limited range of motion. Palpable tenderness will be present over the joint space between the scaphoid and the lunate. Occasionally, the scaphoid can be felt slipping as the wrist is moved, or a painful click may be

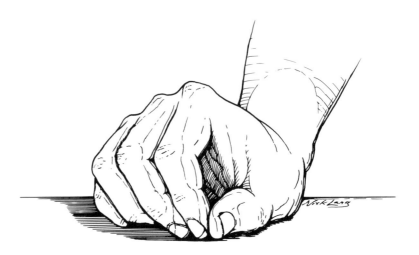

Figure 6.112 The functional position of the hand.

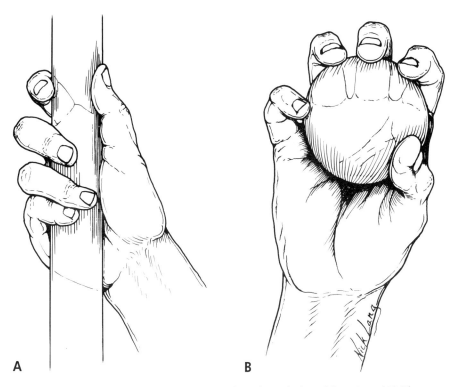

Figure 6.113 The fundamental patterns of prehensile hand function. (**A**) The power grip. (**B**) A precision maneuver.

perceived. A space of more than 3 mm between the scaphoid and lunate may be seen on a closed fist, supinated radiographic view of the wrist.

Trauma to an outstretched hand that is forcefully flexed or extended may cause a fracture to the radius. A Colle's fracture occurs when the wrist is in dorsiflexion and the forearm is in pronation. Local pain and tenderness to palpation and vibration are important physical findings; however, the radiograph is the most important tool for determining the presence of a fracture. Manipulative therapy to this area is then contraindicated.

Singular trauma, such as a fall, or repetitive activities may lead to a sprain to the ligaments of the wrist. Moreover, when the wrist is subjected to sudden increases in work load, such as in gripping or lifting, or racquet games requiring flexion and extension of the wrist, the tendons crossing the wrist can become inflamed, resulting in tendonitis. In addition, a possible response to repeated twisting and straining is a localized, nodular swelling called a *ganglion*. Likely a defense mechanism, the ganglion is characterized by a fibrous outer coat that covers a thick gelatinous fluid derived from the synovium lining the tendon sheaths.

Undoubtedly, the most noted condition affecting the wrist and hand is carpal tunnel syndrome, a peripheral entrapment neuropathy involving the median nerve. The median nerve lies superficial to the flexor tendons beneath the tense transverse carpal ligament (flexor retinaculum), making the carpal tunnel just barely adequate to accommodate these structures. In

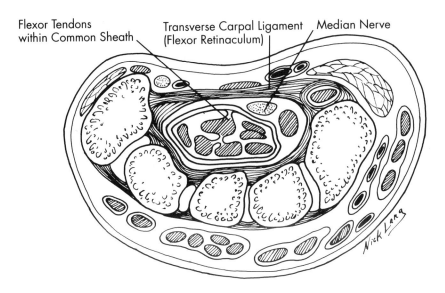

Flexor Tendons within Common Sheath   Transverse Carpal Ligament (Flexor Retinaculum)   Median Nerve

Figure 6.114 Cross-section through the wrist showing the relationship between the carpal bones, tendons, flexor retinaculum, and median nerve.

the act of grasping an object, particularly with the wrist in flexion, the flexor tendons are displaced forward and can compress the nerve against the unyielding ligament. Narrowing of the carpal tunnel can occur through bony deformity after fracture, degenerative joint disease, synovial swelling of a tendon or of the wrist joint ligaments, and thickening of the transverse carpal ligament (Fig. 6-114). Most often, though, no definitive local cause for nerve compression can be detected. Moreover, Upton[13] has identified the possibility that peripheral nerves can be compressed at more than one spot along their course, creating "double-, triple-, and quadruple-crush" syndromes. Therefore, although the patient's clinical picture may be defined as carpal tunnel syndrome, the nerve compression may not necessarily be at the wrist but may be at the elbow, shoulder, and/or neck. This syndrome occurs more often in women, with the common age of onset between 40 and 50. Slight paresthesias may precede the onset of the acute symptoms for several months. Then, paroxysms of pain, paresthesia, and numbness occur in the area of the median nerve distribution. The patient is often awakened at night by pain that can be described as burning, aching, prickly, pins-and-needles, and numbness. Motor weakness of the thumb adductor or opposer may be found. The patient may describe relief from dangling the hand over the side of the bed, shaking the hand vigorously, or rubbing it.

Because the wrist structures are innervated primarily from segments C6 through C8, lesions affecting structures of similar derivation may refer pain to the wrist and vice versa. Symptoms experienced at the wrist and hand must always be suspected as possibly having a more proximal origin (Fig. 6-115).

Observe the wrist and hand for general posture and attitude. In the resting attitude of the hand, the metacarpophalangeal and interphalangeal joints are held in a position of slight flexion. Observe the arm and hand for natural swing when the patient walks. Also note functional activities of the hand and wrist including the firmness of the person's handshake as well as

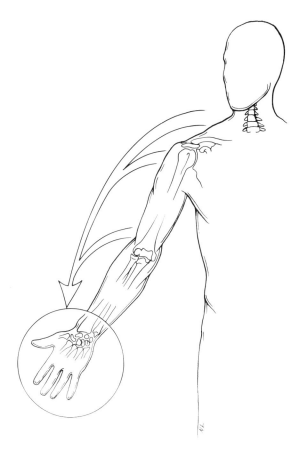

Figure 6.115 Symptoms in the hand and wrist must be suspected of having a more proximal origin.

temperature and moisture of the hand. The dominant hand should be determined. Sometimes this can be done by noting the hand with more developed musculature but is most easily done simply by asking the patient.

To begin the evaluation of the wrist and hand, osseous symmetry, bony relationships, and pain production are identified through static palpation of the wrist and hand (Fig. 6-116). Palpate the radius and ulna distally, identifying each of their styloid processes. Just distal to the radial styloid and in the anatomic snuff box, the scaphoid can be palpated. Wrist flexion will facilitate the palpation of the lunate, which lies next to the scaphoid. The triquetrum and pisiform overlie one another and are just distal to the ulnar styloid. The trapezium can be identified at the base of the first metacarpal. The trapezoid lies at the base of the second metacarpal. The capitate is found between the base of the third metacarpal and the lunate. The hook of the hamate, and hence the hamate, can be found on the palmar surface just distal and to the thumb side of the pisiform. Then palpate the metacarpals through the palm of the hand with the fingers along the shaft of the metacarpal on the palmar surface while the thumb is over the dorsal surface. Finally, palpate the 14 phalanges, 2 for the thumb and 3 for each finger.

Identify tone, texture, and tenderness changes through soft tissue palpation of the flexor and extensor tendons, the thenar eminence, and hypothe-

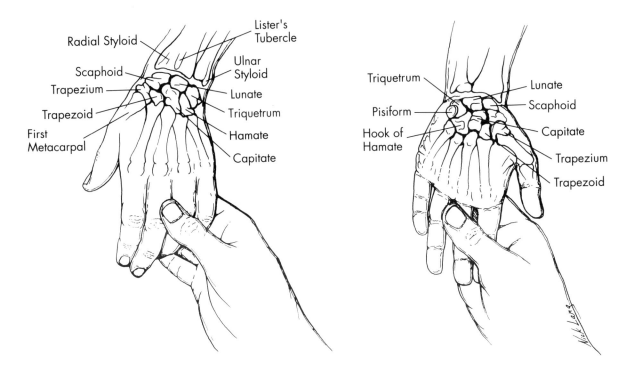

Figure 6.116 Localization of osseous structures of the left wrist.

nar eminence. Determine patency of the radial and ulnar arteries (Allen's test), and take a radial pulse.

Evaluate accessory joint motions for the wrist and hand articulations to determine the presence of joint dysfunction (Table 6-17).

Assess anterior to posterior and posterior to anterior glide of the distal radioulnar joint with the patient supine or sitting. Grasp the distal radius with one hand and the distal ulna with the other. Apply an opposing anterior to posterior and posterior to anterior shearing stress between the radius and ulna (Fig. 6-117).

Conduct medial to lateral compression of the distal radioulnar joint with the patient supine or sitting, and use both hands to encircle the distal radius and ulna. Use both hands to apply a medial to lateral compression stress to the distal radius and ulna (Fig. 6-118).

To evaluate long axis distraction of the intercarpal joint, the patient can be seated or supine. Grasp the distal forearm with one hand and the distal wrist with the other. While stabilizing the forearm, distract the wrist in the long axis (Fig. 6-119).

Perform medial to lateral tilt and glide of the intercarpal joints with the patient seated and the affected arm raised in forward flexion. Stand on the affected side, facing the lateral aspect of the arm. Grasp the distal radius and ulna with your proximal hand, while grasping the patient's distal wrist with your distal hand. Use both hands to create opposing forces, creating a

Table 6.17 Accessory Joint Movements of the Wrist and Hand Joints

Joint	Movement
Distal radioulnar	Anterior to posterior glide Posterior to anterior glide Medial to lateral compression
Intercarpal	Long axis distraction Medial to lateral tilt Medial to lateral glide Anterior to posterior glide Posterior to anterior glide
Individual carpals	Anterior to posterior glide Posterior to anterior glide
Intermetacarpal	Anterior to posterior glide Posterior to anterior glide
Metacarpophalangeal and interphalangeal	Long axis distraction Medial to lateral glide Lateral to medial glide Anterior to posterior glide Posterior to anterior glide Internal rotation External rotation

shearing stress (medial to lateral glide) (Fig. 6-120) and radial and ulnar deviation stress (medial to lateral tilt) (Fig. 6-121).

Assess anterior to posterior and posterior to anterior glide of the intercarpal joint with the patient seated and arm raised in forward flexion. Stand on the affected side. Grasp the distal radius and ulna with your proximal hand while grasping the patient's distal wrist with your distal hand. Using both hands to create opposing forces, stress the intercarpal joints in an

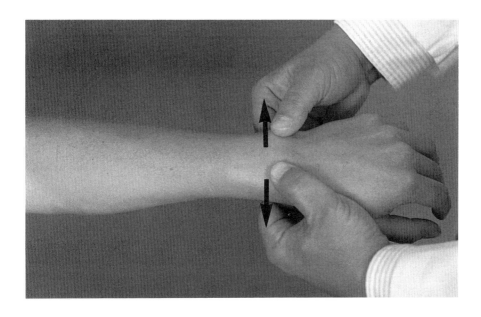

Figure 6.117 Assessment of anterior to posterior and posterior to anterior glide of the distal radioulnar joint.

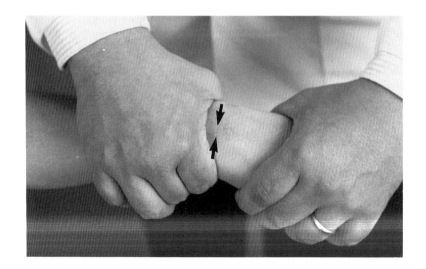

Figure 6.118 Assessment of medial to lateral compression of the distal radioulnar joint.

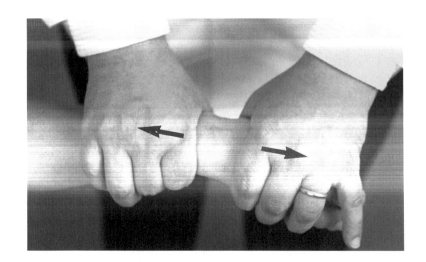

Figure 6.119 Assessment of long axis distraction of the intercarpal joint.

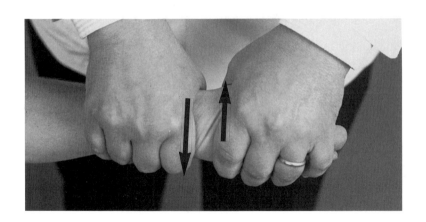

Figure 6.120 Assessment of medial to lateral and lateral to medial glide of the intercarpal joint.

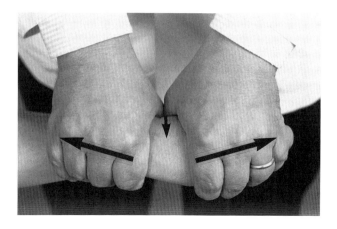

Figure 6.121 Assessment of medial to lateral and lateral to medial tilt of the intercarpal joint.

anterior to posterior and posterior to anterior glide, looking for a springing, joint play movement (Fig. 6-122).

Assess anterior to posterior and posterior to anterior glide of the individual carpal bones with the patient seated and the affected arm raised in forward flexion. Stand facing the patient. Use your thumb and index or middle fingers to contact the anterior and posterior surfaces of the carpal bone to be evaluated, while using your other hand to stabilize the rest of the wrist. Apply an anterior to posterior and posterior to anterior stress to each individual carpal bone, looking for a springing, joint play movement (Fig. 6-123A & B).

Assess anterior to posterior and posterior to anterior glide of the inter-metacarpal joints with the patient seated and the affected arm raised in forward flexion. Stand facing the patient, and grasp the adjacent metacarpals with both hands, stressing them in an anterior to posterior and posterior to anterior glide (Fig. 6-124).

Evaluate the metacarpophalangeal and interphalangeal joints in a similar

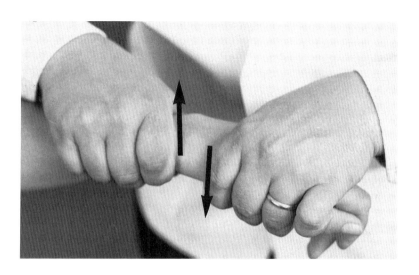

Figure 6.122 Assessment of anterior to posterior and posterior to anterior glide of the intercarpal joint.

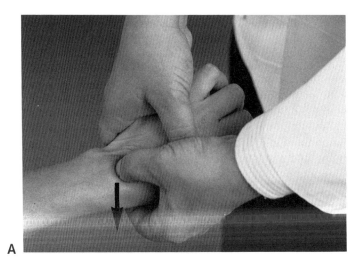

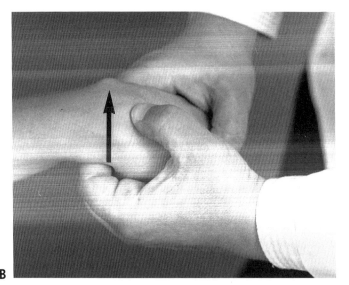

Figure 6.123 Assessment of (**A**) posterior to anterior and (**B**) anterior to posterior glide of the individual carpals.

fashion. With the patient seated, grasp the proximal member of the joint to be tested with one hand while grasping the distal member of the joint being tested with the other hand. Then stress each metacarpophalangeal or interphalangeal joint with long axis distraction, anterior to posterior and posterior to anterior glide, lateral to medial and medial to lateral glide, and internal and external rotation (Figs. 6-125 and 6-126).

Adjustive Techniques

The application of an impulse thrust often can be performed using the accessory joint motion test procedure and adding the impulse thrust at the end. Although this is true of any joint in the body, in the wrist and hand, fewer adjustive procedures are unique or different from the testing procedure.

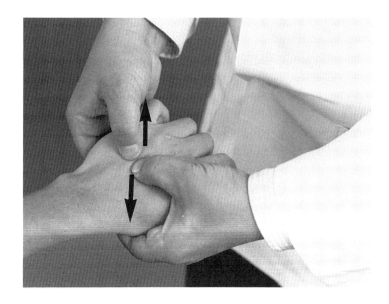

Figure 6.124 Assessment of anterior to posterior and posterior to anterior glide of the intermetacarpal joints.

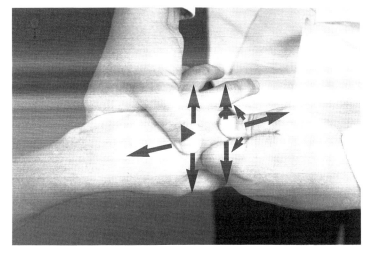

Figure 6.125 Assessment of long axis distraction, internal and external rotation, anterior to posterior, posterior to anterior, lateral to medial, and medial to lateral glide of the metacarpophalangeal joints.

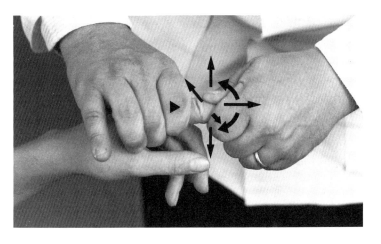

Figure 6.126 Assessment of long axis distraction, internal and external rotation, anterior to posterior, posterior to anterior, lateral to medial, and medial to lateral glide of the interphalangeal joints.

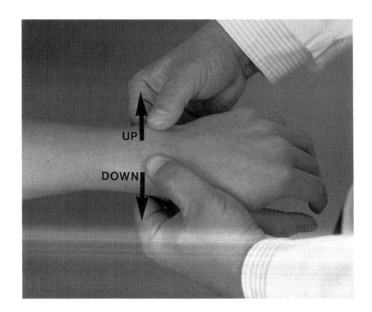

Figure 6.127 Adjustment for anterior to posterior and posterior to anterior glide of the distal radioulnar joint.

Anterior to posterior and posterior to anterior glide, distal radioulnar joint (Fig. 6-127)

IND: Wrist trauma, wrist pain, and loss of anterior to posterior or posterior to anterior glide of the radius and ulnar.

PP: The patient is supine or sitting.

DP: Stand facing the patient on the involved side.

SCP: Distal radius and distal ulna.

CP: Grasp the distal radius with one hand and the distal ulna with the other.

P: Apply an opposing anterior to posterior and posterior to anterior shearing thrust beween the radius and ulna.

Medial to lateral compression, distal radioulnar joint (Fig. 6-128)

IND: Wrist trauma, wrist pain, carpal tunnel syndrome, and loss of radius and ulnar compressibility.

PP: The patient is seated on the adjusting table with the affected arm resting on the headrest, such that the ulnar surface of the forearm is down and the radial aspect is up.

DP: Stand at the head end of the table, facing the patient.

SCP: Distal radius.

CP: Establish a pisiform contact with your cephalad hand over the patient's distal radius.

IH: Place your caudal hand pisiform contact in the contact hand's anatomic snuff box.

VEC: Compressive approximation.

P: With both arms, deliver an extension thrust, creating an impulse movement and compressing the radius and ulna. This procedure can be augmented with the use of a mechanical drop headpiece.

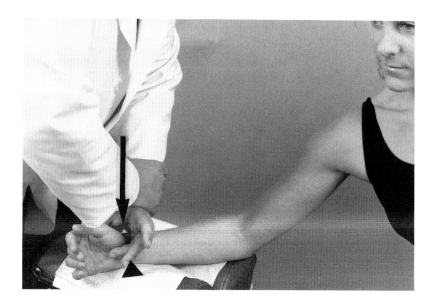

Figure 6.128 Adjustment for lateral to medial compression of the distal radioulnar joint.

Long axis distraction, intercarpal joint (Fig. 6-129)

IND: Wrist pain, decreased or painful flexion and extension movements, compressive trauma to the wrist, and loss of long axis accessory movements.

PP: The patient is seated with the affected arm raised in forward flexion.

DP: Stand facing the patient.

SCP: The hand.

CP: Using your inside hand, grasp the patient's hand as though to give a handshake.

IH: Grasp the distal forearm with your outside hand.

VEC: Long axis distraction.

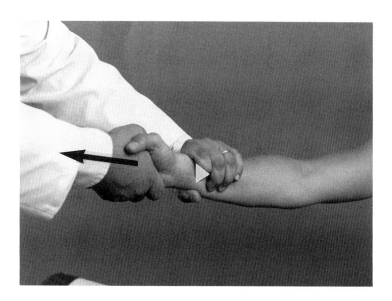

Figure 6.129 Adjustment for long axis distraction of the intercarpal joint.

P: While you stabilize the forearm with your indifferent hand, distract the wrist in the long axis with your contact hand.

Sustained long axis distraction, intercarpal joint (Fig. 6-130)

IND: Wrist pain, decreased or painful flexion and extension movements, compressive trauma to the wrist, and loss of long axis accessory movements.

PP: The patient is seated with the affected arm slightly flexed at the shoulder and slightly flexed at the elbow.

DP: Stand or sit on the affected side.

SCP: Proximal to the hypothenar and thenar eminences.

CP: Position your inside arm so that the inferior aspect of your arm rests in the patient's antecubital fossa and a calcaneal contact can be placed just proximal to the patient's hypothenar and thenar eminences.

IH: With your outside hand, place a calcaneal contact over the dorsal aspect of the metacarpal heads with a palmar contact over the back of the patient's hand.

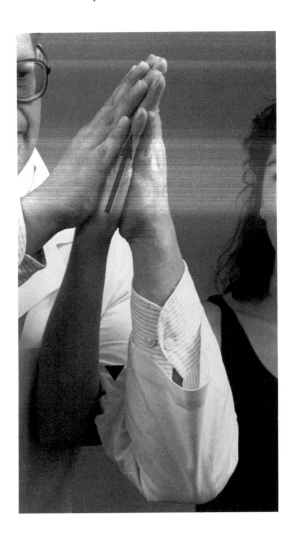

Figure 6.130 Manipulation for sustained long axis distraction of the intercarpal joint.

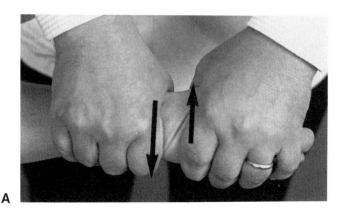

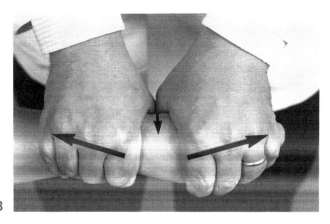

Figure 6.131 Adjustment for (**A**) medial to lateral and lateral to medial glide and (**B**) medial to lateral and lateral to medial tilt of the intercarpal joint.

VEC: Long axis distraction.

   P: Squeeze both contact hand and indifferent hand together to maintain contact while flexing the patient's elbow. The lever action will create and maintain a long axis distraction at the wrist.

Medial to lateral tilt and glide, intercarpal joint (Fig. 6-131)

IND: Decreased or painful radial or ulnar deviation, decreased medial to lateral or lateral to medial glide movements.

  PP: The patient sits with the affected arm raised in forward flexion.

  DP: Stand on the affected side, facing the lateral aspect of the arm.

SCP: Distal radius and ulna.

  CP: Using your proximal hand, grasp the distal radius and ulna.

  IH: With your distal hand, grasp the patient's distal wrist.

   P: Use both hands to develop opposing forces, and deliver an impulse thrust, creating a shearing stress (medial to lateral glide) and/or radial and ulnar deviation stress (medial to lateral tilt).

Anterior to posterior and posterior to anterior glide, intercarpal joint (Fig. 6-132)

IND: Decreased or painful flexion and extension movements, and loss of anterior to posterior and posterior to anterior accessory joint movements.

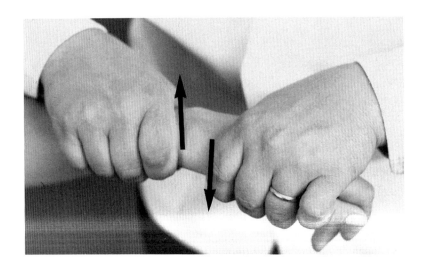

Figure 6.132 Adjustment for anterior to posterior and posterior to anterior glide of the intercarpal joint.

PP: The patient sits with the affected arm raised in forward flexion.
DP: Stand on the affected side.
SCP: Distal radius and ulna.
CP: With your proximal hand, grasp the distal radius and ulna.
IH: With your distal hand, grasp the patient's distal wrist over the metacarpal-carpal joints.
P: Using both hands to create opposing forces, deliver an impulse thrust, stressing the intercarpal joints in either an anterior to posterior or posterior to anterior direction.

Anterior to posterior and posterior to anterior glide, individual carpals (Fig. 6-133)

IND: Palpable point tenderness over the involved carpal, wrist pain, wrist trauma, painful wrist movements, carpal tunnel syndrome (lunate most often), and restricted glide motions of the carpals.
PP: The patient is seated with the affected arm raised in slight forward flexion.
DP: Stand facing the patient.
SCP: Carpal bone.
CP: Establish a thumb contact over the affected carpal.
IH: Using your other hand, apply a thumb contact over the contact hand thumb to reinforce it.
VEC: Anterior to posterior or posterior to anterior.
P: Use both hands to remove articular slack, and deliver an impulse thrust with both thumbs to create anterior to posterior or posterior to anterior glide.

Anterior to posterior and posterior to anterior glide, intermetacarpal joints (Fig. 6-134)

IND: Adhesions between metacarpals, mild degenerative arthritis, and restricted intermetacarpal glide movements.

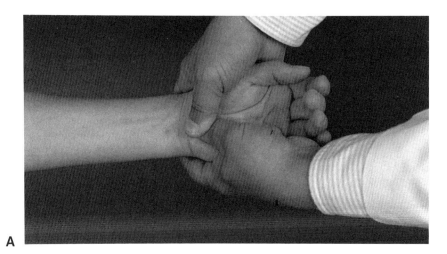

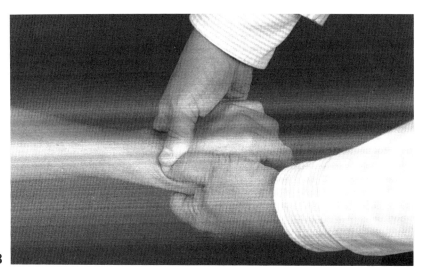

Figure 6.133 Adjustment for (**A**) anterior to posterior and (**B**) posterior to anterior glide of the individual carpals.

PP: The patient is seated with the affected arm in forward flexion and elbow flexed such that the palm of the hand faces outward.

DP: Stand facing the patient.

SCP: Metacarpal bone.

CP: Establish a thumb contact on the palmar aspect of a metacarpal bone. With your fingers, hold the same metacarpal shaft on the dorsal surface of the hand.

IH: Make the same contacts on the adjacent metacarpal.

VEC: Anterior to posterior or posterior to anterior.

P: Use both hands to create an anterior to posterior and posterior to anterior shear between the two metacarpals.

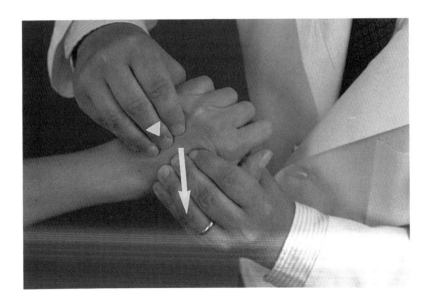

Figure 6.134 Adjustment for anterior to posterior and posterior to anterior glide of the intermetacarpal joints.

Finger joint technique—long axis distraction, posterior to anterior and anterior to posterior glide, lateral to medial and medial to lateral glide, axial rotation of the metacarpophalangeal and interphalangeal joints (Fig. 6-135)

IND: Finger pain, painful finger movement, mild degenerative arthritis, and lack of accessory joint movement in the finger joints.

PP: The patient is seated.

DP: Stand facing the patient.

SCP: Distal component of the affected joint.

CP: Grasp the distal member of the joint to be adjusted with either hand.

IH: With your other hand, grasp the proximal member of the joint being adjusted.

VEC: Long axis distraction, anterior to posterior and posterior to anterior glide, lateral to medial glide, and internal and external rotation.

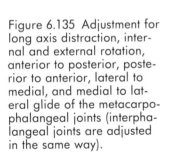

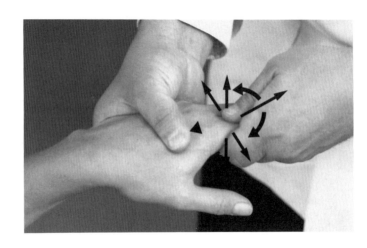

Figure 6.135 Adjustment for long axis distraction, internal and external rotation, anterior to posterior, posterior to anterior, lateral to medial, and medial to lateral glide of the metacarpophalangeal joints (interphalangeal joints are adjusted in the same way).

P: Apply an impulse thrust to the affected metacarpophalangeal or interphalangeal joint using long axis distraction, anterior to posterior and posterior to anterior glide, lateral to medial glide, and internal and external rotation.

THE HIP

The hip joint is one of the largest and most stable joints in the body.[10] In contrast to the other extremity joints and specifically its counterpart in the upper extremity, the shoulder, the hip has intrinsic stability provided by its relatively rigid ball-and-socket configuration (Fig. 6-136). Although dys-

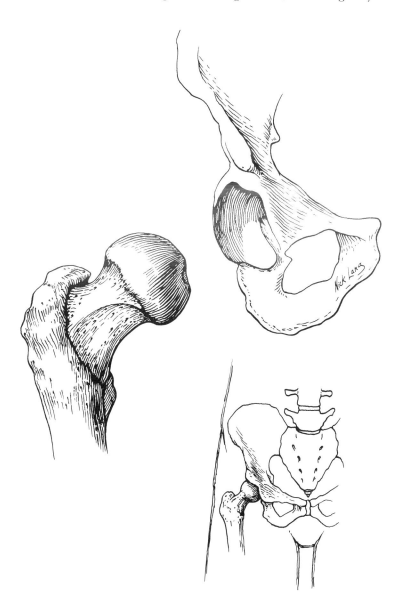

Figure 6.136 The hip joint.

function of the hip is not as frequently encountered as dysfunction in the spine and other extremity joints, its identification and treatment are very important and often overlooked. The hip joint must accommodate the great deal of mobility necessary for gait and the performance of daily activities. Furthermore, the hip joint is a multiaxial articulation that must form a stable link between the lower limb and the spine and pelvis.

Functional Anatomy

Osseous Structures

The hip is a deep ball-and-socket joint with a spherical convex surface on the head of the femur with a concave articular surface formed by the acetabulum of the pelvis. The acetabulum is formed by a fusion of the three bones that make up the innominate, the ilium superiorly, the ischium posteroinferiorly, and the pubic bone anteroinferiorly (Fig. 6-137). A fibro-cartilaginous acetabular labrum surrounds the rim of the acetabulum, effectively deepening it and serving to protect the acetabulum against the impact of the femoral head in forceful movements. Hyaline cartilage lines the horseshoe-shaped surface of the acetabulum. The center of the acetabulum is filled in with a mass of fatty tissue covered by synovial membrane. The cavity of the acetabulum is directed obliquely anterior, lateral, and inferior. The inferior component is important because of the transference of weight from the upper body through the sacroiliac joints, into the head of the femur, and down its shaft.

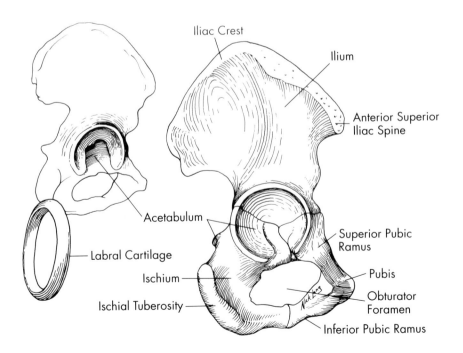

Figure 6.137 The structures of the innominate and acetabulum.

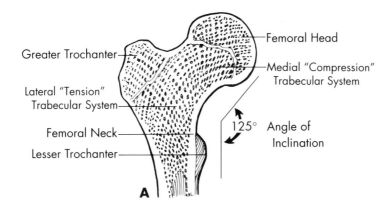

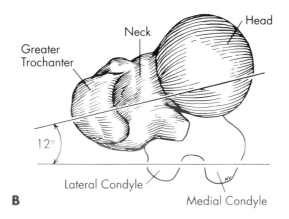

Figure 6.138 The proximal femur. (**A**) A coronal section showing the trabecular patterns and the angle of inclination of the femoral neck. (**B**) An apical view showing the angle of anteversion.

The femur is the longest bone in the body as well as one of the strongest. It must withstand not only weight-transmission forces but also those forces developed through muscle contraction.

The femoral head is completely covered with hyaline cartilage except for a small pit near its center known as the *fovea capitis*. The cartilage is thicker above and tapers to a thin edge at the circumference.

The femoral neck forms two angular relationships with the femoral shaft that influence hip function (Fig. 6-138). The angle of inclination of the femoral neck to the shaft in the frontal plane (the neck to shaft angle) is approximately 125 degrees (90 to 135 degrees). This angle offsets the femoral shaft from the pelvis laterally and facilitates the freedom of motion for the hip joint. An angle of more than 125 degrees produces a coxa valga, whereas an angle of less than 125 degrees results in coxa vara. A deviation in either way can alter the force relationships of the hip joint. The angle of anteversion is the second angle associated with the femoral neck and is formed as a projection of the long axis of the femoral head and the transverse axis of the femoral condyles. This angle should be approximately 12 degrees but has a great deal of variation, of which 10 to 30 degrees is considered within normal limits. Any increase in this anterior angulation is called *excessive anteversion* and results in a toe-in posture and gait. An angle that is less than ideal produces a retroversion and an externally rotated leg posture and gait (toe-out).

The atmospheric pressure holding the head of the femur in the acetabulum amounts to approximately 18 kg. This could support the entire limb without ligamentous or muscular assistance, though capsular ligament and muscular tension do help to keep the head of the femur stabile in the acetabulum.

A unique trabecular pattern corresponding to the lines of force through the pelvis, hip, and lower extremity are developed through the course of the femoral neck (Fig. 6-139). Tension trabeculae are more superior and run from the femoral head to the trochanteric line. Compression trabeculae are more inferior and run from the trochanteric area to the femoral head. The epiphyseal plates are at right angles to the tension trabeculae, which likely places them perpendicular to the joint reaction force on the femoral head. Aging produces degenerative changes, which will gradually cause the trabeculae to resorb, predisposing the femoral neck to fracture.

Ligamentous Structures

The hip joint is completely invested by an articular capsule that attaches to the rim of the acetabulum, to the femoral side of the intratrochanteric line, and to parts of the base of the neck and adjacent areas. The joint capsule is a cylindric structure resembling a sleeve running between its attachment around the peripheral surface of the acetabular labrum to the femoral neck

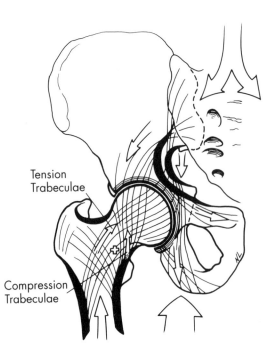

Figure 6.139 The hip joint showing tension and compression trabeculation as well as the forces transmitted from the ground and gravity. (Modified from Kapandji,[9] with permission.)

Tension Trabeculae

Compression Trabeculae

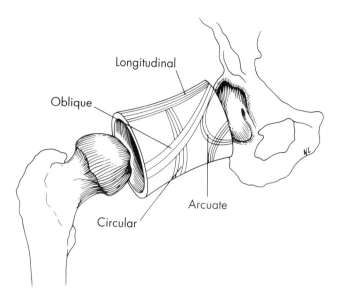

Longitudinal

Oblique

Arcuate

Circular

Figure 6.140 Diagrammatic representation of the cylindric joint capsule showing the orientation of fibers to resist stresses.

(Fig. 6-140). It therefore encloses not only the head of the femur but the neck as well. From its femoral attachments, some of the fibers are reflected upward along the neck as longitudinal bands, termed *retinacula*. The capsule is thicker toward the upper and anterior part of the joint, where the greatest amount of resistance is required. Some deep fibers of the distal portion of the capsule are circular, coursing around the femoral neck and forming the zona orbicularis. They form somewhat of a sling, or a collar, around the neck of the femur.

The joint capsule is reinforced and supported by strong ligaments named for the bony regions to which they are attached (Fig. 6-141). The iliofemoral ligament lies anterior and superior and forms an inverted Y from the lower part of the anteroinferior iliac spine to the trochanteric line of the femur. It prevents posterior tilt of the pelvis during erect standing, limits extension of the hip joint, and is responsible for the so-called "balancing on the ligaments" maneuver that occurs in the absence of muscle contraction.

The ischiofemoral ligament consists of a triangular band of strong fibers extending from the ischium below and behind the acetabulum to blend with the circular fibers of the joint capsule and attaching to the inner surface of the greater trochanter. It reinforces the posterior portion of the capsule and limits excessive medial rotation, abduction, and extension.

The pubofemoral ligament is attached above to the obturator crest and the superior ramus of the pubis, while below, it blends with the capsule and with the deep surface of the vertical band of the iliofemoral ligament. It reinforces the medial and inferior portion of the joint capsule and limits excessive abduction, lateral rotation, and extension.

The apex of the ligamentum teres attaches to the fovea capitis femoris, and its base attaches by two bands, one into either side of the acetabular notch (Fig. 6-142). This ligament does not truly contribute to the support of the joint, though it becomes taut when the thigh is semiflexed and

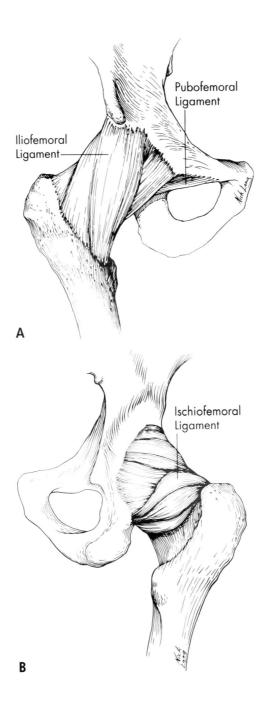

Figure 6.141 The ligamentous structure of the right hip. (A) Anterior view. (B) Posterior view.

then adducted or externally rotated. It sometimes contains and offers some protection for a nutrient artery that supplies the femoral head. The ligamentum teres is lined with synovium and is believed to play a role in assisting with joint lubrication. As such, it may act somewhat like the meniscus in the knee by spreading a layer of synovial fluid over the articular surface of the head of the femur.

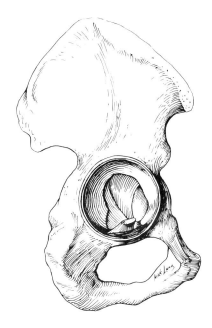

Figure 6.142 The ligamentum teres and transverse acetabular ligaments are not true supportive ligaments.

The transverse ligament crosses the acetabular notch, converting the notch into a foramen through which the artery that will supply the head of the femur can run.

Musculature

The hip is supported by strong muscles on all four sides (Table 6-18). The posterior musculature composed of the gluteus maximus, posterior fibers of the gluteus medius, hamstrings, and piriformis provide posterior stability for the hip joint. Anterior joint stability is provided by the iliopsoas, sartorius, and rectus femoris muscles. The tensor fascia lata, gluteus medius, and gluteus minimus provide lateral stability. Medial stability comes from the pectineus, adductors, and gracilis muscles. With the amount of movement and soft tissues lying in the different planes associated with the hip, many bursa exist; however, only three have important clinical significance. The

Table 6.18 Actions of the Muscles of the Hip Joint

Action	Muscles
Extension	Gluteus maximus, gluteus medius, hamstrings
Flexion	Iliopsoas, sartorius, rectus femoris, tensor fascia lata, gracilis, pectineus
Abduction	Tensor fascia lata, gluteus medius and minimus, piriformis
Adduction	Adductors, pectineus, gracilis
External rotation	Piriformis, gemelli, obturators, quadratus femoris
Internal rotation	Tensor fascia lata, gluteus medius and minimus, gracilis

iliopectineal bursa lies between the iliopsoas muscle and the hip joint capsule. It sometimes communicates with the joint cavity itself, and excess fluid from trauma may spill into it. The combined motions of hip flexion and adduction or excessive extension can compress the inflamed bursa, creating pain. The trochanteric bursa separates the tendon of the gluteus maximus and the iliotibial band from the greater trochanter. Direct trauma to this area or overuse of the joint may irritate the bursa, causing it to become inflamed. A third bursa, the ischiogluteal bursa, lies superficially over the ischial tuberosity. This bursa will become inflamed in persons who sit for prolonged periods of time and need to flex and extend their hip.

Because of the hip's role in posture and gait, the combined actions of many powerful muscles are required. Hip flexion is accomplished primarily by the iliopsoas and is assisted by the rectus femoris, pectineus, adductor longus, gracilis, tensor fascia lata, and sartorius. Hip extension occurs through the contraction of the gluteus maximus muscle, easily one of the most powerful muscles in the body. Hip extension is assisted by the hamstrings and the posterior fibers of the gluteus medius. The gluteus medius and minimus, tensor fascia lata, and to a lesser extent, piriformis create hip abduction. Hip adduction is the primary role of the adductor muscles, the gracilis, and pectineus, with some influence by the hamstrings. External rotation of the hip occurs through contraction of the piriformis, obturators, gemelli, and quadratus femoris muscles. Internal rotation of the hip is accomplished by the tensor fascia lata, gluteus medius, gluteus minimus, and gracilis muscles.

Several of the muscles that act at the hip joint also act with equal or greater effectiveness at the knee joint. These are known as two-joint muscles of the lower extremity. The location and line of pull or action of the muscles make it relatively easy to understand the mechanics of muscle testing any individual muscle.

Biomechanics

The movements of the femur are similar to those of the humerus but not as free because of the depth of the acetabulum. In the standing position, the shaft of the femur slants somewhat in a medial direction and is not straight vertical. This places the center of motion of the knee joint more nearly under the center of motion of the hip joint. Therefore, the mechanical axis of the femur is almost vertical. The degree of slant of the femoral shaft depends on both the angle between the neck and the shaft and the width of the pelvis. Seen from the side, the shaft of the femur bows forward. These orientations of the femur are provisions for resisting the stresses and strains sustained in walking, and jumping and for ensuring proper weight transmission.

Pelvic rotation about the hip accounts for a significant portion of forward bending. Trunk flexion from the erect posture through approximately the first 45 to 60 degrees involves primarily the lumbar spine, with further forward bending occurring as a result of the pelvis rotating about the hip (Fig. 6-143). The iliofemoral and ischiofemoral ligaments twist as they go from the pelvic attachment to the femur. In the erect neutral position, these ligaments are under a moderate tension. Thigh extension "winds" these

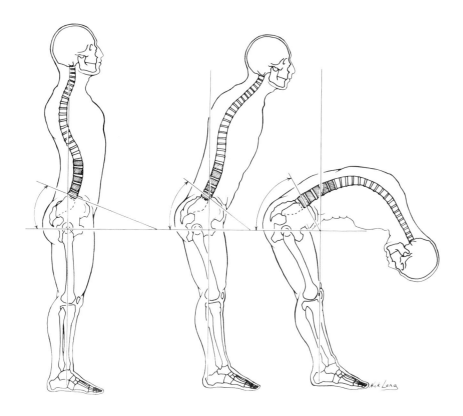

Figure 6.143 Trunk flexion begins with lumbar spine flexion followed by pelvic flexion at the hip joints.

ligaments around the neck of the femur and tightens them. Further, during posterior tilting of the pelvis, these ligaments are taut and therefore are responsible for maintaining optimal pelvic position (Fig. 6-144). Anterior hip and thigh pain may occur, owing to tension in these ligaments from excessive posterior pelvic tilting. In contrast, flexion of the hip "unwinds" these ligaments. Moreover, anterior pelvic tilting is not prevented by these ligaments, and the hip extensors must play an important role in stabilizing the pelvis in the anteroposterior direction. The twisting of these ligaments, as well as the twisting that occurs within the joint capsule, draws the joint surfaces into a close-packed position through a "screw-home" movement of the joint surfaces. The close-packed position of the hip is in extension, abduction, and internal rotation (Table 6-19). According to Kapandji the erect posture tilts the pelvis posterior, relative to the femur, causing these ligaments to become coiled around the femoral neck.[14]

During flexion, a forward movement of the femur occurs in the sagittal plane. If the knee is straight, the movement is restricted by the tension of the hamstrings. In extreme flexion, the pelvis tilt supplements the movement at the hip joint. Extension is a return movement from flexion. Hyperextension, however, is a backward movement of the femur in the sagittal plane. This movement is extremely limited. In most people, this is possible only when the femur is rotated outward. The restricting factor is the iliofemoral ligament at the front of the joint. The advantage of restriction of this movement is that

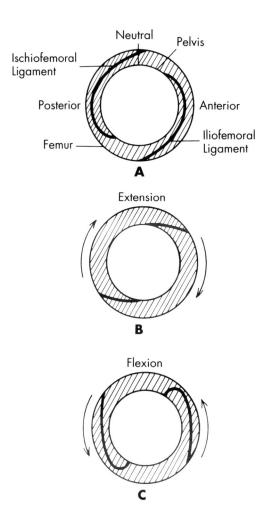

Figure 6.144 Diagrammatic representation of the effects of flexion and extension on the ischiofemoral and ilio-femoral ligament. (**A**) The right hip in the neutral position. (**B**) Extension tightens ligament. (**C**) Flexion slackens ligaments.

it provides a stable joint for weight bearing without the need for strong muscular contraction. The movements are mostly rotary actions. Abduction is described as a sideward movement of the femur in the frontal plane with the thigh moving away from the midline of the body. A greater range of movement is possible when the femur is rotated outward. Adduction is a return movement from abduction, whereas hyperadduction is possible when the other leg is moved out of the way. Abduction and adduction motions are a combination of roll and glide. Internal and external rotation are a

Table 6.19 Close-Packed and Loose-Packed (Rest) Positions for the Hip Joint

Close-Packed Position	Loose-Packed Position
Full extension, internal rotation and abduction	30 degrees flexion, 30 degrees abduction, and slight external rotation

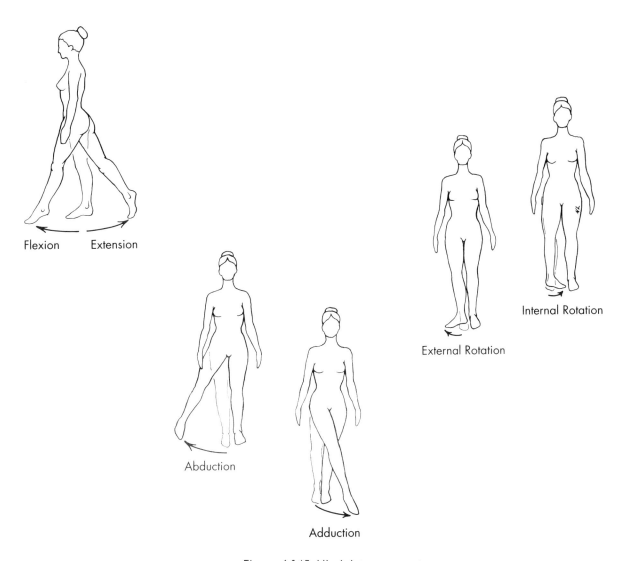

Flexion   Extension

Abduction

Adduction

External Rotation

Internal Rotation

Figure 6.145 Hip joint movements.

rotary movements of the femur around its longitudinal axis, resulting in the knee turning inward and outward, respectively (Fig. 6-145). Circumduction is a combination of flexion, abduction, extension, and adduction performed sequentially in either direction (Table 6-20).

When the hip is externally rotated, the anterior ligaments become taut, while the posterior ligaments relax. The converse is true when the hip is internally rotated (Fig. 6-146). During adduction, the inferior part of the joint capsule becomes slack, while the superior portion becomes taut. The opposite is true during abduction; the inferior part of the capsule becomes taut, while the superior portion relaxes and folds on itself (Fig. 6-147). During abduction, the iliofemoral ligament becomes taut, while the pubo-femoral ligament and ischiofemoral ligament slacken. Again, during adduc-

Table 6.20 Arthrokinematic and Osteokinematic Movements of the Hip Joint

Osteokinematic Movements (Degrees)		Arthrokinematic Movements
Flexion	120	Rotation
Extension	30	Rotation
Abduction	45–50	Roll and glide
Adduction	20–30	Roll and glide
Internal rotation	35	Roll and glide
External rotation	45	Roll and glide

tion, the opposite occurs; the pubofemoral ligament and the ischiofemoral ligament becomes taut, while the iliofemoral ligament slackens.

Pelvic stability in the coronal plane is secured by the simultaneous contraction of the ipsilateral and contralateral adductors and abductors. When these antagonistic actions are properly balanced, the pelvis is stabilized in the position of symmetry (Fig. 6-148). If, however, an imbalance exists between the abductors and the adductors, the pelvis will tilt laterally to the side of adductor predominance. If the pelvis is supported by only one limb, stability is provided only by the action of the ipsilateral abductors. An insufficiency in the abductor muscles, and specifically, the gluteus medius,

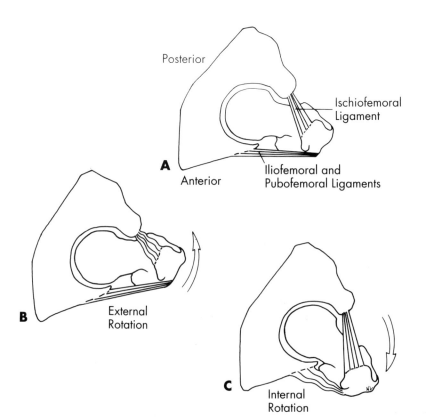

Figure 6.146 Transverse section through left hip demonstrating affects of internal and external rotation on the ischiofemoral, iliofemoral, and pubofemoral ligaments. (A) Neutral position. (B) External rotation slackens posterior ligament and stretches anterior ligaments. (C) Internal rotation slackens anterior ligaments.

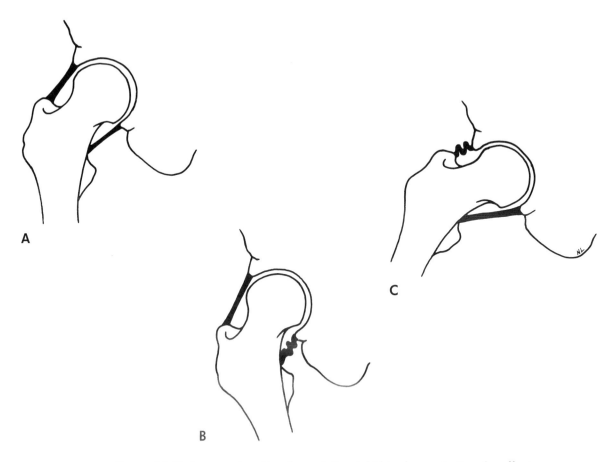

Figure 6.147 A coronal section through the right hip demonstrating the effects of abduction and adduction of the joint capsule. (**A**) Neutral. (**B**) Adduction tightens superior fibers and slackens inferior fibers. (**C**) Abduction tightens inferior fibers and slackens superior fibers.

results in the body weight not being counterbalanced, resulting in a pelvic tilt to the opposite side. The severity of muscular insufficiency relates directly to the degree of lateral pelvic tilting. Furthermore, during standing on one leg, the femoral head must support more than the weight of the body. The total force acting vertically at the femoral head is equal to the force produced by the pull of the abductors plus the force produced by the body weight or up to three times the body weight.[1]

The resting, or loose-packed, position of the hip, or that in which the joint capsule is totally slack, is 10 degrees flexion, 10 degrees abduction, and 10 degrees external rotation. This position will often be assumed to accommodate swelling. Pathomechanical changes and degenerative processes can alter the resting position. A joint posture of flexion, adduction, and external rotation is the classic capsular pattern of the hip.

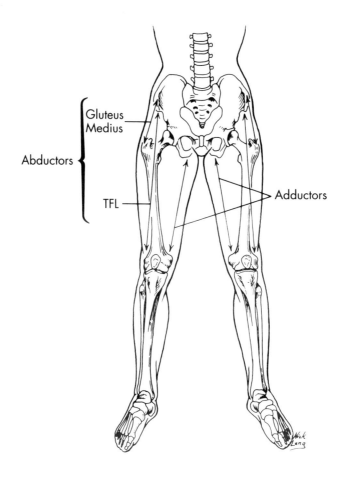

Figure 6.148 Pelvic stability in the coronal plane is produced by a balance between the abductors and adductors.

Evaluation

Though the hip joint exhibits three degrees of freedom of motion and is analogous to the glenohumeral joint, the hip is intrinsically a much more stable joint. The hip, however, is still quite prone to pathomechanical changes and, as such, is often overlooked as a source for mechanical joint dysfunction. Clinically, pain originating in the hip joint is primarily perceived as involving the L3 segment, though derivation of the hip joint is from segments L2 through S1. Hip pain can be due to referral from the facets of the lower lumbar spine. Moreover, the knee also refers pain to the hip area, and the hip can refer pain to the knee (Fig. 6-149).

The muscles working across the hip joint are subjected to strains, either through overuse (chronic strain) or overstress (acute strain, trauma). Tenderness is usually localized to the involved muscle, and the pain increases with resisted contraction. Commonly strained muscles include the sartorius, rectus femorus, iliopsoas, hamstrings, and adductors.

Trochanteric bursitis, due to overuse or direct injury, will present as pain felt primarily over the lateral hip region that is often aggravated by going up stairs. The pain is usually described as deep and aching pain that began insidiously. Getting in and out of a car is sometimes listed as a precipitating

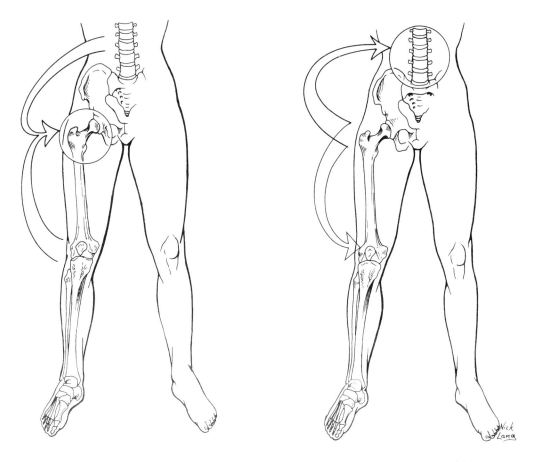

Figure 6.149 Hip pain can be referred from the knee or lumbar spine, and hip disorders can refer pain to the lumbar spine and knee.

factor. Point tenderness is found over the inflamed bursa, at the posterolateral aspect of the greater trochanter.

Entrapment of several peripheral nerves can occur in association with hip dysfunction. The femoral nerve lies close to the femoral head, and trauma or hematoma may produce entrapment, causing weakness of the hip flexors and local tenderness in the groin. The sciatic nerve, which passes deep to or through the piriformis muscle, may be compressed with contraction of the piriformis muscle. A sciatic radiculopathy with concomitant motor and sensory changes may result. The lateral femoral cutaneous nerve is prone to entrapment near the anterior superior iliac spine, where the nerve passes through the lateral end of the inguinal ligament. Entrapment creates a condition called *meralgia paresthetica* and is characterized by a burning pain in the anterior and lateral portions of the thigh. The condition may be associated with a biomechanical dysfunction of the lumbopelvic complex and postural unleveling of the pelvis.[15]

Use radiographic examination of children with hip pain (anteroposterior and frog leg) to evaluate the integrity of the capital femoral epiphysis. A

Table 6.21 Accessory Joint Movements of the Hip Joint

Long axis distraction
Anterior to posterior glide
Posterior to anterior glide
Internal rotation
External rotation
Inferior glide in flexion

slipped capital femoral epiphysis may occur, creating hip and/or knee pain. On examination, the hip will tend to swing into external rotation instead of flexion. A referral for a surgical consult is indicated.

An unrecognized or improperly treated slipped capital femoral epiphysis or a reactive synovitis may occlude the blood supply to the femoral head, and part or all of the femoral head may die, owing to avascular necrosis. These avascular changes usually involve the superior and anterolateral weight-bearing part of the femoral head, and in later stages, this area becomes irregular, collapsed, and sclerotic. Examine radiographs for rarefaction of the femoral head, characteristic of Legg-Calvé-Perthes avascular necrosis.

To begin the evaluation of the hip, observe the hip joint for the presence of any skin lesions associated with trauma, signs of inflammation, and the presence of pelvic obliquity. Observe gait patterns, though usually a pathomechanical hip dysfunction will not be severe enough to create a noticeable change in gait. However, toeing in or toeing out may be identified.

Note osseous symmetry and relationships between the greater trochanters, anterosuperior iliac spine (ASIS) and posterosuperior iliac spine (PSIS),

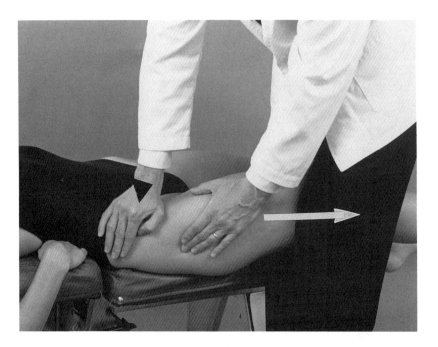

Figure 6.150 Assessment of long axis distraction of the hip joint.

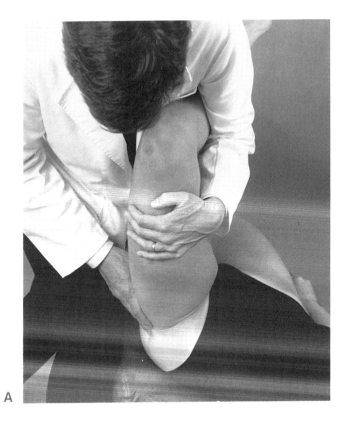

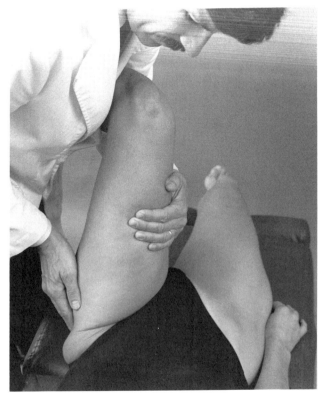

Figure 6.151 Assessment of (**A**) external and (**B**) internal rotation of the hip joint.

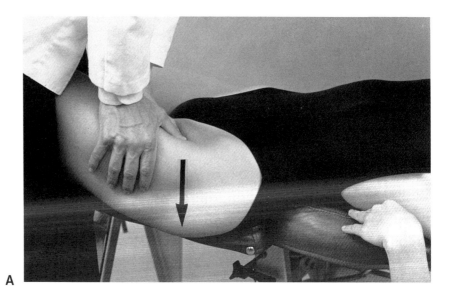

A

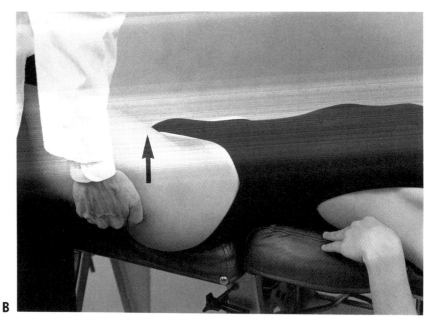

B

Figure 6.152 Assessment of **(A)** anterior to posterior and **(B)** posterior to anterior glide of the hip joint.

iliac crests, ischial tuberosities, and pubic symphysis. Identify tone, texture, and tenderness changes through soft tissue palpation of the bursa, inguinal ligament, hip flexors, hip extensors, hip adductors, and hip abductors.

Evaluate accessory joint motions for the hip joint for the presence of joint dysfunction (Table 6-21).

Evaluate long axis distraction of the iliofemoral joint with the patient supine and the affected side close to the edge of the table. Straddle the patient's distal thigh, grasping just proximal to the epicondyles with your knees. With your outside hand, palpate the greater trochanter, while you stabilize the pelvis at the ASIS with your inside hand. By straightening your legs, you can induce a long axis distraction into the hip joint and perceive a springing joint play movement with the contact on the greater trochanter (Fig. 6-150).

Evaluate internal and external rotation with the patient supine with the affected hip flexed to 90 degrees and the knee flexed to 90 degrees. Stand on the affected side facing headward using your outside hand to palpate the hip joint and greater trochanter while grasping the patient's calf and thigh area with your inside arm. Then induce internal and external rotational stresses while evaluating for the presence of a springy end-feel–type motion (Fig. 6-151).

Determine anterior to posterior and posterior to anterior glide movement with the patient supine and the involved leg slightly abducted. Straddle the patient's thigh just above the knee. Grasp the proximal thigh with both hands, and induce an anterior to posterior and posterior to anterior stress, feeling for the presence of a springing joint play movement (Fig. 6-152).

Evaluate inferior glide of the hip in flexion with the patient supine with the involved knee flexed to 90 degrees and the hip flexed to 90 degrees. Stand on the involved side, facing the patient, bending over such that the patient's calf can rest over your shoulder. Grasp the anterior aspect of the

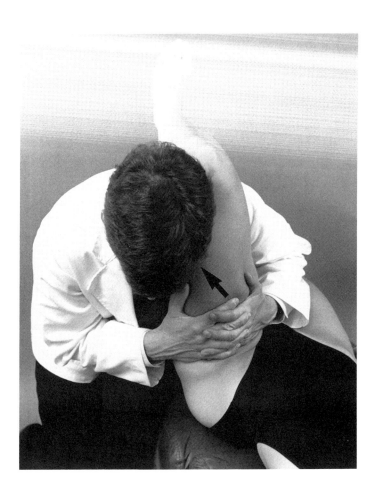

Figure 6.153 Assessment of inferior glide in flexion of the hip joint.

proximal thigh, and create a caudal stress toward the foot end of the table, evaluating for the presence of a springing end-feel movement (Fig. 6-153).

Adjustive Techniques

Long axis distraction—supine (Fig. 6-154)

IND: Hip pain, pain on hip movements, decreased active hip movement, and loss of long axis distraction accessory movement.

PP: The patient is supine with the ischial tuberosities just headward of the slightly raised pelvic piece.

DP: Stand at the foot of the table.

SCP: Distal tibia.

CP: With both hands, grasp the distal tibia just above the ankle.

VEC: Long axis distraction.

P: Use the raised pelvic piece to stabilize the patient's pelvis on the table while using both hands to produce long axis distraction at the hip joint. It is difficult to perceive whether the distraction has affected the hip, the knee or the ankle, and likely affects all three. A modification to this technique is done by wrapping a towel around the patient's ankle and grasping the towel with both hands (Fig. 6-155).

Long axis distraction—side posture (Fig. 6-156)

IND: Hip pain, pain on hip movements, decreased active hip movement, and loss of long axis distraction accessory movement.

PP: The patient lies in a basic side posture position with the involved side up and the hip flexed to about 60 degrees and the knee bent to 90 degrees with the dorsum of the foot in the popliteal fossa of the other leg.

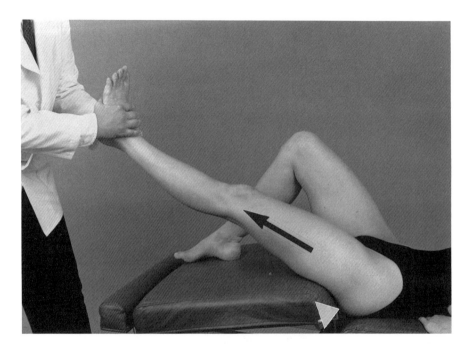

Figure 6.154 Adjustment for long axis distraction of the hip joint.

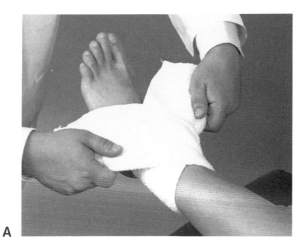

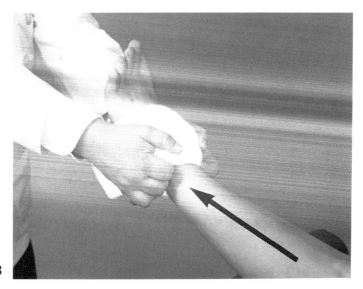

Figure 6.155 Modification for long axis distraction using a towel. (**A**) Wrapping the towel. (**B**) Grasping the towel to apply the thrust.

DP: Stand in front of the patient, straddling the patient's involved leg.

SCP: Posterior and superior aspect of the greater trochanter.

CP: With your caudal hand, establish a pisiform, hypothenar contact on the posterosuperior aspect of the greater trochanter.

IH: Use your cephalad hand to apply a palmar contact over the patient's shoulder.

VEC: Long axis distraction.

P: With your indifferent hand, stabilize the patient's trunk while using your contact hand to create long axis distraction to the hip joint. This same procedure can also be used for a loss of internal rotation and inferior glide in flexion.

Internal rotation (Fig. 6-157)

IND: Hip pain, genu varum, externally rotated femur, and loss of internal rotation accessory joint movement.

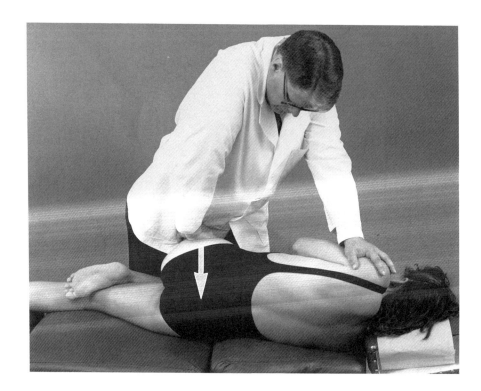

Figure 6.156 Adjustment for long axis distraction (as well as inferior glide in flexion and/or internal rotation) of the hip joint in the side posture position.

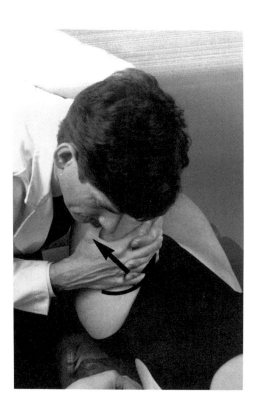

Figure 6.157 Adjustment for internal rotation of the hip joint.

PP: The patient is supine with the affected hip flexed to 90 degrees and the knee flexed to 90 degrees.

DP: Stand on the side of involvement, facing headward.

SCP: Femur–midshaft.

CP: With your cephalad hand, grasp the affected femur at the midshaft area.

IH: With your caudal hand, grasp the patient's calf, holding it against your body.

VEC: Internal rotation.

P: Using your indifferent hand, induce internal rotation, then deliver an impulse-type thrust with the contact hand.

External rotation (Fig. 6-158)

IND: Hip pain, genu valgum, anterior pelvic tilting, internally rotated femur, and loss of external rotational accessory joint movement.

PP: The patient is supine with the affected hip flexed to 90 degrees, abducted slightly, and the knee flexed to 90 degrees.

DP: Stand on the side of involvement, facing outward and between the patient's leg and the adjusting table.

SCP: Medial aspect of the proximal femur.

CP: With your cephalad hand, grasp the medial aspect of the proximal femur.

IH: With your caudal hand, grasp the patient's tibia and hold it against your torso.

VEC: External rotation.

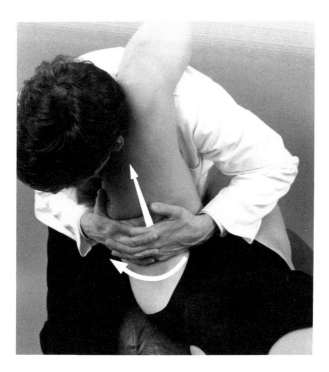

Figure 6.158 Adjustment for external rotation of the hip joint.

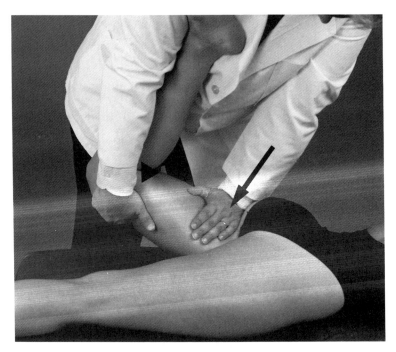

Figure 6.159 Adjustment for posterior to anterior glide of the hip joint.

P: Using your indifferent hand, stress the femur into external rotation, then supply an impulse thrust with the contact hand.

Posterior to anterior glide (Fig. 6-159)

IND: Hip pain, decreased active extension and external rotation, posterior positioned femoral head, loss of posterior to anterior glide accessory joint movements.

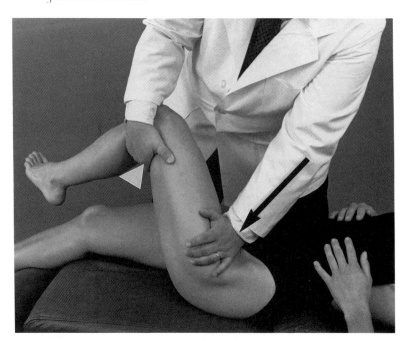

Figure 6.160 Adjustment for anterior to posterior glide of the hip joint.

PP: The patient lies prone.

DP: Stand at the side of the table on the involved side.

SCP: Posterior aspect of the proximal femur.

CP: With your cephalad hand, apply a knife-edge contact to the posterior aspect of the proximal femur.

IH: With your caudal hand, grasp the distal femur from the medial aspect (the patient's knee can be bent and cradled against your indifferent hand and forearm).

VEC: Posterior to anterior.

P: With your indifferent hand, draw the hip into extension by raising the knee off the table. Deliver an impulse thrust posterior to anterior with your contact hand.

Anterior to posterior glide (Fig. 6-160)

IND: Hip pain, restricted active flexion and internal rotational movements, anterior positioned femoral head, and loss of anterior to posterior glide accessory joint movements.

PP: The patient is supine with the hip and knee flexed slightly.

DP: Stand at the side of the table opposite the involved leg.

SCP: Anterior aspect of the proximal femur.

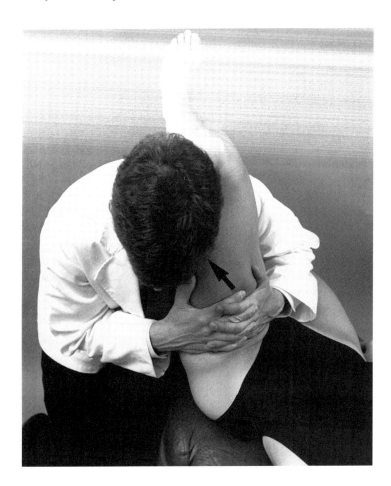

Figure 6.161 Adjustment for inferior glide in flexion of the hip joint.

> CP: With your cephalad hand, establish a knife-edge contact over the anterior aspect of the proximal femur.
> IH: With your caudal hand, grasp the distal femur with the fingers in the popliteal fossa.
> VEC: Anterior to posterior.
> P: Using your indifferent hand, flex the hip while delivering an impulse thrust anterior to posterior to the proximal femur with the contact hand.

Inferior glide in flexion (Fig. 6-161)

> IND: Hip pain, trochanteric bursitis, groin pain, restricted active flexion and internal rotational movements, and loss of inferior glide in flexion accessory joint movements.
> PP: The patient is supine with the involved knee flexed to 90 degrees and the hip flexed to 90 degrees.
> DP: Stand on the involved side, facing the patient, flexed forward with the patient's calf resting over your shoulder.
> SCP: Anterior aspect of the proximal femur.
> CP: Grasp the anterior aspect of the proximal thigh with both hands.
> VEC: Superior to inferior.
> P: With both hands, deliver an impulse thrust caudally.

THE KNEE

The distal end of the femur and proximal end of the tibia are connected by numerous ligaments and stabilized by strong muscles to form the very complicated knee joint. This joint is situated between the body's two longest lever arms and therefore must be able to transmit significant loads as it sustains high forces through upright posture and gait. Three articular complexes are typically discussed in conjunction with the knee. However, only the tibiofemoral articulation and patellofemoral articulation participate in knee joint activity. The tibiofibular articulation does not actually participate in actions of the knee. However, dysfunctional processes in the proximal tibiofibular articulation can affect other knee functions and can be a source of knee pain.

The knee joints are located between the ends of each supporting column of the body and are therefore subjected to severe stress and strain in the combined function of weight bearing and locomotion. For adaptation to the weight-bearing stresses, the knee has large condyles, which are padded by the intra-articular menisci. To facilitate locomotion, the articular structure allows a wide range of motion, and to resist lateral stresses, the knee has strong ligaments on its sides. To combat the downward pull of gravity and to meet the demands of violent locomotor activities such as running and jumping, the knee is provided with powerful musculature.

Functional Anatomy

Osseous Structures

The femoral shaft lies in an oblique alignment to the lower leg, which produces a physiologic valgus angle of approximately 170 to 175 degrees

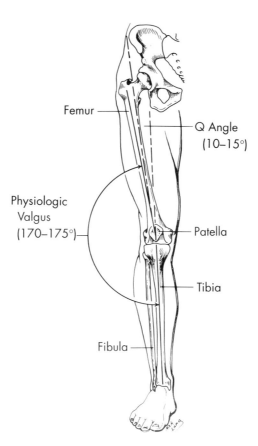

Femur

Q Angle
(10–15°)

Physiologic
Valgus
(170–175°)

Patella

Tibia

Fibula

Figure 6.162 The physio-
logic valgus tilt of the lower
extremity places the knee
under the hip.

(Fig. 6-162). The distal end of the femur is expanded to form a large, convex, U-shaped articular surface (Fig. 6-163). The medial and lateral femoral condyles lie on the end of the U-shape and are separated by the intercondylar fossa. Anteriorly, the articular surface of the femoral condyles form the patellar groove. The proximal end of the tibia is flattened to create a plateau with a bifid, nonarticulating intracondylar eminence dividing the plateau into medial and lateral sections to accommodate the medial and lateral femoral condyles. The tibial tuberosity projects from the anterior surface of the tibia, serving as the point of insertion of the quadriceps tendon (Fig. 6-164). The patella, which is the largest sesamoid bone in the body, lies embedded within the quadriceps tendon. It is triangular in shape, with its apex directed inferiorly. The anterior surface is nearly flat, while a longitudinal ridge divides the posterior surface into medial and lateral articulating facets. The longitudinal ridge fits into the patellar groove of the femur. The proximal head of the fibula is expanded and contains a single facet that corresponds with a facet on the posterolateral aspect of the rim of the tibial condyle.

Ligamentous Structures

Internal to the joint are the cruciate ligaments, arranged in a criss-cross manner providing anterior to posterior as well as medial to lateral stability

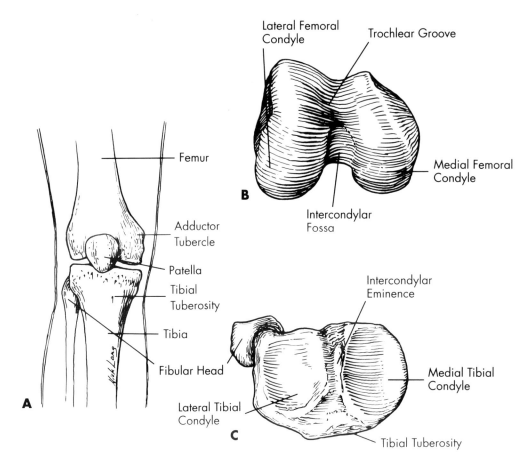

Figure 6.163 Osseous structures of the right knee. (A) Anterior view. (B) Articular surface of the distal femur. (C) Articular surface of the proximal tibia.

at the knee. Secondarily, they prevent excessive medial rotation of the tibia and help to maintain contact beween the articular surfaces of the tibia and femur (Figs. 6-165 to 6-168). The anterior cruciate ligament extends from the anterior aspect of the intercondylar eminence of the tibia and runs posterior and superior to the medial side of the lateral condyle of the femur. The posterior cruciate ligament attaches from the posterior intercondylar eminence of the tibia, extending anterior and superior to the lateral side of the medial condyle of the femur. The anterior cruciate ligament resists anterior displacement of the tibia and checks extension movements. In contrast, the posterior cruciate ligament primarily checks posterior displacement of the tibia and resists internal rotation of the tibia. The posterior cruciate ligament, lying medial to the anterior cruciate ligament, is the strongest of the knee ligaments. It is especially important for providing medial to lateral stability of the knee when in extension.

The collateral ligaments provide medial to lateral stability and support for the knee while also preventing excessive external rotation of the tibia. The medial, or tibial, collateral ligament attaches from the medial epicondyle

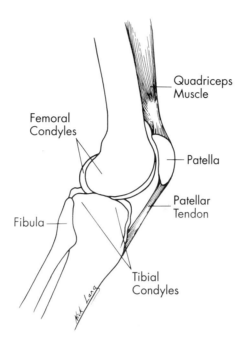

Figure 6.164 Lateral view of the knee.

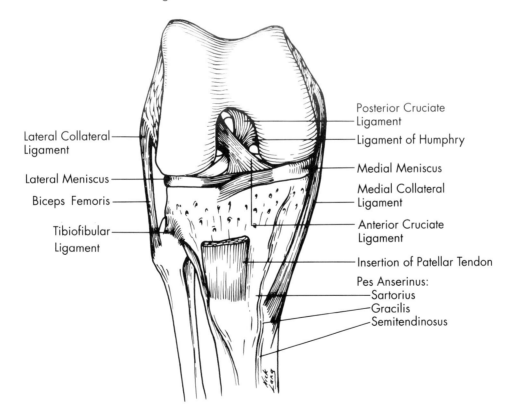

Figure 6.165 Anterior view of the right knee ligaments.

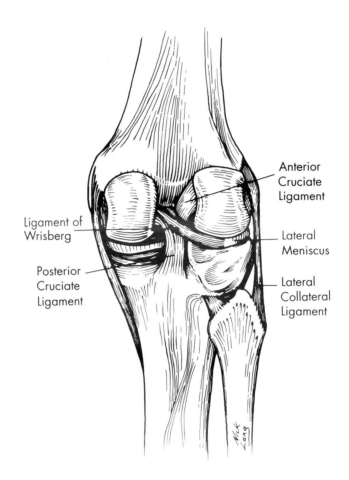

Anterior
Cruciate
Ligament

Ligament of
Wrisberg

Lateral
Meniscus

Posterior
Cruciate
Ligament

Lateral
Collateral
Ligament

Figure 6.166 Posterior view
of the right knee ligaments.

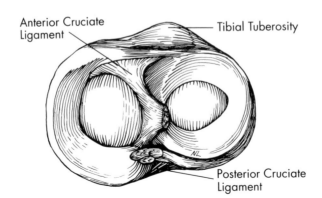

Anterior Cruciate
Ligament

Tibial Tuberosity

Figure 6.167 Superior aspect of the proximal right
tibia showing origin of the
cruciate ligaments.

Posterior Cruciate
Ligament

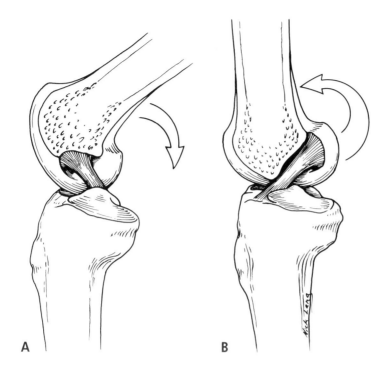

Figure 6.168 On knee extension: **(A)** The anterior cruciate ligament becomes taut while in flexion. **(B)** The posterior cruciate ligament becomes taut.

of the femur to the medial aspect of the shaft of the tibia. This ligament becomes taut on extension of the knee, abduction of the tibia on the femur, and external rotation of the tibia on the femur. The medial collateral ligament provides some help in preventing anterior displacement of the tibia on the femur. The lateral, or fibular, collateral ligament attaches from the lateral epicondyle of the femur to the head of the fibula. This ligament becomes taut on extension, adduction, and external rotation of the tibia on the femur. The tendon of the biceps femoris almost completely covers the lateral collateral ligament, while the popliteus tendon runs underneath it and separates it from the meniscus.

Surrounding the external aspect of the joint is the fibrous joint capsule attaching at the margins of the articular cartilage. The inferior portion of the capsule has been referred to as the coronary ligament. A substantial thickening in the medial portion of the joint capsule has fibrous attachments to the periphery of the medial meniscus, thereby binding it firmly to the femur and loosely to the tibia. The lateral aspect of the joint capsule has a similar thickening and has fibrous attachments to the lateral meniscus.

The posterior fibers of the medial collateral ligament blend with the joint capsule and the attachments to the medial meniscus. The patellofemoral ligaments form as thickenings of the anterior joint capsule and extend from the middle of the patella to the medial and lateral femoral condyles. Their function is to stabilize the patella in the patellar groove. The posterior thickening of the joint capsule arches over the popliteus tendon, attaches to the base of the fibular head, and becomes taut in hyperextension. Also blending with the posterior joint capsule is the oblique popliteal ligament, which forms as an expansion of the semimembranosis tendon and runs

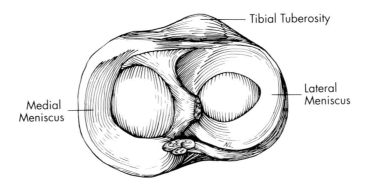

Tibial Tuberosity

Lateral
Meniscus

Medial
Meniscus

Figure 6.169 The menisci of
the knee.

obliquely proximal and lateral to attach to the lateral femoral condyle. It
also becomes tight in hyperextension.

Lying between the femur and the tibia are the two semilunar cartilages
called *menisci* (Fig. 6-169). The menisci are shaped such that the more
peripheral portions are thicker than the central part. This serves to deepen
the articular surface on the tibial plateau, which provides additional stability
to the joint. Because they increase the surface area of the joint, the menisci
help to share the load in weight bearing across the joint by distributing
weight in a broader area. They also aid in the lubrication and nutrition of the
joint and, coupled with their shock-absorbing capabilities, help to decrease
cartilage wear. The periphery of each meniscus attaches to the joint capsule,
while the inner edge remains free. The medial meniscus is C-shaped, with
the posterior portion being larger than the anterior. The anterior horn
inserts on the intercondylar area of the tibia, while the posterior horn inserts
just anterior to the attachment of the posterior cruciate ligament. The lateral
meniscus is almost a complete circle, with the tips of each horn quite close
to one another. The lateral meniscus is more mobile than the medial meniscus.

Musculature

Stabilizing the knee are the many muscles that cross it (Table 6-22). Laterally,
the iliotibial band attaches to the lateral condyle of the tibia, providing
anterolateral reinforcement and stabilization against excessive internal rotation of the tibia on the femur. Crossing the anterior aspect of the knee is
the quadriceps tendon. It is formed by the junction of the four heads of the
quadriceps muscle, which consist of the vastus lateralis, the vastus medius,
the vastus medialis, and rectus femoris. The quadricep musculature function
to extend the knee. Balanced activity between the vastus medialis and lateralis maintains optimum orientation of the patella within the patellofemoral
groove. The sartorius and gracilis muscles provide medial stability to the
joint. The sartorius also assists in knee and hip flexion, external rotation of
the femur, and internal rotation of the tibia, depending on whether the
extremity is weight bearing. The gracilis acts to adduct the femur and
assists in knee flexion and internal rotation of the tibia. Posteromedial
reinforcement of the joint is supplied by the pes anserinus tendons (semi-

Table 6.22 Actions of the Muscles of the Knee Joint

Action	Muscles
Extension	Quadriceps
Flexion	Hamstrings, gracilis, sartorius, tensor fascia lata, popliteus
Internal rotation	Sartorius, gracilis, semitendinosis, semimembranosis, popliteus
External rotation	Biceps femoris, tensor fascia lata (iliotibial tract)

tendonosis, gracilis, and sartorius), and the semimembranosis tendon. These help to prevent external rotation, abduction, and anterior displacement of the tibia. Posterolateral support from the biceps femoris tendon helps to check excessive internal rotation and anterior displacement of the tibia. The hamstring muscle is the primary knee flexor; the biceps femoris also provides some external rotation. Posterior reinforcement of the knee joint is provided by the gastrocnemius muscle and the popliteus muscle (Fig. 6-170). The gastrocnemius is a primary ankle plantar flexor but also assists in knee flexion. The popliteus internally rotates and flexes the tibia when the limb is not weight bearing. The converse occurs with the limb weight bearing.

Because the knee is exposed to a variety of demands in human locomotion, numerous bursas are located in relationship to the knee joint and to the

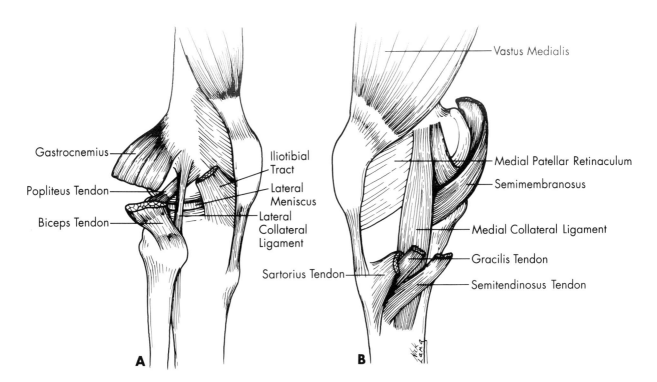

Figure 6.170 **(A)** Lateral and **(B)** medial aspects of the right knee demonstrating muscular attachments.

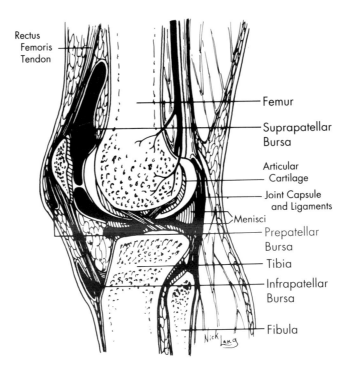

Figure 6.171 Sagittal section through the knee demonstrating numerous bursas.

synovial cavity. The synovial membrane of the knee joint is the most extensive of any in the body. The suprapatellar pouch, or quadriceps bursa, is actually an extension of the synovial sac that runs from the superior aspect of the patella upward beneath the quadriceps tendon and then folds back on itself to form a pouch inserting on the distal femur above the condyles (Fig. 6-171). The prepatellar bursa is a relatively large but superficial bursa that lies between the skin and the patella. It can become inflamed with prolonged kneeling activities. The deep and superficial infrapatellar bursas lie just under and over the patellar tendon, respectively. Bursal sacs also lie between the semimembranosis tendon and the medial head of the gastrocnemius muscle, and two bursas separate the medial lateral heads of the gastrocnemius muscle from the joint capsule. (A Baker's cyst occurs with effusion of the medial gastrocnemius and the semimembranosis bursas.) A bursa also lies under the pes anserine tendon, separating it from the tibial collateral ligament.

Biomechanics

The knee joint must provide a broad range of motion while maintaining its stability. It must react to rotational forces as well as absorb shock and then immediately prepare for propulsion. The knee functions as a modified hinge joint, with flexion and extension being its primary motions. Limited rotation occurs, especially when the joint is not in the closed packed position (extension) (Table 6-23). Flexion and extension of the knee is a combination

Table 6.23 Close-Packed and Loose-Packed (Rest) Positions for the Knee Joint

Close-Packed Position	Loose-Packed Position
Full extension with full external rotation	25 degrees flexion

of roll, slide, and spin movements, which effectively shift the axis of movement posterior as the knee moves from extension into flexion (Fig. 6-172). Similar to the elbow, flexion is limited by soft tissue of the calf and posterior thigh, while extension is limited by the locking of the joint from bony and soft tissue elements in the joint's close packed position. Moreover, the so-called screw-home mechanism, which is a combination of external rotation of the tibia occurring with knee extension, further approximates the osseous structures and tightens the ligamentous structures to stabilize the joint (Fig. 6-173). The marked incongruent positions of the tibiofemoral joint are reduced by the fibrocartilaginous menisci. These also help to distribute the forces of compressive loading over a greater area and reduce compressive stresses to the joint surfaces of the knee. Ranges of motion of the knee are listed in Table 6-24.

The patellofemoral joint plays an active role in flexion and extension of the knee joint. This joint has a gliding motion, moving caudally approximately 7 cm when going from full flexion to full extension. The articular surface of the patella never makes complete contact with the femoral condyles; the joint space decreases with flexion, and at full flexion, the patella sinks into

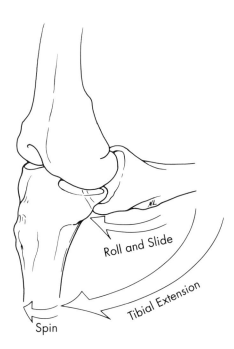

Figure 6.172 Flexion and extension movement are a combination of roll, slide, and spin.

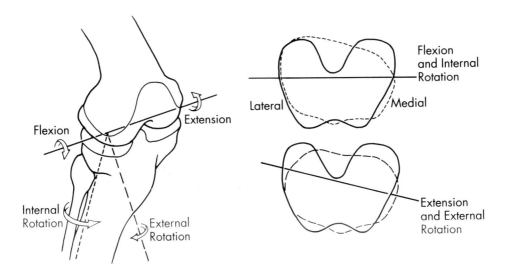

Figure 6.173 The "screw-home" mechanism of the knee combining external rotation with extension, which maximally approximates the joint surfaces. (Modified from Nordin and Frankel,[10] with permission.)

the intracondylar groove (Fig. 6-174). This characteristic is important in helping to increase weight-bearing capabilities in a flexed position (squatting). Therefore, the patella plays two important biomechanical roles for the knee. It primarily aids in knee extension by producing anterior displacement of the quadriceps tendon, thereby lengthening the lever arm of the quadriceps muscle force. Additionally, it allows a wider distribution of compressive force on the femur, especially in a fully flexed position.

The patella has an optimum position in relationship to the knee joint in both the vertical and sagittal planes. On a lateral view of the knee, the length of the patella is compared to the distance from the inferior pole of the patella to the tibial tubercle (Fig. 6-175). If the difference of these two numbers is greater than 1 cm, the position of the patella is either high (alta) or low (baja), depending on which distance is greater. To determine whether the patella is aligned properly in the femoral groove, the Q-angle can be determined. After locating the center of the patella, extend a line up the center of the patellar tendon through the center point. Then draw a line

Table 6.24 Arthrokinematic and Osteokinematic Movements of the Knee Joint

Osteokinematic Movements (Degrees)		Arthrokinematic Movements
Flexion	130	Roll and glide
Extension	10	Roll and glide
Internal rotation	10	Rotation
External rotation	10	Rotation

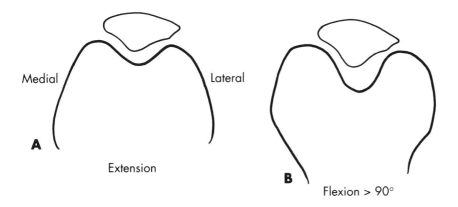

Figure 6.174 The relation of the patella to the femur in (**A**) extension and (**B**) flexion of the knee.

from the center of the patella toward the ASIS (Fig. 6-176). The resultant angle is the Q-angle. The normal Q-angle is 10 to 15 degrees, being slightly greater in females. Muscle imbalance and rotational disrelationships of the tibia and femur produce changes in the Q-angle.

The superior tibiofibular joint is mechanically linked to the ankle, but a dysfunctional process in this joint will present clinically as pain in and about the knee. Therefore, inclusion of it in a discussion of the knee is clinically relevant. The superior tibiofibular joint allows superior and inferior movement as well as internal and external rotation of the fibula. During ankle dorsiflexion, the fibula internally rotates and rises superior. The addition of ankle eversion causes some posterior displacement of the fibular head. Ankle plantar flexion draws the fibula inferiorly and creates external rotation. The addition of ankle inversion will draw the fibular head anterior.

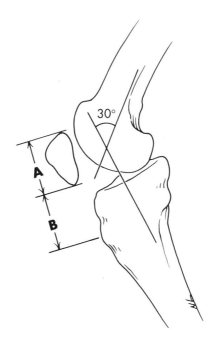

Figure 6.175 Identification of the position of the patella. If A − B > 1 cm, then a low (baja) patella exists; if B − A > 1 cm, then a high (alta) patella exists.

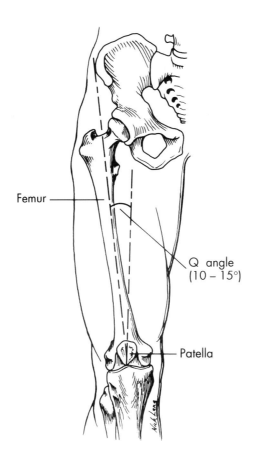

Figure 6.176 The Q-angle: the angle formed from the intersection of lines from the center of the patella to the ASIS and along the quadraceps tendon.

Evaluation

The knee joint is affected by a wide variety of clinical syndromes. Trauma is by far the most common causative agent. Injuries to the collateral ligaments will usually require some type of traumatic force. The mechanism of most medial collateral ligament injuries is a twisting external rotation strain while the knee is flexed or a valgus (abduction) blow to the knee. A lateral collateral ligament injury may occur with a varus (adduction) blow to the knee, and when internal rotation and hyperextension occur with this force, the fibular head may avulse.

The anterior cruciate ligament is commonly injured by forced internal rotation of the femur on a fixed tibia, while the knee is abducted and flexed. The posterior cruciate ligament can be torn when a traumatic force is delivered to the front of the flexed tibia, driving it posterior under the femur. Forced external rotation of the femur on the tibia while the foot is fixed and the knee is abducted and flexed will also injure the posterior cruciate ligament.

Following traumatic injuries to the knee causing ligamentous injury, joint instabilities are likely. The knee can undergo translational or rotational instabilities. Orthopedic stress tests are performed to identify the presence of joint instability.

The menisci are another site of possible injury. A trauma that couples rotation or violent extension of the knee may cause an isolated longitudinal or transverse tear in the meniscus.

Problems involving the patellofemoral joint complex are common and may be more frequent than ligamentous or meniscus disorders. A patient complaining of vague aching pain about the knee that is aggravated by going up or down stairs likely has patellofemoral joint dysfunction. Patellar tracking problems can occur primarily from injuries to the knee and quadriceps mechanism or secondarily in response to problems affecting the ankle or hip. Chondromalacia patella, an erosion and fragmentation of the subpatellar cartilage, may be secondary to trauma, recurrent subluxation, pronated feet, postural instability, short leg syndrome, or excessive femoral torsion with resultant irregular Q-angle.

An avulsion fracture with resulting aseptic necrosis of the tibial tuberosity may occur from a sudden contraction of the quadriceps femoris. This condition is called Osgood-Schlatter's disease and is more common in boys.

The knee joint is innervated by segments L3 through S1, and therefore, in cases of pain of nontraumatic onset, lesions situated elsewhere in the L3 through S2 segments must be ruled out. The lumbar spine, hip, and foot are sources of referred pain to the knee (Fig. 6-177).

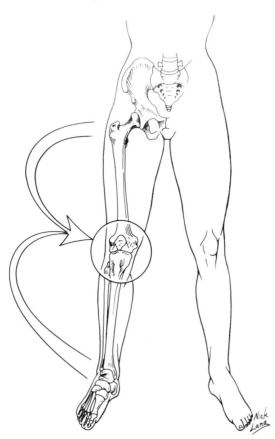

Figure 6.177 The ankle and hip can refer pain to the knee.

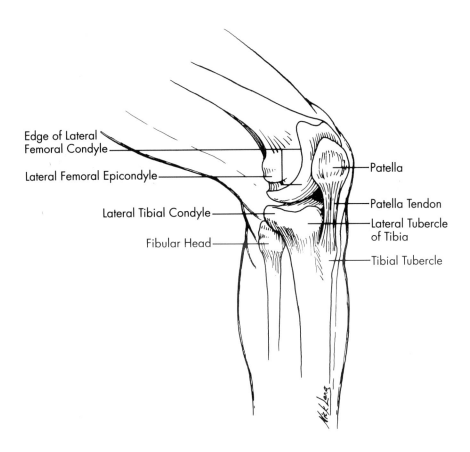

Figure 6.178 Surface anatomy of the right knee.

To begin the evaluation of the knee, observe the knee for evidence of swelling, symmetry of contours, and postural changes (valgus, varus, or recurvatum). Movements of knee during gait should be smooth and rhythmic, with the knee bent during the swing phase and fully extended at heel strike.

Identify osseous symmetry and pain production through static palpation of the tibial plateau, tibial tubercle, adductor tubercle, femoral condyles, femoral epicondyles, fibular head, patella, and trochlear groove (Fig. 6-178). Determine the Q-angle.

Identify tone, texture, and tenderness changes through soft tissue palpation of the quadriceps muscle, infrapatellar tendon, the collateral ligaments, the pes anserine tendons, peroneal nerve, tibial nerve, popliteal artery, hamstring muscles, and gastrocsoleus muscle.

Evaluate accessory joint motions for the knee articulations to determine the presence of joint dysfunction (Table 6-25).

Assess long axis distraction with the patient supine and the affected leg slightly abducted. Stand facing the patient, straddling the affected leg such that your knees can grasp the patient's distal leg just proximal to the malleoli. Use both hands to palpate the knee joint at its medial and lateral aspects an use your legs to create a long axis distraction, while palpating with your

Table 6.25 Accessory Joint Movements of the
Knee Joint

Joint	Movement
Tibiofemoral	Long axis distraction
	Anterior to posterior glide
	Posterior to anterior glide
	Internal rotation
	External rotation
	Medial to lateral glide
	Lateral to medial glide
Patellofemoral	Superior to inferior glide
	Inferior to superior glide
	Lateral to medial glide
	Medial to lateral glide
Tibiofibular	Anterior to posterior glide
	Posterior to anterior glide
	Inferior to superior glide
	Superior to inferior glide

hands for a springy end feel (Fig. 6-179). Alternately, one hand may stabilize
the patient's femur on the table, while the other hand palpates for end feel.

Evaluate anterior to posterior and posterior to anterior glide with the
patient supine and the involved knee flexed to 90 degrees with the foot flat
on the table. Either kneel or sit on the patient's foot for stability, while
grasping the proximal tibia with both hands. Stress the proximal tibia in
an anterior to posterior and posterior to anterior direction, looking for a
springing end feel (Fig. 6-180).

To evaluate internal and external rotation, use the same positions as for
anterior to posterior and posterior to anterior glide. Stress the proximal
tibia internally and externally to feel for a springing end feel (Fig. 6-181).

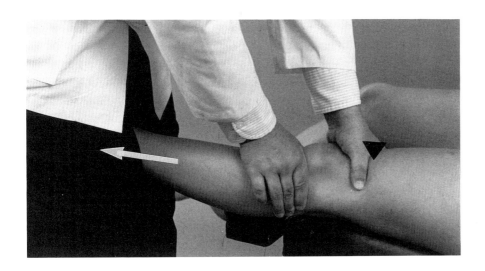

Figure 6.179 Assessment of
long axis distraction of the
tibiofemoral joint.

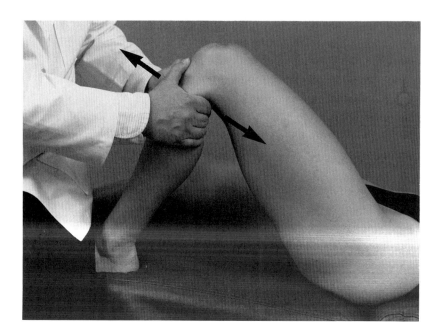

Figure 6.180 Assessment of anterior to posterior and posterior to anterior glide of the tibiofemoral joint.

Evaluate medial to lateral and lateral to medial glide with the patient supine and the involved leg abducted beyond the edge of the table. Then straddle the patient's involved leg just proximal to the ankle, while grasping the proximal tibia with both hands. Apply a medial to lateral and lateral to medial stress to the knee joint to identify a springing end feel. Alternatively, grasp the patient's involved leg with the tibia held between your

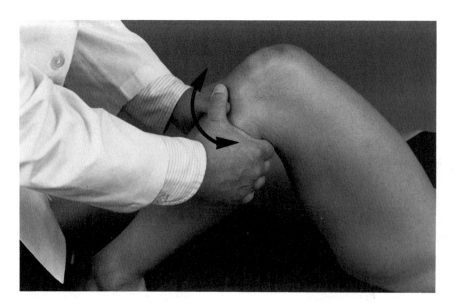

Figure 6.181 Assessment of external and internal rotation of the tibiofemoral joint.

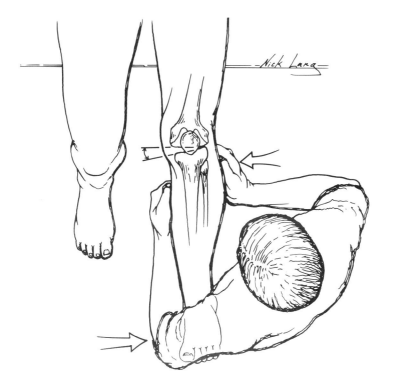

Figure 6.182 Lateral to medial glide of the left knee.

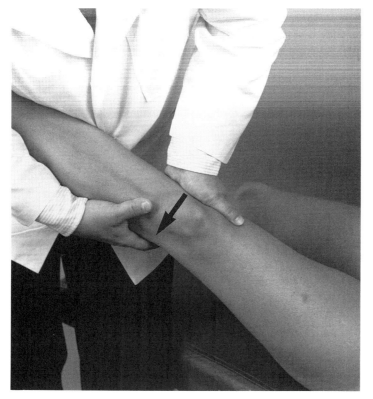

Figure 6.183 Assessment of medial to lateral glide of the tibiofemoral joint.

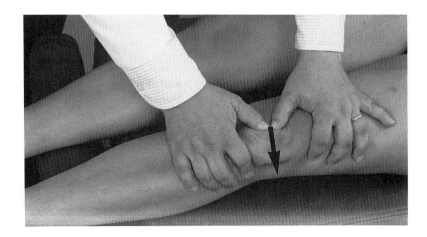

Figure 6.184 Assessment of medial to lateral glide of the patellofemoral joint.

arm and body, with one hand on the tibia and one hand on the femur. The two hands can then create a medial to lateral or lateral to medial stress action (Figs. 6-182 and 6-183).

Evaluate the patellofemoral articulation for medial to lateral glide (Fig. 6-184), lateral to medial glide (Fig. 6-185), superior to inferior glide (Fig. 6-186), and inferior to superior glide (Fig. 6-187) with the patient lying supine and the involved leg straight in passive knee extension. Contact the borders of the patella with both thumbs and apply a stress to the patella medial to lateral, lateral to medial, superior to inferior and inferior to superior, feeling for a comparative amount of movement from side to side as well as a springing quality of movement.

Evaluate anterior to posterior and posterior to anterior glide of the tibio-fibular articulation with the patient supine with the affected knee bent to 90 degrees and the foot flat on the table. Either kneel or sit on the patient's

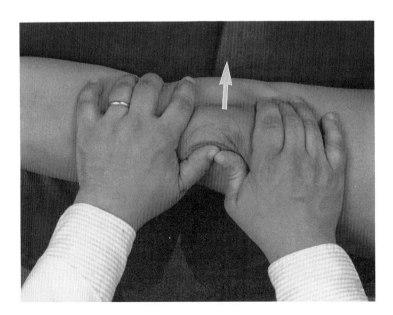

Figure 6.185 Assessment of lateral to medial glide of the patellofemoral joint.

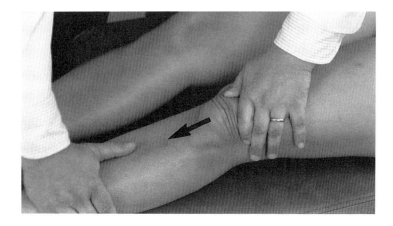

Figure 6.186 Assessment of superior to inferior glide of the patellofemoral joint.

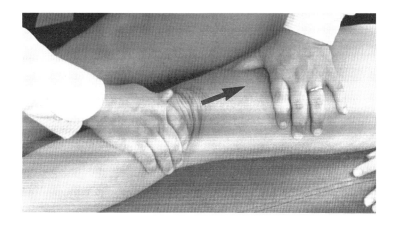

Figure 6.187 Assessment of inferior to superior glide of the patellofemoral joint.

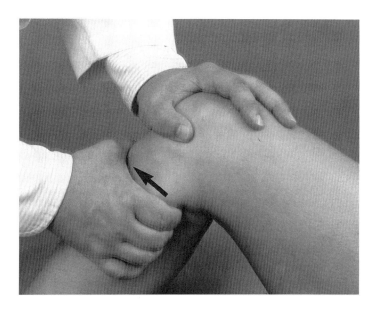

Figure 6.188 Assessment of posterior to anterior glide of the tibiofibular joint.

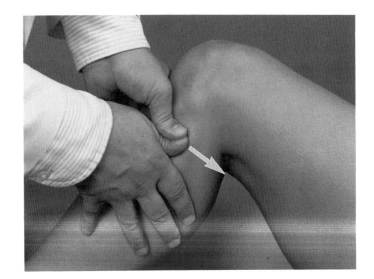

Figure 6.189 Assessment of anterior to posterior glide of the tibiofibular joint.

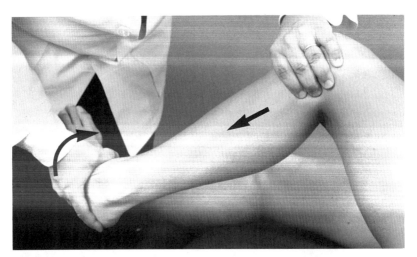

Figure 6.190 Assessment of superior to inferior glide of the tibiofibular joint.

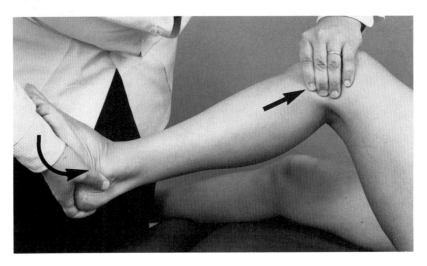

Figure 6.191 Assessment of inferior to superior glide of the tibiofibular joint.

foot to stabilize it, and grasp the proximal fibula with the outside hand while stabilizing the proximal tibia with the inside hand. Then stress the fibula, posterior to anterior and anterior to posterior, looking for a springing end feel (Figs. 6-188 and 6-189).

Perform inferior to superior and superior to inferior glide of the tibiofibular articulation with the patient supine with the affected leg straight and the knee in the relaxed extension. Use a digital contact of the cephalad hand to palpate the proximal fibular while grasping the patient's foot with your caudal hand. Then passively invert (with plantar flexion) and evert (with dorsiflexion) the patient's ankle while palpating for the fibula to move it superiorly and inferiorly (Figs. 6-190 and 6-191).

Adjustive Techniques

Femorotibial distraction (Fig. 6-192)

IND: General mobilization of the femorotibial joint, compressive joint injury, generalized knee pain, restricted active ranges of motion, and loss of long axis distraction accessory movements.

PP: The patient is supine with the involved leg abducted beyond the edge of the adjusting table.

DP: Straddle the patient's involved leg, grasping the patient's distal tibia above the malleoli with your knees. If the adjusting table has an elevating pelvic piece, raise it to form a ledge for the patient's buttocks.

SCP: Proximal tibia.

CP: Use both hands to grasp the proximal tibia.

VEC: Long axis distraction.

P: Straighten your knees while simultaneously using your hands to pull the proximal tibia into a long axis distraction movement.

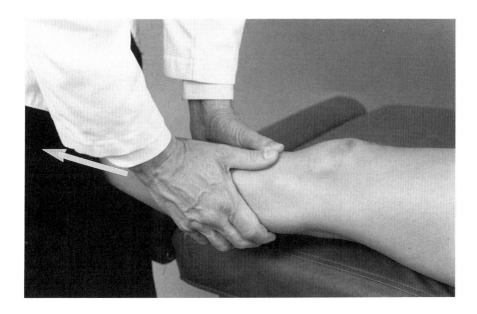

Figure 6.192 Adjustment for long axis distraction of the tibiofemoral joint.

Posterior to anterior tibial glide (Fig. 6-193)

IND: Anterior to posterior tibial trauma; posterior cruciate ligament damage; knee pain and, specifically, popliteal fossa tenderness; posterior displacement of the proximal tibia; and loss of posterior to anterior tibial glide.

PP: The patient lies prone with the involved leg flexed to just less than 90 degrees.

DP: Stand at the foot end of the table and bend over so that the patient's dorsum of the foot can rest on your inside shoulder.

SCP: Posterior aspect of the proximal tibia.

CP: With your inside hand, establish a knife-edge contact on the posterior aspect of the proximal tibia.

IH: Using your outside hand, reinforce the contact hand.

VEC: Posterior to anterior.

P: Use both hands to remove articular slack and thrust in the long axis

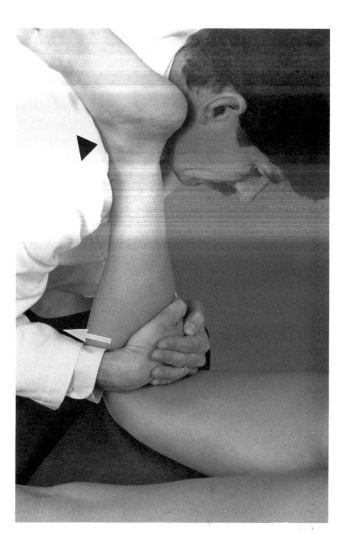

Figure 6.193 Adjustment for posterior to anterior glide of the tibiofemoral joint.

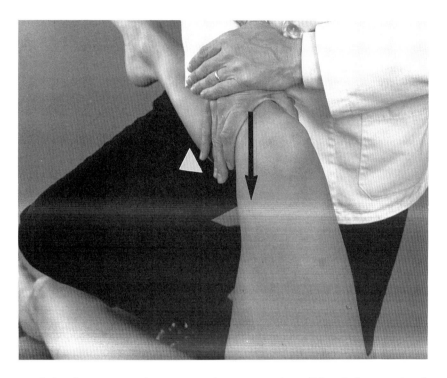

Figure 6.194 Adjustment for anterior to posterior glide of the tibiofemoral joint.

of the femur, creating a posterior to anterior glide of the proximal tibia.

Anterior to posterior tibial glide (Fig. 6-194)

IND: Posterior tibial trauma, anterior cruciate ligament damage, deep anterior and subpatellar tenderness, anterior displacement of the tibia, and loss of anterior to posterior tibial glide.

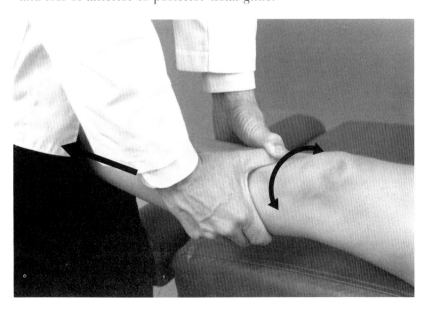

Figure 6.195 Adjustment for external and internal rotation of the tibiofemoral joint in the supine position.

PP: The patient is supine with the affected leg flexed to 90 degrees at the hip and the knee.

DP: Stand on the affected side with your caudal foot placed on the table such that the patient's affected leg will rest over your thigh.

SCP: Anterior aspect of the proximal tibia.

CP: Use your cephalad hand to apply a web contact over the anterior aspect of the proximal tibia.

IH: With your caudal hand, place a knife-edge contact, reinforcing the contact hand.

VEC: Anterior to posterior.

P: Use both hands to create an impulse thrust anterior to posterior on the proximal tibia.

Tibial rotation—supine (Fig. 6-195)

IND: Rotational trauma, capsular ligament pain, patellar tracking problems, rotational misalignment of the tibia, and loss of rotational accessory movements of the tibia.

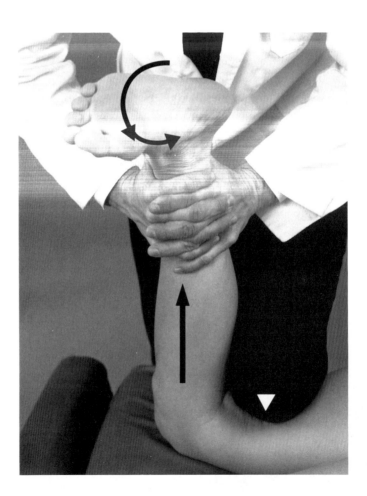

Figure 6.196 Adjustment for external rotation of the tibiofemoral joint in the prone position.

  PP: The patient is in supine position with the affected leg abducted off
       the edge of the table.
  DP: Stand facing the patient and straddling the affected leg, grasping
       the patient's ankle between the knees.
 SCP: Proximal tibia.
  CP: Using both hands, grasp the proximal tibia with the thumbs along
       the sides of the tibial tuberosity.
 VEC: Rotation.
    P: Extend your knees and hop footward to create some long axis distrac-
       tion while simultaneously twisting the proximal tibia, either internally
       or externally, with your hands.

Tibial rotation—prone (Fig. 6-196)

 IND: Rotational trauma, capsular ligament pain, patellar tracking prob-
       lems, rotational misalignment of the tibia, and loss of rotational
       accessory movements of the tibia.
  PP: The patient lies prone with the affected leg flexed to just less than
       90 degrees.
  DP: Stand at the side of the table on the affected side, placing your
       cephalad proximal tibia on the patient's distal femur.
 SCP: Distal tibia.
  CP: Using both hands, grasp the patient's distal tibia with fingers inter-
       laced.
 VEC: Rotation.
    P: Stabilize the patient's thigh on the table, use both hands to apply
       long axis distraction, and then impart an impulse thrust, creating
       internal or external rotation of the tibia.

Medial to lateral tibial glide (Fig. 6-197)

 IND: Lateral tibial trauma, medial collateral ligament pain, medially dis-
       placed tibia, loss of medial to lateral glide movement.
  PP: The patient is supine with the involved hip flexed to approximately
       45 degrees.
  DP: Stand on the side opposite the involved leg, grasping the distal tibia
       with your caudal arm and axilla.
 SCP: Medial aspect of the proximal tibia.
  CP: With your cephalad hand, establish a pisiform–hypothenar contact
       on the medial aspect of the proximal tibia.
  IH: Move your caudal arm under the patient's tibia, and grasp the contact
       hand's wrist.
 VEC: Medial to lateral.
    P: Create articular tension by using your body on the distal tibia as a
       lever, pivoting against the contact hand. When all joint movement
       is removed, deliver a medial to lateral impulse thrust.

Lateral to medial tibial glide (Fig. 6-198)

 IND: Medial tibial trauma, lateral collateral ligament pain, lateral displace-
       ment of the tibia, and loss of lateral to medial tibial glide movement.

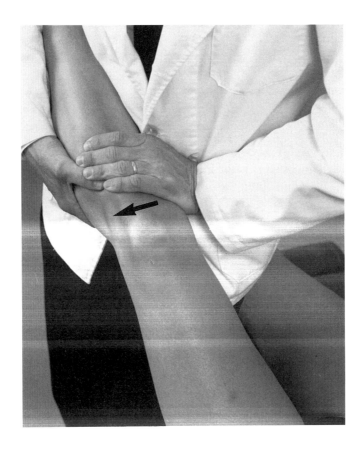

Figure 6.197 Adjustment for medial to lateral glide of the tibiofemoral joint.

PP: The patient is supine with the involved hip flexed to approximately 45 degrees.

DP: Stand on the involved side with your caudal arm grasping the patient's distal tibia in the axilla.

SCP: Lateral aspect of the proximal tibia.

CP: Using your cephalad hand, apply a pisiform–hyothenar contact on the lateral aspect of the proximal tibia.

IH: Move your caudal arm under the patient's tibia, and grasp the wrist of the contact hand.

VEC: Lateral to medial.

P: Using your contact hand as a pivot, tilt the distal tibia with your indifferent arm to remove articular slack, at which point, use the contact hand to deliver a lateral to medial impulse thrust to the proximal tibia.

Patellar dysfunction (Fig. 6-199)

IND: Vague aching pain about the knee, quadriceps tendonitis, chondromalacia patella, patellar tracking problems, and restricted patellar movements.

PP: The patient is supine with the involved knee in relaxed extension.

DP: Stand on the involved side.

SCP: Patella.

CP: Use both hands to apply thumb-web contacts over the borders of the patella.

VEC: Inferolateral, inferomedial, superolateral, and superomedial.

P: Depending on the direction of dysfunctional movement and involved soft tissues, give a thrust to the patella in a down and in, down and out, up and in, or up and out direction.

Posterior to anterior fibular glide—prone (Fig. 6-200)

IND: Lateral knee pain, shin splints, hamstring strain, trauma to the anterolateral aspect of the knee, posterior displaced fibula, and loss of posterior to anterior fibular movement.

PP: The patient lies prone with the knee flexed to just less than 90 degrees.

DP: Stand at the foot end of the table, flexed at the waist so the dorsum of the patient's foot can rest on your inside shoulder.

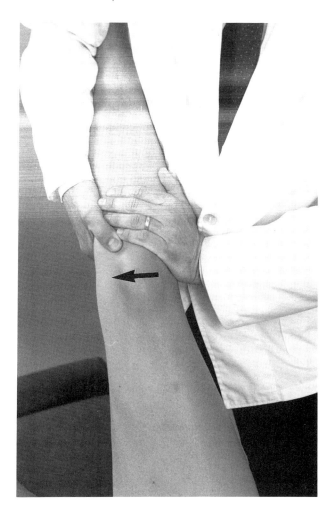

Figure 6.198 Adjustment for lateral to medial glide of the tibiofemoral joint.

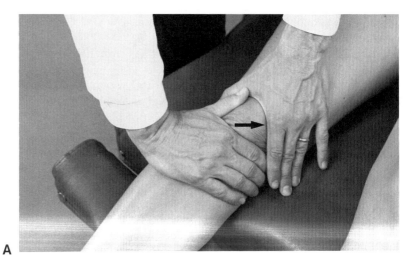

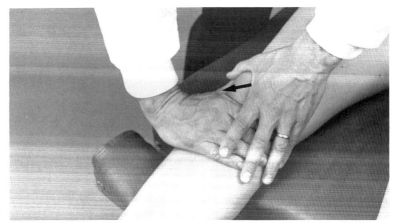

Figure 6.199 Adjustment for (**A**) superior and medial or (**B**) inferior and lateral glide of the patellofemoral joint.

SCP: Posterior aspect of the proximal fibula.
 CP: With your outside hand, establish a pisiform–hypothenar contact on the posterior aspect of the proximal fibula.
 IH: Use your inside hand to reinforce the contact.
VEC: Posterior to anterior.
  P: Using both hands, deliver a posterior to anterior impulse thrust to the proximal fibula.

Posterior to anterior fibular—supine (Fig. 6-201)

IND: Lateral knee pain, shin splints, hamstring strain, trauma to the anterolateral aspect of the knee, posterior displaced fibula, and loss of posterior to anterior fibular movement.
 PP: The patient is supine with the involved leg flexed at the hip and knee.
 DP: Stand on the involved side.

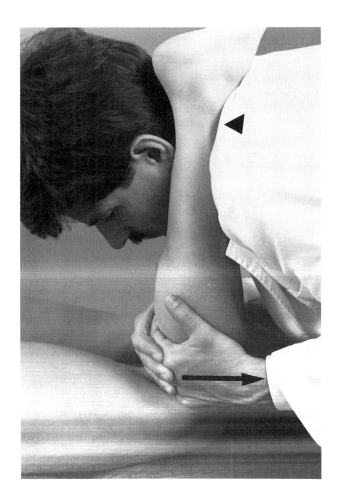

Figure 6.200 Adjustment for posterior to anterior glide of the tibiofibular joint in the prone position.

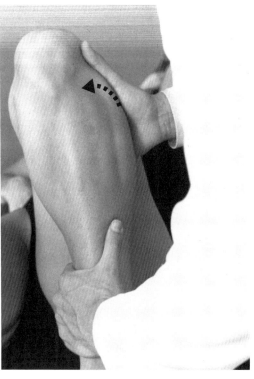

Figure 6.201 Adjustment for posterior to anterior glide of the tibiofibular joint in the supine position.

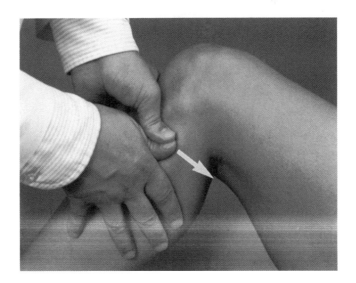

Figure 6.202 Adjustment for anterior to posterior glide of the tibiofibular joint.

SCP: Posterior aspect of the proximal fibula.
CP: Using your superior hand, apply the palmar aspect of the index contact on the posterior aspect of the proximal fibula.
IH: With your caudal hand, grasp the distal tibia.
VEC: Posterior to anterior.
P: Use your indifferent hand to flex the leg while giving a lifting motion with the contact hand, creating posterior to anterior movement of the proximal fibula.

Anterior to posterior fibular glide (Fig. 6-202)
IND: Lateral knee pain, shin splints, hamstring strain, trauma to the anterolateral aspect of the knee, posterior displaced fibula, and loss of posterior to anterior fibular movement.
PP: The patient is supine with the affected knee bent to 90 degrees and the foot flat on the table.
DP: Either kneel or sit on the patient's foot to stabilize it.
SCP: Anterior aspect of the proximal fibula.
CP: With your outside hand, establish a thumb or pisiform–hypothenar contact over the anterior aspect of the proximal fibula.
IH: With your inside hand, grasp the proximal tibia and reinforce your contact.
VEC: Anterior to posterior.
P: Using your indifferent hand, stabilize the tibia while using the contact hand to deliver an impulse thrust anterior to posterior to the proximal fibula.

Inferior to superior fibular glide (Fig. 6-203)
IND: Fibular collateral ligament pain, inversion ankle sprain, inferior displacement of the fibula, and loss of inferior to superior fibular movement.

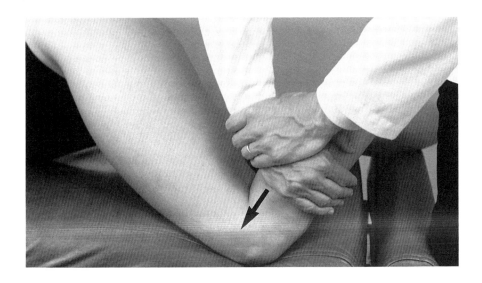

Figure 6.203 Adjustment for inferior to superior glide of the tibiofibular joint.

PP: The patient is side lying with the affected leg up and positioned posterior to the unaffected side. Both knees should be slightly flexed.

DP: Stand at the foot end of the table, such that the patient's involved foot rests against your thigh, maintaining the patient's ankle in eversion.

SCP: Anterior and inferior aspect of the proximal fibula.

CP: Using your anterior hand, establish a knife-edge contact on the anteroinferior aspect of the proximal fibular head.

IH: With your posterior hand, reinforce the contact hand.

VEC: Inferior to superior.

P: While maintaining the ankle in eversion, deliver a thrust to the proximal fibula in an inferior to superior direction. This movement can be achieved in a similar fashion by placing a thenar contact under the inferior aspect of the lateral malleolus, reinforcing the contact with the other hand, and delivering a thrust inferior to superior.

Superior to inferior fibular glide (Fig. 6-204)

IND: Lateral knee pain, eversion ankle sprain, superiorly displaced fibula, and loss of superior to inferior fibular movement.

PP: The patient is side lying with the involved side up and involved leg resting on the table behind the uninvolved leg, such that the ankle of the involved leg can hang in inversion off the edge of the adjusting table.

DP: Stand at the side of the table behind the patient, facing footward.

SCP: Posterior and superior aspect of the proximal fibula.

CP: With your outside hand, establish a knife-edge contact over the posterosuperior aspect of the proximal fibula.

IH: Using your inside hand, reinforce the contact hand.

VEC: Superior to inferior.

P: Using both hands, apply a superior to inferior impulse thrust to the fibular head.

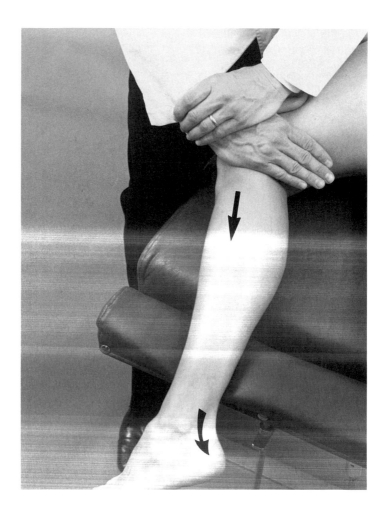

Figure 6.204 Adjustment for superior to inferior glide of the tibiofibular joint.

ANKLE AND FOOT

The ankle and foot can be discussed together because they are intimate components of a very intricately functioning unit. Together, they make up a significant component in a kinetic chain responsible for propulsion and balance. These joints may be viewed as initial supports for the musculoskeletal frame as they form the base on which all other osseous and muscular mechanisms reside. To the contrary, these joints may also be viewed as a *terminal segment,* in that they must translate and carry out the messages from the central nervous system to the hip, knee, and, finally, ankle, and foot. This joint complex must attenuate weight-bearing forces, support and propel the body, and maintain equilibrium.[8] Certainly, this part of the lower extremity is subject to a multiplicity of traumatic and postural disorders, leading to numerous joint dysfunction syndromes.

Functional Anatomy

Osseous Structures

The distal tibia and fibula join with the talus to form a mortice-type hinge joint called the *talocrural joint*. The calcaneus, the largest tarsal bone, articulates with the talus, forming the subtalar joint. The navicular articulates with the talus proximally and cuneiforms distally. The cuboid articulates with the calcaneus proximally and with the fourth and fifth metatarsals distally (Fig. 6-205). It also articulates with the navicular and third cuneiform medially. The first, or medial cuneiform, articulates with the first metatarsal; the second, or intermediate cuneiform, articulates with the second metatarsal; and the third, or lateral cuneiform, articulates with the third metatarsal. Two phalanges complete the structure of the great toe, while three phalanges complete the bony structures of each of the other four toes.

The function of the tibia is to transmit most of the body weight to and from the foot, and though the fibula plays a very important role in ankle stability, it is not directly involved in the transmission of weight-bearing forces. Functionally, the talus serves as a link between the leg and the foot.

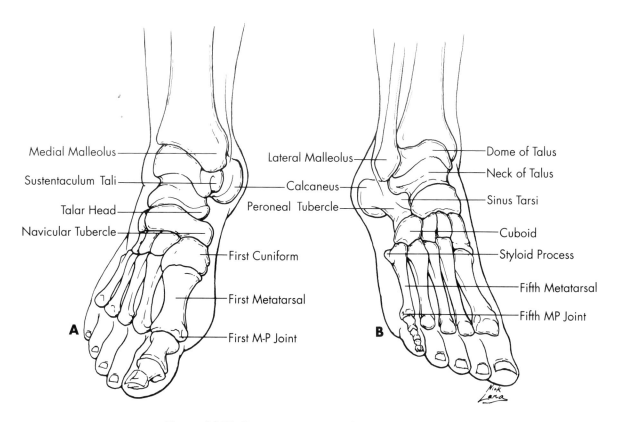

Figure 6.205 Osseous structures of the foot and ankle.

Ligamentous Structures

Although many ligaments and joint capsules are associated with the foot and the ankle, some are more important to localize, palpate, and functionally understand (Figs. 6-206 to 6-208). The deltoid ligament, composed of four parts, provides medial stability to the ankle by attaching from the medial malleolus to the talus anteriorly and posteriorly, as well as to the navicular and calcaneus. Laterally, the ankle is secondarily stabilized by five fibular ligaments: the anterior and posterior tibiofibular, anterior and posterior talofibular, and calcaneofibular ligaments. The plantar calcaneonavicular (spring) ligament attaches from the sustentaculum tali to the navicular (Figure 6-209). The function of this ligament is to keep the medial aspect of the forefoot and hindfoot in apposition and, in so doing, help to maintain the arched configuration of the foot.

Musculature

Similar to the wrist, the muscles of the ankle are located in the calf. Posteriorly, the large gastrocsoleus muscle group attached from the femoral condyles, proximal fibula, and tibia to the calcaneus, providing plantar flexion of the ankle. The tendon of the tibialis posterior passes under the medial malleolus to attach to the plantar surfaces of the navicular, cuneiforms, the cuboid and second, third, and fourth metatarsals. As such, it serves primarily as an inverter and adductor, or supinator, of the foot. The flexor hallucis longus and flexor digitorum longus muscles also have tendons that pass

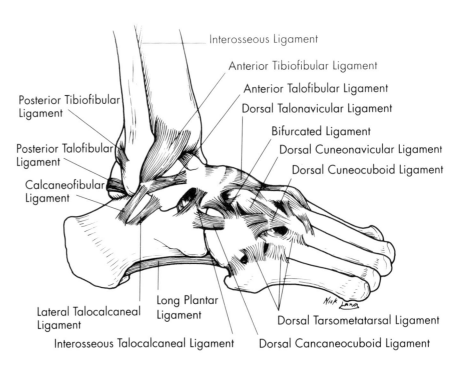

Interosseous Ligament

Anterior Tibiofibular Ligament

Anterior Talofibular Ligament

Dorsal Talonavicular Ligament

Bifurcated Ligament

Dorsal Cuneonavicular Ligament

Dorsal Cuneocuboid Ligament

Posterior Tibiofibular Ligament

Posterior Talofibular Ligament

Calcaneofibular Ligament

Lateral Talocalcaneal Ligament

Long Plantar Ligament

Interosseous Talocalcaneal Ligament

Dorsal Tarsometatarsal Ligament

Dorsal Cancaneocuboid Ligament

Figure 6.206 Ligaments on the lateral aspect of the right ankle.

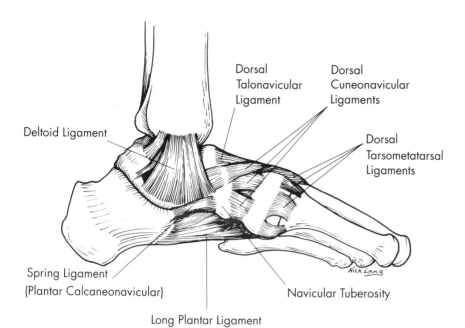

Deltoid Ligament

Dorsal Talonavicular Ligament

Dorsal Cuneonavicular Ligaments

Dorsal Tarsometatarsal Ligaments

Spring Ligament (Plantar Calcaneonavicular)

Navicular Tuberosity

Long Plantar Ligament

Figure 6.207 Ligaments on the medial aspect of the right ankle.

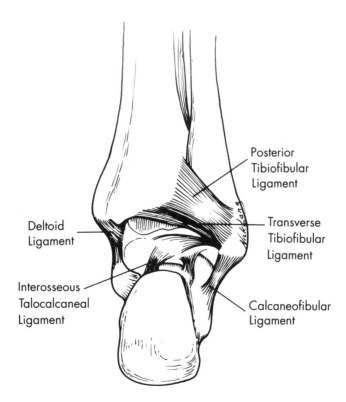

Deltoid Ligament

Posterior Tibiofibular Ligament

Transverse Tibiofibular Ligament

Interosseous Talocalcaneal Ligament

Calcaneofibular Ligament

Figure 6.208 Ligaments on the posterior aspect of the right ankle.

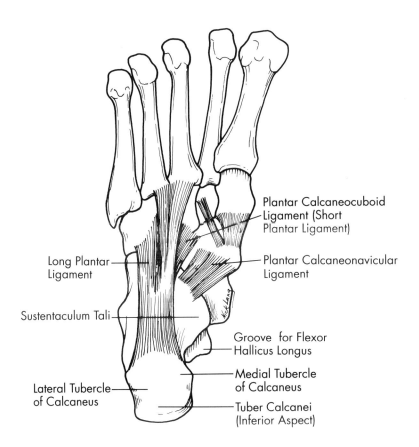

Plantar Calcaneocuboid Ligament (Short Plantar Ligament)

Plantar Calcaneonavicular Ligament

Long Plantar Ligament

Sustentaculum Tali

Groove for Flexor Hallicus Longus

Medial Tubercle of Calcaneus

Lateral Tubercle of Calcaneus

Tuber Calcanei (Inferior Aspect)

Figure 6.209 Ligaments on the plantar aspect of the left foot.

under the medial malleolus, with each inserting on the distal phalanx of each toe, thereby creating flexion of the toes. Anteriorly are the extensor digitorum longus, tibialis anterior, and extensor hallucis longus muscles. The extensor digitorum longus attaches to the dorsal surfaces of each of the distal phalanges, primarily extending the four toes, but also serving to dorsiflex, evert, and abduct the foot. The extensor hallucis longus is the primary extensor of the big toe. The tendon of the tibialis anterior passes over the ankle joint, across the medial side of the dorsum of the foot, and inserts into the medial and plantar surface of the medial cuneiform bone and the base of the first metatarsal. It functions as the primary dorsiflexor of the ankle, but because of its insertion, it will also invert and adduct the foot. On the lateral aspect is the peroneus muscle group. The tendons of the peroneus longus and brevis pass under the lateral malleolus and cross the cuboid to insert in the medial cuneiform and base of the first metatarsal. The chief action, then, of both peronei muscles is to evert the foot. The peroneus tertius is continuous with the origin of the extensor digitorum longus muscle; its tendon diverges laterally to insert into the dorsal surface

Table 6.26 Actions of the Muscles of the Foot and Ankle

Action	Muscles
Ankle plantar flexion	Gastrocnemius, soleus, plantaris
Ankle dorsiflexion	Extensor digitorum longus, tibialis anterior, peroneus tertius, extensor hallucis longus
Ankle inversion (adduction)	Tibialis posterior, tibialis anterior
Ankle eversion (abduction)	Extensor digitorum longus, peroneus longus and brevis, peroneus tertius
Toe flexion	Flexor digitorum longus, flexor hallucis longus
Toe extension	Extensor digitorum longus, extensor hallucis longus

of the base of the fifth metatarsal bone. It works with the extensor digitorum longus to dorsiflex, evert, and abduct the foot.

The ankle musculature can be divided into positional groups and divided according to the actions they perform (Table 6-26). The gastrocnemius, soleus, and plantaris muscles lie posteriorly and are responsible for plantar flexion of the foot and ankle. The extensor hallucis longus, extensor digitorum longus, peroneus tertius, and tibialis anterior muscles lie anteriorly and serve primarily to dorsiflex the foot and extend the toes. The peroneus longus and brevis muscles are situated laterally and pronate and evert the foot. The tibialis posterior, flexor digitorum longus, and flexor hallucis longus muscles are medial and function to invert the foot and flex the toes.

The intrinsic muscles of the foot lie in layers and generally perform the actions indicated by the muscles names.

Biomechanics

The functional biomechanics of the foot and ankle must include the ability to bear weight and allow flexible locomotion. The ankle joint is a uniplanar hinge joint, with talus motion occurring primarily in the sagittal plane about a transverse axis. The lateral side of the transverse axis is skewed posteriorly from the frontal plane (Fig. 6-210). The primary movement at the ankle mortice is dorsiflexion (20 to 30 degrees) and plantar flexion (30 to 50 degrees) (Table 6-27). Through the normal gait pattern, however, only 10 degrees of dorsiflexion and 20 degrees of plantar flexion are required.[16]

The subtalar joint formed between the talus and calcaneus is also a hinge-like joint. The axis of movement passes through all three cardinal planes of movement, thereby allowing movement to some extent in all three planes. Movement of this joint, then, includes the complex movement of supination and pronation of the calcaneus on the talus. Supination is a combination of inversion, adduction, and plantar flexion, while pronation is a combination

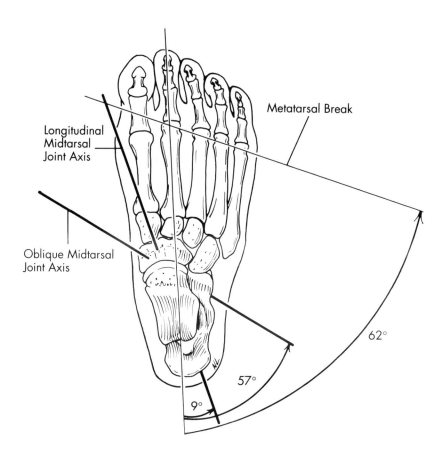

Figure 6.210 Dorsiflexion and plantar flexion in the foot and ankle occur around an oblique axis, while eversion and inversion occur around the longitudinal axis (Modified from Wadsworth,[8] with permission.)

of eversion, abduction, and dorsiflexion (Fig. 6-211). The subtalar joint has the important function to absorb shock at heel strike and rotation of the lower extremity in the transverse plane during the stance phase of gait.

The transverse or midtarsal joint is composed of the talonavicular and calcaneal cuboid articulations. The amount of movement occurring at these joints, which function in unison, depends on whether the foot is in pronation or supination. The supinated position creates a divergence of the axes of

Table 6.27 Arthrokinematic and Osteokinematic Movements of the Ankle and Foot Joints

Osteokinematic Movements (Degrees)		Arthrokinematic Movements
Ankle dorsiflexion	20	Roll and glide
Ankle plantar flexion	50	Roll and glide
Subtalar inversion	5	Roll and glide
Subtalar eversion	5	Roll and glide
Forefoot abduction	10	Roll and glide
Forefoot abduction	10	Roll and glide

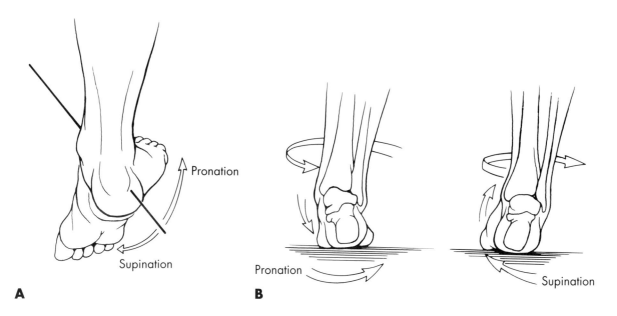

Figure 6.211 Pronation and supination movements **(A)** in free swing action (open kinetic chain) and **(B)** with weight bearing (closed kinetic chain).

movement, which deceases the amount of movement, setting up a rigid bony structure necessary for stability at the heel–strike stage of gait. Pronation, on the other hand, allows for the axes of motion to become aligned, which allows for increased mobility and decreased stability. The ligaments that run on the plantar surface between these tarsal bones are an essential component for absorbing stress and maintaining the longitudinal arch. Table 6-28 identifies the close-packed and loose-packed positions for the ankle and toe joints.

The individual tarsal joints, metatarsal-tarsal joints, metatarsophalangeal joints, and interphalangeal joints enhance the foot's stability or flexibility. They must provide a base for the stance phase, as well as the necessary hinges for flexion and extension during toe-off. Ligaments and tendons

Table 6.28 Close-Packed and Loose-Packed (Rest) Positions for the Ankle and Foot Joints

Joint	Close-Packed Position	Loose-Packed Position
Tibiotalar articulation	Full dorsiflexion	10 Degrees of plantar flexion midway beween full inversion and eversion
Toes	Full extension	Flexion

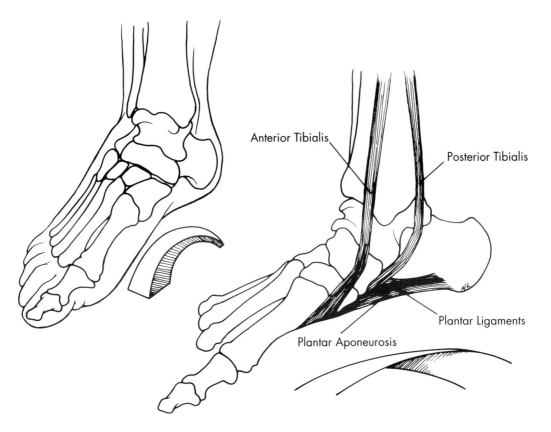

Figure 6.212 The longitudinal arch formed by the tibialis anterior and posterior.

further enhance stability and flexibility by maintaining arches in the foot (Fig. 6-212).

During the gait cycle, two main phases are described. The first occurs with the foot on the ground and is called the *stance phase*, while the second occurs when the foot is not contacting the ground, called the *swing phase* (Fig. 6-213). The stance phase is further divided into a contact component, midstance component, and a propulsive component. Movements of the leg and foot change through the different components. Pronation of the subtalar joint occurs initially at heel strike, while the tibia internally rotates. This is followed by supination of the subtalar joint and external rotation of the tibia through midstance and propulsive stages, as well as through the swing phase of gait. This creates a shifting area of weight bearing across the foot, starting from the posterolateral aspect of the calcaneus and curving over to the first metatarsophalangeal joint. Abnormal supination or pronation of the subtalar joint will result in altered gait patterns, as well as weight-bearing stresses on the plantar surface of the foot.

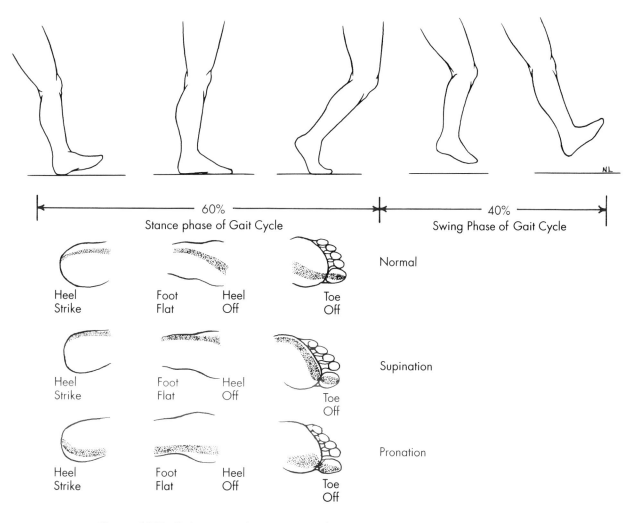

Figure 6.213 Gait pattern demonstrating that 60 percent of the gait is the stance phase, while 40 percent is the swing phase. Also shown is the pattern of weight bearing on the plantar surface of the foot normally and in pronation and supination.

Evaluation

With the concentrated stress that occurs to the foot and ankle during bipedal static and dynamic postures, these areas are susceptible to many injuries. Commonly, ankle injuries have an acute traumatic onset, whereas the foot is more likely to develop chronic and insidious onset disorders from stress overload. Pain and paresthesias arising from the lower lumbar or first sacral nerve roots should not be overlooked (Fig. 6-214). Most foot and ankle pain, however, arises from local disease or pathomechanic processes.

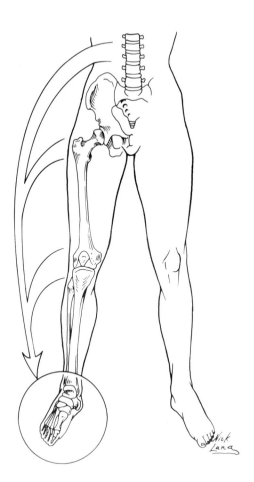

Figure 6.214 The low back, hip, and knee can refer pain to the ankle and foot area.

The most common traumatic injury to this area is the inversion sprain of the ankle, causing a separation to the lateral compartment with damage to the anterior talofibular ligament and possibly to the calcaneofibular ligament. Rarely does inversion occur alone, because usually, plantar flexion of the ankle, as well as external rotation of the leg also occur.

An eversion sprain involving trauma to the medial aspect of the ankle and affecting the deltoid ligament usually occurs when the foot is fixed in an excessive amount of pronation and the individual turns forcefully toward the opposite foot. The stress is applied first to the anterior tibiofibular ligament.

Shin splints refer to a generalized, deep aching, or sometimes, sharp pain along the tibia. It is considered an overuse or abuse syndrome occurring commonly as a result of running or jumping on a hard surface. This activity causes the talus to be driven upward into the mortice, forcing the tibia and fibula to separate. Stress to the interosseous membrane results and may cause a periostitis. Furthermore, activity of the anterior tibialis may result in fluid becoming entrapped within the fascial covering, creating a compartment syndrome.

Plantar fascitis results as a strain to the plantar fascia on the sole of the foot. This may be due to standing on hard surfaces, quick acceleration or deceleration, repeated shocks, standing on ladders, or long periods of pronation. A calcaneal heel spur may eventually occur as the fascitis continues or worsens. The fascia will pull the periosteum off the calcaneus, creating a painful periostitis, and bone will be laid down at the site of stress.

Hallux valgus is a lateral deviation of the big toe usually with a concomitant metatarsal varum. Improperly fitting footwear as well as an unstable and pronated foot have been blamed for this condition.

The evaluation of the foot and ankle begins with observation during static posture as well as gait for symmetry, arches, toe deformities, and soft tissue swelling. Inspect the plantar surface of the foot for signs of weight-bearing asymmetry in the form of callous formation. Identify osseous symmetry and pain production through static palpation of the distal tibia and fibula (malleoli), dome of the talus, navicular, cuboid, calcaneus, cuneiforms, metatarsals and phalanges.

Identify tone, texture, and tenderness changes through soft tissue palpation of the medial and lateral ligaments, Achilles tendon, plantar fascia, as well as the musculature that controls movement of the foot and ankle. Additionally, palpate the posterior tibial artery and dorsalis pedis artery.

Evaluate accessory joint movements for the foot and ankle articulations to determine the presence of joint dysfunction (Table 6-29).

Table 6.29 Accessory Joint Movements of the Foot and Ankle Joints

Joint	Movement
Tibiotalar joint	Long axis distraction Anterior to posterior glide Posterior to anterior glide Medial to lateral tilt (inversion) Lateral to medial tilt (eversion)
Subtalar joint	Anterior to posterior glide Posterior to anterior glide Medial to lateral tilt (inversion) Lateral to medial tilt (eversion)
Tarsals—cuboid, navicular, cuneiforms	Anterior to posterior glide Posterior to anterior glide
Intermetatarsal joints	Anterior to posterior glide Posterior to anterior glide
Metatarsophalangeal and interphalangeal joints	Long axis distraction Anterior to posterior glide Posterior to anterior glide Medial to lateral tilt (inversion) Lateral to medial tilt (eversion) Internal rotation External rotation

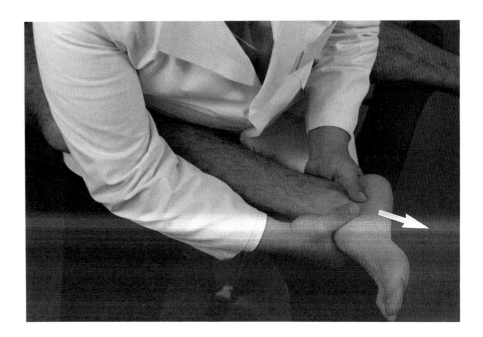

Figure 6.215 Assessment of long axis distraction of the tibiotalar joint.

Assess long axis distraction of the tibiotalar articulation or ankle mortice joint with the patient supine, knee flexed to about 90 degrees, and the hip flexed and abducted. Sit on the table between the patient's legs and face footward. Place web contacts over the dome of the talus and superior aspect of the calcaneus, applying a distraction force through both hands (Fig. 6-215).

Evaluate anterior to posterior and posterior to anterior glide of the ankle mortice joint with the patient supine and the hip and the knee both slightly flexed such that the calcaneus rests on the table. Stand at the side of the table and place a web contact of your cephalad hand over the anterior aspect of the distal tibia, while placing a web contact with your caudal hand over the anterior aspect of the dome of the talus. With both hands, grasp the respective structures and maintain the joint in its neutral position. Apply an anterior to posterior and posterior to anterior translational force through both hands, working in opposite directions, looking for a springing joint play movement (Fig. 6-216).

Assess medial to lateral and lateral to medial glide of the tibiotalar articulation with the patient supine. Stand at the foot of the table, facing headward. Grasp the dome of the talus with the fingers of both hands, using the thumbs to grasp under the plantar surface of the foot. Then stress the talus in a medial to lateral and lateral to medial direction, feeling for a springing joint play movement (Fig. 6-217).

Evaluate subtalar joint glide with the patient lying in the prone position and the knee flexed to approximately 60 degrees. Stand at the foot of the table, facing headward with the plantar surface of the patient's toes resting against your abdomen. Then grasp the calcaneus with palmar contacts while interlacing your fingers in a "praying-hands" position. Use both hands to

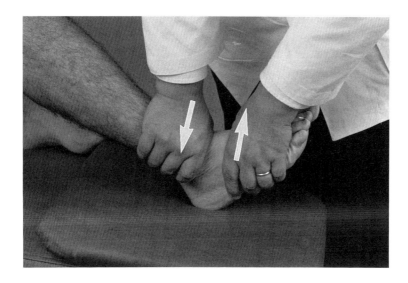

Figure 6.216 Assessment of anterior to posterior and posterior to anterior glide of the tibiotalar joint.

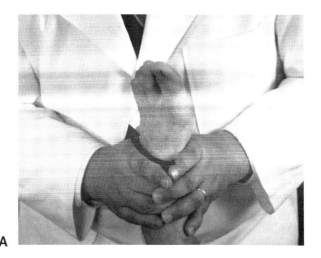

A

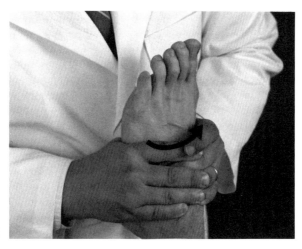

B

Figure 6.217 Assessment of (**A**) medial to lateral and (**B**) lateral to medial glide of the tibiotalar joint.

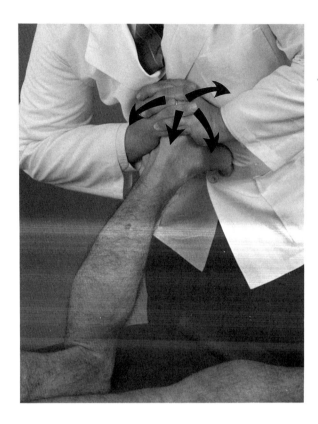

Figure 6.218 Assessment of anterior to posterior, posterior to anterior, medial to lateral, and lateral to medial glide of the subtalar joint.

create anterior to posterior and posterior to anterior glide, as well as medial to lateral and lateral to medial glide movements (Fig. 6-218).

Perform anterior to posterior and posterior to anterior glide of the navicular, cuboid, and cuneiforms by grasping the specific tarsal bone while stabilizing the proximal tarsal and creating an anterior to posterior and posterior to anterior glide movement (Fig. 6-219).

Perform anterior to posterior and posterior to anterior shear of the intermetatarsals by grasping adjacent metatarsals with each hand and creating an anterior to posterior and posterior to anterior shear (Fig. 6-220).

Evaluate the metatarsophalangeal and interphalangeal joints for anterior to posterior and posterior to anterior glide, medial to lateral and lateral to medial glide, axial rotation, and long axis distraction by grasping the metatarsals with one hand for stabilization and placing the specific phalanx between the index and middle fingers of the other hand (Fig. 6-221).

Adjustive Techniques

Long axis distraction (Fig. 6-222)

IND: Generalized ankle pain, generalized joint hypomobility, postacute or subacute inversion sprain, free adhesions in the ankle mortice, and loss of long axis distraction joint play movement.

PP: The patient is supine on the table with the pelvic section raised and the buttocks resting against the raised pelvic piece.

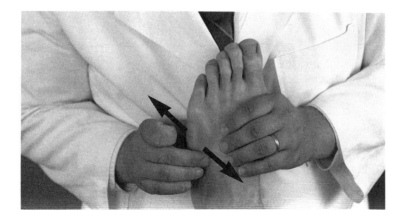

Figure 6.219 Assessment of anterior to posterior and posterior to anterior glide of the cuboid (same procedure used for the navicular and cuneiforms).

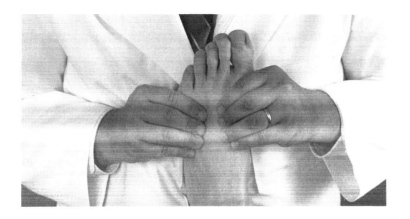

Figure 6.220 Assessment of anterior to posterior and posterior to anterior shear between the metatarsals.

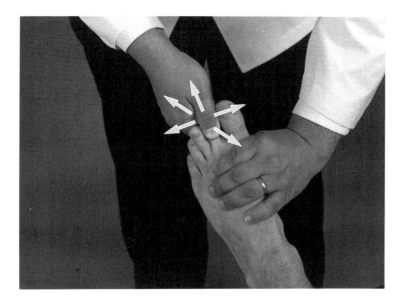

Figure 6.221 Assessment of long axis distraction, internal and external rotation, anterior to posterior, posterior to anterior, lateral to medial, and medial to lateral glide of the metatarsophalangeal joints (same procedure for the interphalangeal joints).

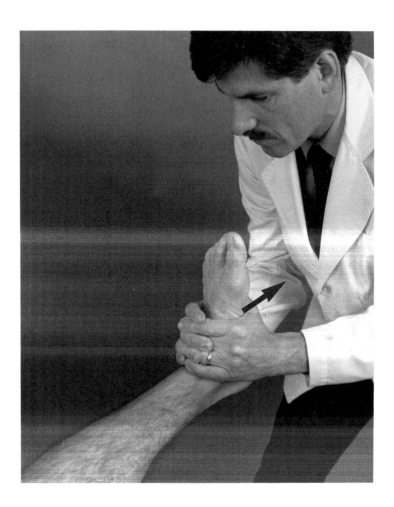

Figure 6.222 Adjustment for long axis distraction of the tibiotalar joint.

DP: Stand at the foot end of the table, facing cephalad.
SCP: Dome of the talus.
CP: Use either hand to apply proximal interphalangeal contact with the middle finger over the dome of the talus.
IH: With your other hand, use a middle-finger contact over the contact hand to reinforce it. With the thumbs of both hands, grasp the plantar surface of the foot.
VEC: Long axis distraction.
P: Maintain the ankle in dorsiflexion, and apply a long axis distraction with both hands. To induce subtalar long axis distraction, move the knife-edge or web contact of your indifferent hand to the posterior superior aspect of the calcaneus.

Anterior to posterior glide—tibiotalar joint (Fig. 6-223)

IND: Decreased dorsiflexion, anterior joint pain on dorsiflexion, loss of anterior to posterior glide, and anterior misalignment of the talus.
PP: The patient is supine on the table with the heel just off the end of the table.

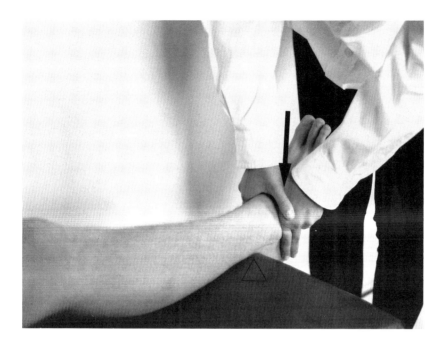

Figure 6.223 Adjustment for anterior to posterior glide of the tibiotalar joint.

DP: Stand at the foot end of the table, facing headward.
SCP: Dome of the talus.
CP: With your outside hand, establish a web contact over the dome of the talus, grasping the foot with your thumb and fingers.
IH: With your other hand, either reinforce the contact hand or grasp the distal tibia for stabilization.
VEC: Anterior to posterior.
P: Apply an anterior to posterior translational thrust to the talus.

Posterior to anterior glide—tibiotalar joint (Fig. 6-224)

IND: Decreased plantar flexion, ankle pain on plantar flexion, posterior misalignment of the talus, and loss of posterior to anterior glide movement.
PP: The patient lies prone, positioned with the distal tibia at the edge of the table.
DP: Stand at the foot end of the table, at the side of the table facing the side of involvement.
SCP: Posterior aspect of the talus.
CP: With your caudal hand, establish a web contact over the posterior aspect of the talus.
IH: With your cephalad hand, grasp the distal tibia for stabilization.
VEC: Posterior to anterior.
P: With your contact hand, apply a thrust, creating posterior to anterior glide of the talus.

Lateral to medial or medial to lateral glide—tibiotalar joint (Fig. 6-225)

IND: Palpable pain over the lateral collateral ligament, perceived pain anterior to the lateral malleolus, inversion ankle sprain, palpable

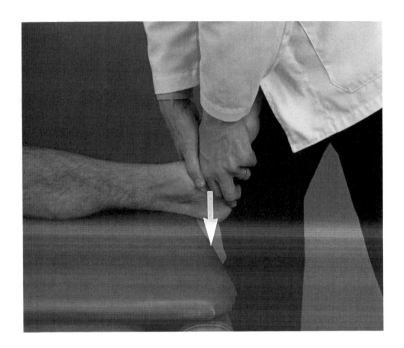

Figure 6.224 Adjustment for posterior to anterior glide of the tibiotalar joint.

pain in the deltoid ligament, eversion ankle sprain, a laterally or medially displaced proximal talus, and loss of medial or lateral glide at the tibiotalar articulation.

PP: The patient is supine with the legs straight and the foot off the end of the table.

DP: Stand at the foot end of the table, facing headward.

SCP: Dome of the talus.

CP: For everting, use your inside hand to establish a middle finger distal interphalangeal contact over the dome of the talus, drawing tissue and articular slack lateral to medial. For inverting, use your outside hand to apply the middle finger contact over the dome of the talus, drawing tissue and medial slack medial to lateral.

IH: With your other hand, grasp the posterior aspect of the calcaneus.

VEC: Lateral to medial or medial to lateral.

P: Use both hands to distract in the long axis and give a thrust, drawing the dome of the talus lateral to medial or medial to lateral.

Tibiotalar distraction (Fig. 6-226)

IND: Generalized ankle pain, generalized joint hypomobility, postacute or subacute inversion sprain, free adhesions in the ankle mortice and subtalar joint, and loss of long axis distraction joint play movement.

PP: The patient is supine on the table with the pelvic section raised and the buttocks resting against the raised pelvic piece.

DP: Stand at the foot end of the table, facing the affected ankle.

SCP: Dome of the talus.

CP: Using your cephalad hand, establish a web contact over the dome of the talus with the forearm along the line of the tibia.

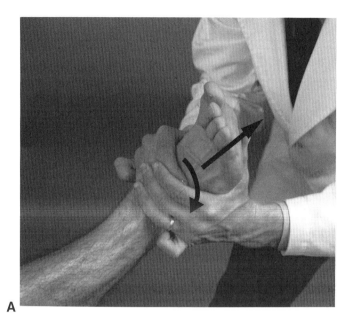

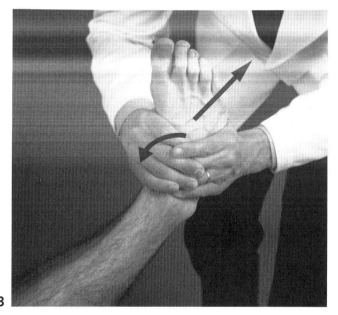

Figure 6.225 Adjustment for
(**A**) lateral to medial and (**B**)
medial to lateral glide of
the tibiotalar joint.

IH: With your caudal hand, grasp the calcaneus while applying a web
     contact over the superior aspect of the calcaneus.

VC: Long axis distraction.

  P: Use both hands to deliver an impulse thrust in the long axis of the
     tibia. Medial to lateral glide (inversion) or lateral to medial glide
     (eversion) can be produced as well.

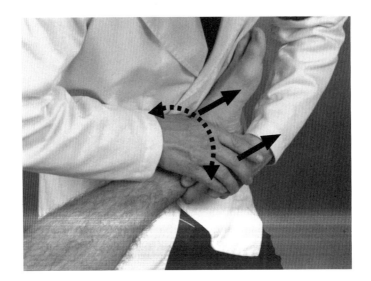

Figure 6.226 Distraction of the tibiotalar joint, which can combine either inversion or eversion.

Subtalar distraction (Fig. 6-227)

IND: Subtalar discomfort, subtalar hypomobility, heel pain, painful inversion or eversion, and plantar fascitis.

PP: The patient lies prone with the dorsum of the foot resting on the edge of the table, maintaining the ankle in plantar flexion.

DP: Stand on the affected side, facing footward in a lunge position.

SCP: Posterior and superior aspect of the calcaneus.

CP: With your cephalad hand, establish a calcaneal contact on the posterior superior aspect of the calcaneus.

IH: With your caudal hand, reinforce the contact hand.

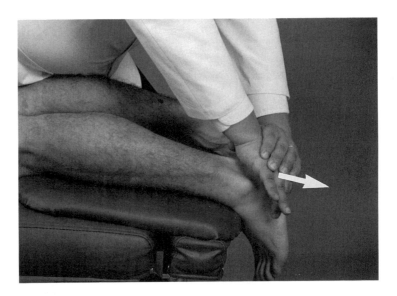

Figure 6.227 Adjustment distraction of the subtalar joint.

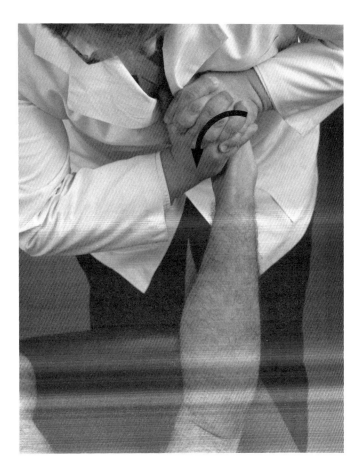

VEC: Distraction.
   P: Use both hands to deliver a thrust footward, drawing the calcaneus away from the talus.

Subtalar glide (Fig. 6-228)

IND: Subtalar discomfort, subtalar hypomobility, heel pain, painful inversion or eversion, and plantar fascitis.
 PP: The patient lies prone with the knee flexed to about 45 degrees.
 DP: Stand at the foot end of the table, facing headward such that the plantar aspect of the patient's foot can rest against your abdomen.
SCP: Calcaneus.
 CP: With both hands, grasp the calcaneus, interlacing the fingers in a "praying-hands" position.
VEC: Anterior to posterior; medial to lateral.
  P: While stabilizing the patient's foot against your abdomen, the calcaneus can be moved medially, laterally, anteriorly, or posteriorly.

Plantar to dorsal glide—cuboid (Fig. 6-229)

IND: Lateral longitudinal arch pain, an inferior misaligned cuboid, loss of plantar to dorsal movement of the cuboid.

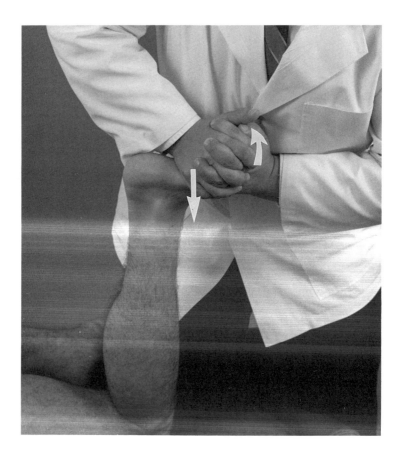

Figure 6.229 Adjustment for plantar to dorsal glide of the cuboid.

PP: The patient lies in the prone position with the knee bent to 90 degrees.

DP: Stand between the patient's legs, facing the affected side at its medial aspect.

SCP: Plantar aspect of the cuboid.

CP: Use your cephalad hand to apply a pisiform contact over the plantar aspect of the cuboid, wrapping your fingers around the lateral aspect of the foot.

IH: With your caudal hand, cradle the dorsum of the foot and/or interlace the fingers with the contact hand.

VEC: Plantar to dorsal.

P: Use your indifferent hand to accentuate the longitudinal arch against the pressure applied to the plantar surface of the cuboid. Then give a thrust through the contact hand in a plantar to dorsal direction on the cuboid.

Plantar to dorsal glide—navicular (Fig. 6-230)

IND: Medial longitudinal arch pain, excessive pronation, inferior misalignment of the navicular, and loss of plantar to dorsal accessory movement.

PP: The patient lies prone with the knee bent to 90 degrees.

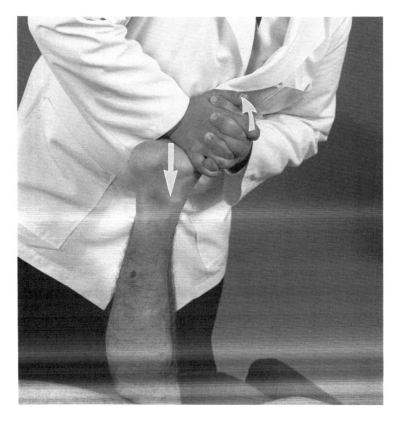

Figure 6.230 Adjustment for plantar to dorsal glide of the navicular.

DP: Stand at the affected side, facing the lateral aspect of the foot.

SCP: Plantar aspect of the navicular.

CP: With your cephalad hand, establish a pisiform contact over the plantar aspect of the navicular, wrapping your fingers around the medial aspect of the foot.

IH: With your caudal hand, cradle the dorsum of the foot and/or interlace fingers with the contact hand.

VEC: Plantar to dorsal.

P: Using your indifferent hand, increase the longitudinal arch against the pressure applied to the navicular while applying a plantar to dorsal thrust to the navicular.

Plantar to dorsal glide—cuneiform (Fig. 6-231)

IND: Palpable arch pain, foot fatigue, ankle sprain, plantar misalignment of the cuneiforms, and loss of plantar to dorsal accessory joint movement of the cuneiforms.

PP: The patient lies prone with the knee flexed to about 45 degrees.

DP: Stand at the foot end of the table facing headward.

SCP: Plantar aspect of a cuneiform.

CP: Use your inside hand to apply a thumb contact over the plantar aspect of the cuneiform, wrapping your fingers around the dorsum of the foot.

IH: With your outside hand's thumb, reinforce the contact.

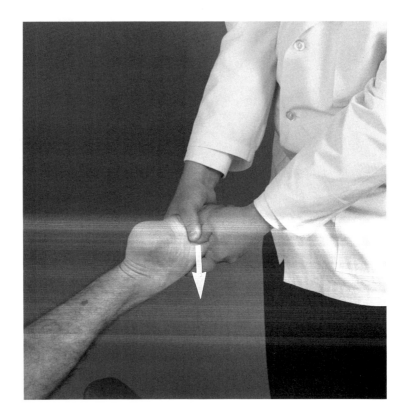

Figure 6.231 Adjustment for plantar to dorsal glide of the first cuneiform.

VEC: Plantar to dorsal.
  P: With both thumbs, deliver a plantar to dorsal snapping type thrust, being careful not to take the ankle into complete plantar flexion. This procedure can also be used for the navicular and cuboid.

Dorsal to plantar glide—tarsal push (Fig. 6-232)

IND: Pain at the anterior aspect of the foot and ankle, longitudinal arch pain, dorsally misaligned tarsal bone, and loss of dorsal to plantar accessory joint movement.
 PP: The patient is supine with the knee and hip flexed so that the plantar aspect of the foot rests on the table.
 DP: Stand at the foot of the table, facing headward.
SCP: Dorsal aspect of a tarsal bone (cuboid, navicular, cuneiforms).
 CP: Use either hand to establish a pisiform contact over the dorsal aspect of the involved tarsal bone.
 IH: With your other hand, reinforce the contact.
VEC: Dorsal to plantar.
  P: Deliver a very quick, impulse or recoil-type thrust, dorsal to plantar. A mechanical drop section can be used to enhance this procedure.

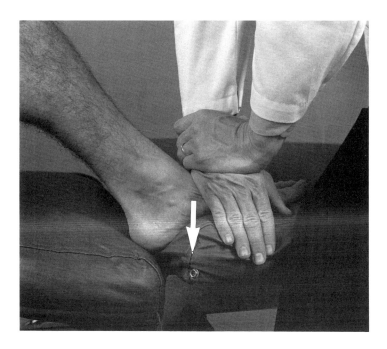

Figure 6.232 Adjustment for dorsal to plantar glide of the tarsals and the navicular shown.

Dorsal to plantar glide—tarsal pull (Fig. 6-233)

IND: Pain at the anterior aspect of the foot and ankle, longitudinal arch pain, dorsally misaligned tarsal bone, and loss of dorsal to plantar accessory joint movement.

PP: The patient is supine with the affected leg straight.

DP: Stand at the foot of the table, facing headward.

SCP: Dorsal aspect of a tarsal bone (cuboid, navicular, cuneiform).

CP: Use either hand to apply a middle-finger distal interphalangeal contact over the dorsal aspect of the affected tarsal.

IH: With your other hand, reinforce the contact, wrapping both hands around the plantar aspect of the foot with the thumbs just distal to the point of contact.

VEC: Dorsal to plantar.

P: Use both hands to apply a dorsal to palmar pressure, while the thumbs apply an opposite plantar to dorsal stress. Then apply a quick thrust through the contact hand, dorsal to plantar.

Plantar to dorsal metatarsal (Fig. 6-234)

IND: Metatarsalgia, foot fatigue, callous formation, plantar misalignment of the metatarsal, and loss of plantar to dorsal accessory joint movement of the metatarsal.

PP: The patient is supine with the leg straight and resting on the table.

DP: Stand at the foot of the table, facing headward.

SCP: Plantar aspect of a metatarsal bone.

CP: Use your outside hand to apply a thumb contact over the plantar aspect of the affected metatarsal.

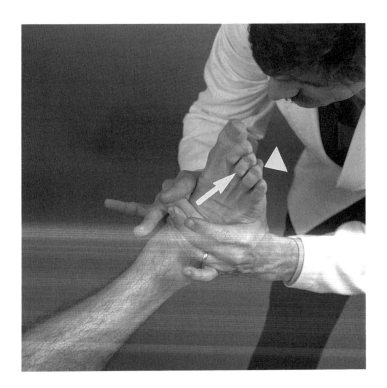

Figure 6.233 Adjustment for dorsal to plantar glide of the tarsals cuneiform shown.

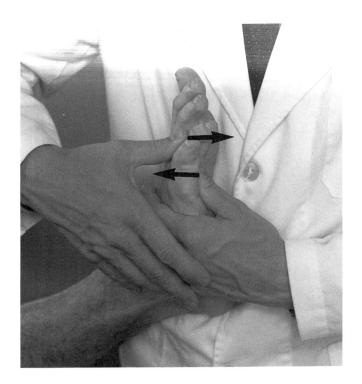

Figure 6.234 Adjustment for plantar to dorsal glide of the metatarsophalangeal joints.

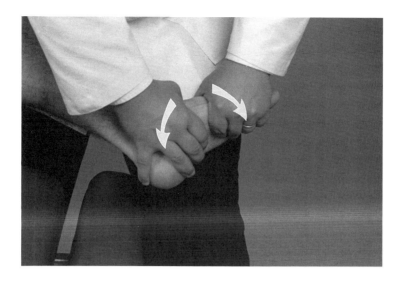

Figure 6.235 Distraction between the navicular, first cuneiform, and first metatarsal
joints.

IH: With your inside hand, establish a thumb contact over the dorsal aspect of the phalanx just distal to the metatarsal contact.

VEC: Plantar to dorsal.

P: Use both thumbs to create a simultaneous shear, emphasizing the plantar to dorsal component on the metatarsal.

Navicular—cuneiform—metatarsal distraction (Fig. 6-235)

IND: Metatarsal varum, medial arch pain, pes planus, and hypomobility of the medial tarsal articulations.

PP: The patient lies supine with the leg externally rotated and abducted off the table.

DP: Stand on the affected side, facing footward with the inside foot on the table, such that the patient's lateral aspect of the affected foot can rest on the doctor's thigh.

SCP: Medial aspect of the navicular.

CP: With your inside hand, establish a web contact over the medial aspect of the navicular.

IH: Use your outside hand to apply a web contact over the medial aspect of the proximal metatarsal.

VEC: Distraction.

P: Using your thigh as a fulcrum, thrust both hands away from one another, effectively separating the navicular from the first cuneiform and the first cuneiform from the proximal metatarsal.

Anterior to posterior and posterior to anterior glide, intermetatarsal joints (Fig. 6-236)

IND: Adhesions between metatarsals, mild degenerative arthritis, and restricted intermetatarsal glide movements.

PP: The patient is supine with the affected leg in slight flexion.

DP: Stand at the foot of the table, facing headward.

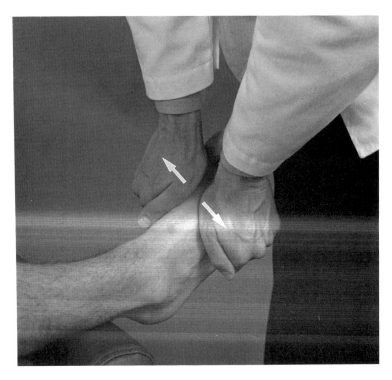

Figure 6.236 Adjustment for anterior to posterior and posterior to anterior glide between the metatarsals.

SCP: Metatarsal bone.
  CP: Establish a thumb/thenar contact on the palmar aspect of a metatarsal bone, and with your fingers, hold the same metatarsal shaft on the dorsal surface of your hand.
  IH: Make the same contacts on the adjacent metatarsal.
VEC: Anterior to posterior or posterior to anterior.
   P: Use both hands to create an anterior to posterior and posterior to anterior shear between the two metatarsals.

Medial to lateral glide of the first metatarsophalangeal joint (Fig. 6-237)

IND: Hallux valgus, bunions, pain at the medial aspect of the first metatarsophalangeal joint, and loss of medial to lateral movement of the first metatarsophalangeal joint.
  PP: The patient is supine with the affected foot off the end of the table.
  DP: Stand at the foot of the table, facing headward.
SCP: Proximal phalanx of the great toe.
  CP: With your outside hand, grasp the proximal phalanx between your index and middle finger.
  IH: Using your inside hand, apply a web contact over the medial aspect of the metatarsophalangeal joint.
VEC: Medial to lateral.
   P: With the contact hand, elevate the foot, using gravity to create long axis distraction at the metatarsophalangeal joint. Induce side to side rocking with the contact hand to mobilize the joint initially. A very shallow medial to lateral thrust can then be applied by the indifferent hand.

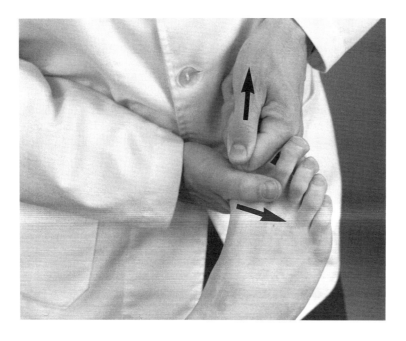

Figure 6.237 Adjustment for medial to lateral glide of the first metatarsophalangeal joint.

Phalangeal metatarsal and interphalangeal distraction (Fig. 6-238)

IND: Decreased or painful toe movement, foot fatigue, and loss of accessory joint movement in the phalangeal metatarsal or interphalangeal joints.

 PP: The patient is supine with the affected foot extending off the end of the table.

DP: Stand at the foot of the table, facing cephalad.

SCP: Individual phalanges.

 CP: Use either hand and loosely curl the index finger, applying its radial aspect against the plantar surface of the metatarsophalangeal joint. With the thumb, then grasp the phalanges from above (dorsal aspect) and distal to the index contact on the plantar surface.

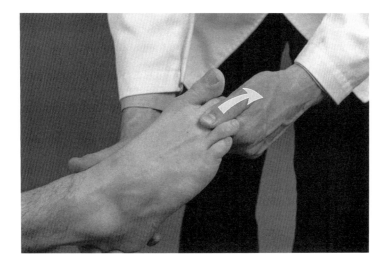

Figure 6.238 Adjustment for long axis distraction of the metatarsophalangeal joints (same procedure for the interphalangeal joints).

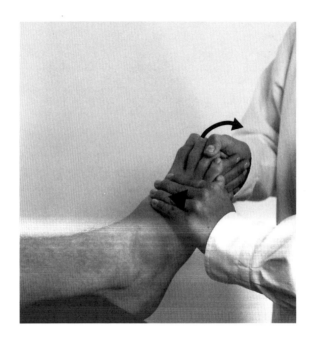

Figure 6.239 Adjustment for internal and external rotation, anterior to posterior, posterior to anterior, lateral to medial, medial to lateral glide of the metatarsophalangeal joints (same procedure for the interphalangeal joints).

IH: With the other hand, grasp the foot to stabilize it.
VEC: Long axis distraction.
P: With the thumb, draw the phalanges over the index contact, and apply a dorsal to plantar distractive thrust.

Toe joint technique: posterior to anterior and anterior to posterior glide, lateral to medial glide, axial rotation of the metatarsophalangeal and interphalangeal joints (Fig. 6-239).

IND: Toe pain, painful toe movement, mild degenerative arthritis, and lack of accessory joint movement in the toe joints.
PP: The patient is seated.
DP: Stand facing the patient.
SCP: Distal component of the affected joint.
CP: Grasp the distal member of the joint to be adjusted with either hand.
IH: With the other hand, grasp the proximal member of the joint being adjusted.
VEC: Anterior to posterior and posterior to anterior glide, lateral to medial glide, and internal and external rotation.
P: Apply an impulse thrust to the affected metatarsophalangeal or interphalangeal joint using anterior to posterior and posterior to anterior glide, lateral to medial glide, and internal and external rotation.

REFERENCES

1. Hertling D, Kessler RM: Management of Common Musculoskeletal Disorders: Physical Therapy Principles and Methods. 2nd Ed. JB Lippincott, Philadelphia, 1990

2. Pinto OF: A new structure related to temporomandibular joint and the middle ear. J Prosthet Dent 12:95, 1962

3. Ermshar CB: Anatomy and neurology. In Morgan DH, House LR, Hall WP et al (eds): Diseases of the Temporomandibular Apparatus. 2nd Ed. CV Mosby, St Louis, 1985

4. Farrar WB, McCarty WL: A Clinical Outline of the Temporomandibular Joint: Diagnosis and Treatment. Montgomery AL, Walter Printing, 1983

5. Curl D: Acute closed lock of the temporomandibular joint: manipulative paradigm and protocol. J Chiro Tech 3(1):13, 1991

6. Kraus SL (ed): TMJ Disorders: Management of the Craniomandibular Complex. Churchill Livingstone, New York, 1987

7. Schoenholtz F: Conservative management of temporomandibular joint dysfunction. J Am Chiro Assoc suppl. 12:57, 1978

8. Wadsworth CT: Manual Examination and Treatment of the Spine and Extremities. Williams & Wilkins, Baltimore, 1988

9. Kapandji IA: The Physiology of the Joints. Vol. 1, 2nd Ed. Churchill Livingstone, Edinburgh, 1970

10. Nordin M, Frankel VH: Basic Biomechanics of the Musculoskeletal System. 2nd Ed. Lea & Febiger, Philadelphia, 1989

11. Donnatelli R, Wooden MJ (eds): Orthopedic physical therapy. Churchill Livingstone, New York, 1989

12. Hoppenfeld S: Physical examination of the spine and extremities. Appleton-Century-Crofts, Norwalk, CT, 1976

13. Upton ARM, McComas AJ: The double crush hypothesis in nerve entrapment syndromes. Lancet 2:359, 1973

14. Kapandji IA: The Physiology of the Joints. Vol. 2, 2nd Ed. Churchill Livingstone, Edinburgh, 1970

15. Ferezy JS: Chiropractic management of meralgia paresthetica: a case report. J Chiro Tech 1(2):52, 1989

16. Kotwich JA: Biomechanics of the foot and ankle. Clin Sports Med 1:19, 1982

BIBLIOGRAPHY

The following citations represent sources for the majority of the evaluative procedures and techniques discussed in this chapter. Although some procedures have been modified in our presentation, most are described in one or more of these texts. They are presented in alphabetical order with chiropractic material first, followed by other professions.

1. Burns, JR: Extremities: Adjusting and Evaluation. Self-published, Davenport, IA, 1984

2. Christensen KD: Illustrated Manual of Common Extremity Adjustments. 2nd Ed. Self-published, Milwaukie, Oregon, 1980

3. Donatelli R, Wooden MJ (eds): Orthopedic Physical Therapy. Churchill Livingstone, New York, 1989

4. Gertler L: Illustrated Manual of Extra-vertebral Technic. 2nd Ed. Oak Bay Chiropractic, Oak Bay, California, 1978

5. Greenman PE: Principles of Manual Medicine. Williams & Wilkins, Baltimore, 1989

6. Hertling D, Kessler RM: Management of Common Musculoskeletal Disorders: Physical Therapy Principles and Methods. 2nd Ed. JB Lippincott, Philadelphia, 1990

7. Kaltenborn FM: Mobilization of the Extremity Joints—Examination and Basic Treatment Principles. 3rd Ed. Olaf-Norlis-Bokhandel, Oslo, Norway, 1980

8. Kirk CR, Lawrence DJ, Valvo NL: States Manual of Spinal, Pelvic and Extravertebral Technic. 2nd Ed. National College of Chiropractic, Lombard, IL, Waverly Press, Baltimore, 1985

9. Schafer RC, Faye LJ: Motion Palpation and Chiropractic Technic—Principles of Dynamic Chiropractic. Motion Palpation Institute, Huntington Beach, CA, 1989

10. Stierwalt DD: Extremity Adjusting. Self-published, Davenport, IA, 1976

11. Wadsworth CT: Manual Examination and Treatment of the Spine and Extremities. Williams & Wilkins, Baltimore, 1988

7
Research and Validation

Dana J. Lawrence

The future health and acceptance of the chiropractic profession rests in part on the use of research to validate and show reliable the procedures used by chiropractors in the specific management of clinical conditions. This entails examination not only of the adjustive procedures but also many of the diagnostic procedures; further, studies need be undertaken to delineate which conditions respond favorably to chiropractic care.

In one sense, research within the chiropractic profession is still very much in its infancy. Much of the early research performed by the profession was "lost to science," because it was published outside the normal scientific channels of indexed scientific journals. Before 1978, when the *Journal of Manipulative and Physiological Therapeutics* (JMPT) was created, very few citations concerned the chiropractic profession within indexed bioscientific data bases. In the eyes of the scientific community, research that is not indexed does not exist, because it is not retrievable from computerized data bases such as Index Medicus. When the JMPT became indexed, for the first time, research performed by the chiropractic research community could be reviewed by any interested party. Since it received indexation, the JMPT has accounted for over half of all indexed articles concerning the chiropractic profession.

The chiropractic profession has only recently begun to perform tests of reliability and validity, and there are far more reliability than validity tests. It is important to understand the difference. A procedure is said to be *reliable* if it gives similar results when applied more than once to the same object it is measuring or when it gives similar results when applied to a series of objects with similar qualities. For example, a motion palpation procedure is reliable if an examining doctor can repeatedly identify the same spinal fixation on an individual during a blinded trial. This is termed *intrarater reliability. Interrater reliability* occurs when a series of doctors all can locate the same spinal fixation using the same procedure in blinded trials. One way of looking at reliability is in terms of repeatability. Reliability tests within the chiropractic profession are commonly used to evaluate specific diagnostic procedures, such as the aforementioned motion palpation.

Validity is far more difficult to assess. *Validity* is the extent to which a measurement actually measures what it is said to measure. It is entirely possible for a reliable measurement to have no validity; the procedure is repeatable between examiners but does not measure what it is supposed to measure. Radiographic line-drawing procedures used by chiropractors potentially suffer from this problem. It may be possible to repeatedly draw a specific line on an x-ray film; concluding that the presence of an abnormality in a specific line is proof positive of the presence of subluxation is going too far. We have at present no way to categorically demonstrate the presence of subluxation, and thus, our reliable procedure may not have any validity. Any research using the presence of subluxation as a measure is potentially flawed in this manner; whether or not subluxation exists as a clinically measurable phenomenon is still under intense debate.

The controlled clinical trial represents potentially the most fruitful area for future direction in research. Performing clinical research trials will allow the chiropractic profession to better identify those conditions most amenable to chiropractic care and can also help to identify which of the many chiropractic procedures will produce the best response for a given condition. To date, virtually no clincial trials have been performed by the chiropractic profession for any condition; however, several are now under way, and the future bodes well.

Clinical trials examining the use of manipulation for managing conditions such as low back pain most certainly exist. Because the treatment methods used in these studies are at times identical to those used by chiropractors, extrapolation of the data to the chiropractic profession is certainly appropriate. In addition, clincial trials of manipulation for the treatment of other forms of orthopedic pain have been conducted, and a wide range of studies examines the use of manipulation in the diagnosis and management of many organic conditions. These latter experiments support the use of manipulation in the treatment of somatovisceral conditions.

Many reliability studies have investigated chiropractic diagnostic methodologies. Many studies have examined the reliability of motion palpation procedures and leg length mensuration techniques. Other studies, though fewer in number, have investigated the reliability of radiographic interpretation and line-drawing techniques. This chapter examines the work accomplished in these different areas of investigation.

CLINICAL TRIALS OF MANIPULATION FOR LOW BACK PAIN

Literature Review

In 1984, David Brunarski identified 50 clinical trials of spinal manipulation.[1] Brunarski's article, in essence a meta-analysis, attempted to determine if evidence within the scientific literature supported the contention that manipulative care both was effective for the treatment of painful neuromuscular conditions and was more effective than standard medical care. It also provided an excellent review of the literature.

Brunarski compiled data from all the articles mentioned in his review.[1] The work reported spanned more than 50 years and 8,000 patients. Most

Table 7.1 Criteria for a Strong Randomized Clinical Trial

1. A clearly stated hypothesis
2. Strict guidelines for the description of patient selection and inclusion and exclusion criteria
3. A sample size sufficient to achieve adequate clinical and statistical significance with case and power
4. Randomization allocation
5. Assessments that are blinded
6. A few, objective, quantitative, and statistically manageable outcomes
7. Precise treatment algorithms that may be replicated by subsequent studies
8. Long-term follow-up periods with as few dropouts and losses as possible
9. Data control and analysis by independent methodologists and statisticians
10. Results that are published in refereed journals.

(Adapted from Brunarski,[1] with permission.)

of the patients in these studies had suffered from acute bouts of pain, meaning that the pain had been present for less than 6 weeks. The most common method of measuring response to therapy was, as might be expected, percentage reduction in the subjective perception of pain. The improvement in the manipulated group averaged above 70 percent, while in the nonmanipulated group, it was 50 percent. Patients with chronic pain did not fare as well. These results need to be tempered by the fact that Brunarski pointed out various design flaws in many of the studies, rendering their conclusions weaker than these percentages might indicate. The full explanation of the various biases in the cited work can be found in Brunarski's article.[1] In conclusion, Brunarski listed 10 criteria he felt a randomized controlled trial needed to best demonstrate a significant finding. These are listed in Table 7.1. The interested reader may wish to apply these criteria to the articles discussed later in this chapter.

Meta-analysis was also performed by Ottenbacher and DiFabio.[2] Their intent was to reexamine the existing data on the efficacy of joint mobilization and manipulation as well as demonstrate the methods of quantitative reviewing of previously published data. Their initial data search retrieved 57 papers on the use of manipulation, but only 9 of those met the strict inclusion requirements for the review. As a result, the article analyzed 718 subjects from these tests.

Ottenbacher and DiFabio noted many interesting findings.[2] Studies in which random assignment was not used tended to show more favorable results than those that used a strict randomization process. Patients responded more favorably when the manipulation or mobilization was used in conjunction with other forms of treatment rather than when it was used as a stand-alone therapy. When patient response was measured right after therapy, results were quite favorable; they were less so when measured some time frame further away from therapy. The authors also showed a potential publication bias; articles published in English language journals outside the United States in general demonstrated more favorable results than those published within the United States. The authors called this "empirical favoritism" and felt that it might be a result of mobilization and manipulation receiving higher priority as a therapeutic option outside the United States.

The authors ultimately concluded that the studies showed some support for the use of manipulation to treat spinal pain, but owing to a combination of factors, a great deal more work needed to be done; one definitive article to resolve the issues was not realistic.[2]

DiFabio later published a second literature review on the clinical assessment of manipulation and mobilization of the lumbar spine.[3] That article examined both noncontrolled and controlled studies of manipulation. Many confounding factors help to muddy the waters concerning the results of the studies cited. One chief problem is that it is well known that a large portion of patients suffering from low back pain will spontaneously recover; it is quite difficult to factor into any research study the natural history of the low back patient. With this bias, it becomes hard to claim that the results noted are totally the result of therapy; obviously, this must be the case for the noncontrolled group. With a proper randomization of similar patients into a control and an experimental group, that particular bias is better handled. For the controlled studies, the major confounding issues revolve around experimental design and protocol. Not only randomization is important (so that both control and experimental groups are identical in terms of age, sex, symptoms, etc.); also critical is blind assessment of the outcome measure. The issue of placebo is also quite real; it is difficult to set an appropriate sham procedure to use in such studies, and so placebo can occur in both a positive and negative manner. DiFabio raised as many questions as he answered, if not more.

Research Reports

In a significant report, Waagen and colleagues performed the first double-blind clinical trial of chiropractic adjustment for the relief of low back pain.[1] They used a manual control group; *manual* in this case meaning that the control also had some sort of manual therapy, but one substantially different from the procedure used as the treatment technique.

Waagen et al. included 19 patients in the study, with 9 placed in the experimental group.[4] Patient status was assessed using a global index scale generated from eight different objective tests of function as well as a subjective measure using a Visual Analogue Scale (VAS). The VAS scores were measured both before and after adjustment. The control group received a sham adjustment procedure that simulated an adjustment of the low back by contacting the posterior superior iliac spines. The experimental group received a specific high-velocity adjustment directed to a lesion in the spine that had been determined by palpation, radiographic examination, and consultation. Data were analyzed using nonparametric tests to compare the ordinal changes in pain between the groups; these included the use of the Wilcoxen paired sample signed rank test and the Mann-Whitney U test.

When Waagen and co-workers examined the immediate results of therapy, the experimental patients had a significantly greater relief of pain than did the control group patients; both groups showed relief from pain when measured immediately after therapy. After 2 weeks of therapy, the experimental group exhibited a significant reduction in pain, but the control group now had a nonsignificant response. These results used the VAS as the outcome measure. Using the global index measure, which assessed primarily change in spinal mobility, the experimental group improved significantly when compared to the control group.[4]

These encouraging results are mitigated by the small sample size, but the importance of this report cannot be overemphasized. This represents the first true double-blind, controlled clinical trial of chiropractic adjustment for the therapy of low back pain.[4]

Hadler et al. found somewhat conflicting results.[5] They studied 54 patients randomly stratified into two groups, based on symptom duration. One group had suffered from symptoms for less than 2 weeks, while the second group had symptoms that had lasted longer than 4 weeks. Treatment outcome was assessed using the Roland-Morris questionnaire, which itself had been adapted from the much lengthier Sickness Impact Profile. Patients were either mobilized (which did not use a high-velocity thrust) or manipulated (which did).

The authors noted a difference between the groups receiving manipulation when compared to those who received only a mobilization, especially for those who had suffered for the longer period of time (greater than 4 weeks).[5] The patients who received manipulation achieved a 50 percent reduction in their Roland-Morris scores much more rapidly than those who received a mobilization. This was felt to be quite important, because alleviating the presence of back pain even by just a few days has major ramifications. The authors felt compelled to act cautiously with their results. Their study population was between the ages of 18 and 40 years, so the authors felt that the results might not be generalizable to different patient populations, especially older ones who may have other, confounding conditions. The protocol used in this study, however, could be used for other groups of patients.

Mathews et al. performed a trial that examined manipulation, traction, sclerosant, and epidural injections.[6] The patients in this study suffered from sciatica in addition to their low back pain. This single article reported on four different clinical trials. In the first part of the study, only the use of sclerosant injection was examined. The authors found no significant difference in the responses of patients who received the injection when compared to those receiving alternative therapies.

The second part of the article dealt with the use of manipulation.[6] The authors used a prospective, controlled, single-blind study design, which also subdivided the patients into groups that had a limited straight leg raise and those that did not. The third part examined the use of traction for back pain and compared it to the use of heat, finding no significant difference. The final part of the study examined epidural injection compared to injection of saline into the interspinous ligament.

The patient age range was 18 to 60 years.[6] Symptoms had occurred within the last 3 months (except for the trial using sclerosant; symptoms had to have been present for over 3 months). Ultimately, 513 patients were included in the study and were assigned to the various control or experimental groups. In the manipulation part of the study, the manipulation was given daily for

2 weeks. Different types of thrusts were given, depending on where pain occurred with spinal motion. Some patients might receive a rotational thrust, while others received a straight posteroanterior thrust. The control group received infra-red heat treatments three times per week.

Within 2 weeks, 62 percent of the experimental patients and 70 percent of the controls had recovered, forcing the authors to use survival data techniques to analyze an 18-day period.[6] The results of this analysis showed that the experimental group had a 10 percent better response rate than the controls. This was not found to be significant, because the numbers were small for such an analysis. In a second and larger repeat of the study, the recovery rate was 80 percent experimental versus 67 percent control, and the authors noted a nearly 30 percent better response in the manipulated group. Statistical significance was stronger here, because the numbers were much greater.

For patients with negative straight leg raise tests, daily examination showed that in the second to fifth day of therapy, over twice as many of the experimental group had recovered compared to control.[6] For those with positive signs, the response was even better, and by the second week a significant reduction in pain was seen overall. (The other components of the study will not be examined because they have no bearing on manipulation per se.)

Godfrey et al. performed a single-blind, randomized trial within a medical setting.[7] They based their initial design on some of the competing theories concerning the pathogenesis of low back pain, including the formation of scar tissue between the lamellae of the disc, muscular contracture at the involved joint, deformation of articular surfaces causing inhibited motion, and disc protrusion. They reasoned that because these causes were mechanical in nature, a mechanical correction might benefit for the patients. The study included 81 patients, most of whom had suffered from back pain for 3 to 7 days. The control therapy included massage and electrostimulation at a low level. Outcomes were assessed using scales that quantified a variety of symptoms and signs, including mobility, pain on palpation, and aggravation of the pain when coughing and that also examined activities of daily living and so forth. Much of the assessment procedure had previously been described by Maigne.[8]

Interestingly, the manipulations for this study were performed in part by a chiropractic physician.[7] Under analysis, both groups of patients improved quickly during the first 2 weeks; Godfrey et al. found no statistical significance between the two groups across all the scales used for assessment. The authors were careful to point out that the negative results may have been due to several different factors, such as the style of manipulation, the presence of type II error (false acceptance of the null hypothesis), placebo use, etc.

In a widely cited paper published in 1975, Doran and Newell performed a study with 456 subjects suffering from low back pain.[9] They assigned the patients to one of four groups: receiving either manipulation, a corset, analgesics, or a physiotherapeutic regimen. Outcomes were assessed using a pain questionnaire and doctor commentary, with reevaluations at 3 weeks, 3 months, and 3 years after therapy. Results noted some immediate improvement in the group receiving manipulation, but over a longer period of time, the four groups performed fairly equally (with the analgesic group lagging somewhat behind in effectiveness). Many criticisms have since been leveled at this paper, which may reduce its overall impact.

Evans and colleagues performed a trial using 32 patients suffering from back pain of at least 3 weeks' duration.[10] The patients received either manipulation or codeine (as the control). Evans et al. assessed the outcomes using several different parameters, including pain scores, an index that measured patient satisfaction with the therapy, radiographic measurement of flexion of the lower spine, and the amount of codeine ingested by the control patients. Here, there was a reduction of the pain suffered by the patients receiving manipulation, with the greatest reduction occurring during the first week of therapy and then gradually decreasing into the fourth week. There was also noted a concomitant increase in spinal flexion during the period when the manipulation was applied. Finally, again, the patients who responded best were noted to have suffered from the low back pain for the shortest period of time and, in this case, also tended to be somewhat older in age.

Other significant research papers have been published. Bergquist-Ullman and Larsson performed a study that compared manipulation, back school, and placebo.[11] Their results showed similar decreases in pain in all three groups at all the times assessed; sick days lost from work were also similar. Sims-Williams et al. noted that pain reduction and spinal motion improved in both their experimental and control groups; however, those patients who had suffered from shorter episodes of pain did report more of an improvement in symptomatology in the short term.[12] After 1 year, however, both groups were again similar in measures of improvement. A list of other articles discussing manipulation and low back pain can be found in the Suggested Readings List.

Implications of Research in Low Back Pain

The information generated by these various reports is confusing and contradictory. It is apparent that there is no single answer to the question concerning the best use of manipulation for low back pain. Certain trends do appear; patients who have suffered from short episodes of acute low back pain tend to show positive responses within the first few days or weeks of therapy using manipulation. More heartening is patient perception of these therapies. Cherkin and MacCornack showed that patients receiving care from chiropractors for low back pain were three times as likely to report that they were satisfied with the care they received when compared with a group receiving medical care from a health maintenance organization (at a ratio of 66 : 22 percent).[13] These patients were also satisfied with the information given them by their chiropractor and felt that their chiropractic doctor both cared about them and was confident and capable of handling their problem. Although Cherkin and MacCornack theorized that the reason for this may have more to do with the nature of the interaction between the chiropractor and the patient, in light of the preceding research, the answer may be more complicated.

One of the most significant trials of manipulation and low back pain is that of Meade and colleagues.[14] This trial, which lasted nearly 10 years, compared chiropractic care to outpatient care. The study included 741 patients, one of the largest such studies ever done. The authors' essential conclusions were that chiropractic care was significantly more effective than the other care, especially so for patients with chronic or severe pain. Surprisingly, in light of other studies showing that manipulation had its greatest effects early in care, the most significant results here were demonstrated nearly 2 years after initial care. Placebo was accounted for. The authors concluded that chiropractic must be given serious consideration in the British health-care system. This trial, although controversial and subject to certain design flaws, stands as the most significant clinical trial of chiropractic.

Great problems exist in attempting to determine the best use of manipulation not only for the treatment of low back pain but also any possible condition. In the case of low back pain, complicating factors include specificity of diagnosis (after all, there are a great many causes of low back pain; which are amenable to treatment?), the ability to correlate diagnostic criteria with clinical status, selecting the proper therapeutic option, and prognosis.[15] Recommendations have been made concerning how best to design clinical back pain trials. Bloch presented seven criteria that will assist in designing appropriate methodologies for these trials[16]:

1. Generalizability, bias, and noise
2. Study architecture
3. The population
4. The intervention
5. The outcome
6. Statistical considerations
7. Critical appraisal

Careful attention to these criteria when designing chiropractic clinical low back (or other) trials will enable the profession to better determine the best situations for use of manipulative procedures. The final question must always be, "What is best for the patient?"

CLINICAL TRIALS OF MANIPULATION FOR PAIN OTHER THAN LOW BACK PAIN

The body of literature regarding the use of manipulation for pain conditions outside the low back is less complete than for those discussing low back pain itself.

Barker presented a case of thoracic pain syndrome that was successfully managed using manipulation.[17] He collected data on 20 separate cases of thoracic disc syndrome, and using manipulative procedures originally described by Bourdillon,[18] claimed improvement in 18, with the other 2 made temporarily worse. He concluded that manipulation of the thoracic joints can benefit patients suffering from thoracic pain and that such tools should be made part of the typical medical therapeutic arsenal.

Molea et al. studied the effectiveness of manipulative techniques for treating postexercise muscle soreness.[19] The authors induced muscular soreness in the flexor muscles of the elbow of 27 otherwise healthy individuals. After waiting for the soreness to increase to a maximal point, they then treated the patients with one of three procedures: a muscle energy manipulative technique, a myofascial manipulative technique, or a placebo technique contacting the patient's occiput. The authors made no attempts at structural diagnosis. Design was single-blind. Pain measures were rated using a 4-point pain scale. In addition, range of motion measurements were made of the neck and upper extremities. The authors found no significant differences between the experimental and control groups.

Molea and co-workers viewed the induced postexercise muscle soreness as a corollary of somatic dysfunction as defined by the osteopathic profession.[19] With the soreness, alterations in joint and muscle function occur, as well as swelling, indicating involvement of vascular or lymphatic structures. The authors do note that there are some potential flaws in their research design. They used student physicians to administer the treatments; they also felt that the very method of measurement may subtly alter the measurement being made. They also studied a small population of patients.

The chiropractors Terrett and Vernon examined the effect of spinal manipulation on paraspinal cutaneous pain tolerance.[20] To perform this study, the authors had to construct a model of experimental pain, using three standardized criteria: a target tissue, a method of pain induction that could be measured using an interval scale; and, a treatment variable that acted as an independent variable on each subject. Here, the model developed used the paraspinal cutaneous tissue, electrical induction of pain, and spinal manipulation. They included 50 patients in the study. Pain was induced by a Siemans Neurotron stimulator. After current was applied to the patient's back, zones of most intense pain were elicited as described in the experimental protocol. The control treatment procedure in this experiment consisted of a springing of both thumbs placed on the paraspinal tissues. The spinal manipulative procedure used entailed a crossed bilateral pisiform contact on an involved vertebra.

Results from this study showed a significant difference in the reduction of pain between the experimental and control groups.[20] The authors felt that their findings corroborated the presence of a "silent somatic dysfunction" and suggested an underlying subclinical facilitation of cutaneous sensory reflex pathways coupled with a biomechanical fault in an adjacent spinal motion segment.[20] Finally, a neurologic rationale is proposed to attempt to explain some of the effects demonstrated. This article points to important implications for the role of spinal manipulation in relieving spinal pain.

In yet another study, a series of patients suffering from back pain after surgical procedures were treated using manipulation.[21] Several of the 28 patients had pain that referred into an extremity as well. All suffered from back pain occurring after surgery and had no other causative factors for the pain. Assessment measures included appearance of distortion of normal spinal curves when in different positions, leg length measurements (done supine), palpatory tests, passive mobility tests, straight leg raise, and neurologic tests.

All the patients received manipulation as their therapy.[21] The types of manipulations used vary by patient, dependent on their particular condition and the results of the assessment procedures. Over half of the patients became symptom free after only one treatment. Over 70 percent of the patients ultimately became symptom free; only two of the patients failed to respond to therapy. The authors then discussed the possible and proposed mechanisms for back pain following surgery, and they postulate a rationale for the benefits of manipulative therapies. Although the study's methodologic design contains some obvious biases and potential errors, it does indicate a need to examine the phenomenon more completely and to consider a more rigorous test.

In a rather extensive review of the literature, Vernon[22] reports on several trials involving the use of manipulation for the management of headache. Some of these were descriptive, such as one by Vernon himself.[23] One group of patients was investigated using a mail questionnaire, while the second group of patients was studied while visiting the college clinic. Both groups were asked to rate several variables, such as how long a headache lasted, whether they experienced (subjective) improvement, the severity of symptoms, and so forth. Both groups demonstrated reduced symptomatology after treatment with manipulative procedures. This particular study suffered from having small sample populations.

Jirout studied 200 patients who showed signs of fixation at an upper cervical region (in this case, C2–C3) and most of whom also suffered from headache.[24] When manipulation was directed to the fixated vertebral segment, relief from headache occurred in over 80 percent of the patients.

At present, the only randomized clinical trial of manipulation for chiropractic adjustment and migraine headache is the one performed by Parker and colleagues.[25] The doctors examined 85 patients, most of whom had suffered from migraine headache for about 19 years. They separated the patients in three different treatment groups: a control group that received a mobilization from a physiotherapist, a second experimental group that received a medical manipulation, and a third experimental group that received the chiropractic adjustment. The study lasted 6 months; only the middle 2 months were used for treatment, while the first 2 months were for pretreatment, and the final 2 months were used for follow-up. Of several hypotheses tested by this work, the only one that was found to have any statistical significance was that pain intensity would be reduced in the chiropractic-treated group. The authors then attributed this particular finding to placebo effect arising from unreasonably high expectations of both the treating doctors and from the patients. This report later received fairly widespread criticism arising from several fronts. For example, it was noted that the control group itself did receive a form of manipulation as the treatment used, some potentially inappropriate statistical procedures were used, and the power of the experiment overall was low.[26]

Other trials and research into the use of manipulation for headache also exist (see the Suggested Readings List).

CLINICAL TRIALS OF MANIPULATION AND SOMATOVISCERAL DISORDERS

One of the most intriguing areas for future development of chiropractic procedures is in the management of organic disorder, referred to as "type O" disorders to distinguish them from the more commonly seen "type M," or musculoskeletal disorders that make up the basis of most chiropractic practice. Drawing on basic research from several sources, an elegant approach to the management of some organic disorders is now being developed. Much of this research was brought about by research performed by far-thinking osteopaths, who then had the wherewithal to subject their theories to clinical testing. However, the work accomplished by these osteopaths has immediate applicability to the chiropractic profession.

One of the obvious major problems that exist in designing a test to determine whether manipulation can affect a given organic condition is identifying the location to be adjusted. In chiropractic terminology, this involves locating either a subluxation or fixation; in osteopathic terminology, this involves locating the area of somatic dysfunction. The nature of the research in this area is to locate a locus of somatic dysfunction in patients suffering from organic dysfunction, to locate a specific somatic dysfunction by the use of various criteria, and then finally to manipulate an area and see if an effect is noted.

Somatic Dysfunction in the Cervical Region

Johnston et al.[2] and Vorro and Johnston[28] studied clinical signs of somatic dysfunction in the cervical region using both kinematic instrumental measurement and electromyographic assessment. In these studies, the examiners first palpated a group of subjects and assessed the symmetry or asymmetry of cervical motion in side bending. They then examined motion using an instrumental recording system.[27] The examiners noted a distinct decrease in all primary ranges of motion in groups that had palpated with asymmetric motion when compared to those with symmetric motion.[27] They concluded that "during physical examination, the palpable clinical sign of asymmetry in response to passive cervical sidebending appears to be an early indicator of a measurable impairment in cervical function."[27]

The authors then examined the subjects electromyographically.[28] The muscles of the group that had been noted to have asymmetric motion on palpation were found to be slower to initiate action and were also reduced in strength of action and time. By combining the findings from the two studies, the authors advanced a method for determining the presence of somatic dysfunction, at least as it concerned the cervical spine. This was a significant step to using such methods in a clinical setting or trial.

Johnston later furthered this work in a series of reports dealing with segmental definition.[29–31] The first of these articles provided a scientific foundation for the use of palpatory diagnosis. It described specific palpatory tests and gave information about how to judge the results of those tests. In this case, Johnston identified a primary segmental dysfunction as "asymmetric responses to opposing directions of each motion test and the presence of mirror image asymmetries."[29] The location of any somatic dysfunction would be determined by the comparison of these asymmetries in up to a three spinal segment location and thus could provide an examining physician with a specific location for the use of manipulative therapy when the somatic dysfunction was present.

In part 2, Johnston describes how, once the location of the somatic dysfunction was determined by the presence of mirror-image asymmetries, various manipulative procedures might be used to restore normal, symmetric motion.[30] Johnson felt that this was due to the addition of sensory input of somatic origin resulting from the procedure, which also implied the presence of an adaptive somatosomatic reflex.

The third report in this series then synthesized the finding from the first two parts to apply it to the task of locating somatic dysfunction directly owing to a visceral reflex pathway.[31] Johnston examined criteria for recognizing linkages between vertebral and costal asymmetries in the thoracic spine as a motor component of a visceral reflex. One such linkage Johnston discussed is a lesion of the tenth thoracic vertebra with the right tenth rib in patients suffering from cholelithiasis. Mirror asymmetries then also exist at T9 and T11. In patients suffering from a recurrent acute upper gastritis, the linkage has been found to be at T5 and the left fifth rib. This exciting work is only the start in defining a role for manipulative therapy in the management of visceral conditions because it provides a means to locate a vertebral area for both diagnosis and treatment.

In an earlier study, Johnston and Hill had begun to investigate location of somatic dysfunction relating to possible visceral reflex pathology.[32] The doctors selected 60 patients to participate in the study; they divided the patients into three experimental groups based on their hypertensive status and the presence or absence of a pattern of segmental dysfunction. Each patient had palpation of the cervical and upper thoracic spine performed, which was administered according to a set of criteria delineated in the body of the article. One question asked was whether there would be any difference in palpation between the normotensive and hypertensive groups relating to the cervicothoracic spine. Outside of the region of the somatic pattern, the incidence of findings of segmental dysfunction was insufficient to characterize one group as being different from any other. In neither of the two pattern-positive groups of 20 normotensive and 20 hypertensive patients was there consistent dysfunction at a noncriterion level. There was a higher incidence of involvement at the T2 and T4 thoracic regions, which is perhaps not surprising.

Johnson prepared some clinical notes on the use of osteopathic manipulative therapy for patients suffering from cardiac disease, specifically, coronary artery disease.[33] The technique involves the use of a contact on the second rib on the left, at its sternal end. He believes that the reflex effect on the contact will help to decrease respiratory distress and increase chest expansion and aeration. Dr. Johnson then discusses five cases that benefited from his particular form of therapy. Although this is obviously not a clinical trial, the presence of apparently repeatable positive results can form the basis of a more in-depth study.

Hypertension Management

Attempts at managing various manifestations of cardiac disease have been common in the osteopathic profession. Morgan et al. attempted an in-depth study of the management of hypertension[34] with 29 hypertension patients placed into one of two groups. The patients in the first group received a series of manipulations directed to the atlanto-occipital joint, T1 to T5, and T11 to L1 (which was considered the experimental treatment), while the second group received sham manipulation (soft tissue massage) of T6 to T10 and L4 to sacrum. This series of treatments continued for 6 weeks, and then the two groups were crossed over so that the therapies in each group were reversed; again, the treatments continued for 6 weeks. After the twelfth week, therapy was halted in both groups. In this study, the results did not demonstrate that the experimental group fared any better than the control; in point of fact, the experiment did not prove that either of the manipulative therapy regimens used had any effect on lowering blood pressure or controlling blood pressure.

Many possible biases exist within this study. No questions were asked the patient concerning life-styles, and patients were not controlled for weight and height. There may also be some concern about the broad-based areas selected for adjustment. It may have been better to select the single best area to adjust; e.g., many chiropractors might have selected T2 as the likely area to have the greatest effect on hypertension.

The work of Morgan et al.[34] stands in direct contrast to that of Fichera and Celander.[35] Their study examined 35 normotensive and 22 hypertensive individuals. Each patient was instructed to lie supine for 15 minutes. An electrosphygmograph recorded a rectilinear graph of systolic and diastolic pressures on the patient, recording 10 measurements during that 15-minute rest. Then a 20-cc blood sample was withdrawn, and the patient was instructed to lie prone for 5 minutes. The experimental group was manipulated in both left and right cervical and thoracic regions; the control group received no manipulation. Then the patient turned supine again, and a series of blood pressures were taken over a 15-minute period, ending with a second tube of drawn blood.

The rationale for the drawn blood concerns the fact that one of the most sensitive indicators of changes in the autonomic nervous system is in the fibrinolytic enzyme system and fibrinogen level.[35] This enzyme system is involved in determining blood viscosity, which is affected by autonomic tone. A decrease in fibrinolytic activity with a decrease in the level of fibrinogen is associated with an increase in autonomic tone of the parasympathetic nervous system; an increase of these parameters is associated with an increase in sympathetic activity. Thus, they form a way to directly note autonomic nervous system response.

This study noted a statistically significant decrease ($P < .01$) in both the systolic and diastolic pressures of the hypertensive group of patients.[35] In addition, hematocrit decreased 86 percent in the hypertensive group and only 37 percent in the normotensive group. This was significant at $P < .01$. The same was true for plasma fibrinogen concentration. The authors conclude by offering a rationale for the observed effects. In an earlier paper, they had already laid the groundwork for the clinical study represented by this work.[36]

Somatic Dysfunction in Coronary Artery Disease

Cardiac disease continues to attract the notice and efforts of the osteopaths. Beal and Kleiber tackled the role of somatic dysfunction in attempting to identify patients suffering from coronary artery disease.[37] Dr. Beal felt that if somatic dysfunction was associated with cardiac disease, then perhaps a way might be found to help identify and even predict patients suffering from that disabling and potentially fatal disease. He studied 99 patients scheduled to undergo a cardiac catheterization test, examining each for evidence of somatic dysfunction found by palpatory methods. The doctors doing the palpation had no knowledge of the patients' health status; they did not know that any patient suffered from cardiac disease.

Of all the patients examined, 70 were found to have somatic dysfunction located from T1 to T5 on the left side. The sensitivity of this test, for patients with left-sided somatic dysfunction in the T1 to T5 region with true-positive results for diagnosis of cardiac disease was 92 percent. The efficiency of the palpatory test for both positive and negative prediction was 79 percent. These compared favorably with previously reported results.[38] Palpation was considered to be a very positive and potentially useful diagnostic tool.

Somatic Dysfunction and Kidney Disease

A similar study was performed examining the somatic manifestations found in patients suffering from kidney disease.[39] In this controlled trial, three groups of patients were tested to determine whether somatic manifestations of renal disease could be repeatably found in the region of T9 to T12. There was one experimental group, made up of patients suffering from advanced renal disease; there were two control groups, one of normotensive individuals without renal disease and one of hypertensive individuals without renal disease. The examining doctors recorded both palpatory findings and thermographic findings in the thoracic spine. Both of these procedures showed that the patients suffering from renal disease had a higher incidence of involvement in the area of T9 to T12. This was true for palpation demonstrating somatic dysfunction and for thermography, demonstrating heat emission.

The authors concluded that their findings supported the presence of somatomotor and vasomotor changes as a reflex component of renal disease.[39] They pointed out several potential problems that might impact on categorical diagnosis, such as nonrenal visceral stimuli affecting the same spinal regions.

Effects of Manipulation on Cardiac and Respiratory Parameters

Manipulation may effect many different physiologic parameters in the body, though the precise mechanisms are not understood and remain theoretical. Clymer et al. examined the effect of manipulation on segmental pulsatile blood volume, systemic blood pressure, heart rate, and respiratory rate.[40] They measured pulsatile blood volume by electrical impedance plethysmography using four electrodes. The changes were monitored for 10 seconds every 2 minutes during a 10-minute warm-up period, every 1 minute during a 5-minute manipulation period, and then again every 2 minutes during the 16 minute post-treatment period. The area manipulated was from T12 to L3.

Cardiac and respiratory rates were monitored via a recording polygraph machine.[40] Blood pressure was measured at the outset, right before manipulation, right after manipulation, and at the end of the entire process. Two groups of patients were tested. The control group of 10 patients underwent the preceding process but without a manipulation. The experimental group consisted of 30 subjects, all of whom received the manipulative therapy. The results showed a significant decrease in pulsatile blood volume in the experimental group; no significant changes occurred in either respiratory rate or systemic blood pressure. The heart rate did decrease in the experimental group. The effect is believed to be due to activation of sympathetic nerve fibers of the paravertebral sympathetic ganglia.

Howell and Kapler present a case report concerning a positive experience in using manipulation to treat a patient suffering from advanced cardiopulmonary disease.[41] The patient in this case was suffering from both chronic obstructive lung disease and cor pulmonale. The patient received a course of therapy that lasted 16 months and that used both manipulation and a brief course of diuretics. The area selected for manipulation was T4 and T5, because on palpatory examination, these areas were felt to be restricted in motion. After the course of therapy, improvement was noted in levels of dyspnea, fatigue, oxygen tension, and oxygen percent saturation; however, decreases occurred in flow rate volumes, demonstrating that some deterioration may yet have occurred.

Northrup has provided a protocol for the manipulative management of hypertension.[42] The protocol centers on specific palpatory assessment of lesions in the spine, though he also suggests that some cranial palpation may be beneficial. He also suggests paying attention to blood pressure measurements in various positions, coupled with the location of palpatory lesion. He then discusses proposed mechanisms of treatment, centering on autonomic effects relating to the carotid sinus.

Examination and diagnosis of a patient suffering from a possible viscerosomatic reflex pathology can be very confusing. Not only may a visceral pathology have somatic manifestations, a somatic problem may have visceral manifestations. Sandford and Barry eloquently demonstrate this.[43] Their article presents the case of a patient suffering from a latissimus dorsi muscle strain, which manifested itself as a recurrence of a chronic abdominal pain. A regular course of medical therapy had been unsuccessful at relieving the "abdominal problem"; further examination ultimately revealed the latissimus strain. Therapy then consisted of spray and stretch procedures. The authors believe the confounding diagnosis occurred because of the convergence–projection theory; that is, that pain signals of visceral and somatic origin converge somewhere in their afferent paths. The cortex then perceives these signals as arising from afferents that had previously excited that pathway.

Implications of Research Reports

The majority of research examining somotovisceral and viscerosomatic manifestations of disease has been performed by osteopaths. As mentioned, research in the chiropractic profession is still in its infancy; however, the research noted here has direct applicability to the chiropractic profession. Though most chiropractors are aware of continuing calls for further clinical research within the profession, we are by no means unique in that regard.[44] Clinical research must be always a high priority for the chiropractic profession so that we may better identify where our procedures have their best use.

One report that amply demonstrates this is the important work by Nansel et al. in which the first triple-blind test of the chiropractic adjustment was studied.[45] Using a highly controlled protocol, the authors showed a dramatic reduction in the degree of asymmetry in subjects who received a cervical chiropractic adjustment; this reduction was not achieved by the control group. Though the authors studied a time frame only 30 to 45 minutes after the adjustment, they felt that the study protocol could be adapted to longer time frames and provide a means whereby the chiropractic adjustment could be better studied. This is exciting work with many implications for future study.

RELIABILITY STUDIES

Clinical trials are simply not possible unless the assessment procedures used by those studies have themselves been tested and found reliable. As an example, the chiropractic profession faces a particular difficulty when using the presence or absence of subluxation as an indicator in a research study. First, there are several different accepted definitions of *subluxation*; thus, any research must use a operational definition only. Second, procedures for identifying the presence of subluxation have not themselves been tested for reliability. Any research using presence or absence of subluxation as the indicator will be subject to question.

It thus becomes necessary to subject routine diagnostic procedures to tests designed to see whether they are indeed reliable procedures. This entails the implementation of both intraexaminer and interexaminer studies. Not only must a given doctor reliably find the same parameter in a single patient of a class of patients (intraexaminer reliability); a series of doctors must also reliably find similar findings in a patient or series of patients (interexaminer reliability). Therefore, many chiropractic procedures have been subject to intense investigations of their reliability.

Motion Palpation

With the development of motion palpation as a diagnostic tool, the need to examine the method has become very important. Gonnella et al. developed a 7-scale system to try to evaluate the intraexaminer and interexaminer reliability of palpating intervertebral motion.[46] This scale graded intervertebral motion using seven descriptions of motion: ankylosed, considerable restriction (hypomobility), slight restriction (hypomobility), normal, slight increase (hypermobility), considerable increase (hypermobility), and unstable. Criteria for these descriptors were provided. Five therapists examined five patients in the spinal regions of T12 to S1. The maneuvers used included forward bending, side bending to the left and right, and rotation to both the left and the right. The patients were examined twice over a 2-week period. Examinations were performed both under blinded and normal conditions.

Intraexaminer results were considered reasonably good both among and between sessions; consistency among therapists was not demonstrated. Further, each therapist tended to show a particular bias in his measurements. The results here are perhaps not surprising; it is understood that intraexaminer scores are usually much more favorable than interexaminer; also, a therapist does use many other visual and tactile clues to aid in diagnosis than simply palpation.

Beattie et al. examined the reliability of the attraction method of measuring motion in patients suffering from back pain.[47] The method under study used a tape measure to measure the distance between two preestablished points on the lumbar spine before and after the patients underwent extension of the low back without bending their knees. Two groups of 100 patients were used: One group suffered from low back pain while the second did not. Intraexaminer and interexaminer studies were done on the procedure, with agreement studies using intraclass correlation coefficients.

The study demonstrated a high degree of intraexaminer reliability for measuring backward bending of the lumbar spine, seen in both the painful and nonpainful groups.[47] The authors also noted a high degree of interexaminer reliability in the nonsymptomatic group. The symptomatic group was not studied, so no conclusions can be drawn regarding the use of the procedure in this regard.

A second report also examined the reliability of using a flexible rule for measurement in the lumbar spine. In this case, the authors used a flexible ruler to assess the lumbar lordosis.[48] This study used a total of 80 patients; 40 had low back pain and 40 did not. The examiners asked patients to stand in a relaxed position with their lower back and buttocks exposed. Positioning of the feet was standardized to allow for repeated measurement. A flexible ruler was placed into the lumbar lordosis between the L3 spinous process and the second sacral spinous process, and the outline of this curve was then traced onto paper. An angle, θ, was measured by calculating θ equal to 4 times the arctangent of $2H/L$, where L and H equal length and height measured from the tracing. This measurement provided the magnitude of the lordotic curve.

The intratester reliability measurements were high for both groups and for each examiner.[48] However, again, the intertester measurements were not much higher than would be suggested by chance. The authors note that in several areas error and bias may have occurred; the examiners might have not used exactly the same landmarks for measurement, patient stance might differ, and so on. They concluded that the results of such measurements may be reliable if taken by the same physical therapist.

Johnston et al. studied procedures designed to establish palpatory criteria for finding spinal segmental dysfunction in the thoracic spine.[49] They studied 30 subjects. The examiner lightly tapped over each spinous process to determine variations in tension of the thoracic paravertebral tissues. This was repeated using a deeper tapping bilaterally to determine increased illness or decreased rebound as a positive sign of deep muscular tension. This was rated using an intensity scale and was recorded on a sheet draped over the spine of each subject.

For each of the five examiners, the agreement levels surpassed 79 percent in distinguishing between two marked segments, one with relatively normal tissue tension and one with increased deep tissue tension. There was also a good degree of interexaminer agreement in the smaller scale study examining this question.

Many other reliability tests of motion palpation have been performed (see the Suggested Readings list).

Leg Length Deficiency

Lawrence has examined many reliability studies investigating leg length deficiency.[50] Procedures for assessing the length of the leg have long intrigued the chiropractic profession and in fact form the basis for many analytic adjustive systems such as Activator Technique, Thompson Terminal Point Technique, and Upper Cervical Specific Technique. Yet a close examination of the reliability studies covering the main method of assessment leaves a rather large question concerning whether the measurement procedure is either reliable or valid; most seem to show little reliability, leaving the question of validity rendered moot.

Orthopedic and Radiographic Examination

Even standard orthopedic and radiographic examination has been subject to testing for reliability of interpretation. Frymoyer et al. examined the differences between how medical physicians and chiropractic physicians read and interpret radiographs.[51] The authors used 99 anteroposterior and lateral lumbar radiographs of patients suffering from low back pain. These were subject to interpretation both by chiropractors, who examined 56 different radiographic variables, and by a medical physician, who performed a standard medical interpretation of the same films. Only 6 of the 56 variables examined showed a high degree of interexaminer reliability; 16 variables showed a fair degree of reliability. However, there was virtually no agreement between the chiropractic analysis and the medical interpretation, save for the measure of disc space height at the L3–L4 and L4–L5 regions. The authors concluded that spinal radiographs, whether analyzed by a medical radiologist or a chiropractic physician, have little value in determining the presence or absence of low back complaints and, more important, have no value for epidemiologic studies.

Such studies make very confusing the interpretation of both diagnostic and therapeutic interventions. Such a situation is not unique to the chiropractic profession by any means, and it is a measure of intellectual honesty that such studies are performed. Only by continual testing, retesting, and refining our analytic, diagnostic, and therapeutic procedures will we best serve our public.

CONCLUSION

The research efforts of the chiropractic profession need to be directed in several different directions. One direction is toward basic science, with a goal of gaining knowledge of the physiologic and anatomic underpinnings of our clinical processes. If a subluxation does exist, how will it manifest itself on a physiologic level? Will it produce anatomic change? How will it affect the body on a microscopic level? Once such questions are answered, we are that much closer to knowing how pathology will manifest itself.

A second direction is to continue with small-scale reliability studies designed to determine which of the many analytic and diagnostic procedures we use are worthwhile. Once we can determine the reliability of a procedure, it becomes easier to then make decisions regarding the validity of that procedure. Does it measure what we believe it is measuring? To make that determination, we need to know that the procedure itself is at the least repeatable.

A final and most important direction for our research is the controlled clinical trial. We need to determine which techniques are best used to treat which problems and under what circumstances. If we can do this, we set standards of care that will answer how chiropractors may best serve a hurting public.

We face many difficulties in meeting this challenge. Research takes a great deal of money, and the chiropractic profession has not been able to tap federal monies with any great amount of success. We are fortunate that funding agencies now exist within the profession, a prime one being the Foundation for Chiropractic Education and Research (FCER). But groups such as FCER are not enough in and of themselves. There has traditionally been an antiscientific attitude among many chiropractors, an attitude that has equated the proper use of science and the scientific method as being medical. Anything medical is anathema to such individuals. This attitude hampers the scientific progress of the chiropractic profession. The tools of science are available to anyone who wants to use them. To tap future funding sources, the profession will need to be better educated in the scientific method and to have a better understanding of research design, biostatistics, grant writing, and the publication process.

The new generation of chiropractors is being trained well to handle these challenges. A cadre of qualified researchers are being developed who have the requisite skills and who are developing competent publication records. The implications for the future are interesting to speculate on. The future does indeed look bright.

REFERENCES

1. Brunarski DJ: Clinical trials of spinal manipulation: a critical appraisal and review of the literature. J Manipulative Physiol Ther 7:243, 1985

2. Ottenbacher K, DiFabio RP: Efficacy of spinal manipulation/mobilization therapy: a meta-analysis. Spine 10:833, 1985

3. DiFabio RP: Clinical assessment of manipulation and mobilization of the lumbar spine: a critical review of the literature. Phys Ther 66:51, 1986

4. Waagen GN, Haldeman S, Cook G et al: Short term trial of chiropractic adjustments for the relief of chronic low back pain. Manual Med 2:63, 1986

5. Hadler NM, Curtis P, Gillings DB et al: A benefit of spinal manipulation as adjunctive therapy for acute low-back pain: a stratified controlled trial. Spine 12:703, 1987

6. Mathews JA, Mills SB, Jenkins VM et al: Back pain and sciatica: controlled trials of manipulation, traction, sclerosant and epidural injections. Br J Rheum 26:416, 1987

7. Godfrey CM, Morgan PP, Schatzker J: A randomized trial of manipulation for low-back pain in a medical setting. Spine 9:301, 1984

8. Maigne R: Doulers d'Orgine Vertebrale et Traitements par Manipulations. Expansions Scientifiques Francais, Paris, 1968

9. Doran DML, Newell MS: Manipulation in the treatment of back pain: a multicentre study. Br Med J 2:161, 1975

10. Evans DP, Burke MS, Lloyd KN et al: Lumbar spinal manipulation on trial, part 1—clinical assessment. Rheumatol Rehabil 17:46, 1978

11. Bergquist-Ullman M, Larsson U: Acute low back pain in industry. Acta Orthop Scand (Suppl) 170:1, 1977

12. Sims-Williams H, Jayson MIV, Young SMS et al: Controlled trial of mobilisation and manipulation for patients with low back pain in general practice. Br Med J 5:1338, 1978

13. Cherkin DC, MacCornack FA: Patient evaluations of low back pain care from family physicians and chiropractors. West J Med 150:351, 1989

14. Meade TR, Dyer S et al: Low back pain of mechanical origin: randomised comparison of chiropractic and hospital outpatient treatment. Br Med J 300:1431, 1990

15. Swezey RL: Editorial: low back pain treatment: Is a "Yank" in King Arthur's court or elsewhere as effective as traction, epidural injections or what else? Br J Rheumatol 26:401, 1987

16. Bloch R: Methodology in clinical back pain trials. Spine 12:430, 1987

17. Barker ME: Manipulation in general medical practice for thoracic pain syndromes. Br Osteopathic J 15:95, 1983

18. Bourdillon JF: Spinal Manipulation. Heinemann, London, 1970

19. Molea D, Murcek B, Blanken C et al: Evaluation of two manipulative techniques in the treatment of postexercise muscle soreness. JAOA 87:477, 1987

20. Terrett ACJ, Vernon H: A controlled study of the effect of spinal manipulation on paraspinal cutaneous pain tolerance levels. Am J Phys Med 63:217, 1984

21. Miller R: A clinical study of post-surgical joint symptoms treated by manipulation. Br Osteopathic J 14:113, 1982

22. Vernon H: Spinal manipulation and headaches of cervical origin. J Manipulative Physiol Ther 12:455, 1989

23. Vernon H: Manipulative therapy in the chiropractic treatment of headaches: a retrospective and prospective study. J Manipulative Physiol Ther 5:109, 1982

24. Jirout J: Comments regarding the diagnosis and treatment of dysfunctions in the C2–C3 segment. Manual Med 2:62, 1985

25. Parker GB, Tupling H, Pryor DS: A controlled trial of cervical manipulation for migraine. Aust NZ J Med 8:589, 1978

26. Commission of Inquiry into Chiropractic: Chiropractic in New Zealand. Hasselberg, New Zealand PD 1978

27. Johnston WL, Vorro J, Hubbard RP: Clinical/biomechanic correlates for cervical function: part 1. A kinematic study. JAOA 85:429, 1985

28. Vorro J, Johnston WL: Clinical/biomechanic correlates of cervical function: part 2. A myoelectric study. JAOA 87:353, 1987

29. Johnston WL: Segmental definition: part 1, a focal point for diagnosis of somatic dysfunction. JAOA 88:99, 1988

30. Johnston WL: Segmental definition: part 2. Application of an indirect method in osteopathic manipulative treatment. JAOA 88:211, 1988

31. Johnston WL: Segmental definition: part 3. Definitive basis for distinguishing somatic findings of visceral reflex origin. JAOA 88:347, 1988

32. Johnston WL, Hill JH: Spinal segmental dysfunction: incidence in cervico-thoracic region. JAOA 81:67, 1981

33. Johnson FE: Some observations on the use of osteopathic therapy in the care of patients with cardiac disease. JAOA 72:799, 1972

34. Morgan JP, Dickey JL, Hunt HH et al: A controlled trial of spinal manipulation in the management of hypertension. JAOA 85:308, 1985

35. Fichera AP, Celander DR: Effect of osteopathic manipulative therapy of autonomic tone as evidenced by blood pressure changes and activity of the fibrinolytic system. JAOA 68:1036, 1969

36. Celander E, Koeniog AJ, Celander DR: Effect of osteopathic manipulative therapy on autonomic tone as evidenced by blood pressure changes and activity of the fibrinolytic system. JAOA 67:1037, 1968

37. Beal MC, Kleiber GE: Somatic dysfunction as a predictor of coronary artery disease. JAOA 85:302, 1985

38. Cox JM: Palpable musculoskeletal findings in coronary artery disease. Results of a double blind study. JAOA 82:832, 1983

39. Johnston WL, Kelso AF, Hollandsworth DL et al: Somatic manifestations in renal disease: a clinical research study. JAOA 87:22, 1987

40. Clymer DH, Levin FL, Sculthorpe RH: Effects of osteopathic manipulation on several different physiological functions: part III. Measurement of changes in several different physiological parameters as a result of osteopathic manipulation. JAOA 72:204, 1972

41. Howell RK, Kappler RE: The influence of osteopathic manipulative therapy on a patient with advanced cardiopulmonary disease. JAOA 73:322, 1973

42. Northrup TL: Manipulative management of hypertension. JAOA 60:973, 1961

43. Sandford PR, Barry DT: Acute somatic pain can refer to sites of chronic abdominal pain. Arch Phys Med Rehabil 69:532, 1988

44. D'Alonzo GE: Clinical research in osteopathic medicine. JAOA 87:113, 1987

45. Nansel DD, Cremata E, Carlson J et al: Effect of unilateral spinal adjustments on goniometrically assessed cervical lateral-flexion end-range asymmetries in otherwise asymptomatic subjects. J Manipulative Physiol Ther 12:419, 1989

46. Gonnella C, Paris SV, Kutner M: Reliability in evaluating passive intervertebral motion. Physical Therapy 62:436, 1982

47. Beattie P, Rothstein JM, Lamb RL: Reliability of the attraction method for measuring lumbar spine backward bending. Physical Therapy 77:364, 1987

48. Lovell FW, Rothstein JM, Personius WJ: Reliability of clinical measurements of lumbar lordosis taken with a flexible ruler. Physical Therapy 69:96, 1989

49. Johnston WL, Allan BR, Hendra JL et al: Interexaminer study of palpation in detecting location of spinal segmental dysfunction. JAOA 82:839, 1983

50. Lawrence DJ: Chiropractic concepts of the short leg: a critical review. J Manipulative Physiol Ther 8:157, 1985

51. Frymoyer JW, Phillips RB, Newberg AH et al: A comparative analysis of the interpretations of lumbar spinal radiographs by chiropractors and medical doctors. Spine 11:1020, 1986

SUGGESTED READINGS

Papers Discussing Low Back Pain and Manipulation Not Cited in Text

Buerger AA: A controlled trial of rotational manipulation in low back pain. Manuelle Medizin 2:17, 1980

Cassidy JD, Kirkaldy-Willis WH, McGregor M: Spinal manipulation for the treatment of chronic low back and leg pain. A five-year experience. Department of Orthopaedics, University of Saskatchewan. In: Proceedings of the International Society for the Study of the Lumbar Spine. Toronto, June 1982.

Chrisman OD, Mittnach A, Snook GA: Study of the results following rotatory manipulation in the lumbar intervertebral disc syndrome. J Bone Joint Surg [Am] 46:517, 1964

Coyer AB, Curwen IHM: Low back pain treated by manipulation. Br Med J 19:344, 1955

Edwards BC: Low back pain and pain resulting from lumbar spine conditions: a comparison of treatment results. Aust J Physiotherapy 15:104, 1969

Farrell JP, Twomey LT: Acute low back pain. Comparison of two conservative approaches. Med J Aust 1:160, 1982

Fisk JW: A controlled trial of manipulation in a selected group of patients with low back pain favoring one side. NZ Med J 74:288, 1971

Glover JR: Back pain: a randomized clinical trial of rotational manipulation of the trunk. Br J Ind Med 31:59, 1974

Hoehler FK, Tobis J: Low back pain and its treatment by spinal manipulation: measures of flexibility and asymmetry. Rheumatol Rehab 21:21, 1982

Jayson MIV, Sims-Williams H, Young S et al: Mobilization and manipulation for low back pain. Spine 6:409, 1981

Kane RL, Fisher FD, Leymaster C et al: Manipulating the patient. A comparison of the effectiveness of physician and chiropractor care. Lancet 1:1333, 1974

Nwuga VCB: Relative therapeutic efficacy of vertebral manipulation and conventional treatment in back pain management. Am J Phys Med 61:273, 1982

Parson WB, Cumming JDA: Manipulation in back pain. Can Med Assoc J 79:103, 1958

Potter GE: A study of 744 cases of neck and back pain treated with spinal manipulation. J Can Chiro Assoc 2:154, 1977

Rasmussen GG: Manipulation in the treatment of low back pain. A randomized clinical trial. Manuelle Medizin 1:8, 1979

Siehl D, Olson DR, Ross HE, Rockwood EE: Manipulation of the lumbar spine with the patient under general anesthesia: an evaluation of EMG and clinical-neurologic examination of its use for lumbar nerve root compression. J Am Osteopathic Assoc 70:43, 1971

Sims-Williams H, Jayson MIV, Young SMS, et al: Controlled trial of mobilization and manipulation for patients with low back pain: hospital patients. Br Med J 2:1318, 1979

Zylbergold RS, Piper MC: Lumbar disc disease: comparative analysis of physical therapy treatments. Arch Phys Med Rehab 62:176, 1981

Research on Manipulation and Headache

Beckwith C: Migraine pathophysiology and manipulative treatment. Yearbook Am Assoc Osteopath 14:508, 1953

Droz JM, Crot F: Occipital headaches: statistical results in the treatment of vertebragenous headache. Swiss Annals 8:127, 1985

Parker GB, Pryor DS, Tupling H: Why does migraine improve during a clinical trial? Further results from a trial of cervical manipulation for migraine. Aust NZ J Med 10:192, 1980

Mannen EM: The use of cervical radiographic overlays to assess the response to manipulation. J Can Chiro Assoc 24:108, 1980

Miller B, Maxwell JL, DeBoer K: Chiropractic treatment of tension headache: a case report. J Am Chiro Assoc 21:62, 1984

Turk RZ, Ratkolb O: Mobilization of the cervical spine in chronic headaches. Manual Medizin 3:15, 1987

Wright JS: Migraine: a statistical analysis of chiropractic treatment. J Am Chiro Assoc 12:363, 1978

Reliability Test of Motion Palpation

Boline PD, Keating JC, Brist J, Denver G: Interexaminer reliability of palpatory evaluations of the lumbar spine. Am J Chiro Med 1:5, 1988

DeBoer KF, Harmon R, Tuttle CD, Wallace H: Reliability study of detection of somatic dysfunctions in the cervical spine. J Manipulative Physiol Ther 8:9, 1985

Kaltenborn F, Lindahl D: Reproducibility of the results of manual mobility testing of specific intervertebral segments. Swed Med J 66:962, 1969

Love RM, Brodeur BR: Inter- and intraexaminer reliability for motion palpation of the thoracic spine. J Manipulative Physiol Ther 10:1, 1987

Mior SA, King RS, McGregor M, Bernard M: Intra- and interexaminer reliability of motion palpation in the cervical spine. J Can Chiro Assoc 29:195, 1985

Mootz RD, Keating JC, Kontz HP et al: Intra- and interobserver reliability of passive motion palpation of the lumbar spine. J Manipulative Physil Ther 12:440, 1989

Nansel DD, Peneff AL, Jansen RD, Cooperstein R: Interexaminer concordance in detecting joint-play asymmetries in the cervical spines of otherwise asymptomatic patients. J Manipulative Physiol Ther 12:438, 1989

Russell R: Diagnostic palpation of the spine: a review of procedures and assessment of their reliability. J Manipulative Physiol Ther 6:181, 1983

Wiles MR: Reproducibility and interexaminer correlation of motion palpation findings of the sacroiliac joints. J Can Chiro Assoc 24:59, 1980

APPENDIX 1
Forms of Chiropractic Technique

The few systems described briefly here are designed to provide only a flavor of the wide diversity of chiropractic technique systems. This list is by no means all inclusive, nor is inclusion of a given technique an indication of its potential importance or acceptance by the chiropractic profession at large.

DIVERSIFIED TECHNIQUE

One of the most frequently used procedures and taught at most of the chiropractic colleges, the roots of Diversified Technique are hard to trace. Although it appears that the body of procedures grew out of the work of Janse, Hauser, and Wells,[14] procedures in their book can be traced to the work of the medical manipulator John McMillan Mennell. Mennell is credited with developing an analytic system for determining the presence of joint play in the human body. From the procedures outlined by Mennell, Janse adapted a series of chiropractic adjustive procedures now well used.

The collected procedures also drew on work by the osteopathic profession; the term *diversified* relates to the fact that the sources for these techniques are diverse. Wells himself was an osteopath in addition to a chiropractor.

Today, Diversified Technique is associated mainly with the National College of Chiropractic, where it forms their core technique curriculum, though, as noted, the procedure is in partial use at most other chiropractic colleges. Most of the procedures of Diversified Technique have been delineated in the book *The States Manual of Spinal, Pelvic and Extravertebral Techniques.*[15]

Diversified Technique is not based on any particular analytic system. Rather, it can be used with any analytic system (i.e., with both Sacro-Occipital Technique as well as Thompson Terminal Point). Diversified Technique uses the normal biomechanics of the spine and extremities to create motion at a vertebra or extremity joint. Thus, its application becomes nearly universal, which may account for its widespread use within the chiropractic profession.

BASIC TECHNIQUE

Basic Technique is also referred to as *Logan Basic procedure,* in honor of Hugh B. Logan, who did much to advance the central concepts of this form of technique. Basic Technique notes that the body must have normal structure to have normal function. In part, this system takes into account the effects of gravity on the spine and its related structures. Logan and others noted that if the spine were posturally deficient as a result of the effects of gravity, it placed a greater energy demand on the body, which over time could lead to more serious effects on the human body.

Logan himself noted differences in the positioning of the fifth lumbar vertebra when he lay down and when he stood during a period of illness. He began to look for patterns, which he subsequently noted followed certain characteristics. From these patterns, Logan hypothesized that the body of the lowest freely movable vertebra will rotate toward the low side of the sacrum (or the vertebra on which it rests), that is, that the body of that vertebra rotates toward the side of least support. This is usually the low side of the sacrum.

The initial impetus for these ideas started as early as 1919 but became more codified with the creation of the college in 1930. Logan adapted the light contact from work done by Dr. Francis Dillon. Logan felt that the sacrum was the biomechanical keystone of the body, because it supported the spine and also allowed for locomotion, and he felt that the spine would respond to changes in the sacrum. Thus, returning the sacrum to normal relations with its articulating bones was essential to reduce spinal involvements. He felt this required little force to accomplish.

The system that built up around Logan's initial concepts was fairly simple, requiring specific types of contacts in and around the sacrum. Pressure is applied steadily to these contacts with no true thrust.

THOMPSON TERMINAL POINT TECHNIQUE

Thompson Terminal Point Technique grew out of initial work by Derefield in Detroit, Michigan, many years ago. As has been the case so often in chiropractic, Derefield began noticing certain clinical patterns in his patients. In large measure, he began using leg length assessment (today known as the Derefield leg check) before deciding how to adjust his patients. For example, he might notice regularly that a posteroinferior ilium would always have a certain leg check pattern. After adjusting, the pattern that had existed might be changed, which was seen as presumptive evidence of a successful adjustment.

Initially, Derefield's procedures focused on the pelvic region and subluxations in that area. Derefield later drew the cervical spine into his analytic system. He altered the assessment of leg length by having patients rotate their heads to one side or the other. He then used the patterns of such leg length changes to determine the presence of subluxation and thus the choice of an adjustive procedure. J. Clay Thompson later expanded on this initial work, and with a Dr. Niblo was able to solve other problems arising from the analytic system. Many of the concepts relating to short leg assessment are still controversial.

Thompson feels the basic procedures of Thompson Terminal Point Technique fit well with most other forms of chiropractic technique. He developed a mechanical drop-section table; the table section drops a small distance on the delivery of a chiropractic thrust and then stops suddenly. He feels this allows Newton's laws of motion to develop a certain amount of kinetic energy not seen in other forms of chiropractic and thus may have elements of correction not seen. As well, the table helps to relieve stress on the doctor and can be set to adjust for differences in patient weight.

PIERCE-STILLWAGON TECHNIQUE

Pierce-Stillwagon Technique was developed by Drs. Walter Pierce and Glenn Stillwagon. It uses a combination of radiographic mensuration with the recent addition of cineradiographic procedures, thermographic sensor, and specific chiropractic technique to decide where and when to adjust a patient. In particular, the technique emphasizes the location of bilateral anterosuperior (AS) or posteroinferior (PI) pelvic misalignment. It is felt the AS misalignment will cause a lumbar hyperlordosis with accompanying postural defects and that the PI misalignment will cause a flattened lumbar curve. Moreover, Pierce has specifically singled out the C5 segment as being the area to adjust for a decreased cervical curve. This is primarily a systems approach.

PALMER UPPER CERVICAL TECHNIQUE

The Palmer Upper Cervical Technique is a direct descendent of the "hole-in-one" technique developed by B.J. Palmer. It uses a combination of skin temperature analysis, leg length measurement, motion and static palpation, along with x-ray analysis. Adjustments are applied only to the upper cervical complex and use a recoil thrust procedure. Typically, the patient lies in a side posture position, and a mechanical drop head piece can be employed.

SPINAL TOUCH TECHNIQUE

Spinal Touch seems to be an outgrowth, either directly or indirectly, of Logan Basic Technique in that it is based on the effects of gravity on the human body. It pays especially close attention to the sacrum, in recognition of its importance in weight bearing and locomotion. Spinal Touch analyzes both the center of gravity of the body, as well as the center of gravity of the sacrum, to analyze imbalances in the body and sacrum. It applies its therapy by using the "all or none law," a light-amplitude contact on the skin over certain noted areas. Plumb-line analysis is an important evaluation tool for this technique.

APPLIED KINESIOLOGY

Applied kinesiology is largely due to the work of George Goodheart, a Michigan chiropractor. Goodheart noticed a relationship between muscular weakness and possible organic weakness and developed an entire procedure to "systematize" his findings. In essence, he allows the body to aid in its own diagnosis. Applied kinesiology has received a lot of attention and remains a controversial system, with many practitioners using some or all of its methods. Although many findings have long been published in proceedings and research reports in the field, reports in other publications has been decidedly mixed.[16–18]

It is beyond the scope of this text to examine the procedures used by applied kinesiologists, because the system is so extremely complex. It is mainly an analytic procedure, however, using manual muscle testing as an indicator for dysfunction.

DIRECTIONAL NONFORCE TECHNIQUE

Directional Nonforce Technique (DNFT) is due to the work of Richard Van Rumpt, an early graduate of National College of Chiropractic. To quote Van Rumpt, the basic postulate of DNFT is "that innate [intelligence] can be contacted by visualization—thought projection—thought materialization—conscious thought forming—activated thought transmission—projection of mental energy or mind power, to make a chiropractic and subluxation analysis or listing."[19] This procedure is based on more esoteric considerations of metaphysical constructs.

The analytic system uses a special leg reflex. There is a consideration that subluxation in certain body locations cannot occur singly (e.g., that an atlas subluxation must also involve axis or occiput and that a thoracic subluxation must also involve a rib, etc.). The adjustment attempts to remove nerve interference and uses low-force techniques. This is a more marginal chiropractic technique.

ACTIVATOR TECHNIQUE

Activator Technique was the brainchild of W.C. Lee and Arlan W. Fuhr. Their emphasis from the start was on body mechanics and how to use light-force contacts to effect changes in those mechanics. They were attempting to use their system to determine where in the body a subluxation occurred. Their analysis centered on predominantly the cervical and lumbar regions. According to the system, when there is a lumbar syndrome, nine possible subluxations may occur; these may be identified using a leg check procedure. Similar findings held true for the cervical spine. This basic premise has been expanded to include other areas of the spine.

Activator Technique is known for its use of mechanical adjusting device, generally the "Activator Adjusting Instrument" or even "Activator" for short. The device produces a percussion when it is triggered and so induces a known force into the human body. This device has now begun to be examined via more rigorous research.[20] As well, efforts have been made to place it into a basic science model.

NIMMO RECEPTOR-TONUS THERAPY

Ray Nimmo was one of the first chiropractic pioneers to apply the research of individuals, such as Travell and Simon regarding trigger points, to a chiropractic foundation. Nimmo Receptor-Tonus Therapy looks at the use of known physiologic laws and then asks how these laws operate in purely chiropractic situations. Emphasis is placed on posture and muscular involvement as well as the neurologic involvements that may then occur. This system of therapy is built on these initial circumstances. No thrust is given, and there is no specific or direct mechanical goal for the spinal or extremity joints.

GONSTEAD TECHNIQUE

Clarence Gonstead devised a chiropractic system that uses full spine radiography, line drawing, motion palpation, and thermocouple instrumentation. In a sense, the Gonstead system is based on the level foundation, in this case, that of a level pelvis. If the pelvis is stable and level, then Gonstead notes, the spinal column will achieve maximum balance and stability (because it is supported by the pelvis).

Much of the theoretical underpinnings of Gonstead Technique are based on the biomechanics of the intervertebral disc. Thus, analysis of the intervertebral disc space on radiographic films is paramount. These are taken using two full spine radiographic images: an anterior to posterior (AP) and a lateral film. Great care is also taken with regard to patient positioning and protection. Initial analysis involves looking carefully at the pelvis and then attempting to determine what may happen as a result.

SACRO-OCCIPITAL TECHNIQUE

Major Bertrand DeJarnette developed the Sacro-occipital Technique (SOT) system, which is purported to restore normal functioning to the central and peripheral nervous systems through the effects on the meninges by the mechanical relationship between the cranium and pelvis. Padded wedges, called "blocks," are placed between the patient's pelvis and the table with the patient in either the prone or supine position, and gravity is allowed to affect the relationship of the innominates to the sacrum. Occipital fibers that apparently represent texture changes in the upper trapezius muscles are evaluated and treated. Cranial manipulative procedures based on the work of the osteopaths Sutherland and Upledger are also used. Evaluation is based on postural assessment as well as some reflex phenomenon (the arm fossa test, dollar sign, and heel tensions).

APPENDIX 2
Named Chiropractic Techniques

(Many of the following techniques are not described in Appendix 1-A.)

Diversified Technique
Sacro-occipital Technique
Gonstead Technique
Activator Technique
Pierce-Stillwagon Technique
Receptor-Tonus Technique (Nimmo Technique)
Spinal Touch Technique
Applied Kinesiology
Chiropractic Spinal Biophysics
Applied Spinal Biomechanical Engineering
Logan Basic Technique
Palmer Upper Cervical Technique
National Upper Cervical Technique
Pettibon Technique
Spinal Stress
Spears Painless System
Thompson Terminal Point Technique
Toftness Technique
Motion Palpation and Chiropractic Technique
Endonasal Technique
Perianal Postural Reflex Technique
Von Fox Combination Technique
Blair Technique
Bioenergetic Synchronization Techique
King Concept
CHOK-E System
Chiropractic Neurobiochemical Analysis
Polarity Technique
Concept Technique
Chiroenergetics
Mears Technique
Craniopathy
Reinert Technique

Directional Nonforce Technique (DNFT)
Flexion Distraction Therapy (Cox Technique)
Leander Technique
Grostic Technique
Freeman Chiropractic Procedure
Atlas Orthogonality Technique
Neuro-emotional Technique
Neuro-organizational Technique
Micromanipulation
Network

APPENDIX 3

Chiropractic Glossary Of Commonly Used Terms

Active Movement Movement accomplished without outside assistance; the patient moves the joint unassisted.

Adaptation The adjustment of an organism to its environment. A compensatory reaction of the body to a mechanical distortion.

Adhesion A fibrous band or structure by which parts adhere abnormally.

Adjustment The chiropractic adjustment is a specific form of direct articular manipulation utilizing either long or short leverage techniques with specific contacts. It is characterized by a dynamic thrust of controlled velocity, amplitude and direction.

Agonistic Muscles Muscles or portions of muscles so attached anatomically that when they contract they develop forces that reinforce each other.

Alignment To put in a straight line; arrangement of position in a straight line.

Amplitude Greatness of size, magnitude, breadth, or range.

Analysis Separation into component parts; the act of determining the component parts of a substance.

> **Spinal Analysis** Examination of the spinal column to determine the relationship of vertebrae to each other and adjcent structures.

Angiothlipsis Pressure on an artery, direct or indirect (e.g., in the I.V.F. through pressure generated by a discopathy, in the foramina transversarii through osteogenic reactions.

Anomaly Congenital or developmental deviation from the normal, standard.

Antagonistic Muscles Muscles or portions of muscles so attached anatomically that when they contract they develop forces that oppose each other.

Anterior Pelvic Tilt A position of the pelvis in which the vertical plane through the anterior superior iliac spines is anterior to the vertical plane through the symphysis pubes. It is associated with hyperextension of the lumbar spine and flexion at the hip joints.

Anterolisthesis Anterior translation of the vertebral body.

Arthrosis Degenerative joint disease of the truly movable joints of the spine or extremities.

Articular Strain The result of forces acting on a joint beyond its capacity to adapt. Refers to stretching of joint components beyond physiologic limits, causing damage.

Asymmetry Lack or absence of symmetry of position or motion. Dissimilarity in corresponding parts or organs of opposite sides of the body that are normally alike.

Axis A line around which rotatory movement takes place or along which translation occurs. The three-dimensional description of motion of an object with three axes perpendicular to one another. The right handed Cartesian orthogonal system has three axes designated X, Y, and Z.

> **X Axis** A line passing horizontally from side to side. May also be referred to as the coronal axis or the frontal axis. Movement around the X axis is said to be in the sagittal plane.
> **Y Axis** A line perpendicular to the ground. May also be referred to as the vertical axis. Movement around the Y axis is said to be in the horizontal or transverse plane.
> **Z Axis** A line passing horizontally front to back. May also be referred to as the sagittal axis. Movement around the Z axis is said to be in the coronal plane.

Axoplasmic Flow The flow of neuroplasm along the axon between synapses and toward and away from end organs.

Barrier Limit of impeded motion.

> **Anatomic Barrier** The limit of anatomic integrity: the limit of motion imposed by an anatomic structure. Forcing the movement beyond this barrier would produce tissue damage.
> **Elastic Barrier (physiologic)** The elastic resistance that is felt at the end of passive range of movement; further motion toward the anatomic barrier may be induced passively.

Biomechanics The study of structural, functional, and mechanical aspects of human motion. It is concerned mainly with external forces either of a static or dynamic nature dealing with human movements.

Body Mechanics The study of the static and dynamic human body to note the mechanical integration of the parts and to endeavor to restore and maintain the body in as nearly as possible normal mechanical condition.

Bogginess A tissue texture abnormality characterized principally by a palpable sense of sponginess in the tissue interpreted as resulting from congestion owing to increased fluid content.

Bucket Handle Rib Motion Movement of the lower ribs during respiration such that with inhalation the lateral aspect of the rib elevates, resulting in an increase of transverse diameter of the thorax.

Caliper Rib Movement Movement of lower ribs during respiration such that the rib moves anterior in inhalation.

Center of Gravity The point in a body where the body mass is centered.

Chiropractic

> **Chiropractic Practice** A discipline of the scientific healing arts concerned with the pathogenesis, diagnostics, therapeutics, and prophylaxis of functional disturbances, pathomechanical states, pain syndromes, and neurophysiological effects related to the statics and dynamics of the locomotor system, especially of the spine and pelvis.
>
> **Chiropractic Science** Concerned with the investigation of the relationship between structure (primarily the spine) and function (primarily the nervous system) of the human body that leads to the restoration and preservation of health.

Compensation Changes in structural relationships to accommodate for foundation disturbances and to maintain balance.

Contact Point The area of the adjustive hand that makes contact with the patient in the delivery of the chiropractic adjustment. There are 12 contact points.

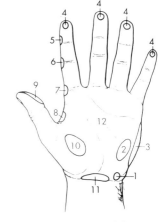

1. pisiform
2. hypothenar
3. metacarpal (knife-edge)
4. digital
5. distal interphalangeal (DIP)
6. proximal interphalangeal (PIP)
7. metacarpophalangeal (MP or index)
8. web
9. thumb
10. thenar
11. calcaneal
12. palmar

Contraction A shortening or reduction in size; in connection with muscles, contraction implies shortening and/or development of tension.

Contracture A condition of fixed high resistance to passive stretch of a muscle resulting from fibrosis of the tissues supporting the muscle or joint.

Coupling A phenomenon of consistent association of one motion (translation or rotation) about an axis with another motion (translation or rotation) about a second axis. One motion cannot be produced without the other.

Creep Deformation of a viscoelastic material with time when it is subjected to a constant, suddenly applied load.

Curvature Deviation from a rectilinear direction. An abnormal bending of the spine in any direction away from the natural contour that involves three or more vertebrae.

Curve An anatomic term for a normal bending of the spine in the sagittal plane (e.g., primary dorsal and sacral curves, secondary cervical and lumbar curves).

Deformation A change in length or shape.

Degrees of Freedom The number of independent coordinates in a coordinate system required to completely specify the position of an object in space. One degree of freedom is rotation around one axis or translation along one axis. The spine is considered to have six degrees of freedom because it has the capability of rotatory movement around three axes as well as translatory movement along three axes.

Diagnosis The art of distinguishing one disease from another. The use of scientific and skillful methods to establish the cause and nature of a person's illness.

Discogenic Caused by derangement of an intervertebral disc.

Discopathogenic Abnormal action or function of a disc resulting in a disorder or condition; originating because of disc degeneration.

Discopathy Any pathologic changes in a disc.

Disc Herniation Extrusion of nucleus pulposus into a defect in the annulus fibrosus.

Displacement State of being removed from normal position; as pertaining to vertebral displacement, it refers to a disrelationship of the vertebra to its relative structure.

Distortion Distortion in the body framework includes any mechanical departure from ideal or normal symmetry.

Distraction The movement of two surfaces away from each other.

Dynamics A branch of mechanics that consists of the study of the loads and motions of interacting bodies.

Dysarthrosis The strict meaning of joint motion restriction without the neurologic connotations. It refers to kinetics.

Dyskinesia Impairment of the power of voluntary movement, resulting in fragmentary or incomplete movements, aberrant motion.

Eccentric Work or Contraction Work produced by a muscle when its length is increasing.

Effleurage A form of massage employing slow rhythmic stroking executed with a minimum of force and light pressure.

Elasticity The property of a material or structure to return to its original form following the removal of the deforming load.

End Play (End Feel) Discrete, short range movements of a joint independent of the action of voluntary muscles, determined by springing each vertebrae at the limit of its passive range of motion.

Equilibrium State of a body at rest in which the sums of all forces and movements are zero.

Extension The separation of two embryologically ventral surfaces; movement away from the fetal position; the return movement from flexion.

Facilitation An increase in afferent stimuli so that the synaptic threshold is more easily reached; thus there is increase in the efficacy of subsequent impulses in that pathway or synapse. The consequence of increased efficacy is that continued stimulation produces hyperactive responses.

Fibrosis The formation of fibrous tissue.

Fibrositis Inflammatory hyperplasia of the white fibrous tissue of the body, especially of the muscle sheaths and fascial layers of the locomotor system.

Fixation (Dynamic Fault) The state whereby an articulation has become temporarily immobilized in a position which it may normally occupy during any phase of physiologic movement. The immobilization of an articulation in a position of movement when the joint is at rest, or in a position of rest when the joint is in movement.

Flexibility The ability of a structure to deform under the application of a load.

Flexion The approximation of two embryologically ventral surfaces; movement toward the fetal position.

Foundation Any structure that supports or participates in the support of any part of the body framework.

Friction Massage A form of deep circular or transverse massage in which the skin is moved over the subcutaneous tissue.

Functional a) Of or pertaining to the function of an organ. Not structural; affecting functions only. b) Of, or pertaining to a function; affecting the functions but not the structure.

Gliding Movement in which the joint surfaces are flat or only slightly curved and one articulating surface slides on the other.

Gravitational Line A vertical line through the body where body mass is centered. In the theoretical, laterally viewed ideal posture, it starts at the external auditory canal, passes through the lateral head of the humerus at the tip of the shoulder, across the greater trochanter, the lateral condyle of the knee, and slightly anterior to the lateral malleolus.

Health A state of optimal physical, mental, and social well-being and not merely the absence of disease and infirmity.

Homeostasis a) Maintenance of static or constant conditions in the internal environment. b) The level of well-being of an individual maintained by internal physiologic harmony.

Hyper Beyond excessive.

Hypo Under or deficient.

Impinge To press or encroach upon; to come into close contact; an obstructive lesion causing pressure on a nerve.

Inhibition Effect of one neuron upon another tending to prevent it from initiating impulses.

Innate Inborn; hereditary.

Innate Intelligence The intrinsic biologic ability of a healthy organism to react physiologically to the changing conditions of the external and internal environment.

Instability Quality or condition of being unstable; not firm, fixed, or constant.

Inversion A turning inward, inside out, upside down, or other reversal of the normal relation of a part. Often used to describe passive inverted traction.

Instrumentation The use of any tool, appliance, or apparatus; work performed with instruments.

Ischemic Compression Application of progressively stronger painful pressure on a trigger point for the purpose of eliminating the point's tenderness.

Isokinetic Exercise Exercise using a constant speed of movement of the body part.

Joint Dysfunction Joint mechanics showing area disturbances of function without structural change. Subtle joint dysfunctions affecting quality and range of joint motion. They are diagnosed with the aid of motion palpation, and stress and motion radiography investigation.

Joint play Discrete, short range movements of a joint independent of the action of voluntary muscles, determined by springing each vertebrae in the neutral position.

Kinematics The division of mechanics that deals with the geometry of the motion of bodies, displacement velocity, and acceleration without taking into account the forces that produce the motion.

Kinesiology The science or study of movement and the active and passive structures involved.

Kinesthesia The sense by which movement, weight, position, etc., are perceived; commonly used to refer specifically to the perception of changes in the angles of joints.

Kinesthetic Pertaining to kinesthesia.

Kinetic Chain A combination of several successively arranged joints constituting a complex unit, as links in a chain.

> **Closed Kinetic Chain** A system in which motion of one link has determinate relations to every other link in the system.
>
> **Open Kinetic Chain** A combination of links in which the terminal joint is free.

Kinetics A branch of mechanics that studies the relation between the force system acting on a body and the changes it produces in the body motion.

Klapping Tapotement (clapping, cupping).

Kneading A form of massage employing forceful circular and transverse movement of a large raised fold of skin and underlying muscle.

Kyphoscoliosis Backward and lateral curvature of the spinal column.

Kyphosis Abnormally increased convexity in the curvature of the thoracic spine.

Kyphotic Affected with or pertaining to kyphosis.

Lateral Flexion Bending to the side within the coronal plane.

Laterolisthesis Lateral translatory excursion of the vertebral body.

Lesion Any pathologic or traumatic discontinuity of tissue or loss of function.

Lever A rigid bar moving on a fixed fulcrum.

Listing (Dynamic) Designation of the abnormal movement characteristic of one vertebra in relation to subadjacent segments.

    A. Dynamic Listing Nomenclature
        1. Flexion restriction
        2. Extension restriction
        3. Lateral flexion restriction (right or left)
        4. Rotational restriction (right or left)

Listing (Static) Designation of the spatial orientation of one vertebra in relation to adjacent segments.

    A. Static Listing Nomenclature
        1. Flexion malposition
        2. Extension malposition
        3. Lateral flexion malposition (right or left)
        4. Rotational malposition (right or left)
        5. Anterolisthesis
        6. Retrolisthesis
        7. Laterolisthesis

Lordosis The anterior concavity in the curvature of the lumbar and cervical spine.

Lordotic Anterior spinal curve.

Malposition Abnormal or anomalous position.

    A. Static Listing Nomenclature
        1. Flexion malposition
        2. Extension malposition
        3. Lateral flexion malposition (right or left)
        4. Rotational malposition (right or left)
        5. Anterolisthesis
        6. Retrolisthesis
        7. Laterolisthesis

Manipulation Therapeutic application of manual force. Spinal manipulative therapy broadly defined includes all procedures where the hands are used to mobilize, adjust, manipulate, apply traction, massage, stimulate, or otherwise influence the spine and paraspinal tissues with the aim of influencing the patient's health.

Massage The systematic therapeutic friction, stroking, and kneading of the body. Maneuvers performed by hand on the skin of the patient and through the skin of the patient upon the subcutaneous tissue.

There may be variables in intensity of pressure exerted, surface area treated, and frequency of application.

Meric System The treatment of visceral conditions through adjustment of vertebrae at the levels of neuromeric innervation to the organs involved.

Misalignment Not in proper alignment.

Mobilization The process of making a fixed part movable. A form of manipulation applied within the physiologic passive range of joint motion characterized by non-thrust passive joint manipulation.

Motion The relative displacement with time of a body in space with respect to other bodies or some reference system.

Myofascial Syndrome Pain and/or autonomic phenomena referred from active myofascial trigger points with associated dysfunction. The specific muscle or muscle group that causes the symptoms should be identified.

Myofascial Trigger Point A hyperirritable spot, usually within a taut band of skeletal muscle or in the muscle's fascia, that is painful on compression and that can give rise to characteristic referred pain, tenderness, and autonomic phenomena. A myofascial trigger point is to be distinguished from cutaneous, ligamentous, periosteal, and nonmuscular fascial trigger points. Types include active, latent, primary, associated, satellite, and secondary.

Myofascitis a) Inflammation of a muscle and its fascia, particularly of the fascial insertion of muscle to bone. b) Pain, tenderness, other referred phemomena, and the dysfunction attributed to myofascial trigger points.

Myofibrosis Replacement of muscle tissue by fibrous tissue.

Nerve Interference A chiropractic term used to refer to the interruption of normal nerve transmission (nerve energy).

Nerve transmission The transmission of information along a nerve cell.

Impulsed Based Nerve transmission involving the generation and transfer of electrical potentials along a nerve axon.

Non-Impulsed Based The transfer of chemical messengers along a nerve axon (i.e., axoplasmic flow).

Neurodystrophic The disease process within a nerve resulting from trauma, circulation disorders, or metabolic diseases (e.g., a neurodystrophic factor (diabetes and pernicious anemia).

Neurogenic Originating in nerve tissue.

Neuropathogenic A disease within a tissue resulting from abnormal nerve performance (e.g., Barré-Lieou syndrome resulting from neuropathogenic reflexes caused by pathomechanics of the cervical spine).

Neuropathy A general term denoting functional disturbances and/or pathologic changes in the peripheral nervous system.

Neurophysiologic Effects A general term denoting functional or aberrant disturbances of the peripheral or autonomic nervous systems.

The term is used to designate nonspecific effects related to a) motor and sensory functions of the peripheral nervous system; b) vasomotor activity, secretomotor activity and motor activity of smooth muscle from the autonomic nervous system (e.g., neck, shoulder, arm syndrome [the extremity becomes cool with increased sweating]); c) trophic activity of both the peripheral and autonomic nervous system (e.g.,muscle atrophy in neck, shoulder, arm syndrome).

Neurothlipsis Pressure on a nerve, direct or indirect (e.g., in the intervertebral foramen through congestion of perineural tissues; in the carpal tunnel through direct ligamentous pressure).

Nutation Motion of the sacrum about a coronal axis in which the sacral base moves anteriorly and inferiorly and the tip of the coccyx moves posteriorly and superiorly; nodding, as of the head.

> **Counter Nutation** Motion of the sacrum about a coronal axis in which the sacral base moves posteriorly and superiorly and the tip of the coccyx moves anteriorly and inferiorly; nodding, as of the head.

Osteophyte A degenerative exostosis secondary to musculotendinous stress.

Palpation a) The act of feeling with the hands. b) The application of variable manual pressure through the surface of the body for the purpose of determining the shape, size, consistency, position, inherent motility, and health of the tissues beneath.

> **Motion Palpation** Palpatory diagnosis of passive and active segmental joint range of motion.
>
> **Static Palpation** Palpatory diagnosis of somatic structures in a neutral static position.

Palpatory Diagnosis The process of palpating the patient to evaluate neuromusculoskeletal and visceral systems.

Palpatory Skills The sensory and tactile skills used in performing a physical examination.

Palpitation A subjective sensation of an unduly rapid or irregular heart beat.

Passive Movement Movement carried through by the operator without conscious assistance or resistance of the patient.

Pathomechanical States Joint pathomechanics with structural changes—those architectural changes are the scars of imbalanced motion and weightbearing, trauma, and biochemical changes associated with aging and deficiency states. These tissue changes may be revealed by static radiography and biopsy and definitely diagnosed with surgical exposure, e.g.,

1) arthrosis
2) spondylolisthesis
3) disc degenerations

Pelvic Lateral Shift A movement in the coronal plane of the pelvis in which one anterior-superior spine moves closer to the midline while the opposite anterior-superior spine has moved further away from the midline. It is associated with adduction and abduction of the hip joints.

Pelvic Lateral Tilt A position of the pelvis in which it is not level in the horizontal plane (i.e., one anterior-superior iliac spine is higher than the other). It is associated with lateral flexion of the lumbar spine and adduction and abduction of the hip joints.

Pelvic Rotation A position of the pelvis in which one anterior-superior iliac spine is anterior to the other. Pelvis rotation is a rotatory movement around the Y or vertical axis.

Pelvic Tilt A deviation of the pelvis in the sagittal plane from neutral position.

Petrissage Same as kneading.

Physiologic Motion Normal changes in the position of articulating surfaces during the movement of a joint or region.

Plane A flat surface determined by the position of three points in space.

> **Coronal Plane** Frontal plane.
>
> **Frontal Plane** A plane passing longitudinally through the body from one side to the other, and dividing the body into anterior and posterior portions.
>
> **Sagittal Plane** A plane passing longitudinally through the body from front to back and dividing it into right and left portions. The median or midsagittal plane divides the body into approximately equal right and left portions.
>
> **Transverse Plane** A plane passing horizontally through the body perpendicular to the sagittal and frontal planes, dividing the body into upper and lower portions.

Plastic Deformation A non-recoverable deformation.

Plasticity The property of a material to permanently deform when it is loaded beyond its elastic range.

Plumb Line Weighted, true vertical line utilized for visual comparison with the gravitational line.

Posture a) The attitude of the body. b) The relative arrangement of the parts of the body. Good posture is that state of muscular and skeletal balance that protects the supporting structures of the body against injury or progressive deformity irrespective of the attitude (erect, lying, squatting, stooping) in which these structures are working or resting.

Prophylaxis That branch of applied biology that seeks to reduce or eradicate disease by removing or altering the responsible etiologic factors. The prevention of disease; preventive treatment.

> **1)** To prevent occurrence of lesions because of poor postural hygiene, physical fitness, and faulty body mechanics.
>
> **2)** The prevention of recurrence with follow-up care (e.g., exercise).
>
> **3)** Many lesions are not curable and become quiescent with treat-

ments; therefore, follow-up care to prevent further pathology, or at least to retard the pathomechanical process, is necessary.

Proprioception   Sensory perception of movement or position within the body.

Range of Motion   The range of translation and rotation of a joint for each of its six ranges of freedom.

Reciprocal Innervation   The inhibition of antagonistic muscles when the agonist is stimulated.

Rectilinear Motion   Motion in a straight line.

Referred Pain   Pain felt in a part other than that in which the cause that produced it is situated.

Reflex   The result of transforming an ingoing sensory impulse into an outgoing efferent impulse without an act of will.

Reflex Therapy   Treatment that is aimed at stimulating afferent impulses and evoking a given response (i.e., neuromuscular).

Relaxation   The decrease in stress in a deformed structure with time when the deformation is held constant.

Resilience   The property of returning to the former shape, size, or state after distortion.

Restriction   Limitation of movement. Describes the direction of limited movement in subluxated and/or dysfunctional joints.

Retrolisthesis   Posterior translation of the vertebral body.

Roentgenometrics   The direct measurement of structures shown in the roentgenogram/radiograph.

Rolfing   A 10-hour cycle of deep manual intervention in the soft tissue structure of the body, formerly called structural integration, designed by Ida P. Rolf, Ph.D. Deep effleurage is used to strip tendons and to stretch myofascial tissues to achieve both postural and psychological effects. See Effleurage.

Ropiness   A tissue texture abnormality characterized by a cord or stringlike feeling.

Rotation   Motion of a body around an axis.

Sacroiliac Fixation (Sacroiliac Joint Locking)   The absence of normal motion at the sacroiliac joint demonstrable by motion palpation in which the axis of rotation has shifted to either the superior or inferior portion of the sacroiliac joint, or rarely a situation in which there is total joint locking with no axis of rotation.

Sacroiliac Extension Fixation (AS)   A state of the sacroiliac joint in which the posterior-superior iliac spine is fixed in an anterior-superior position with the innominate bone on that side fixed in extension in relation to the sacrum. The axis of rotation then shifts inferior and the superior joint remains mobile.

Sacroiliac Flexion Fixation (PI)   A state of the sacroiliac joint in which the posterior-superior iliac spine is fixed in a posterior-inferior position with the innominate bone on that side fixed in flexion in relation to the sacrum. The axis of rotation then shifts superiorly and the inferior joint remains mobile.

Scan An intermediate screening palpatory examination designed to focus the clinician on regional areas of joint dysfunction.

Scoliosis An appreciable lateral deviation in the normally straight vertical line of the spine.

> **Functional Scoliosis** Lateral deviation of the spine resulting from poor posture, foundation anomalies, occupational strains, etc., that are still not permanently established.
>
> **Structural Scoliosis** Permanent lateral deviation of the spine such that the spine cannot return to neutral position.

Shear An applied force that tends to cause an opposite but parallel sliding motion of planes within an object.

Short Leg An anatomic, pathologic, or functional leg deficiency leading to dysfunction.

Side Bending See Lateral Flexion.

Somatic Dysfunction Impaired or altered function of related components of the somatic (body framework) system: skeletal, arthrodial, and myofascial structures and related vascular, lymphatic and neural elements.

Spinography Roentgenometrics of the spine.

Spondylitis Inflammation of the vertebrae.

Spondyloarthrosis Arthrosis of the synovial joints of the spine.

Spondylolisthesis Anterior slippage of a vertebral body on its caudal fellow.

Spondylolysis An interruption in the pars interarticularis, either unilateral or bilateral.

Spondylophytes Degenerative spur formation arising from the vertebral end plates and usually projecting somewhat horizontally.

Spondylosis Degenerative joint disease as it affects the vertebral body end plates.

Spondylotherapy The therapeutic application of percussion or concussion over the vertebrae to elicit reflex responses at the levels of neuromeric innervation to the organ being influenced.

Sprain Joint injury in which some of the fibers of a supporting ligament are ruptured but the continuity of the ligament remains intact.

Spur A projecting body, as from a bone.

Statics The branch of mechanics that deals with the equilibrium of bodies at rest or in motion with zero acceleration.

Stiffness A measure of resistance offered to external loads by a specimen or structure as it deforms.

Strain An overstretching and tearing of musculotendinous tissue.

Stress The sum of the biologic reaction to any adverse stimulus—physical, mental, and/or emotional, internal or external—that tends to disturb the organism's homeostasis; should these compensating reactions be inadequate or inappropriate, they may lead to disorders.

Stretching Separation of the origin and insertion of a muscle or attachments of fascia or ligaments by applying a constant pressure lengthening the fibers of muscle or fascia.

Stringiness A palpable tissue texture abnormality characterized by fine or stringlike myofascial structures

Subacute Less than acute, between acute and chronic.

Subluxation An aberrant relationship between two adjacent articular structures that may have functional or pathologic sequelae, causing an alteration in the biomechanical and/or neurophysiologic reflections of these articular structures, their proximal structures, and/or body systems that may be directly or indirectly affected by them.

Symmetry The similar arrangement in formand relationship of parts around a common axis or on each side of a plane of the body.

Syndesmophyte An osseous excrescence or bony outgrowth from a ligament. Usually projecting vertically in the spine.

Tapotement A tapping or percussing movement in massage; it includes clapping, beating, and punctation.

Technique Any of a number of physical or mechanical chiropractic procedures used in the treatment of patients.

Thrust The sudden manual application of a controlled directional force upon a suitable part of the patient, the delivery of which effects an adjustment.

Tonus The slight continuous contraction of muscle, which in skeletal muscles aids in the maintenance of posture.

Torsion A type of load that is applied by a couple of forces (parallel and directed opposite to each other about the axis of a structure).

Traction The act of drawing or exerting a pulling force.

Translation Motion of a rigid body in which a straight line in the body always remains parallel to itself.

Trigger Point See Myofascial trigger point.

Trophic Of or pertaining to nutrition.

Vertebral Motion Segment a) Two adjacent vertebral bodies and the disc between them, the two posterior joints and the ligamentous structures binding the two vertebrae to one another; b) the consideration of the anatomic and functional relationships of two vertebrae, the mechanical integration of their articular processes and the related musculature, ligaments and synovial membranes.

Viscoelasticity The property of a material to show sensitivity to the rate of loading or deformation. Two basic components are viscosity and elasticity.

Viscosity The property of materials to resist loads that produce shear.

APPENDIX 4

Chiropractic Treatment Procedures Categorization Algorithm

A

Nonmanual procedures do not require direct contact of the doctor to the patient. Examples are nonmanual physiologic therapeutics (manual physiologic therapeutics fall under "Extra-Articular Procedures"), exercise programs, braces, supports, nutrition, counseling, and so on.

B

Does the procedure affect the anatomic joint? *Anatomic joint* in this context means "The junction or union between two or more bones, especially one that admits motion of one or more bones" (*Dorland's*). The anatomic joint includes such structures as the bone ends, articular cartilage, ligaments, synovial membrane, or capsular fibers.

C

Does the procedure affect the physiologic joint? *Physiologic joint* in this context pertains to those structures responsible for the functioning of the joint: the anatomic joint structures as well as the nerves, muscles, tendons, blood vessels, and so on.*

D

Indirect visceral procedures affect a nonphysiologic joint structure when the contact is made distant to that structure. Examples include foot reflexology, ear reflexology, sysmpathetic stimulation by percussion over the thoracic transverse processes, and pressure over the carotid sinus.

* Randolph KM: Management of Common Musculoskeletal Disorders. Harper & Row, New York, 1983

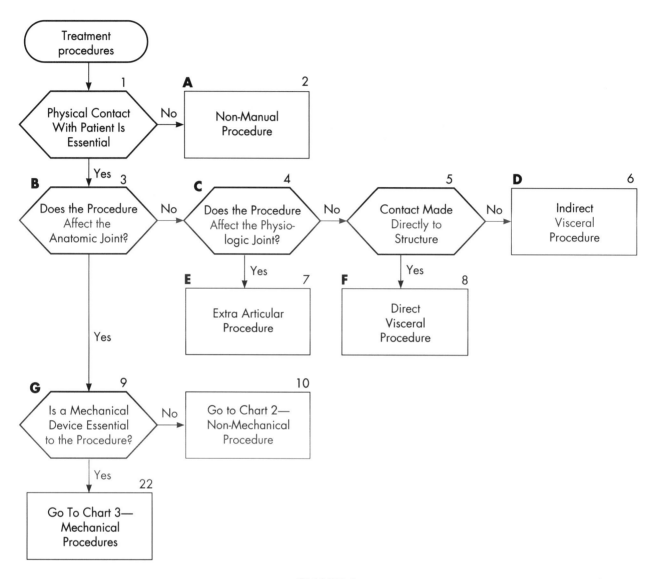

CHART 1

E

Extra-articular procedures affect the structures making up the physiologic joint and thus the anatomic joint indirectly but do not include those procedures that have a direct effect on the anatomic joints. Extra-articular technic procedures include proprioneurofacilitation, transverse friction massage, trigger-point therapy, as well as manual physiologic therapeutic procedures.

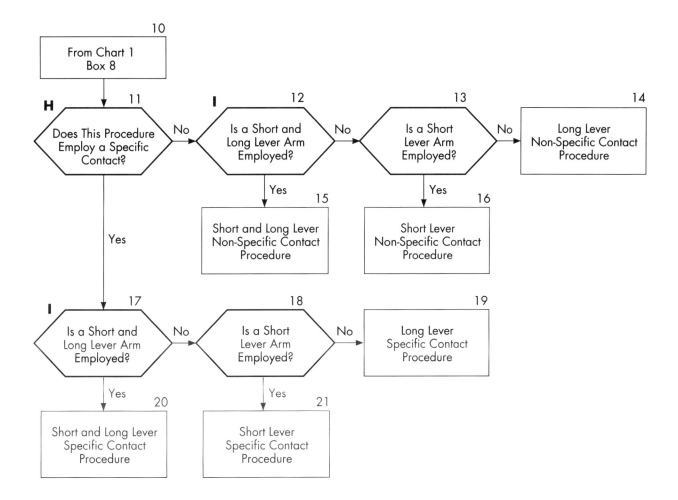

CHART 2—NON–MECHANICAL PRODEDURES

F

Direct visceral procedures are those technic procedures during which a contact is made directly on a nonphysiologic joint structure. Examples may include milking the gall bladder, colon massage, diaphragm release, pelvic diaphragm release, and milking the tonsils.

G

Is a mechanical device essential to the procedure? *Mechanical device* in this context means any device used to augment or deliver the adjustment but not including a general table or chair.

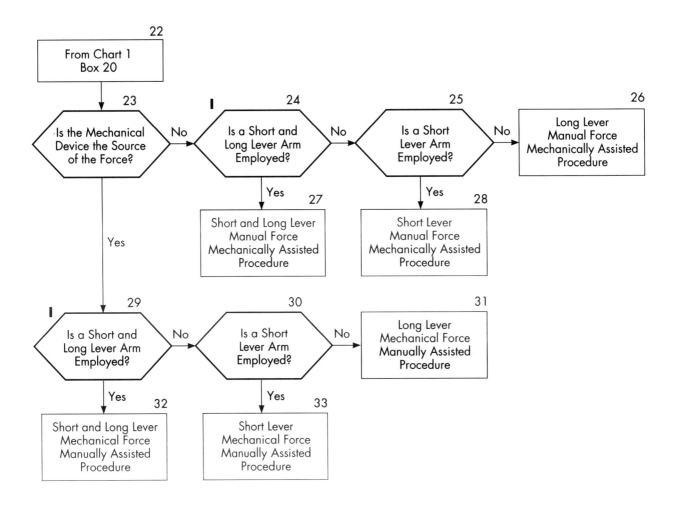

CHART 3—MECHANICAL PROCEDURES

H

Does this procedure employ a specific contact? *Specific contact* in this context means a contact as proximal to the articulating joint surfaces as possible, with as small a contact point as possible.

I

Is a short- and long-lever arm employed? During a short-lever arm technic, the impulse is intended to cause a translatory glide, whereas during a long-lever arm technic, the impulse is intended to cause a hingelike motion.

(From Bartol KM: Algorithm for the categorization of chiropractic technic procedures. J Chiro Tech 4(1):8, 1992, with permission.)

APPENDIX 5

Controlled Trials of Spinal Manipulation for Treatment of Back Pain: Summary of Salient Features

Author[1,2] (Year) (Country of Origin)	Duration of Pain[3]	Sciatic[4,5] Pain/SNI	Minor[6] Neurologic Findings	Palpatory[7] Findings	Manipulation Defined (Type)	# Manipulated/ Total Sample[8] (# of Manip.)[9]	Results
Coyer (1955) (Britain)	A	Excluded	Excluded	None	Yes (Cyriax)	76/136 (1)	50% of manipulated group pain free at 1 week compared to 27% of controls treated with bedrest; values for 6 weeks were 88% and 72%, respectively
Edwards (1969) (Australia)	Not defined	Included/ presumably included	Presumably included	None	Yes (Maitland)	92/184 (13 max.)	No overall difference between manipulation and heat/massage, but manipulation improved those with sciatic pain and provided relief in half (4.8 vs. 9.7) the number of treatments
Glover (1974) RCT (Britain)	A/S + C	Included/not stated	Included	Yes	Yes (Rotational)	43/84 (1)	In general no difference between manipulation and diathermy vs. diathermy alone, manipulation provided better pain relief for those with <7 days of pain and first attack of back pain (61% vs. 42% mean pain relief at 3 days)
Doran (1975) RCT (Britain)	A, S, C	Excluded	Excluded	No	No	116/456 (6 avg.)	No difference between manipulation, physiotherapy, corset, and analgesics, using chi-square; later reanalysis by Hoehler (1987) showed statistical benefit for manipulation (45% vs. 35% improved at 3 weeks)
Bergquist (1977) RCT (Sweden)	Mainly A, some S	Included/ included	Presumably excluded	Yes	Yes (Janda)	72/217 (variable)	"Combined physiotherapy" including manipulation or "back school" better than diathermy (time to recovery 15.8, 14.8, and 28.7 days, respectively)
Evans (1978) RCT (Britain)	S, C	Included/ excluded	Probably excluded	No	Yes (Rotational)	32 (3 weeks)	Statistically significant improvement for manipulation vs. codeine in overall pain score for each group, older patients did better than younger, but crossover design, randomization failure make conclusions questionable
Sims-Williams (1978) RCT (Britain)	Not specified	Included/not stated	Included	Yes	Yes (Maitland)	47/94 (14 max.)	Significant improvement for manipulation vs. diathermy in return to light work at one month; effect was gone by three months; pain <1 month responded better
Rasmussen (1979) RCT (Denmark)	A	Excluded	Probably excluded	No	Yes (Rotational)	12/24 (2 weeks)	Distinct benefit for manipulation vs. diathermy, though non-blinded assessment (10/12 improved with manipulation vs. 3/12 in control group)

Study	Type						Comments
Hoehler (1981) RCT (USA)	52% A 17% C	Not stated	Not stated	Yes	Yes (Rotational)	56/95 (5 avg.)	Immediate benefit of manipulation vs. sham (84% vs. 68% pain relief); gone by 3 weeks; sophisticated control group
Coxhead (1981) RCT (Britain)	Mainly S	Only/presumably included	Presumably included	No	Yes (Maitland)	155/322 (14 max.)	Manipulation possibly slightly better than corset, back school, or traction; certainly better than no treatment, at 4 weeks; gone at 4 months. Later reanalysis by Hoehler (1987) showed statistically significant benefit of manipulation (82% vs. 73% improved) at 4 weeks
Zylbergold (1981) RCT (Canada)	Not stated	Not stated	Excluded	No	No	8/28 (2/week for 4 wk)	Manipulation no better than heat and physical therapy or traction in functional status at 4 weeks
Nwuga (1982) RCT (Nigeria)	A	Only/presumably included	Included	No	Yes (Oscillatory rotation)	26/51 (12 max.)	Significant benefit for manipulation vs. diathermy for total rotation and straight leg raising compared to baseline for each group, NOT between groups. Significantly shorter time to pain relief for manipulated group (121 min. vs. 160 min. combined total treatment time)
Farrell (1982) RCT (Australia)	A	Included/presumably included	Excluded	No	Yes (Maitland)	24/48 (9 max.)	Short term benefit for manipulation vs. diathermy, exercises, and instructions; shorter time to pain relief (3.5 vs. 5.8 treatments); no difference in groups at 3 weeks
Godfrey (1984) RCT (Canada)	A	Not stated	Not stated	Yes	Yes (Maigne)	22/81 (5 max.)	Trend toward benefit from manipulation vs. massage; later reanalysis by Hoehler (1987) showed statistically significant benefit for manipulation for back mobility (30% vs. 15%), but not overall symptomatology at 2 weeks; chiropractor and M.D. manipulator
Gibson (1985) RCT (Britain)	S, C	Probably excluded	Excluded	No	Yes (Minimal rotation)	41/109 (4 max.)	No benefit in subjective or objective outcomes immediately and at 2, 4, and 12 weeks; control groups received diathermy
Arkuszewski (1986) (Poland)	C	Included/included	Included/included	No	No	50/100 (6 avg., 10 max.)	Time to pain relief improved for manipulation vs. massage (3.1 vs. 3.8 weeks); at 6 months, 60% of manipulated group vs. 36% of control group had returned to old job; results limited by nonblinded assessment

Author[1,2] (Year) (Country of Origin)	Duration of Pain[3]	Sciatic[4,5] Pain/SNI	Minor[6] Neurologic Findings	Palpatory[7] Findings	Manipulation Defined (Type)	# Manipulated/ Total Sample[8] (# of Manip.)[9]	Results
Waagen (1986) RCT (USA)	S, C	Excluded	Excluded	No	Yes (Chiropractic adjustments)	9/19 (4 avg.)	Benefit for manipulation vs. sham on Visual Analogue Scale measurements of pain immediately and at 2 weeks (0.6 and 1.7 difference between groups on VAS immediately and at 2 weeks, respectively); manipulations were given by chiropractor; 10 dropouts from enrollees
Meade (1986) RCT (Britain)	A, S, C	Not excluded/ excluded	Included	No	No	23/50 (unknown)	Mean improvement in Oswestry Score between 0 and 6 weeks was 3.0 for those treated at medical clinic with exercises, traction, hydrotherapy, and possibly manipulation vs. 10.7 for those treated at chiropractic clinic; chiropractic manipulation
Ongley (1987) RCT (USA)	C	Excluded	Not excluded	No	Yes (Sacroiliac lumbar roll)	40/81 (1)	Experimental group had significantly better outcomes on validated questionnaire; addition of injection of "proliferant" to experimental subjects makes interpretation of effect of manipulation alone difficult
Hadler (1987) RCT (USA)	Mainly A, some S	Included/ presumably included	Included	No	Yes (Lumbar rotation)	28/54 (1)	No overall difference in validated back pain questionnaire between manipulation and mobilization, but patients with pain of 2 to 4 weeks duration achieved a 50% reduction in pain score more rapidly with manipulation than with mobilization
Mathews (1987) RCT (Britain)	A, S	Included/ included	Excluded	Yes	Yes (Rotation; straight thrust)	165/291 (up to 10)	Benefit for manipulation in patients with straight leg raising signs both subjectively and objectively at 2 weeks (30% difference in recovery rate); controls were given infrared heat. Patients without straight leg raising signs improved greatly in all groups, trend favoring manipulation but not significant; no difference at one year

| Meade (1990) RCT (Britain) | A, S, C | Not excluded/ excluded | Presumably included | No | No | No | 375/717 (9 avg.) | Comparison of "chiropractic care" vs. "medical clinic care" for patients with back pain; 99% of chiropractic patients were manipulated, some medical patients were manipulated as well. Significantly greater improvement in Oswestry Score in chiropractic group at 6, 12, and 24 months; improvement in physiologic variables greater for chiropractic group as well. Patients with subacute and chronic pain improved similarly to those with acute pain. |

NOTES:
[1] First author and year of publication are provided for each study.
[2] Studies designated RCT had random allocation of subjects.
[3] A = Acute; S = Subacute; C = Chronic.
[4] Inclusion or exclusion of patients with typical sciatic pain is listed; "only" refers to studies which included only patients with sciatic pain.
[5] SNI means sciatic nerve root irritation, defined as typical sciatic pain and a positive ipsilateral straight leg raising sign (positive = pain distal to knee).
[6] Minor neurologic findings are one of the following: decreased ankle reflex, dermatomal sensory deficit, or nonprogressive motor weakness.
[7] Palpatory findings refers to the use of specific physical findings thought to be indicative of joint fixation as a criterion for entry.
[8] "# Manipulated" refers to the number of subjects in the manipulation group.
[9] "# of Manip." refers to the number of manipulative sessions during the study.

(From Shekelle PG, Adams AH: The Appropriateness of Spinal Manipulation for Low-Back Pain: Project Overview and Literature Review. RAND Corp, Santa Monica, CA, 1991, with permission.)

Index

Note: Page numbers followed by *f* indicate figures and those followed by *t* indicate tables.

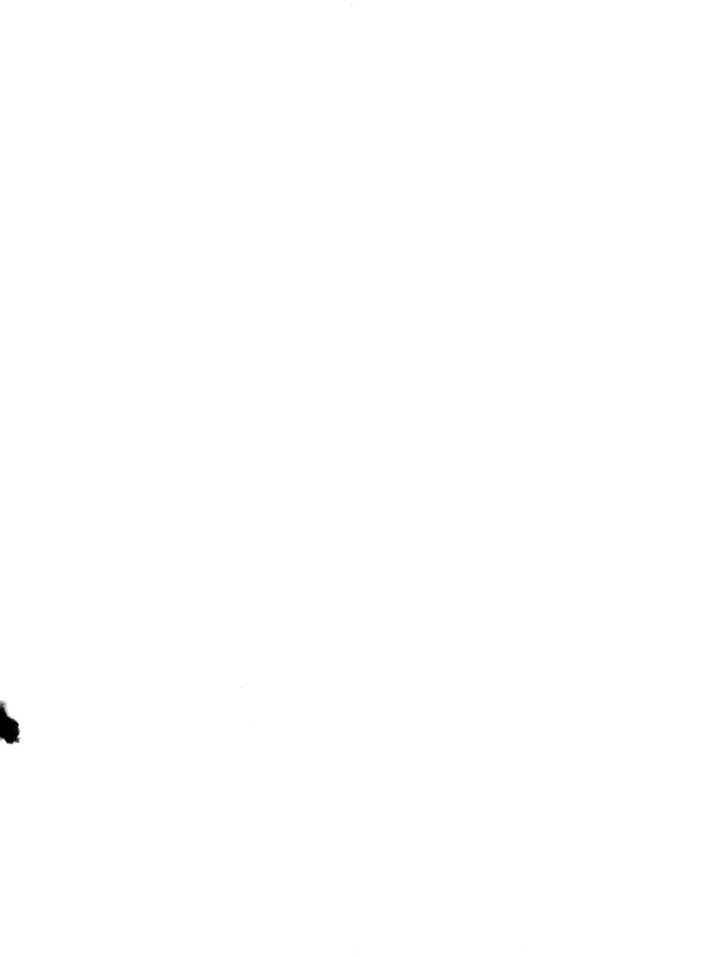